KU-526-516

# COMPLEMENTARY THERAPIES for PHYSICAL THERAPY

## A Clinical Decision-Making Approach

# COMPLEMENTARY THERAPIES for PHYSICAL THERAPY

## A Clinical Decision-Making Approach

Judith E. Deutsch, PT, PhD

Professor and Director, Rivers Lab
Department of Rehabilitation and Movement Sciences
Doctoral Programs in Physical Therapy
University of Medicine and Dentistry of New Jersey
Newark, New Jersey

Ellen Zambo Anderson, PT, MA, GCS

Associate Professor
Department of Rehabilitation and Movement Sciences
Doctoral Programs in Physical Therapy
University of Medicine and Dentistry of New Jersey
Newark, New Jersey

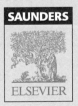

SAUNDERS

ELSEVIER

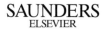

11830 Westline Industrial Drive
St. Louis, Missouri 63146

COMPLEMENTARY THERAPIES FOR PHYSICAL THERAPY:
A CLINICAL DECISION-MAKING APPROACH

ISBN-13: 978-0-7216-0111-3
ISBN-10: 0-7216-0111-1

**Copyright © 2008 by Saunders, an imprint of Elsevier Inc.**

**All rights reserved.** No part of this publication may be reproduced or transmitted in any form or by any means, electronic or mechanical, including photocopying, recording, or any information storage and retrieval system, without permission in writing from the publisher. Permissions may be sought directly from Elsevier's Rights Department: phone: (+1) 215 239 3804 (US) or (+44) 1865 843830 (UK); fax: (+44) 1865 853333; e-mail: healthpermissions@elsevier.com. You may also complete your request on-line via the Elsevier website at http://www.elsevier.com/permissions.

### Notice

Neither the Publisher nor the Authors assume any responsibility for any loss or injury and/or damage to persons or property arising out of or related to any use of the material contained in this book. It is the responsibility of the treating practitioner, relying on independent expertise and knowledge of the patient, to determine the best treatment and method of application for the patient.

The Publisher

ISBN-13: 978-0-7216-0111-3
ISBN-10: 0-7216-0111-1

*Vice President and Publisher:* Linda Duncan
*Senior Editor:* Kellie White
*Associate Developmental Editor:* Kelly Milford
*Publishing Services Manager:* Julie Eddy
*Project Manager:* Rich Barber
*Design Direction:* Julia Dummitt

Printed in the United States

Last digit is the print number:  9  8  7  6  5  4  3  2  1

Working together to grow
libraries in developing countries

www.elsevier.com | www.bookaid.org | www.sabre.org

ELSEVIER    BOOK AID International    Sabre Foundation

# Contributors

**Ellen Zambo Anderson, PT, MA, GCS**
Associate Professor
Department of Rehabilitation and Movement
    Sciences
Doctoral Programs in Physical Therapy
University of Medicine and Dentistry of New Jersey
Newark, New Jersey

**Glenna Batson, PT, DSc**
Assistant Professor
Winston-Salem State University
Director, Wellness Partners in the Arts, Inc.
Durham, North Carolina

**Judith E. Deutsch, PT, PhD**
Professor and Director, Rivers Lab
Department of Rehabilitation and Movement
    Sciences
Doctoral Programs in Physical Therapy
University of Medicine and Dentistry of New Jersey
Newark, New Jersey

**Chantel Dickinson, PT**
Certified Pilates Instructor
Energy Balancing Pilates Studio
Englewood, New Jersey

**Mary Lou Galantino, PT, PhD**
Professor
Doctoral Program in Physical Therapy
The Richard Stockton College of New Jersey
Pomona, New Jersey
Adjunct Research Scholar
Center for Clinical Epidemiology and Biostatistics
University of Pennsylvania School of Medicine
Philadelphia, Pennsylvania

**Bill Gallagher, PT, CMT, CYT**
Director
The East West Rehab Institute
New York, New York

**Susan Gerik, MD**
Associate Professor of Pediatrics and Family
    Medicine
Director of Children's Special Services
University of Texas Medical Branch
Galveston, Texas

**Gary L. Goldberg, PhD**
Clinical Psychologist, Siegler Center for
    Integrative Medicine
St. Barnabas Ambulatory Care Center, Livingston,
    New Jersey
Assistant Professor, ICAM and Department of
    Medicine
University of Medicine and Dentistry of New Jersey
Newark, New Jersey

**Susan Gould Fogerite, PhD**
Director of Research, Institute for Complementary
    and Alternative Medicine (ICAM)
Associate Professor, Department of Clinical Lab
    Sciences
School of Health-Related Professions University
    of Medicine and Dentistry of New Jersey
Newark, New Jersey

**Richard Lund**
Director
Wellness Through Tai Chi
Woodbridge, New Jersey

**Ellen D. Mandel, MS, PA-C, RD**
Assistant Professor
Department of Physician Assistant
Seton Hall University
South Orange, New Jersey

**John Maypole, MD**
Assistant Professor of Pediatrics
Boston University School of Medicine
Chief of Pediatrics
South End Community Health Center
Boston, Massachusetts

**Suzanne McDonough, PT, PhD**
Professor
School of Health Sciences
University of Ulster
Belfast, Ireland

**Patricia Quinn McGinnis, PT, PhD**
Associate Professor
Doctoral Program in Physical Therapy
The Richard Stockton College of New Jersey
Pomona, New Jersey

**Sheelagh McNeill PhD, LicAc, BAC, SMISCP**
Senior Orthopaedic Physiotherapist
Physiotherapy Department
Sligo General Hospital
The Mall
Sligo, Ireland

**John Musser, MD**
Center for Clinical Epidemiology and Biostatistics
University of Pennsylvania School of Medicine
Philadelphia, Pennsylvania

**Diane Rigassio Radler, PhD, RD**
Assistant Professor
Graduate Programs in Clinical Nutrition
University of Medicine and Dentistry of New
    Jersey
School of Health-Related Professions University
    of Medicine and Dentistry of New Jersey
Newark, New Jersey

**Cathy Caro Scarpito, PT**
Owner, ProCare Physical Therapy
Piscataway, New Jersey

**James Stephens, PT, PhD**
Clinical Assistant Professor
Department of Physical Therapy
Temple University
Philadelphia, Pennsylvania

**Cindy Wolk-Weiss, BSW**
Director and Integrated Holistic Counselor
Center for Healing Journeys
Bound Brook, New Jersey

**Perry Wolk-Weiss, DC**
Director and Chiropractor
Get Well Center
Bound Brook, New Jersey

**Lori Zucker, PT, DPT**
Private Practice
Livingston, New Jersey

# Reviewers

**John A. Astin, PhD**
Research Scientist
California Pacific Medical Center
San Francisco, California

**Simona Cipriani**
Pilates, Massage Therapy, Feldenkrais
The Art of Control
Mount Kisco, New York

**John Cottingham, PT, MS**
Christie Clinic in Rantoul
Department of Physical Therapy
Rantoul, Illinois

**Nancy Davidson, PT, MPH, Pac, LAc**
Traditional Acupuncture and Rehabilitation
Raleigh, North Carolina

**Moshe Frenkel, MD**
Associate Professor
University of Texas, Medical Branch
Family Medicine
CAM Education Project
Galveston, Texas

**Mary Lou Galantino, PT, PhD**
Professor
Doctoral Program in Physical Therapy
The Richard Stockton College of New Jersey
Pomona, New Jersey
Adjunct Research Scholar
Center for Clinical Epidemiology and Biostatistics
University of Pennsylvania School of Medicine
Philadelphia, Pennsylvania

**Earlene Gleisner, RN**
Reiki Master, Author, Publisher
Private Practice
Laytonville, California

**Martha Hinman, PT, EdD, MHEd**
Professor, Department of Physical Therapy
Director, Transitional DPT Program
Hardin-Simmons University
Abilene, Texas

**Shoshanna Katzman, MS, LAc**
Acupuncturist, Qigong Professional, and Energy
    Medicine Specialist
Director
Red Bank Acupuncture and Wellness Center
Tinton Falls, New Jersey

**David M. Kietrys, PT, MS, OCS**
Associate Professor
Doctoral Program in Physical Therapy
University of Medicine and Dentistry of New
    Jersey-SHRP
Stratford, New Jersey

**Sandy Matsuda, PhD, OTR/L**
Assistant Professor
Occupational Therapy
University of Missouri-Columbia
Columbia, Missouri

**Diane Miller, JD, MS**
Legal and Public Policy Director
National Health Freedom Action
St. Paul, Minnesota

**Jim Oschman, PhD**
Nature's Own Research Association
Dover, New Hampshire

**Adam Perlman, MD, MPH**
Hunterdon Endowed Professor of
    Complementary and Alternative Medicine
Executive Director and Associate Professor
Institute for Complementary and Alternative
    Medicine
School of Health-Related Professions University
    of Medicine and Dentistry of New Jersey
Newark, New Jersey

**Carla Oswald Reed, PT**
Guild Certified Feldenkrais Practitioner, Physical
    Therapist
Movement to Wholeness
Sterling, Virginia

**Ellen C. Ross, PT, PhD**

Professor and Program Director Post-Professional
  Physical Therapy
Department of Rehabilitation and Movement
  Sciences
University of Medicine and Dentistry of New
  Jersey
Newark, New Jersey

**Judith C. Stern, MA, PT, Certified Teacher of
the AT**

Senior Faculty
American Center for the Alexander Technique
Private Practice
Rye, New York

**Dalia Zwick, PT, PhD**

PT Senior Rehabilitation Supervisor
Premier Health Care
New York, New York

JUDITH E. DEUTSCH

*In loving memory of my father,* Hans P. Deutsch, *who taught me to value intellectual pursuits, hard work, and perseverance—but more importantly, kindness and love*

*To my husband, Joel Stern, and our children, Sarah and Daniel, whose love and joy make my life whole*

ELLEN ZAMBO ANDERSON

*To my husband, Scott, and our children, Kevin, Derek, and Taylor, whose laughter and love have complemented my life in immeasurable ways*

In memory of our beloved colleague and friend
Ellen Christina Ross, PT, PhD (1956-2007)

# Foreword

Complementary and alternative medicine (CAM) is maturing. Increasingly, it is being integrated into the mainstream of health care. This book is an excellent illustration of that. Physical therapy is an established allied health science with an integral role in many areas of medicine, ranging from assistance in managing congenital deformities to sports medicine to the aged. Its focus is on the whole person, a variety of symptoms and functions, and on healing. Therefore, it is not surprising that it has a philosophical and practical affiliation with CAM. When I was director of The Office of Alternative Medicine at the National Institutes of Health (NIH) from 1995 to 1999, I found the most use of complementary medicine within the physical therapy department. As a military physician interested in integrative medicine in the Department of Defense, I found that practices such as acupuncture and manipulation were already integrated into the PM & R clinics at places like Walter Reed and the National Naval Medical Center.

Physical therapy has taken the lead in the integration and establishment of standards for use of complementary and alternative medicine within health care. This book takes the next step by providing clear approaches to the use of evidence-based medicine and step-by-step clinical decision making for complementary medicine. Drs. Deutsch and Anderson have done an admirable job in providing a blueprint for the integration of CAM and physical therapy that other health professionals can emulate. The CCC and PICO approach that they have provided form a rational framework for developing standards of care in integrative medicine.

Evidence-based medicine processes can be complex. A single approach (e.g., using only "top of the hierarchy" evidence for making clinical decisions) is often not adequate in day-to-day practice.

The use of randomized controlled trials is important in clinical decision making. Judy Deutsch and Ellen Anderson have taken the "top of the hierarchy" evidence-based approaches and merged them with practical step-by-step approaches useful for health care delivery. In addition, this book provides a useful description of the context of practice, including legal and ethical issues, medical malpractice, professional standards, and quality of care issues—all important components of delivering appropriate integrative medicine. Especially interesting are the case examples, in which the discussion is framed both theoretically and through specific illustrations of how the principles outlined in the book are applied in real life. From these, any practitioner with appropriate training can understand how to integrate these practices for their own use.

After the smoke has cleared from the debate on science and complementary medicine, the suffering patient still stands before us. The patient is our primary audience—the customer we serve. In the midst of conflicting agendas driven by economics, new devices, family and social forces, professional turf, and reimbursement, it is the patient and service to the patient that we must always keep in mind. Many allied health practices and especially physical therapy, have emphasized patient-centered care. With this book, physical therapy leads the way in the practical integration of CAM into practice. This book is a guide for physical therapists on integrative medicine. The hope is that others will also read it, use it, and improve on it in the years ahead.

**Wayne B. Jonas**
President and CEO
Samueli Institute
Alexandria, Virginia

# Foreword

Sensing a mounting interest in alternative or "complementary" medicine, the National Institutes of Health (NIH) established an Office of Alternative Medicine in 1992. The grand sum of $3 million was allocated from the total NIH budget that exceeded many billions of dollars to fund $50,000 grants to explore some of these alternatives. This effort appeared somewhat meager when one considers that by 1993, up to 34% of American adults were using alternative therapies, and 72% of them were not informing their physicians about such usage.[1] By 1998, the NIH had established a Center on Complementary and Alternative Medicine (NCCAM) whose current budget is approximately $121.4 million.[2] This amount, while substantially greater than initial support for the Office of Alternative Medicine, offers opportunities to study mechanisms and effectiveness of approaches that hardly match the spending habits of adults in the United States who paid more than $34 billion for complementary medicine in 2004.[3] When one digests these data using a global perspective, the value of better understanding and implementing alternative forms of treatment in any medical milieu becomes important. Imagine yourself levitating 5 miles above the earth . . . just high enough to gather a spherical perspective. At that height, a glance to the West would reveal a population far less than what one would encounter when looking to the East. More compelling, however, is the reality that what we call "alternative" as we gaze easterly represents practice patterns administered to the majority of our globe's populace. What we consider conventional medicine when facing west is offered to fewer of our inhabitants. This fact raises the somewhat rhetorical if not cynical question, "What form of medical practice truly is "alternative?"

If one carefully examines the NCCAM website,[4] complementary and alternative medicine (CAM) is divided into five categories with their respective components: biological based practices (botanical, functional food, whole diet therapy); energy medicine (biofield, ayurvedic medicine, magnetic therapy, homeopathy, light therapy); manipulative and body-based practices (chiropractic, massage, osteopathic manipulation, spinal manipulation); mind-body medicine (meditation, placebo effect, relaxation, immunity); and whole medical systems (ayurveda, homeopathy, naturopathy, botanical, acupuncture, moxibustion). Whether intended or not, the contents of *Complementary Therapies for Rehabilitation: A Clinical Decision-Making Approach* dovetails nicely into the categorization developed by NCCAM and arguably can be used as a yardstick against which to measure complementary applications based upon clinical decision making. Such an undertaking, in turn, necessitates a compilation and analysis of existing evidence upon which to render such decisions. Clearly this book, like our federally supported centerpiece (NCCAM), strives to interdigitate the science underlying alternative procedures with the art of administering them. In this context, the value of the text indeed "complements" the value placed by our own biomedical enterprise in validating the importance of alternative treatments.

The chapters on acupuncture and therapeutic touch fall within the CAM classification of whole medical systems, and a case can be easily made that presentations on Reiki, manual body-based therapies, Rolfing, Feldenkrais, Alexander, and craniosacral therapy fall within the manipulative and body-based practices. The contributions on arnica, ginkgo biloba, and glucosamine chondroitin would be considered parts of biologically based practices, while energy therapy and magnets would be considered aspects of energy medicine. Tai chi, qi gong, and yoga could consume several categories but would most likely fall within the mind-body complement; however, there are many individuals who would be less inclined to consider tai chi as an alternative form of treatment because of its vastly accumulated literature within the past 15 years.

Against this background, the critical question that students and clinicians alike should explore is, "Why is this text important and unique?" First, along with several other emerging areas of interest such as genomics, biomedical interfaces (including robotics and virtual environments), alternative treatments are gaining greater exposure and use— both of which appear to be expanding exponentially. Since all the alternative topics covered in this text can directly affect the unique professional attributes of physical therapists (i.e., the identification, treatment, and amelioration of movement pathology, or of occupational therapists whose skill sets also embrace optimization of patient quality of life, activities of daily living and maximized utilization of the living/working environment), it stands to reason that these professionals rather than ancillary (and at times unlicensed) personnel be trained in the administration of these approaches, especially as we gain greater evidence for their efficacy. In fact, many physical therapy educational programs have now incorporated several of these procedures within existing, more traditional courses, as new courses, or as electives. At Emory University, for example, an elective course on creative therapies encompasses tai chi, qi gong, pilates, yoga, and a host of other relevant, but currently not identified as "mainstream" concepts, such as robotics, virtual environments, and genomics-rehabilitation interfaces. These contributions are provided by physical therapists who employ these approaches or by colleagues with specialized interests committed to collaborating with physical therapists in establishing or administering the techniques for which they have gained expertise. Moreover, the interactions with students are by no means purely didactic. Students actually experience and apply procedures as part of the learning process. During the exit interview process for such a course, students are required to not only critique the experience but to discuss prospective ways in which they visualize and can justify application of alternative treatments to patients with specific diagnoses. Collectively, the momentum highlighted above lays testimony to the growing utilization of complementary treatment. Second, the treatments presented by Judy Deutsch, Ellen Anderson, and their contributors are specific to those aspects of alternative treatment that are compatible with existing directives and intentions of rehabilitation treatments. The text does not attempt to engage in concepts and constructs that fall within the purview of alternative therapy, but outside the scope of physical therapy practice. Third, all the presenters possess substantial experience in the areas about which they write. Fourth, a decision-making model is uniformly employed that is not only timely, but structures the learner's thinking processes in a manner that is compatible with defending and justifying use of procedures for payment under existing (or potentially new) reimbursement codes by absorbing not just procedure but evidence to support its use. In this context, a fifth value to this text can be gained from recognizing that not only are case scenarios presented, but they are constructively critiqued as well, thus permitting the learner to "tap into" the thinking processes of the writer while creating an association between the examples and present or future patients.

The fact that alternative and complementary approaches to health care are now integral to consumer knowledge and acquisition is beyond dispute. Physicians are often encouraged to learn about complementary pharmacy, lest the non-prescription herbals and substances ingested or topically applied by their patients might antagonize or reverse the action of prescription medications. The extent to which physician involvement or interest transcends this primary concern is debatable, although alternative medicine has entered the curriculum of some medical schools. The majority of non-pharmacological alternative approaches, particularly those that deal with specific entities, such as magnets or movement, are left to the understanding of other members of the health care team, including non-physician rehabilitation specialists. We do not have the luxury of ignoring these approaches or devices, lest unlicensed or untrained individuals administer alternative treatments that might actually harm a patient.

I recall in vivid detail how an older adult in one of our tai chi studies complained of exaggerated pain emanating from his osteoarthritic knee because his instructor insisted that he follow the movement form in great detail, thereby necessitating the generation of substantial torque about that joint as the patient was instructed to transition from one tai chi movement form to the next. The discomfort and pain could have easily been avoided through a simple modification that would require the person to pick up the entire lower extremity and gently externally rotate at the hip before resuming foot contact. Whether the student or clinician wishes to be a provider of alternative treatments or to assist in a collaborative, consultative capacity with the non-clinician "expert" is a matter of self-determination. However, the time has arrived for us to take responsibility for such engagement. We are rapidly approaching a decision point with potential ethical ramifications. Will not becoming enmeshed in such dialogue and advice be considered an injustice to our patients? Given that more and more of our patients are choosing to use their resources to seek alternative treatment, the future is now, and we should seriously consider embracing it. An ancient proverb states, "That which is escaped now is pain to come." This outstanding text speaks to this double entendre . . . we can help to reduce our patients' pain now while potentially reducing our own future discomfort by becoming active participants in the CAM movement. Absorbing the content of this text positions the student and clinician to do just that.

**Steven L. Wolf, PhD, PT, FAPTA, FAHA**
Professor, Department of Rehabilitation Medicine
Professor of Geriatrics, Department of Medicine
Associate Professor, Department of Cell Biology
Emory University School of Medicine
Professor of Health and Elder Care
Nell Woodruff Hodgson School of Nursing at
Emory University
Senior Scientist, Atlanta VA Medical Center
Rehabilitation Research & Development Center
Atlanta, Georgia

## REFERENCES

1. Eisenberg DM et al: Unconventional medicine in the United States: Prevalence, costs, and patterns of use, *New Engl J Med* 328:246-252, 1993.
2. MacLennan AH, Wilson DH, Taylor AW: The escalating cost and prevalence of alternative medicine, *Preventative Med* 35:166-173, 2002.
3. Herman PM, Craig BM, Caspio O: Is complementary and alternative medicine (CAM) cost-effective? A systematic review, *BMC Complement Altern Med* 3:11-26, 2005.
4. http://nccam.nih.gov/health/backgrounds/energymed.htm (September 1, 2007).

# Preface

## WHO WILL BENEFIT FROM THIS BOOK?

The purpose of the book is to provide physical therapy students and clinicians with a book on complementary therapies (CAM) that are most likely encountered in rehabilitation. We feel it is important that the reader practice a clinical decision-making approach that incorporates principles of evidence-based practice. The process to evaluate the appropriateness of a complementary therapy based on evidence, patient preferences, and their clinical experience is modeled and reinforced throughout the book. Given the rapid rate of discovery in CAM, the evidence-based content may become outdated, but the general principles of CAM and the process to evaluate it will not.

## WHY IS THIS BOOK IMPORTANT TO THE PROFESSION?

Why write another book on complementary and alternative medicine (CAM) or therapies? Clearly, the public, not only in the United States but around the world, is interested in and seeking these therapies. Our clients are performing their own web searches and arriving for physical therapy sessions with pointed questions. We are being asked to serve as consultants, advisors, and in some instances, as providers of the so-called complementary therapies. It is important to do this in an educated manner.

In parallel with the public's interest in CAM is the development of evidence-based practice. Tools for evaluating efficacy of therapies are available. The evidence-based approach, with its triad of patient values, clinician expertise, and evidence, offers an excellent model for evaluating complementary therapies.

The ability to address our client's queries using an evidence-based approach is the reason we have written this book. We have placed the evidence-based approach into the larger context of physical therapist clinical decision making to offer the reader a framework for making those important clinical decisions. Our goal is to provide not only content information on CAM, but much more importantly, to suggest a process by which CAM can be evaluated.

## ORGANIZATION

The book is organized into two parts. Chapters 1 to 3 describe CAM, the clinical decision-making model that is used throughout the book, and potential modifiers of the clinical decision-making approach. The second part has five sections. Each section is defined by the domain of CAM as established by NCCAM. They are as follows: Whole Medical Systems, Mind Body Interventions, Biologically Based Therapies, Energy Therapies, and Manual Body-Based Therapies. An overview of the domain is provided in each section, followed by chapters that include a case scenario for which a complementary therapy is investigated, described, and either included or not, in the plan of care. For example, in the Mind-Body Interventions section, there are specific chapters on Yoga and Tai Chi. In the Manual Body-Based Therapies, there are chapters on The Ida Rolf Method of Structural Integration, Feldenkrais, Alexander, Craniosacral Therapy, and Pilates.

## DISTINCTIVE FEATURES OF THIS BOOK

In this book the reader will find:
- A background and description of CAM use and research
- A clinical decision-making process for incorporating complementary therapies into a rehabilitation plan of care
- Legal, ethical, and cultural modifiers that influence clinical decision-making for CAM
- Overview chapters on each of the National Center on Complementary and Alternative Medicine's (NCCAM) five domains of complementary and alternative medicine
- Specific therapy chapters that model the clinical decision-making process
- Case scenarios for which the integration of a complementary therapy into a plan of care is considered
- A review of complementary therapy and its scientific literature as it relates to the case scenario
- Clinical hypothesis generation, examination, intervention, and evaluation of addition of CAM to the plan of care
- Resources for identifying practitioners, additional reading, and patient education materials

# Acknowledgments

As with the writing of most books, the work and credit for this book is shared with many individuals. We are fortunate to be surrounded by colleagues, peers, friends, and students who have inspired, directed, and supported our work. There are many people to thank.

We are indebted to our contributors, who represent physical therapy, medicine, chiropractic, dietetics, clinical sciences, and complementary therapies. Their expertise and knowledge have provided the breadth and enriched the content of the book. We value the reviewers, who provided excellent feedback to clarify and enhance the text. Many thanks go to our photographers, Joel Stern and Karen Clarkson, and models Soraya Zahedi and Taylor Anderson. Their images made this book more attractive and complete. We appreciate the publishing staff consisting of Kellie White, Kelly Milford, Teri Zak, Marion Waldman, and Andrew Allen for their tireless support, patience, and gentle prodding. Finally, we are deeply grateful for our colleagues and students of the Doctoral Program in Physical Therapy at the University of Medicine and Dentistry of New Jersey-School of Health-Related Professions. The supportive environment that we work in has made this book possible.

# Contents

# COMPLEMENTARY THERAPIES for PHYSICAL THERAPY

## A Clinical Decision-Making Approach

# CHAPTER 1

## CAM Use in Illness and Wellness

*Judith E. Deutsch*

Over the past 15 years complementary and alternative medicine (CAM) or therapies have exploded in their popularity and use.[1-3] In the United States, people across the lifespan are reporting use of CAM for wellness and illness.[1,4] Efforts to characterize and study CAM were formalized in the United States through the Office of Alternative Medicine (OAM) and now the National Center for Complementary and Alternative Medicine (NCCAM).[5] Research to determine the efficacy and effectiveness of CAM also has exploded (Figure 1-1).[6] Given the population's increased use of CAM in addition to the mounting efforts to study CAM, physical therapists ought to be aware of CAM use and the evidence to support it.

This chapter provides some definitions for the terms *alternative, complementary,* and *integrative*; reviews the formation of the National Institute of Health's (NIH's) efforts to categorize and study CAM; summarizes the use of CAM for illness and wellness in the United States; comments on the U.S. government's efforts to study and fund CAM; and provides some background on clinical decision making and evidence-based practice that form the

basis of the book. The book is intended to provide physical therapists with enough foundational knowledge about CAM and a process of clinical decision making that involves evaluation of the evidence to make a decision about incorporation of CAM into a physical therapy plan of care.

## DEFINITIONS OF COMPLEMENTARY AND ALTERNATIVE MEDICINE

Complementary and alternative therapies have been defined in various ways. These definitions have evolved as our understanding and study of the field have been refined. The definitions of complementary and alternative therapies vary with the organization that defines them and shift over time. In 1999 NCCAM described CAM as treatments and health care practices not taught widely in medical schools, not generally used in hospitals, and not usually reimbursed by medical insurance companies."[7] This definition was acknowledged to be broad and evolving.[8] For that reason, in 2007 NCCAM defined CAM "... as a group of diverse medical and health care systems, practices, and

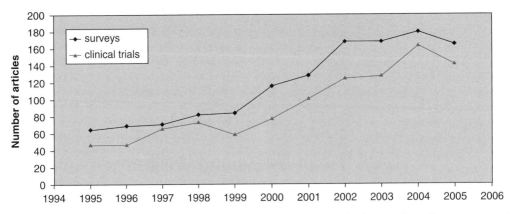

**Figure 1-1** Clinical trials and review studies in CAM. The volume of literature in CAM has increased over the past 10 years. Notice the fourfold increase in clinical trials from 1995 to 2005. Ernst et al.[6]

products that are not presently considered to be part of conventional medicine. Conventional medicine is medicine as practiced by holders of M.D. (medical doctor) or D.O. (doctor of osteopathy) degrees and by allied health professionals, such as physical therapists, psychologists, and registered nurses."

NCCAM is not the only organization or group endeavoring to define CAM. Other definitions of CAM include therapies for which the underlying model of action is different from standard Western scientific understanding; therapies that usually lie outside the official health sector (World Health Organization); and therapies practiced by unregistered (nonlicensed) practitioners (General Medical Council). What these definitions have in common is the distinction between complementary and alternative: the alternative therapy is provided in place of traditional health care management, whereas complementary therapies are adjuncts to traditional therapies.

Integrative medicine is the third term that requires a definition. It was described by Weil in 2000 as healing-oriented medicine that draws upon all therapeutic systems to form a comprehensive approach to the art and science of medicine. Integrative practices are the appropriate use of conventional and alternative methods to facilitate the body's innate healing response in consideration of all factors that influence health, wellness, and disease. Weil's 2000 definition, originally posted

on the University of Arizona Integrative Medicine website in September 2000, is no longer available. More recently, in 2007, the following definition can be found: "Healing-oriented medicine that takes account of the whole person (body, mind, and spirit), including all aspects of lifestyle. It emphasizes the therapeutic relationship and makes use of all appropriate therapies, both conventional and alternative."[9] Integrative medicine neither rejects conventional medicine nor accepts alternative medicine uncritically. As mentioned earlier, definitions of CAM change as the field develops.

The Samueli Institute advises health care professionals and health policy planners on important research questions regarding complementary, alternative, and integrative medicine. As an independent scientific adviser, the Institute strives to provide research that is unbiased, based on evidence, and grounded in science. The Institute sponsored a conference to address definitions and standards of healing. The goal was to focus on establishing sound definitions to operationalize terms for research. The unifying construct of their work was using the term *healing*. Their work provides an additional dimension along which we can define, study, and integrate across healing practices.[10]

The process of defining CAM is an evolving one. Therapies previously considered alternative may move along the continuum to become complementary and then integrative. For example, 15 years ago, acupuncture may have been considered an alternative therapy based on a definition not taught or commonly found in hospitals. Today acupuncture theory and rationale for referral are taught in medical schools[11] and offered in hospitals. The reason for this change is partially a landmark report by a consensus panel convened by the NIH that concluded that clear evidence exists of acupuncture efficacy for postoperative and chemotherapy-related nausea and vomiting, for nausea of pregnancy, and for postoperative dental pain. The NIH panel also cited other conditions for which acupuncture may be effective as a stand-alone or an adjunct therapy, but for which less convincing scientific data exist. These other conditions included drug addiction, stroke rehabilitation, headaches, menstrual cramps, tennis elbow, low back pain, carpal tunnel syndrome, and asthma. This consensus report has served as one of the most significant government statements that has contributed to increased acceptance of acupuncture and Oriental medicine by the biomedical profession in the United States.[12]

For purposes of this book CAM therapies are referred to as complementary. The rationale for this orientation is that the authors believe that in physical therapy practice the decision to include CAM in the plan of care is likely to be a complement rather than an alternative to physical therapy. Abundant evidence to support the efficacy and effectiveness of these therapies may result in the evolution of a physical therapist integrating practice of CAM. In fact the term *CAM* could be changed to *CAT*, with the term *therapies* replacing *medicine*.

## CATEGORIES OF CAM

In addition to defining CAM, the NCCAM has ordered the different therapies into four domains. Like the definitions of CAM this cataloging scheme has evolved and been refined. Although imperfect, the categorization does provide a framework for organization of the multitude of therapies considered under CAM. Because whole medical systems (formerly called *alternative medical systems*) contain many of the domains they are grouped separately. The four domains are mind-body therapies, biologically based therapies, energy therapies, and manipulative and body-based therapies.

A definition and example of each domain follows, but for more detail the reader is referred to the specific chapters in this book or the NIH NCCAM Backgrounder Series, found on the NCCAM website. Whole medical systems (see Chapter 4) "involve complete systems of theory and practice that have evolved independently from or parallel to allopathic (conventional) medicine."[13] Examples of whole medical systems are traditional Chinese medicine (TCM), Ayurvedic medicine, Native American medicine, homeopathy, and naturopathy. Mind-body therapies (see Chapter 7) "focus on the interactions among the brain, mind, body, and behavior, and on the powerful ways in which emotional, mental, social, spiritual, and behavioral factors can directly affect health. They regard as fundamental an approach that respects and enhances each person's capacity for self-knowledge and self-care, and it emphasizes techniques that are grounded in this approach."[14] Biologically based practices (see Chapter 10) use substances found in nature that include, but are not limited to, botanicals, animal-derived extracts, vitamins, minerals, fatty acids, amino acids, proteins, prebiotics and probiotics, whole diets, and functional foods. Some examples include herbal products and the use of other so-called natural but as yet scientifically unproven therapies (e.g., using shark cartilage to treat cancer).[15] Energy-based therapies (see Chapter 13) deal with veritable (can be measured) and putative (have not yet been measured) energy fields for healing. Examples of veritable energy fields are sound, light, and electromagnetic forces. Putative, also called *biofield energies*, are subtle energy forms that can be found in nature and people. Examples of putative energy fields originate from whole medical systems such as qi in TCM and prana in Ayurveda.[16] Manipulative and manual body-based therapies (see Chapter 18) deal with modification of the structure of the human body to improve function. Examples of manual body-based therapies are osteopathy, chiropractic, massage, and body work.[17]

The second part of this book is organized into these five categories (whole medical systems and the four domains). Each category has an overview chapter, in which the therapies or systems are defined and evaluated and then individual chapters are dedicated to selected therapies in each category.

## REPORTED USE OF CAM

Prevalence of CAM use in addition to the specific conditions and reasons people chose to use CAM are relevant information for the physical therapist. Incorporating questions about CAM use into the client's interview seems essential given the widespread use of CAM for recovery from illness and promotion of wellness. The belief about various types of CAM serves as a window into the client's perspectives about health that may affect the outcome of the physical therapy intervention. For example, a client may use glucosamine/chondroitin sulfate as a supplement for knee osteoarthritis (OA). Proper education about nutrition and supplements in relation to the degree of OA is important to address during the course of physical therapy.

Reports of CAM use in the United States and many other Western countries have proliferated. Use is reported for the population at large[1-4] and for specific groups such as the elderly[18] and client populations such as people with multiple sclerosis,[19,20] Parkinson's disease,[21] and children with asthma.[22] Reported CAM use in the United States grew from a prevalence of 34% to 47% of the population between 1990 and 1997.[2] According to Tindle et al, that growth stabilized in 2002.[3] However, data from the CDC survey suggest otherwise, with reports of 62% prevalence.[4] Use of specific therapies has either increased from 12.1% to 18.6% for herbals or decreased from 9.9% to 7.4% for chiropractic.[3]

Whether prevalence of use is increasing or not, millions of Americans are reporting use of CAM (Figure 1-2).

Prevalence for specific therapy use varies. Results from the NCCAM, Centers for Disease Control (CDC) survey indicate that the 10 most frequently used therapies in the United States were as follows: prayer for an individual's own health (43%), prayer by others for an individual's own health (24%), natural products (18.9%), deep breathing exercises (11.6%), participation in a prayer group (9.6%), meditation (7.6%), chiropractic care (7.5%), yoga (5.1%), massage (5%), and diet-based therapies (3.5%).[4] These findings are relevant information for physical therapists who will need to interview their clients for CAM use.

The conditions for which people chose to go to a CAM practitioner were surveyed.[4] CAM was used most often to treat back pain (16.8%); head or chest colds (9.5%); neck pain (6.6%); joint pain or stiffness (4.9%); arthritis, gout, lupus, or fibromyalgia (4.9%); and anxiety or depression (4.5%). Although this survey focused on the use of CAM for specific illness, a more recent survey of people who were older than 50 years of age in the United States asked questions about CAM use in illness and health.[19] Interestingly, older adults chose to use CAM for treatment of a specific condition (66%) about the

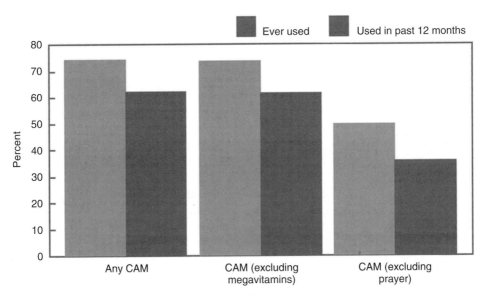

NOTE: CAM is complementary and alternative medicine.
DATA SOURCE: National Health Interview Survey, 2002.

**Figure 1-2** Use of CAM in the United States.

same as for wellness (65%). Therefore physical therapists interviewing their clients should consider inquiring about use of CAM for illness and wellness.

The reasons why people chose to use CAM also have been surveyed extensively.[3,20,23] In a group of people who had used CAM in the previous year, Astin found that factors that predicted CAM use were more education, poorer health status, a holistic orientation, a transformational experience that changed a person's world view, any of a specific group of health problems (back or chronic pain or urinary tract problems), classification as a group committed to environmentalism, feminism, an interest in spirituality, and personal growth psychology.[23] Interestingly, dissatisfaction with conventional health care was not found in the Astin study, although it has been reported as a factor by others.[24] Dissatisfaction with the conventional health care system may be a more important concern for people with chronic illness who deal with the system that is not well designed to address issues of health and wellness related to chronic disease.

## STUDY AND FUNDING OF CAM IN THE UNITED STATES

Following the history of the U.S. government's funding and study of CAM is a useful approach to understanding part of the CAM literature. The OAM was established by order of the U.S. Congress in 1992.[25] The U.S. government allocated $2 million to fund the institute: an amount that did not increase for several years (Figure 1-3). The OAM's mandate was to investigate, evaluate, and validate promising unconventional medical practices and serve as an information clearinghouse and research training program for CAM investigators. Eleven centers with specialty areas were formed to address this mandate (Table 1-1). Some of these centers are still active today. A search of the Computer Retrieval of Information on Scientific Projects (CRISP) database identified that in the fiscal year 1996 (FY 96) $43.7 million was allocated in CAM-related research at the NIH. This involved more than 140 projects in 16 categories, which were primarily in diet, nutritional supplements and herbalism (45%), and mind-body medicine (25%). Manipulative medi-

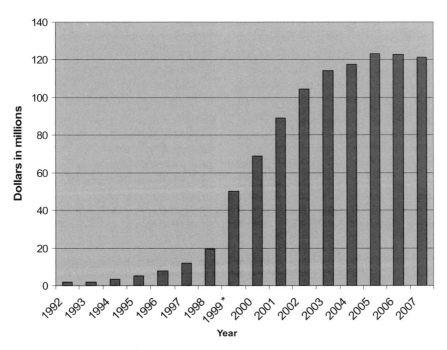

**Figure 1-3** NIH funding for CAM-related activities. Note the more than doubling in funding in 1999, the year that NCCAM was formed.

| Table 1-1 | Office of Alternative Medicine Centers | |
|-----------|---------------------------------------|--|
| FOCUS | LOCATION | PRINCIPAL INVESTIGATOR |
| Cancer | University of Texas Health Science Center | Guy S. Parcel, PhD |
| Women's health | Columbia University College of Physicians | Fredi Kronenberg, PhD |
| Stroke and neurorehabilitation | Kessler Institute for Rehabilitation | Samuel C. Shiflett, PhD |
| HIV and AIDS | Bastyr University | Leanna J. Standish, ND, PhD |
| Pain (two centers) | University of Virginia School of Nursing | Ann Gill Taylor, RN, EdD |
| | University of Maryland School of Medicine | Brian M. Berman, MD |
| Aging | Stanford University | William L. Haskell, PhD |
| Addictions | Minneapolis Medical Research Center | Thomas J. Kiresuk, PhD |
| Internal medicine | Beth Israel Hospital, Harvard School of Medicine | David M. Eisenberg, MD |
| Asthma and allergy | University of Dayton, Davis | M. Enc Gershwin, MD |
| Chiropractic | Palmer College of Chiropractic | William Meeker, CD, MPH |

cine including massage (4%), and whole medical systems (4%), received the smallest amount of funding.

NCCAM was formed in 1999, becoming the twenty-fifth independent component of the NIH.[25] Two strategic plans have shaped the direction of the institute. The most recent strategic plan reflects a refinement of the classification of CAM in addition to a more elaborate research agenda organized by CAM category that spans the continuum from validation and mechanistic studies to large clinical trials.[8] Major achievements of NCCAM include the launch of *CAM on PubMed*, a comprehensive Internet source of research-based information on CAM; the funding of three new types of research centers: Centers of Excellence for Research on CAM, Developmental Centers for Research on CAM, and Planning Grants for International Centers for Research on CAM; dissemination of the findings from the largest representative survey on Americans' use of CAM,[4] and most recently the dissemination on the use of CAM by older adults in the United States.[18]

Funding amounts and allocations changed between 1996 and 2006. The total amount of research money spent in FY 2006 was $106,079,000. The balance of the portfolio relative to 1996 is as follows: biologically based therapies (56%), whole medical systems (22%), mind-body therapies (19%), manipulative body-based practices (6%), and energy medicine (3%). These percentages are approximate and are based on total research dollars as the denominator. Also, some projects are included in more than one category, so percentages and dollars are not additive.

Funding for CAM research has grown tremendously since the formation of NCCAM. As can be seen in Figure 1-3, funding increased dramatically from $10 million per year to $50 million per year in the transition from the OAM to NCCAM. Funding continued to rise and reached a plateau over the past 3 years at the $120 million mark. The NCCAM portfolio now includes funding of therapies not funded in FY 96, such as energy therapies. Funding allocation for biologically based therapies continues to be the highest percentage of total funding. Funding for the manual body-based therapies increased by only 2% (details on how that is allocated can be found in Chapter 18). In total, funding for CAM has increased across all the categories.

This chapter of the book has focused on CAM research in the United States. However, other countries have had similar efforts. The research infrastructures for CAM in the United Kingdom and Canada, for example, were summarized recently.[26] In the United Kingdom the research council for complementary medicine was established in 1982, 10 years before the OAM. Research on whole medical systems has originated in the countries in which that health system prevails. For example, the Chinese litera-ture includes many publications on acupuncture, and the Indian literature includes publications on yoga that predate the recent strong interest and organized research efforts in the West. Similarly German pharmacopeia is a longstanding establishment of homeopathy and use of herbs and botanicals, to which access in the United States may be a barrier because of language.

## CLINICAL DECISION MAKING TO EVALUATE CAM

The primary goal of this book is to enable the reader to use a client-centered, evidence-based practice (EBP) approach to make a clinical decision about incorporation of CAM into a physical therapy plan of care. For this reason the specific therapy chapters are written in a case-based format. The clinical decision-making process emanates from the client's goals and needs for the particular episode of care.

### Client-Centered Care

Client-centered care[27-30] anchors the *Guide to Physical Therapist Practice,*[31] which organizes steps to client management from the initial encounter through development and implementation of the plan of care. The hypothesis-oriented algorithm for clinicians (HOAC)[32,33] is used to guide development and testing of hypotheses at each step of the management process. Both of these models are incorporated into the clinical decision-making algorithm for evaluation of CAM described in detail in Chapter 2 and are used in all the therapy-based chapters. Because clinical decision making is considered an art and a science,[34] elements of precision and interpretation may be found throughout the book.

Because CAM is used for illness and wellness the clinical decision making in the book also is informed by enablement[35,36] and disablement models.[37-39] Therefore the cases are written to take into account the client's goals relative to participation and fulfillment of life roles in addition to the sources of impairment related to pathology.

### Evidence-Based Approach to Evaluating CAM

The uses and limitations of a CAM in illness and wellness should be grounded in the evidence to support them.[40] The process proposed in this book uses an evidence-based practice approach as defined by Sackett et al, which is the integration of best research evidence with clinical expertise and client values.[41] In each of the therapy-specific cases the therapist makes clinical decisions based on the triad of sources identified in EBP. The clinical decision may differ for similar individuals, even if the evidence is identical.

Another consideration is that indications for the use of CAM may be affected by the therapist's decision to use the therapy as an alternative or as a complement to traditional health care management. In evaluating the literature to support the use of a therapy, the therapist should note if the therapy has been demonstrated as effective when used as an alternative or as complement to traditional therapies.

The discussion of how rigorous CAM research should be has been extensive.[42-44] Health care professionals agree that the research should be held to the same standards as other biomedical research,[11,44] while acknowledging the particular challenges of research in this area.[44,45] These challenges include building the infrastructure to support CAM research,[27] operationally defining and validating CAM practices,[44] minimizing bias,[46] and the dissociation of effectiveness and efficacy findings.[47]

The evidence base in CAM is growing. It is a challenge to read and synthesize all of the available literature. Efforts have been made to synthesize the existing research in evidence-based textbooks. The *Desktop Guide to Complementary and Alternative Medicine* is one such resource already in its second edition.[48] These resources can aid the reader by synthesizing the literature. The challenge of course is that the literature is still evolving. For example, changes were reported on the effectiveness of acupuncture between 2000 and 2005, where for seven of the applications the results were positive, but for six applications they were not.[49] The use of sound textbooks alone may not be enough to evaluate the evidence base of CAM relative to a specific case.

This book provides the reader with a system of decision making to decide whether CAM is indicated. This process incorporates all available resources for obtaining evidence as they relate directly to the client case. Therefore the book is not a comprehensive text on CAM but rather a guide to learn how to evaluate CAM to decide if it should be incorporated into the plan of care. The authors acknowledge constraints to an exhaustive review of the literature each time a client presents with CAM with which the therapist may not be familiar. For this reason, the authors have included, in addition to a more comprehensive evidence evaluation system, the PICO (population, intervention, comparison, and outcome) process as a mechanism for formulating targeted searches most relevant to the client.

The application of the PICO process is described in Chapter 2. Briefly the PICO question outlines the essential elements of a clinically relevant question. The format provides the user with the key words that will streamline a search process relative to the case. This targeted approach will select, in princi-ple, the essential references to answer the clinical question. What it will not do is offer background reading or context for a specific inter-vention, which in the case of this book is a complementary or alternative therapy. A PICO is included in each of the therapy-specific chapters to allow readers to compare what knowledge they would obtain from a targeted search relative to a more comprehensive search on the case presented in the chapter.[41]

Whether the therapist chooses a targeted search strategy such as a PICO or to read more broadly about CAM in the context of a particular case, the goal is always the same: to provide sound care based on the client's preferences, the therapist's clinical judgment, and the best available evidence.

## SUMMARY

The increased interest and use of CAM by the U.S. public and across the world, coupled with the explosion of research on the topic, formed the impetus for writing this book. The strategy of the book is to model for the reader a process for evaluation of the literature to make a decision on including CAM in the plan of care. Practice and rein-forcement of this process are provided throughout the therapy chapters. The client-centered approach to the book emphasizes the importance of evidence relevant to the client.

## REFERENCES

1. Eisenberg DM et al: Unconventional medicine in the United States: prevalence, costs and patterns of care, *N Engl J Med* 328(4):246-52, 1993.
2. Eisenberg DM et al: Trends on alternative medicine use in the United States, 1990-1997, *JAMA* 280(18):1569-74, 1998.
3. Tindle HA et al: Trends in use of complementary and alternative medicine by US adults: 1997-2002, *Altern Ther Health Med* 11(1):42-9, 2005.
4. Barnes PM et al: Complementary and alternative medicine use among adults: United States, 2002, *Advance Data* 343:1-19, 2004.
5. Becker N: Straus focuses NCCAM Directives. *Altern Ther Health Med* 6(2):24-5, 2000.
6. Ernst E: Prevalence surveys: to be taken with a pinch of salt, *Complement Ther Clin Pract* 12(4):272-5, 2006.
7. NCCAM: Classification of Alternative Medicine Practice. nccam.nih.gov, last updated November 1990.
8. NCCAM: Expanding Horizons of Health Care: Stra-tegic Plan 2005-2009: U.S. Department of Health and Human Services, National Institutes of Health, 2005.
9. University of Arizona Integrative Medicine Center: Understanding Integrative Medicine. Available at: *http://www.integrativemedicine.arizona.edu/about2. html.* Accessed June 20, 2007.
10. Jonas WB, Chez RA: Recommendations regarding definitions and standards in healing research, *J Altern Complement Med* 10(1):171-81, 2004.
11. Wetzel MS, Eisenberg DM, Kaptchuk TJ: Courses involving complementary and alternative medicine at US medical schools, *JAMA* 280(9):784-7, 1998.
12. NIH Consensus Conference: Acupuncture, *JAMA* 280(17):1518-24, 1998.
13. NCCAM: Whole Medical Systems: An Overview. *Backgrounder.* Available at: *http://nccam.nih.gov/ health/backgrounds/wholemed.htm.* Accessed Novem-ber 20, 2006.
14. NCCAM: Mind Body Medicine: An Overview. *Back-grounder* Available at: *http://nccam.nih.gov/health/ backgrounds/mindbody.htm.* Accessed June 20, 2007.
15. NCCAM: Biologically Based Practices: An Over-view. *Backgrounder* Available at: http://nccam. nih.gov/health/backgrounds/biobasedprac.htm. Accessed June 20, 2007
16. NCCAM: Energy Medicine: An Overview. *Back-grounder* Available at: *http://nccam.nih.gov/health/ backgrounds/energymed.htm.* Accessed June 20, 2007.
17. NCCAM: Manipulative and Body Based Practices: An Overview. *Backgrounder* Available at: *http:// nccam.nih.gov/health/backgrounds/manipulative. htm.* Accessed June 20, 2007.
18. AARP: Complementary and Alternative Medicine: What People 50 and Older Adults Are Using and Discussing with their Physicians. In NCCAM, 2007:21.
19. Shinto L et al: Complementary and alternative med-icine in multiple sclerosis: survey of licensed naturo-paths, *J Altern Complement Med* 10(5):891-7, 2004.
20. Huntley A, Ernst E: Complementary and alternative therapies for treating multiple sclerosis symptoms: a systematic review, *Complement Ther Med* 8(2):97-105, 2000.
21. Rajendran PR, Thompson RE, Reich SG: The use of alternative therapies by patients with Parkinson's disease, *Neurology* 57(5):790-4, 2001.
22. Shenfield G, Lim E, Allen H: Survey of the use of complementary medicines and therapies in children with asthma, *J Paed Child Health* 38(3):252-7, 2002.
23. Astin JA: Why patients use alternative medicine: results of a national study, [see comment] *JAMA* 279(19):1548-53, 1998.
24. Wootton JC, Sparber A: Surveys of complementary and alternative medicine: part III. Use of alternative

and complementary therapies for HIV/AIDS, *J Altern Complement Med* 7(4):371-7, 2004.

25. NCCAM's History and Chronology, *The NIH Almanac—Organization*, 2007. http://www.nih.gov/about/almanac/organization/NCCAM.htm

26. Lewith G et al: Developing CAM research capacity for complementary medicine, *Evidence-Based Complement Altern Med eCAM* 3(2):283-9, 2006.

27. Platt F, Gasper D, Coulehan J: "Tell me about yourself": the patient-centered interview, *Ann Intern Med* 134:1079-85, 2001.

28. Smyth F: The place of humanities and social sciences in education of physicians, *J Med Ed* 37:495-9, 1962.

29. Kravitz R et al: Prevalence and sources of patients' unmet expectations for care, *Ann Intern Med* 125:730-7, 1996.

30. Delbanco T: Enriching the doctor-patient relationship by inviting the patient's perspective, *Ann Intern Med* 116:414-8, 1992.

31. Guide to physical therapist practice, ed 2, *Physical Therapy* 81:9-744, 2001.

32. Echternach J, Rothstein J: Hypothesis-oriented algorithms, *Phys Ther* 69:559-64, 1989.

33. Rothstein J, Riddle DL, Echtemach JL: The Hypothesis-Oriented Algorithm for Clinicians II (HOAC II): a guide for patient management, *Phys Ther* 83:455-70, 2003.

34. Watts N: Decision analysis: a tool for improving physical therapy practice and education. In Wolf SL, editor: *Clinical decision making in physical therapy*, Philadelphia, 1985, FA Davis, pp 7-23.

35. Quinn L, Gordon J: *Functional outcomes documentation for rehabilitation*, Philadelphia, 2003, WB Saunders, pp 6-7.

36. *Enabling America: assessing the role of rehabilitation science and engineering*, Washington, DC, 1997, National Academic Press.

37. Nagi S: Some conceptual issues in disability and rehabilitation. In Sussman, MB, editor: *Sociology and rehabilitation*, Washington, DC, 1965, American Sociological Association, pp 100-13.

38. Verbrugge L, Jette A: The disablement process, *Soc Sci Med* 38:1-14, 1994.

39. International Classification of Impairments, Disabilities, and Handicaps: *A manual of classification relating to the consequences of disease*, Geneva, Switzerland, 1980, World Health Organization.

40. Dossey L: How should alternative therapies be evaluated? An examination of fundamentals, *Altern Ther Health Med* 1(2):6-10, 1995.

41. Sackett D et al: *Evidence-based medicine,* ed 2, New York, 2000, Churchill Livingstone.

42. Panel on Definition and Description CRMC, April 1995: Defining and describing complementary and alternative medicine, *Altern Ther Health Med* 3(2):49-57, 1997.

43. Vickers A et al: How should we research unconventional therapies? A panel report from the conference on Complementary and Alternative Medicine, *Int J Technol Assess Health Care* 13(1):111-21, 1997.

44. Jonas WB: Methodological Challenges to Research in CAM: New Jersey's Institute for Complementary and Alternative Medicine, 2003.

45. Jonas WB, Wayne B, Jonas MD: Supporting the scientific foundation of integrative medicine, Interviewed by Karolyn A. Gazella and Suzanne Snyder, *Altern Ther Health Med* 11(5):68-74, 2005.

46. Ernst E: Methodological aspects of traditional Chinese medicine (TCM), *Ann Acad Med Singapore* 35(11):773-4, 2006.

47. Ernst E, Pittler MH: Efficacy or effectiveness?, *J Intern Med* 260(5):488-90, 2006.

48. Ernst E, Pittler MH, Wider B: *The desktop guide to complementary and alternative medicine,* ed 2, Philadelphia, 2006, Elsevier.

49. Ernst E et al: Acupuncture: its evidence-base is changing, *Am J Chinese Med* 35(1):21-5, 2007.

# CHAPTER 2

## Conceptual Framework for Clinical Decision Making in Complementary and Alternative Medicine

*Judith E. Deutsch, Ellen Zambo Anderson*

This chapter describes a system for the investigation and evaluation of complementary and alternative therapies (CAM) integrated with clinical decision making. In the first part of the chapter, the nine steps of the clinical decision-making process are identified and defined. In the second part of the chapter, the process is applied to a case scenario in which the therapist considers the incorporation of a complementary therapy into a client's plan of care. Because many of the CAM approaches are not well documented in the literature, the clinical decision-making process described in this chapter highlights the investigation of the literature related to CAM. The generation of a clinical hypothesis for the inclusion of CAM into a plan of care is also presented. In subsequent chapters, in which individual CAM approaches are described, the same clinical decision-making process is applied to evaluate the appropriateness of that CAM for a specific individual.

## THE CLINICAL DECISION-MAKING PROCESS

The clinical decision-making process (Figure 2-1) incorporates principles of evidence-based practice[1] to help therapists decide whether CAM is indicated

| | |
|---|---|
| **Step 1:** | Identify client's goals |
| | ↓ |
| **Step 2:** | Identify relevant impairments and abilities |
| | ↓ |
| **Step 3:** | Formulate plan of care |
| | ↓ |
| **Step 4:** | Investigate the literature |
| | ↓ |
| **Step 5:** | Generate a clinical hypothesis |
| | ↓ |
| **Step 6:** | Select and collect the relevant clinical outcome measures |
| | ↓ |
| **Step 7:** | Intervene |
| | ↓ |
| **Step 8:** | Evaluate the outcome of the intervention |
| | ↓ |
| **Step 9:** | Report the results in the appropriate venue |

**Figure 2-1** Clinical decision-making process.

in a plan of care. The *Guide to Physical Therapist Practice*[2] and disablement and enablement models of rehabilitation[3,4] are the conceptual frameworks on which this process is based. The clinical decision-making process consists of sequential steps, beginning with the identification of the client's goals and abilities in addition to impairments that interfere with achieving these goals.

## Step 1: Identify Goals

Interviewing clients to identify their goals is the first step of the clinical decision-making process. The interview is the first part of the client examination, in which a history of the current medical condition or health interest and information obtained from a chart review are used to frame the subsequent selection and administration of tests and measures. This approach is consistent with a client-centered model and is advocated in the Hypothesis-Oriented Algorithm for Clinicians.[5]

## Step 2: Identify the Relevant Abilities and Impairments

Administration of the appropriate tests and measures allows the therapist to identify clients' relevant abilities and impairments. Identification of abilities is consistent with an enablement model.[4]

The hypothesized relationship between impairments and abilities may then guide the therapist in evaluation of the client's condition and methods of intervention. Using the information from the client's history and the tests and measures allows the therapist and client to formulate the physical therapy goals.

## Step 3: Formulate the Plan of Care

A plan of care, which includes the frequency, intensity, and duration of selected interventions, flows from the examination and evaluation process.[6] This process is familiar to physical therapists. In this text the formulation of the plan of care includes an additional component: the decision of whether inclusion of CAM in the plan of care is appropriate.

## STEP 4: INVESTIGATE THE LITERATURE

The main focus of this chapter is on step 4, investigating the literature. A detailed process of investigating the literature is proposed for the therapist who has the luxury of time as well as desire for comprehensive knowledge of the CAM. A targeted approach is also presented as an alternative to a comprehensive approach in order to efficiently evaluate the literature. Often a hybrid of the approaches is applied because targeted searches may not yield any information and a more comprehensive approach will. To evaluate the appropriateness of use of CAM for a particular client, it is recommended that therapists become familiar with the approach by investigating the literature. The following are the three parts of investigating the literature:

1. Preliminary reading of textbooks
2. Search of databases for review articles to gain an overview of the literature and search of databases for specific articles that relate to the clinical question
3. Evaluation of the literature (evaluation of the evidence) by identification of the rigor of the study design and the validity for a specific client scenario

These parts are proposed in a specific order, and some can be eliminated if the therapist feels comfortable with a topic. For example, after taking a post-professional course on CAM, the therapist may go directly to parts 2 and 3 of the process.

### Preliminary Reading

Reading general references such as textbooks before searching for primary sources is a recommended first step. Obtaining this type of reference is relatively easy, and general knowledge on a topic may be summarized well in a book. Although reading a book on the topic may not contain the most current information, it does provide an overview of an area. This overview may include a description of the CAM approach, the assumptions or theoretical basis of the approach, and the recommended indications or contraindications. Preliminary reading also helps identify important terminology that will be used to guide a search. Excellent CAM-specific resources are available for therapists with a thumbnail of the most recent evidence,[7] or a more in-depth description of selected CAMs.[8]

### Searching Databases

Textbooks are useful as a first resource but often are outdated. Searching the literature for review articles and meta-analyses is a recommended second step to gain an overview of a topic and begin to survey the literature. A review article is a description of one or more studies written by someone other than the original author. A meta-analysis is a type of review article in which a statistical method of combining results of a series of independent, previously published studies carried out for the same general purposes is used to summarize the literature.[9] Many choices of databases to search

exist, and an individual's starting point may depend on their ability to access different resources. One route is through paid subscription services, such as Ovid, which offer a constellation of databases to select from; the other is through public access to PubMed. Both search routes are described here and an order is recommended.

Regardless of the search route one chooses, three suggestions exist for searching databases. First, each database has its own configuration and rules for including citations, and it is worth taking the time to learn them to become efficient at searching. This is especially the case for the way terms are organized in the database. In MEDLINE, for example, using the medical subject headings (MeSH terms) more efficiently extracts the relevant references than use of other terms. Useful references provide an overview of different databases and search strategies.[10] Second, key words are selected based on the preliminary reading and the client's condition or goals. A good start is to use the CAM as the keyword and then refine the search by including keywords related to client scenario. The usefulness of the key words may vary by database. Third, the reader may benefit from a survey of the literature and categorizing studies as they relate to outcome or mechanism. Mechanism studies validate an intervention by demonstration or description of how an intervention may work. Outcome studies address the efficacy of an intervention by a description of the changes that occur. The distribution of mechanism and outcome studies varies with the state of the literature. A well-developed literature, such as that of acupuncture, has a large number of outcome and mechanism studies.

### Searching in a Paid Subscription Database (Ovid and VALE)

In the Ovid collection specific databases may contain CAM-based information. They are the following: MEDLINE, CINAHL, PsycINFO, and the EBM Reviews (evidence-based medicine databases). An additional database of potential use is Alt-Health Watch, which is in the VALE collection. These databases are recommended because they encompass the medical, nursing, allied health, psychology, and alternative therapy literatures.

The recommended order for searching these databases is to start with the EBM Review databases. Currently in Ovid there are four EBM Review databases: ACP Journal Club, Cochrane Controlled Trial Reviews (CCTR), Cochrane Data Base of Systematic Reviews, and the Database of Abstracts of

Reviews of Effectiveness (DARE). The descriptions of each database are in Appendix 1 as they appear in the Ovid menu.

If the EBM Review search does not produce articles specific enough for a particular client scenario, other databases available in the Ovid collection should be searched. Databases such as MEDLINE, CINAHL, and PsycINFO contain medically related references, which may provide the specific references needed to address a client's problems or goals.

*MEDLINE.* MEDLINE is an international bibliographic database that includes the fields of medicine, nursing, dentistry, veterinary medicine, the health care system, and the preclinical sciences. MEDLINE cites approximately 5000 biomedical journals published in 37 languages. Between 2000 and 4000 citations are added each day.[11]

*CINAHL.* Cumulative Index to Nursing & Allied Health (CINAHL) is a bibliographic database that includes the fields of nursing and allied health professions, including cardiopulmonary technology, physical therapy, emergency service, physician assistant, health education, radiological technology, medical/laboratory technology and therapy, medical assistant, social service/health care, medical records, surgical technology, and occupational therapy. In addition, selected journals are indexed in the areas of consumer health, biomedicine, and health sciences librarianship with access to books, nursing dissertations, educational software, select conference proceedings, and standards of professional practice. Citations are from approximately 2593 journals, and abstracts are available for 70% of the records.[12]

*PsycINFO.* PsycINFO is an international bibliographic database that includes the field of psychology and the psychological aspects of related disciplines such as medicine, psychiatry, nursing, sociology, education, pharmacology, physiology, linguistics, anthropology, business, and law. In addition to journal article citations, PsycINFO contains summaries of book chapters, books, dissertations, and technical reports. Journal citations are from 2150 periodicals dating back to 1887. Chapter and book citations are available from 1987 to the present.[13]

*Alt HealthWatch.* The Alt HealthWatch database includes complementary, holistic, and integrated approaches to health care and wellness. This database provides full text for articles from more than 170 international and often peer-reviewed reports, proceedings, and association and consumer newsletters. Some of these journals are not indexed in the other databases and occasionally may provide a useful reference.

### Searching a Free Access Database (PubMed)

An alternative database if you do not have access to a paid subscription is to use PubMed, specifically the section on CAM on PubMed, which can be accessed through the NCCAM web page. (*http://www.nlm.nih.gov/nccam/camonpubmed.html*). This database is specific to CAM and free and available to the public. The instructions on how to search the database are found here: *http://www.ncbi.nlm.nih.gov:80/entrez/query/static/help/pmhelp.html*. As in Medline and the other databases, it may be helpful to check how terms are organized within CAM on PubMed using the MeSH browser available here: *http://www.nlm.nih.gov/mesh/MBrowser.html*

The same process of gaining an overview of the literature and evaluating the literature that was described in the paid subscription service can be repeated on the PubMed search.

---

## PICO BOX

The search process and evaluation described above is comprehensive but time intensive. It is especially useful if you know little about the CAM approach. A more targeted approach to searching is the use of a PICO question to generate search terms. The PICO approach is a tool in evidence-based medicine and each term is defined below:

P: Population (client, problem, person, condition, or group attribute)
I: Intervention (the CAM therapy or approach)
C: Comparison (standard care or comparison intervention)
O: Outcome (the measured variables of interest)

Often a standard of care or comparison therapy does not exist, so the question is asked in a PIO format.
Note that each specific therapy chapter in this book contains a PICO or a PIO box.

---

P = **Population** (patient/client, problem, person condition or group attribute)
I = **Intervention** (the CAM therapy or approach)
C = **Comparison** (standard care or comparison intervention)
O = **Outcomes** (the measured variables of interest)

From Center for Evidence Based Medicine: Focusing clinical questions. Available at: *http://www.cebm.net/focus_quest.asp*. Accessed September 15, 2006.

### Targeted Search

A search using a PICO (population, intervention, comparison, and outcome) outlines the essential elements of a clinically relevant question. The format provides the user with the key words that will streamline a search process relative to the case. This targeted approach will select, in principle, the essential references to answer the clinical question. What it will not do is offer background reading or context for a specific intervention, which in the case of this book, is a complementary or alternative therapy. A PICO is included in each of the therapy-specific chapters to allow the reader to compare what knowledge they would obtain from a targeted search relative to a more comprehensive search on the case presented in the chapter.

Whether one chooses a targeted search strategy, such as a PICO, or to read more broadly about CAM in the context of a particular case, the goal is always the same—to provide sound care based on the patient's preferences, one's clinical judgment, and the best available evidence.

### *Evaluating the Literature*

After looking at review articles and then performing a more targeted search by narrowing it with key words, the therapist must evaluate the selected literature. There are many approaches to evaluating the literature. Hierarchies of evidence have been proposed by several authors.[1,14] These allow the reader to determine the levels of control as well as the ability to generalize the findings.

The balance of outcome and mechanism studies is another method to evaluate the literature. In some literatures, many studies may investigate the outcome of an intervention, such as pain reduction, but no studies may investigate how or why (mechanism) an intervention may effect change.

Another tool to evaluate the literature is to review the research designs used in the studies. This allows the health care clinician to understand the development of a particular area of research. Early on, an area may contain descriptive articles, consisting primarily of case studies; more developed literature may have articles with experimental designs (such as randomized clinical trials), in which questions of an inferential nature are asked. The latter is a more rigorous literature from which generalizations can be made. For example, in the well-developed pharmacological literature—preclinical (mechanistic) studies may form the basis for controlled clinical efficacy and effectiveness studies. In contrast, the study of CAM botanicals may contain anecdotal descriptions of botanical use

before well-characterized preclinical studies are designed. In some instances, efficacy studies may precede the preclinical trials.

Analyzing the results of a search that uses multiple databases provides the therapist with an overview of the literature. The results of this search highlight the differences in number and type of references for each database. Using several databases helps identify which disciplines are studying questions of interest. Repeating a search over time allows the therapist to observe how the literature evolves. Additional citations and new areas of study may exist.

## Step 5: Generate a Clinical Hypothesis

Typically hypothesis testing is considered a research tool. However, the HOAC model offers the hypothesis generation and testing approach as an integral part of clinical decision making.[5] The clinical hypothesis may be applied in several ways. It can guide selection of examination tools, be generated as an outcome of the evaluation process, or guide the formulation of the plan of care.

Once the literature has been evaluated and a decision to include CAM in the plan of care is made, a clinical hypothesis must be generated regarding the effect of the CAM on the outcome of the intervention. As with any intervention, a clear rationale must explain why CAM is an appropriate intervention and in addition how the therapy will be implemented.

## Step 6: Select the Relevant Outcome Measures

To test the validity of the clinical hypothesis the appropriate outcome measures must be selected. This requires reading some of the articles for the outcome of the intervention and for the measures used to capture the outcome. The literature also is useful to guide the parameters of the intervention.

## Step 7: Intervene

Including CAM as an intervention in the management of a specific case requires several considerations. First, the therapist must decide if use of CAM as an alternative to physical therapy or as a complement is appropriate. In general, we recommend that these therapies be used as a complement to standard physical therapy practice.

A second consideration is whether the therapist is qualified to provide the CAM. Depending on the training or credentialing involved with being competent in CAM, therapists may either provide it directly or refer to an appropriately trained practitioner.

The frequency, intensity, and duration of the CAM and how it is incorporated into the existing plan of care must be determined. Information from the database search results and the preliminary reading can be used to specify these parameters.

## Step 8: Evaluate the Outcome

Consistent with the *Guide to Physical Therapist Practice*, outcomes of a plan of care are evaluated. When CAM is introduced into the plan of care, evaluation is especially important because the therapist must carefully monitor and justify the inclusion of CAM in the plan of care. This would be true if the therapist administered the CAM or referred the client to a CAM practitioner. Therefore a follow-up visit for reexamination is essential.

## Step 9: Report the Outcome

Many of the CAM approaches are not well documented in the literature. Therefore reporting on the outcomes of their application is important. Those who choose to apply CAM approaches should determine the value of reporting their findings. This most often would take the form of a case report. Dissemination could be done in the clinical setting as an in-service or case presentation with colleagues, or at a conference in the form of a platform or poster, which would have a published abstract. Even better is the submission of a paper. Guidelines for publishing case reports should be consulted.[15]

The process of clinical decision making for the integration of CAM into practice and the report on the outcome of the intervention is complete. The steps of this process allow the health care practitioner to move from a clinical question to investigate the literature to apply the intervention and ultimately to document the results. The process of researching complementary therapies is integrated with clinical decision making, which we propose is accessible for therapists who are considering the use of CAM in their practice. The next section presents a client scenario to illustrate how a licensed health care provider can apply this clinical decision-making process.

## AN EXAMPLE OF THE CLINICAL DECISION-MAKING PROCESS

The case of a 48-year-old college professor for whom the clinician considers the use of imagery as an intervention is used to illustrate the clinical decision-making process. The client scenario and the first three steps (identify goals, identify relevant abilities and impairments, and formulate the plan of care) of the process are described in Box 2-1.

## Step 4: Investigate the Literature

To evaluate the appropriateness of using CAM to treat a particular client, clinicians need to become familiar with the approach by an investigation of the literature. The therapist uses two strategies to investigate the literature. The first is a detailed approach in which preliminary background reading is performed on imagery. This is followed by a search of databases and evaluation of the literature using reviews and primary sources for imagery, cancer, anxiety, and relaxation. The second is the use of the PICO format for a focused search to answer the clinical questions generated by the case.

### Preliminary Reading

For this client, the therapist uses preliminary reading about imagery using CAM[16] and motor learning textbooks[12] to identify the assumptions of the approach, the physiology, and proposed benefits. Reading from the textbooks provides the background information about imagery, which the therapist learns has been described and classified in a variety of ways depending on its application and the literature in which it is described. The therapist creates three main categories to organize the information on imagery: motor imagery and mental practice, cellular and physiological imagery, and psychotherapeutic imagery.

Motor imagery is a rehearsal procedure in which individuals imagine themselves performing a motor skill in either the first or third person.[17] Mental practice involves the rehearsal of cognitive, symbolic, or procedural aspects of a motor task without overt movement.[17,18] The goal of cellular and physiological imagery is to modify the function of the immune system and to affect the sympathetic nervous system, especially the autonomic regulation of the cardiovascular system.[19,20] The purpose of psychotherapeutic imagery is to modify the underlying dimensions of illness such as fear, stress, and lifestyle to improve health. Examples of psychotherapeutic applications of imagery include desensitizing fears and retraining behaviors.[16] These categories are not mutually exclusive. They are useful, however, in organizing a search of the very extensive literature on imagery.

| Box 2-1 | Patient Scenario and Steps of the Process |
| --- | --- |

### STEP 1: IDENTIFY CLIENT'S GOALS
**Case**

A 48-year-old college professor had an anterior cerebral artery stroke 2 years ago and was diagnosed with a Stage I squamous cell lung carcinoma 1 month ago. She will undergo excision of the single nodule followed by radiation. She was referred to physical therapy to evaluate and intervene with her decline in functional status.

### Initial Examination

*Client Report:* She reports that she is easily fatigued and feels nervous. She was ambulating independently in the community and is now having difficulties with long distances and ascending and descending stairs. When she walks or climbs stairs, she becomes short of breath. This makes her nervous, so she limits her outings in the community, which is beginning to interfere with her ability to get around the university campus where she teaches.

*Client Goals:* To be in an optimal state for surgery, identify strategies to manage her nervousness about her condition, and improve community mobility.

*Medications:* Low-dose Inderal; Altace

### STEP 2: IDENTIFY RELEVANT ABILITIES AND IMPAIRMENTS
**Tests and Measures**

*Cardiovascular and Pulmonary: Vitals:* HR: 72; BP: 110/70; *Auscultation*: decreased breath sounds both bases

*Endurance:* 6-minute walk test limited because of shortness of breath observed at 2 minutes of walking

*Musculoskeletal:* Intact

*Neuromuscular: Cognition:* intact in all domains; *Affect:* Appears composed, reports distress with community ambulation (scored 41 on state-trait anxiety scale);

*Motor function:* active isolated movement throughout with residual weakness at the right ankle and foot; *Balance:* relies on vision to maintain balance

*Integumentary:* Intact

### Evaluation

Based on the examination the therapist determines that impairments that interfere with the client's mobility in the community are the following: neuromuscular and cardiopulmonary endurance, nervousness about community mobility, balance, and residual right ankle weakness. The goals for physical therapy will be as follows:

1. Ambulate in the community without dyspnea
2. Manage dyspnea with an independent home program
3. Ascend and descend two flights of stairs without dyspnea

### STEP 3: FORMULATE THE PLAN OF CARE

The plan of care will be implemented two times per week for 1 month and includes the following: neuromuscular and cardiopulmonary conditioning using the treadmill (in the clinic) and walking outside as a home exercise program, lower extremity strengthening, and dynamic balance activities that decrease reliance on vision. This plan of care is consistent with the Guide to Physical Therapist Practice Pattern 6C.[2]

### INCORPORATING CAM INTO THE PLAN OF CARE

The therapist has read some articles on the use of imagery for movement rehabilitation post stroke and would like to explore imagery to decrease the client's nervousness. It is the therapist's impression that the nervousness is associated with shortness of breath and limits community ambulation mobility.

---

### Searching the Databases

In this scenario the therapist chooses the word *imagery* because it appeared consistently in the preliminary reading and is likely to capture the most references. The therapist can then narrow the search by looking for review articles or by combining key words.

The therapist chooses to do an Ovid search because she has access to those resources. She selects MEDLINE, CINAHL, PsycINFO, and Alt-Health-Watch. The databases encompass the medical, allied health, psychology, and alternative therapy literatures and, based on the preliminary reading, appear to be relevant for the topic of imagery.

The therapist searches the EBM Reviews in the Ovid database first because imagery has been studied for a long time and in different literatures. Therefore the therapist anticipates that imagery may have been reviewed critically.

To determine if imagery has been reviewed, the clinician selects the Cochrane Database of Systematic Reviews and finds 17 articles. The reviews are not exclusively about imagery but rather critique the evidence to support a variety of interventions for different diagnoses ranging from infertility to low back pain. Imagery is one of these interventions supported. She repeats the search on DARE to identify critical assessments that summarize the literature and again finds 17 references for imagery. Two of the references are related to clients with cancer (CA)[21,22] or chronic obstructive pulmonary disease (COPD)[23] and describe psychoeducational care or psychological interventions but do not include imagery as part of the care. A fourth article about autogenic training for stress and anxiety directly relates to the client's complaints of stress and anxiety, but again, imagery was not identified as a specific intervention.[24]

The last EBM database searched for clinical trials specifically on imagery is the CCTR database. The key word *imagery* yielded 432 references, which is too large a set to browse. The therapist then enters three more key words: *relaxation, anxiety,* and *dyspnea.* She combines the terms in several ways to narrow the search. The most narrow search combining *imagery, anxiety,* and *dyspnea* yields only one reference,[25] which is not relevant to the case. The same article was found when limiting the search to *imagery, relaxation,* and *dyspnea.* Combining *imagery* and *relaxation* yields 148 references, and *imagery* and *anxiety* 101 references. Browsing the *imagery* and *anxiety* set yields several potentially relevant references in which the relationship between imagery and reduction of anxiety is studied in a variety of ways.

An overview of the *imagery* and *anxiety* search revealed that imagery was found to reduce anxiety, length of stay, and pain medication cost for clients undergoing cardiac surgery.[26] Imagery was also helpful for reduction of anxiety in clients undergoing radiation therapy for breast cancer,[27] elective colorectal surgery,[28] and a variety of other conditions.[29-34] These articles, in which the use of imagery decreased anxiety in a variety of client populations, may be described as *outcome studies.* Examples of the outcome tools used in these studies are mood-rating scales, visual analog scales, length of stay,

state-trait anxiety, and symptom checklists. Although the primary purpose of many of these articles was to report on the outcome of imagery as an intervention, several of the authors also speculated on the mechanism underlying the intervention.[31-37] For example, Gruber et al[32] studied individuals with breast cancer during 18 months while they practiced imagery for relaxation. Positive changes in the natural killer cells, mixed lymphocyte responses, and the number of blood peripheral lymphocytes were found.

The *imagery and relaxation* search contained many articles identified in the previous search with an overlap in the populations studied. Similarly the literature appears to support the use of imagery to promote relaxation, with outcome studies.[35-39] Articles that emphasized the physiological correlates of imagery and relaxation, mechanism studies, also were identified.[40-43] Interestingly, more articles were found using the term *relaxation* than the term *anxiety.* The therapist thinks the difference can be attributed to the outcome measures used to measure relaxation, which may be more global than the outcome measures used to determine anxiety.

Although the EBM databases yielded generally positive information for the use of imagery to promote relaxation and decrease nervousness, the therapist has still not found an article that specifically addresses her client scenario. Therefore she proceeds to use some of the other databases that are available in the Ovid system, such as MEDLINE, CINAHL, PsycINFO, and Alt-Health Watch. The results of this search are presented in Table 2-1.

| Table 2-1 | Summary of Search Results | | | |
|---|---|---|---|---|
| KEY WORDS | MEDLINE 1966-2002 | CINAHL 1982-2002 | PSYCINFO 2002 | ALT-HEALTH 2002 |
| Imagery MeSH and mp | 3,126 | 453 | 12,773 imagery | 62 (limit to peer review articles) |
| Limit reviews | 346 | 40 | 266 (literature review and research review journal article) | NA |
| Anxiety MeSH and mp | 57,284 | 6,663 | 69,969 | 210 |
| Relaxation MeSH/mp | 42,706 | 1,397 | 9,199 | 148 |
| Dyspnea | 7,917 | 1,152 | 1,831 | 7 |
| Imagery and anxiety | 256 | 81 | 840 | 4 |
| Imagery and relaxation | 320 | 122 | 922 | 13 |
| Imagery and dyspnea | 4 | 6 | 16 | 0 |
| Imagery-anxiety reviews | 37 | 8 | 15 | NA |
| Imagery-relaxation reviews | 45 | 15 | 22 | NA |

*MeSH,* Medline search structure; *mp,* key word.

## MEDLINE

Before searching MEDLINE the therapist inputs the term *imagery* into the MeSH browser. *Imagery* is a subheading under *complementary therapies* and *mind/body interventions* and is defined based on principles of psychotherapy. The MeSH term *imagery* was included in 1996. Before that the term was *relaxation therapy. Imagery* is used as a term that includes guided imagery, imagery, guided, directed reverie therapy, and imagery. The search using *imagery* as a MeSH term yields 315 references; adding *imagery* as a key word increases the number of references to 3126. Limiting the search to review articles reduces the number of references to 346 references. This number is still too large to browse, so the therapist searches three additional key words—*anxiety, relaxation,* and *dyspnea*—and combines each term with *imagery.* The numbers are still high, so she limits those searches to reviews and gets 37 (imagery/anxiety/reviews) and 45 (imagery/ relaxation/reviews) articles, which she then browses. She identifies a total of seven articles[44-50] that seem related to the topic.

## CINAHL

Most of the useful articles are in the nursing literature, and many of them deal with persons with cancer. The articles identified in this database describe the use of imagery for clients after surgery or those who had a psychiatric or cancer diagnosis. In the review articles, imagery is grouped with other relaxation techniques, in which the outcomes are relaxation of anxiety and reduction of pain. As with the other databases searched not a single article specific to the scenario is found, and the therapist is beginning to see an overlap of the general references related to her scenario.[44,45,49]

## PsycINFO

Only four articles in this database appear to be related to the case scenario. The imagery and relaxation search contains articles in which imagery and relaxation form a part of a cognitive-behavioral therapy of anxiety.[51] From the imagery and dyspnea search, articles mainly about pediatric asthma are found. Only two references are relevant to this case: in one dyspnea was managed with imagery[52] and in the other CAM approaches to manage dyspnea are described.[53] The imagery and anxiety search had only general references about imagery. The one that was most relevant to the case[54] addressed the role of relaxation before the use of imagery. As with the EBM Reviews not a single article addresses all aspects of the case scenario; however, articles found

in the PsycINFO database were not found in other database searches.

## Alt-HealthWatch

Use of this database yields only two general references on imagery, which are written by the same author.[55,56] One of these references may be useful because it summarizes tools for communication and intervention.[56]

## CAM on PubMed

Free public access may be the reason the therapist chooses to use this database instead of the paid subscription services. Using the word *imagery* the search yields 1782 references. This search includes citations found using imagery as a MeSH term and as a text (key) word. To obtain an overview of how imagery is described in the literature and decrease the number of references the therapist has to browse, the search is limited to review articles. This results in 219 references, which is still a large number of references to review. The key word *imagery* is then combined with *relaxation, anxiety,* and *dyspnea* to narrow the search. The therapist identifies review articles that may be relevant to the client scenario, such as the use of complementary therapy by persons with cancer,[44,49] imagery to reduce cancer pain,[57,58] and the use of imagery in neurorehabilitation.[59] Three of the articles found in the CAM on PubMed search were not found in the MEDLINE search.

A final limit of meta-analyses is placed on the CAM on PubMed search, and this yields four articles. The meta-analyses were selected because in this type of article a statistical method of combining results of independent, previously published studies that were carried out for the same general purposes is used to summarize the literature.[9] From the meta-analysis search, one reference[53] is related to the physiological application of imagery for individuals with dyspnea and may be useful in directing the therapist to specific articles on the use of imagery for dyspnea. This reference already had been identified in the PsycINFO search.

### *Evaluating the Literature*

In this exercise, the search of EBM databases and discipline-specific databases does not yield a single article that specifically addressed the case scenario. However, from the first part of the search using the EBM Reviews, the therapist learns that imagery was used for a variety of client populations. The CCTR database in particular was useful in helping the therapist identify the breadth of studies on imagery and the specific instruments used to measure it. In the second part of the search, using other Ovid databases, related articles were found in which imagery was used for relaxation in the management of clients with either cancer (mostly in MEDLINE) or dyspnea (mostly in PsycINFO). The CINAHL search did not produce articles that were different from the other discipline-specific databases, possibly because most of the articles referenced in MEDLINE were from the nursing literature and overlap with the CINAHL citations. The majority of the studies the therapist identified were outcome studies, and in most instances imagery was used as a complement to another intervention.

In review of the designs found in the search, the therapist finds that the literature on imagery appears to contain a large number of controlled trials that have demonstrated efficacy. In addition, in some articles issues about the method of administering imagery and the appropriate dose are discussed.[23] The exact nature of imagery is evaluated by determination of whether a relaxation response can be compared with imagery[27] and whether clients are complying.[57] The therapists determines that the quality of the literature is fairly good. She bases this decision on the number and quality of the efficacy studies. The therapist may not always have time to do such an extensive search. Instead she may use a targeted PICO approach.

---

### PICO BOX

The therapist performs a targeted search using the PICO approach as outlined below. The search is conducted on September 15, 2006. (Note the 4-year gap from the original search in the chapter.)

P: Cancer
I: Imagery
O: Anxiety, dyspnea

Combining all of the search terms yields no references. Using only the dyspnea outcome for the search yields an article that was identified in the previous search.[53] Using only anxiety for the search yields two additional articles[60,61] that were relevant for this case. In all instances some support exists for the use of imagery to reduce dyspnea and anxiety for people with breast cancer.

P = **Population** (patient/client, problem, person condition or group attribute)
I = **Intervention** (the CAM therapy or approach)
C = **Comparison** (standard care or comparison intervention)
O = **Outcomes** (the measured variables of interest)

---

## Steps 5 and 6: Generate a Clinical Hypothesis and Select the Relevant Clinical Outcomes

Having decided to include imagery as an intervention, the therapist must generate a clinical hypothesis. In this case the therapist hypothesizes that a reduction in nervousness will result in a reduction in dyspnea and in turn will improve the client's ability to ambulate in the university community environment. The therapist will therefore examine the client with measurement tools that will capture these predicted changes. These tests include the state-trait anxiety test, a visual analog scale, community ambulation distance, and dyspnea during ambulation in the relevant context for this client. Given the lack of information on imagery and dyspnea for a client with a diagnosis of cancer and stroke, the therapist anticipates that it may be appropriate to document this experience. The therapist consults books and articles about writing case studies to ensure collection of information in a consistent and valid manner.[15,62]

## Step 7: Intervene

The therapist must determine if she is qualified to use imagery as an intervention or knows enough about imagery to direct the client to identify a suitable imagery practitioner. The therapist has read that imagery is indicated for the person who exhibits interest in assuming personal responsibility for health management; has no secondary gains from the disease state under treatment; and believes that this form of intervention may be beneficial. It is contraindicated for individuals with severe seizure disorder, diabetes, and chronic depression.[8] Based on the literature review, the therapist determines that it would be appropriate for her to administer and recommend some imagery strategies to be included in the client's plan of care. To confirm her plan of care she decides to consult a colleague who was trained as a clinical psychologist.

The therapist recommends that the client consider incorporation of imagery prior to attempting her community ambulation. This includes a tape that guides her through the rehearsal of the walking activities that she finds stressful with specific attention to regulation of her breathing. A practice session during therapy is introduced to refine the details of the script. The therapist then produces an audiotape to which the client can listen. The client is instructed to monitor her breathing rate during the imagery and the ambulation. During ambulation if breathing rate exceeds a specific threshold she is to pause and use imagery to reduce the dyspnea and then proceed.

## Steps 8 and 9: Evaluate the Outcome and Report the Results

Before the inclusion of imagery in the plan of care the therapist has collected some baseline measures on dyspnea, stress, and functional mobility. The therapist collects the same measures after the client has completed 4 weeks of training. For this particular client, the integration of imagery as part of a wellness program has resulted in decreases in stress and improvements in well-being. Because in the therapist's original search little was reported on imagery and dyspnea for individuals who have had both a stroke and cancer, she decides to write a case report. In addition she invites the client to return for a follow-up visit in 2 months to determine if the intervention has had a long-term effect.

Several choices exist for selection of a journal to which to submit the case study, including the complementary therapy literature or the allied health literature. In the physical therapy literature she identifies two section journals: *The Journal of Neurologic Physical Therapy (JNPT)*, which is the official peer-reviewed journal of the Neurology Section of the American Physical Therapy Association (APTA) and the *Cardiopulmonary Physical Therapy* journal. Readers of this literature would be interested in an article on the application of imagery for wellness. Journals in these areas of literature already have published articles about complementary therapies, which indicates an interest and willingness to publish in the area of CAM.

## SUMMARY

This chapter details the process of clinical decision making regarding the inclusion of CAM in the plan of care. The clinical decision-making process integrates principles from the disablement and enablement models, the HOAC algorithm, the *Guide to Physical Therapist Practice*, and evidence-based practice. The process was applied to a case of an individual post stroke who also had cancer to determine if the use of imagery could complement the existing physical therapy plan of care. The approach described here is used throughout the book in the therapy-specific chapters.

## REFERENCES

1. Sackett DL et al: *Evidence-based medicine: how to practice and teach EBM,* ed 2, London, 2000, Churchill Livingstone.
2. American Physical Therapy Association: *American Physical Therapy Association: guide to physical therapist practice,* ed 2, Alexandria, Va, 2001, The Association.
3. Nagi S: Some conceptual issues in disability and rehabilitation, *Sociol Rehabil* 100-13, 1965.
4. Quinn L, Gordon J: *Functional outcomes documentation for rehabilitation,* Philadelphia, 2003, WB Saunders Co, pp. 6-7.
5. Rothstein JM, Echternach JL, Riddle DL: The Hypothesis-Oriented Algorithm for clinicians II (HOAC II): a guide for patient management, *Phys Ther* 83:455-70, 2003.
6. Schenkamn M, Deutsch JE et al: An integrated framework for clinical decision making in neurologic physical therapist practice, *Phys Ther* 86: 1681-1702, 2006.
7. Ernst E, Pittler MH et al: *The desktop guide to complementary and alternative medicine,* Philadelphia, 2006, Elsevier.
8. Jonas WB, Levin JS: *Essentials of complementary and alternative medicine,* Philadelphia, 1999, Lippincott Williams and Wilkins.
9. Portney LG, Watkins MP: *Foundations of clinical research: applications to practice,* ed 2, Upper Saddle River, NJ, 2000, Prentice-Hall Health.
10. Helewa A, Walker JM: *Critical evaluation of research in physical rehabilitation: towards evidence-based practice,* Philadelphia, 2000, WB Saunders.
11. MEDLINE (2006). NLM Fact Sheet, retrieved July 21, 2007, from http://www.nlm.nih.gov/pubs/factsheets/medline.html.
12. CINAHL (2007): Journals Indexed. CINAHL. 2007.
13. APA (2007): PsycInfo Fact Sheet, APA.
14. Jadad AR, Moore RA et al: Assessing the quality of reports of randomized clinical trials: is blinding necessary? *Control Clin Trials* 17:1-12, 1996.
15. McEwen I, editor: *Writing case reports: a how-to manual for clinicians,* Alexandria, Va, 1996, American Physical Therapy Association.
16. Freeman LW: Imagery. In Freeman LW, Lawlis GF, editors: *Mosby's complementary and alternative medicine: a research-based approach,* St Louis, 2001, Elsevier, pp 260-83.
17. Schmidt RA, Wrisberg CA: *Motor learning and performance,* ed 2, Champaign, Ill, 2000, Human Kinetics, pp 222-7.
18. Richardson A: Mental practice: a review and discussion. Part I, *Res Q* 38:95-107, 1967.
19. Naparstek B: *Staying well with guided imagery,* New York, 1994, Time Warner.
20. Zahourek RP: Imagery. In Zahourek RP, editor: *Relaxation and imagery: tools for therapeutic commu-*

*nication and intervention,* Philadelphia, 1988, WB Saunders, pp 53-83.

21. Devine EC, Westlake SK: The effects of psychoeducational care provided to adults with cancer: meta-analysis of 116 studies, *Oncol Nurs Forum* 22:1369-81, 1995.

22. Sheard T, Maguire P: The effect of psychological interventions on anxiety and depression in cancer patients: results of two meta-analyses, *Br J Cancer* 8:177-1780, 1999.

23. NHS Centre for Reviews and Dissemination: Meta-analysis of the effects of psychoeducational care in adults with chronic obstructive pulmonary disease, *Database of Abstracts of Reviews of Effectiveness* 4, 2002.

24. Knji N, Ernst E: Autogenic training for stress and anxiety: a systematic review, *Complement Ther Med* 8:106-10, 2000.

25. Simberkoff MS et al: Efficacy of pneumococcal vaccine in high-risk patients: results of a Veterans Administration cooperative study, *N Engl J Med* 315:1318-27, 1986.

26. Halpin LS, Speir AM, CapoBianco P, Barnett SD: Guided imagery in cardiac surgery, *Outcomes Manag* 6:132-7, 2000.

27. Kolcaba K, Fox C: The effects of guided imagery on comfort of women with early stage breast cancer undergoing radiation therapy, *Oncol Nurs Forum* 26:67-72, 1999.

28. Tusek DL et al: Guided imagery: a significant advance in the care of patients undergoing elective colorectal surgery, *Dis Colon Rectum* 40:172-8, 1997.

29. Thompson MB, Coppens NM: The effects of guided imagery on anxiety levels and movement of clients undergoing magnetic resonance imaging, *Holistic Nurs Pract* 8:59-69, 1994.

30. Forbes D et al: Imagery rehearsal in the treatment of posttraumatic nightmares in Australian veterans with chronic combat-related PTSD: 12-month follow-up data, *J Trauma Stress* 16:509-13, 2003.

31. Manyande A et al: Preoperative rehearsal of active coping imagery influences subjective and hormonal responses to abdominal surgery. *Psychosom Med* 57:177-82, 1995.

32. Gruber BL et al: Immunological responses of breast cancer patients to behavioral interventions, *Biofeedback Self Regul* 18:1-22, 1993.

33. Holden-Lund C: Effects of relaxation with guided imagery on surgical stress and wound healing, *Res Nurs Health* 11:235-44, 1988.

34. Cupal DD, Brewer BW: Effects of relaxation and guided imagery on knee strength, re-injury anxiety, and pain following anterior cruciate ligament reconstruction, *Rehabil Psychol* 46:28-43, 2001.

35. Eller LS: Effects of cognitive-behavioral interventions on quality of life in persons with HIV, *Int J Nurs Stud* 36:223-33, 1999.

36. Walker LG et al: Psychological, clinical and pathological effects of relaxation training and guided imagery during primary chemotherapy, *Br J Cancer* 80:262-8, 1999.

37. Coote D, Tenenbaum G: Can emotive imagery aid in tolerating exertion efficiently? *J Sports Med Phys Fitness* 38:344-54, 1998.

38. Syrjala KL et al: Relaxation and imagery and cognitive-behavioral training reduce pain during cancer treatment: a controlled clinical trial, *Pain* 63:189-98, 1995.

39. Maguire BL: The effects of imagery on attitudes and moods in multiple sclerosis patients, *Altern Ther Health Med* 2:75-9, 1996.

40. McKinney CH et al: Effects of guided imagery and music (GIM) therapy on mood and cortisol in healthy adults, *Health Psychol* 16:390-400, 1997.

41. Gregerson MB, Roberts IM, Amiri MM: Absorption and imagery locate immune responses in the body, *Biofeedback Self Regul* 21:149-65, 1996.

42. Zachariae R et al: Changes in cellular immune function after immune specific guided imagery and relaxation in high and low hypnotizable healthy subjects, *Psychother Psychosom* 61:74-92, 1994.

43. Jasnosky ML, Kugler J: Relaxation, imagery, and neuroimmuno-modulation, *Ann N Y Acad Sci* 496:722–30, 1987.

44. Van Fleet S: Relaxation and imagery for symptom management: improving patient assessment and individualizing treatment, *Oncol Nurs Forum* 27:501-10, 2000.

45. Eller LS: Guided imagery interventions for symptom management, *Ann Rev Nurs Res* 17:57-84, 1999.

46. Clark DM: Anxiety disorders: why they persist and how to treat them, *Behav Res Ther* 37(Suppl 1):S5-S27, 1999.

47. Stephens R: Imagery: a strategic intervention to empower clients. Part I—Review of research literature, *Clin Nurse Spec* 7:170-4, 1993.

48. King JV: A holistic technique to lower anxiety: relaxation with guided imagery, *J Holist Nurs* 6:16-20, 1988.

49. Spiegel D, Moore R: Imagery and hypnosis in the treatment of cancer patients, *Oncol (Hunting).* 11:1179-89, 1997.

50. Harding S: Relaxation: with or without imagery? *Int J Nurs Pract* 2:160-2, 1996.

51. Borkovec TD, Ruscio AM: Psychotherapy for generalized anxiety disorder, *J Clin Psychiatry* 62(Suppl 11):37-42, 2001.

52. Hanley GL, Chinn D: Stress management: an integration of multidimensional arousal and imagery theories with case study, *J Ment Imagery* 13:107, 1989.

53. Pan CX et al: Complementary and alternative medicine in the management of pain, dyspnea, and nausea and vomiting near the end of life: a systematic review, *J Pain Symptom Manage* 20:374-87, 2000.

54. Levine RB, Gross AM: The role of relaxation in systematic desensitization, *Behav Res Ther* 23:187-96, 1985.

55. Zahourek RP: Imagery, *Altern Health Pract* 4:203-31, 1998.

56. Zahourek RP: Overview: relaxation and imagery tools for therapeutic communication and intervention, *Altern Health Pract* 3:89-110, 1997.

57. Wallace KG: Analysis of recent literature concerning relaxation and imagery interventions for cancer pain, *Cancer Nurs* 20:79-87, 1997.

58. Redd WH, Montgomery GH, DuHamel KN: Behavioral intervention for cancer treatment side effects. *J Natl Cancer Inst* 93:810-23, 2001.

59. Jackson PL et al: Potential role of mental practice using motor imagery in neurologic rehabilitation, *Arch Phys Med Rehabil* 82:1133-41, 2001.

60. Hosaka T et al: Effects of a modified group intervention with early-stage breast cancer patients, *Gen Hosp Psychiatry* 23:145-51, 2001.

61. Hosaka T et al: Effects of a structured psychiatric intervention on immune function of cancer patients, *Tokai J Exp Clin Med* 25(4-6):183-8, 2000.

62. Lukoff D, Edwards D, Miller M: The case study as a scientific method for studying alternative therapies, *Altern Ther Health Med* 4:44-52, 1998.

# APPENDIX 1

## EBM Databases

The ACP Journal Club (1991-2002) contains enhanced abstracts and commentaries of methodologically sound and clinically relevant articles from top clinical journals. The editors of the ACP Journal Club screen the top clinical journals, write an enhanced abstract of the chosen articles, and provide a commentary on the value of the article for clinical practice. Using this source, clinicians can understand quickly and apply to their practice important changes in medical knowledge without having to read and synthesize for themselves thousands of journal articles.

The Cochrane Controlled Trials Reviews (CCTR) contains enhanced abstracts and commentaries of methodologically sound and clinically relevant studies from top clinical journals. It is considered the bibliographical database of definitive controlled health care and contains more than 300,000 bibliographical references.

The Cochrane Database of Systematic Reviews (COCH) includes the full text of the regularly updated systematic reviews of the effects of health care prepared by The Cochrane Collaboration. The reviews are presented in two types:

- Complete reviews: regularly updated Cochrane Reviews, prepared and maintained by Collaborative Review Groups

- Protocols: protocols for reviews currently being prepared (all include an expected date of completion). Protocols are the background, objectives, and methods of reviews in preparation.

DARE is a full-text database that contains critical assessments of systematic reviews from a variety of medical journals. DARE is produced by the expert reviewers and information staff of the National Health Services' Centre for Reviews and Dissemination (NHS CRD) at the University of York, England, and consists of structured abstracts of systematic reviews from all over the world. DARE records cover topics such as diagnosis, prevention, rehabilitation, screening, and treatment.

The recommended order for searching these databases is to start with the EBM Review databases. Currently in Ovid there are four EBM Review databases: ACP Journal Club, Cochrane Controlled Trial Reviews (CCTR), Cochrane Data Base of Systematic Reviews, and the Database of Abstracts of Reviews of Effectiveness (DARE). The descriptions of each database are in Appendix 1 as they appear in the Ovid menu.

# CHAPTER 3

# Modifiers of Complementary Therapy: Legal, Ethical, and Cultural Issues

*Ellen Zambo Anderson*

As consumers seek complementary and alternative medicine (CAM) approaches to health and wellness and researchers increase their efforts to investigate scientifically and rigorously these therapies, health care providers need to consider when and how to address their clients' use of CAM. Physicians, therapists, nurses, and licensed health care providers also may want to consider the potential legal, ethical, and cultural issues related to integration of complementary therapies into a plan of care or referral to a practitioner credentialed in a particular approach of CAM or therapy.

This chapter is not intended to be a comprehensive guide to the legal, ethical, and cultural issues of CAM. Instead, the purpose of this chapter is to highlight important considerations for health care providers as they intervene, recommend, and consult with their clients regarding complementary and alternative therapies.

Several books have been written about legal and ethical issues relevant to medicine, allied health, and nursing.[1-6] Terms such as *negligence, malpractice, abandonment,* and *informed consent* are defined,

and examples within the practice of allopathic medicine are provided and examined.[1-5] A discussion of ethics or *bioethics*, a term used to describe ethics that concern clients and health care, often includes issues inextricably linked with the law and legislation, such as withdrawal of life support, assisted suicide, and fertilization/reproduction.[3,5-7] Many textbooks written about culture and health care are primers on the health traditions of different ethnic groups and how their customs and culture influence their view of illness and use of health care services.[8-12] Understanding and accepting these health care traditions is thought to be the first step to provide culturally competent health care within a traditional or allopathic health care system.[10-12] Books written about legal, ethical, and cultural issues relevant to the practice of alternative medical systems such as homeopathy and traditional Chinese medicine or the integration of complementary therapies into a traditional medical model are less available than texts written for the practice of allopathic medicine and focus primarily on the legal aspects of complementary care.[13-17] This chapter will provide definitions of relevant legal and ethical terms and their relationship to CAM and offer a discussion of how these issues might be integrated with concerns about cultural issues and cultural competence.

## LEGAL ISSUES

Law is the foundation of rules, regulations, and statutes that govern the behaviors of individuals and members of institutions and their interactions with others. The rules of law are the formal rules of conduct that provide the basis for conflict resolution between individuals, corporations, the state, and other organizations. The law applies to all people, regardless of education, position, income, or personal philosophy. Therapists, seamstresses, physicians, and actors must obey the laws of their jurisdictions or face some form of punishment, such as fines or imprisonment. In general, the intention of law is to resolve conflict peacefully and protect citizens' health, safety, and welfare.[3] Lawsuits against health care providers can be classified as criminal or civil.

Criminal law is concerned with violations against society's criminal codes or statutes.[3] Practice without a license, falsification of records, and fraud are examples of criminal charges that can be waged against a licensed health care provider by the state or federal government. Defendants are found either guilty or not guilty of breaking the law. Individuals found guilty in a criminal court often face imprisonment as punishment.

Civil law pertains to actions that have caused harm to a person or a person's property. An individual or an entity other than the government wages civil suits. Most civil violations in health care involve malpractice, although health care providers have been charged with other civil wrongs or "tort," such as assault, battery, and breach of confidentiality. In civil cases, the defendant is found either liable or not liable for the harm realized by the plaintiff. Health care providers found liable for harm typically incur monetary damages as their punishment.[1]

Civil malpractice liability can occur when care or services are determined to be substandard or fail to meet minimally acceptable practice standards and/or have violated legal or ethical standards.[1] Professional negligence, breach of a contractual promise made to a client, and intentional conduct that resulted in client harm are examples of actions that can result in malpractice liability claims. Health

care professionals also may be found at least partially liable for client injuries if they occurred by poorly maintained or faulty equipment or if the treatment or practice environment was deemed unsafe.

The practice of CAM raises both criminal and civil legal issues. Medical licensing laws, enacted to protect the public from unqualified physicians, identify the activities and procedures included in the practice of medicine and the criteria that individuals must meet to legally perform those activities and procedures. Licensure provides the highest level of assurance to the public that providers have the authority and capability to practice within a legally sanctioned boundary.[13] Like physicians, physical therapists are licensed in all 50 states and must adhere to their respective state medical or physical therapy practice acts. Although the definition of "practice of medicine" or "practice of physical therapy" may vary among states, all state statutes include statements about a professional scope of practice, including the provision of services that can be rendered legally.

Within a medical practice act, licensed physicians are permitted (and expected) to diagnose, prevent, treat, and cure disease through the administration and interpretation of diagnostic testing, client education and referral, and the provision of pharmaceuticals and/or surgery. Physical therapy practice acts typically include the definition of physical therapy. They also list or describe activities consistent with physical therapy practice, such as client examination, evaluation, and prognosis for the amelioration of physical and movement-related impairments through client education, manual therapy, joint mobilization, electrical and thermal modalities, exercise, splinting, and home or worksite modifications. In all states scopes of practice of physical therapists, nurses, and other licensed health care providers are narrower than the authority given to licensed physicians. Activities such as diagnosis and treatment of biological pathology and the curing of diseases usually are found only in medical practice acts.

Although the National Center for Complementary and Alternative Medicine (NCCAM) has defined CAM as "a group of diverse medical and health care systems, practices and products that are not presently considered to be part of conventional medicine,"[18] no single definition of CAM exists within the law.[13] Nevertheless, nearly 30 states have added various definitions into law that allow physicians to use and practice various forms of complementary, alternative, and traditional cultural medicine. In general, laws that govern CAM are the same laws that govern medicine and health care. Therefore physicians and licensed health care providers who integrate CAM into their conventional practices should be aware of how the law may be applied to issues of scope of practice, licensure, and malpractice when procedures and interventions are considered to be complementary or alternative.

Nonmedical doctors who practice CAM may be regulated in different ways depending on the CAM approach or the state in which the therapy is being offered. Chiropractors, for example, are licensed in all 50 states, but only Nevada, Arizona, and Connecticut license homeopaths, who are also physicians. The practice of naturopathy is illegal in Tennessee and South Carolina, yet 15 other states license naturopaths. Laws governing massage therapy vary across states and may or may not include different approaches of manual body-based therapy, such as Rolfing (see Chapter 19) and Trager Bodywork.[19]

To stay current with changing regulations and interpretations of complementary treatment that is integrated into a traditional medical plan of care such as acupuncture, or as a distinct profession, as in the case of chiropractics, therapists should search state practice laws and the literature. Table 3-1 represents the results of a literature search when the key term *complementary and alternative medicine* was combined with *legal, ethical,* and *cultural,* respectively. A review of this literature highlights current and important considerations for practitioners who practice CAM exclusively and for health care professionals who integrate CAM approaches and therapies into a practice of traditional medicine and rehabilitation.

All states have broad definitions of medicine and prohibit the practice of medicine without a license.

In states where no separate licensure or registration exists for providers of CAM such as herbalists and traditional naturopaths, CAM practitioners may be vulnerable to criminal prosecution for the practice of medicine without a license.[20] Health care providers who are licensed by state legislatures such as physicians, nurses, chiropractors, and physical therapists and who add CAM to the array of interventions they offer clients may be vulnerable to disciplinary action by professional boards for practicing outside the accepted standards of care and/or risk suspension of their licenses depending on the interpretations of their respective practice acts. Several states, however, have enacted laws that permit the practice of CAM by medical doctors thereby reducing their risk of liability for practicing outside their scope of practice. One state, Florida, permits all licensed health care professionals to practice CAM within the defined parameters of the law. Knowledge of changes to laws governing the practice of medicine and health care in a therapist's jurisdiction is important for managing practice and related risk.

Many CAM providers not otherwise licensed as health care providers argue that the practice of CAM falls outside the definition of medicine and the biomedical model of health care because interventions are offered to promote health and healing rather than cure a disease. They suggest that massage therapists, Reiki masters (see Chapter 17), and Rolfers (see Chapter 19) provide services that fall outside the scope of medical practice. Nevertheless, practitioners prosecuted for offering health care services interpreted as the "practice of medicine" include midwives, faith healers, nutritionists, and those who provide ear piercings.[15] Similar to the changes in state laws that have affected licensed health care professionals, several states have enacted laws that affect the practice of unlicensed CAM practitioners. For example, under the Consumer

| Table 3-1 | Literature Search Results | | |
| --- | --- | --- | --- |
| DATABASE KEYWORD | MEDLINE (1966-JULY 2006) | CINAHL (1982-JULY 2006) | CAM ON PUBMED (JULY 2006) |
| "Complementary and alternative medicine" and "legal" | 38 | 19 | 19 |
| "Complementary and alternative medicine" and "ethical" | 36 | 22 | 31 |
| "Complementary and alternative medicine" and "cultural" | 80 | 40 | 41 |

*CAM,* complementary and alternative medicine.

Freedom of Choice laws that have been passed in a few states, unlicensed practitioners can practice CAM as long as they provide consumers with proper disclosure and avoid prohibited acts spelled out in the exemption laws. In addition, some practitioner groups have sought state registration or licensure to be exempt from criminal violations and to obtain a designated scope of practice consistent with their training and credentials. Knowing a state's medical practice act, all other practice acts, and scopes of practice relative to complementary approaches and therapies is an important step toward understanding the risks and liability that may exist in provision of CAM.

## Malpractice

Standard medical dictionary or glossary definitions of "malpractice" are somewhat limited. *Taber's Cyclopedic Medical Dictionary* defines malpractice as "incorrect or negligent treatment of a client by persons responsible for health care,"[21] whereas Aiken[3] describes malpractice as a "dereliction of professional duty through negligence, ignorance or criminal intent." More useful than these definitions, however, is an appreciation of what conditions or situations can be used as a basis for liability and malpractice. Scott[1] suggests that health care providers can be held liable for client injury if any of the following conditions exist:

- A therapeutic promise regarding treatment is breached.
- Substandard or abnormally dangerous care is rendered.
- The provider intends to harm the client or uses dangerously defective products.
- The provider is professionally negligent.

When this definition of malpractice is applied to CAM, Cohen[20] and Green[22] suggest that liability may exist in cases of substandard care and in situations in which the health care professional fails to conform to a standard of care and injury occurs. The definition of standards of care has developed over time through scientific inquiry, dissemination of research findings, and the interaction of physicians and health care leaders. Taught in medical schools, standard medical care includes practices widely accepted across medically based disciplines. Historically, CAM had not been taught in medical schools and was considered care that was not used in U.S. hospitals.[23] Based on these definitions, health care professionals who provide complementary or alternative interventions and do not conform to a standard of care may increase their risk for malpractice liability.

Today, however, instruction in CAM and integrative medicine is finding its way into U.S. medical schools,[24] and hospitals are establishing centers of complementary and integrative health care[25,26] in part because of client demands and in part because of a surge in CAM research.[26-28] A standard of care for CAM is far less developed than the standards of conventional medicine, so courts may assess whether the particular standard of care has been met and whether the CAM therapy or approach contributed to client harm based on medical consensus of the therapy's safety and efficacy.[23] Just as basic science and outcome-based clinical research has challenged or supported standards of care over time, the same is expected in CAM. Cohen[15] suggests that once research in alternative medical systems and complementary therapies has demonstrated safety and efficacy, CAM, or at least specific CAM therapies or approaches, should gain general medical acceptance and fall within a standard of care. This acceptance would decrease the risk of liability for health care providers who practice CAM either by integration of a particular CAM therapy or approach into their practice or by referral of clients to CAM practitioners.[31]

Despite the public's huge interest and use of CAM,[23] research in this area is in its infancy. Some interventions such as acupuncture have a robust literature and is now a recommended intervention for several conditions, including postoperative nausea and vomiting.[30] Other interventions such as polarity therapy and colon therapy have not been investigated extensively for safety and efficacy. As CAM research continues and specific CAM therapies change position on the spectrum of risk and effectiveness, standards of care will change accordingly. Physicians and other licensed health care providers who seek to appraise their potential liability risk for incorporation of CAM into a standard of care will find suggestions from Cohen and Eisenberg[29] in Figure 3-1.

CAM practitioners such as Reiki masters and reflexologists similarly can appraise their potential liability risk based on the research outcomes known for their specific interventions or approaches. When research of a specific CAM therapy provides evidence that supports efficacy for that therapy and client safety, the CAM therapy should achieve general acceptance in the medical community and be included within standards of care. Inclusion in standards of care would then decrease a health care

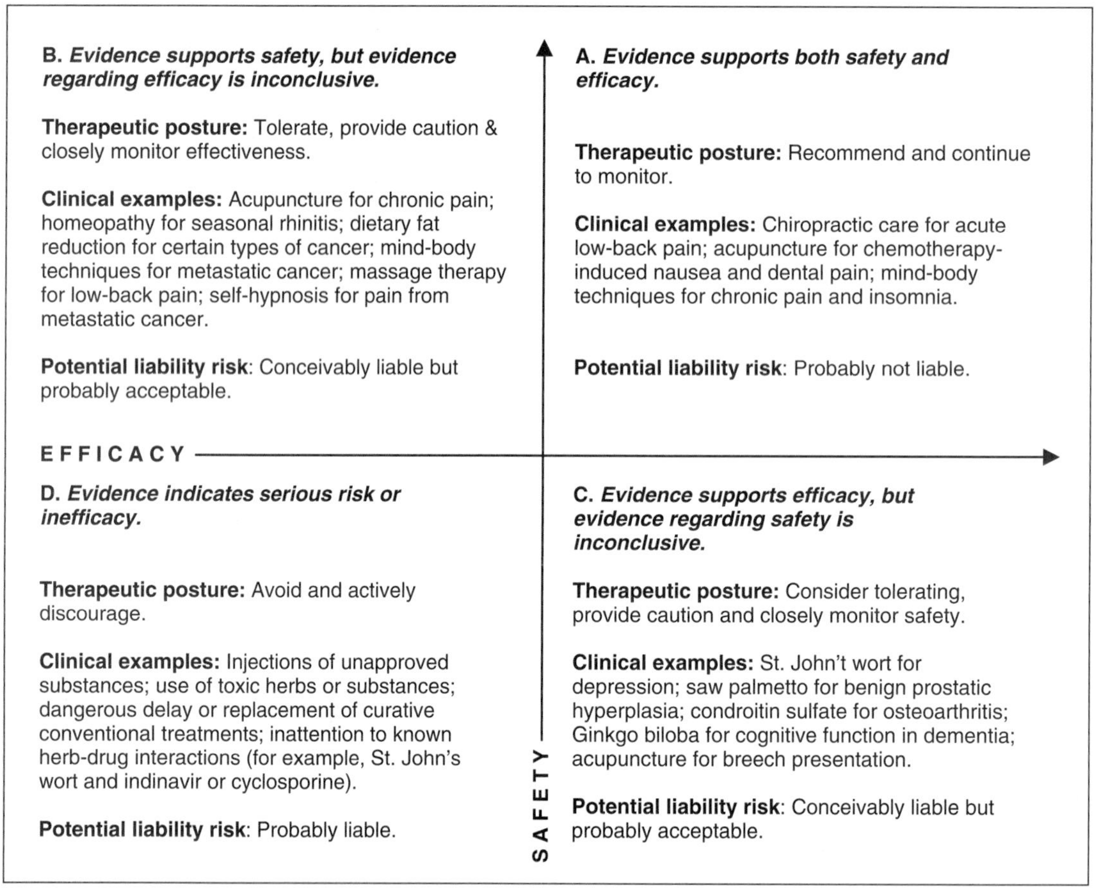

**B.** *Evidence supports safety, but evidence regarding efficacy is inconclusive.*

**Therapeutic posture:** Tolerate, provide caution & closely monitor effectiveness.

**Clinical examples:** Acupuncture for chronic pain; homeopathy for seasonal rhinitis; dietary fat reduction for certain types of cancer; mind-body techniques for metastatic cancer; massage therapy for low-back pain; self-hypnosis for pain from metastatic cancer.

**Potential liability risk:** Conceivably liable but probably acceptable.

**A.** *Evidence supports both safety and efficacy.*

**Therapeutic posture:** Recommend and continue to monitor.

**Clinical examples:** Chiropractic care for acute low-back pain; acupuncture for chemotherapy-induced nausea and dental pain; mind-body techniques for chronic pain and insomnia.

**Potential liability risk:** Probably not liable.

E F F I C A C Y

**D.** *Evidence indicates serious risk or inefficacy.*

**Therapeutic posture:** Avoid and actively discourage.

**Clinical examples:** Injections of unapproved substances; use of toxic herbs or substances; dangerous delay or replacement of curative conventional treatments; inattention to known herb-drug interactions (for example, St. John's wort and indinavir or cyclosporine).

**Potential liability risk:** Probably liable.

**C.** *Evidence supports efficacy, but evidence regarding safety is inconclusive.*

**Therapeutic posture:** Consider tolerating, provide caution and closely monitor safety.

**Clinical examples:** St. John't wort for depression; saw palmetto for benign prostatic hyperplasia; condroitin sulfate for osteoarthritis; Ginkgo biloba for cognitive function in dementia; acupuncture for breech presentation.

**Potential liability risk:** Conceivably liable but probably acceptable.

S A F E T Y

**Figure 3-1** Potential malpractice liability risk associated with complementary and integrative medical therapies. Reproduced with permission from Cohen MH, Eisenberg DM: *Ann Intern Med* 136(8):59, 2002.

provider's risk of liability for providing the therapy because it would no longer be viewed as CAM. Negative research outcomes for a specific CAM regarding efficacy and client safety therapy would suggest that inclusion into a medical plan of care is unwarranted and that inclusion of that therapy may increase substantially the health care provider's malpractice liability risk (see Figure 3-1).

Knowledge of one's own professional scope of practice and the standards of care expected within that profession is necessary for risk management of malpractice liability. Adding CAM to a client's plan of care also requires that health care providers review and evaluate the scientific literature to determine the therapy's safety and efficacy. Chapter 2 of this text describes a decision-making process for including CAM into a client's plan of care that includes a detailed review and evaluation of the scientific literature. If the evidence supports a

potential benefit from the CAM intervention with low risk for injury or negative effects, health care professionals can further minimize their risk for liability through careful documentation of informed consent.

## Informed Consent

Standard practice requires that clients give informed consent for all diagnostic and therapeutic procedures. The implication of this requirement is that clients receive an explanation about all procedures, including their potential risks and benefits and any information that may influence their decision regarding the proposed treatment. With therapies thought to be complementary or alternative, health care professionals also should consider informing clients what is not known about the intervention and what has not been evaluated so that clients are able to include this information in their decision to give or not give consent for treatment.[13] Further discussions also should include the risks and benefits of combining standard care with a complementary therapy versus providing just the standard care or just the CAM approach.[31] Documentation of such discussions in the client's chart can help to decrease the risk of malpractice liability for the health care professional.

## Assumption of Risk

Some experts[29,31] suggest that a written agreement to use CAM, signed by the client, further minimizes liability resulting from the legal doctrine "assumption of risk." Assumption of risk is a defense in which plaintiffs, or in this case clients, voluntarily and knowingly assume the risks of the intervention, relieve the health care professional of malpractice liability, and are not entitled to compensation if harm occurs.

Some jurisdictions have distinguished express assumption of risk from implied assumption of risk.[13] For example, in some jurisdictions *express assumption of risk* has been interpreted so that health care providers are released from their duty to abide by widely accepted standards of care and are protected from liability provided the nontraditional test or therapy was performed safely and correctly. Such a situation may occur when clients initiate unconventional treatment against the advice of their licensed health care providers or when clients choose an alternative approach for disease and symptom management when standard care is available.

Implied assumption of risk is based on a client's consent to the risk of harm from the health care provider's actions. Although the client voluntarily and intelligently consents to a complementary or alternative plan of care, implied assumption of risk triggers comparative negligence so that the client and health care provider accept relative liability.[13] Regardless of whether the assumption of risk is express or implied, this doctrine does not minimize the risk for malpractice liability if, while providing CAM, the licensed health care provider fails to monitor the client's health and functional status or ignores signs and symptoms that may indicate a new or worsening condition.

Monitoring clients conventionally even as they engage in CAM is important for many reasons. By maintaining therapeutic relationships, clients may be appropriately dissuaded from use of potentially harmful or useless therapies. Continuing to monitor the client also allows the health care provider to direct the client toward helpful conventional diagnostic procedures or treatments as the client's health and functional status improve or decline. Conventional monitoring is important for determination of appropriate care and may be helpful in reducing liability risk.[29,32]

## Referral for CAM

In some states, physicians credentialed in acupuncture may choose to integrate this specific CAM approach into a traditional medical practice. Similarly, in some states, physical therapists with credentials in complementary therapies such as the Feldenkrais method (see Chapter 20), Therapeutic Touch (see Chapter 14), or Alexander technique (see Chapter 21) may choose to integrate these therapies into the client's plan of care along with standard interventions such as progressive resistive exercise, balance training, and transelectrical nervous stimulation (TENS). In these situations, the primary health care provider is also the provider of CAM. In this text, examples can be found in the chapters on magnets (Chapter 16), Feldenkrais method (Chapter 20), acupuncture (Chapter 5), craniosacral therapy (Chapter 22), ginkgo biloba (Chapter 11) and Alexander technique (Chapter 21).

In other situations, physicians or therapists may need to counsel a client regarding CAM but are not qualified to provide those therapies or interventions. When this circumstance arises, health care providers may feel compelled to refer their clients to CAM practitioners. Examples can be found in chapters about qigong (Chapter 15), Pilates (Chapter 23), tai chi (Chapter 9), arnica (Chapter 6), and Therapeutic Touch (Chapter 14). Malpractice liability rules regarding referrals differ from rules governing direct client care and can raise ques-tions of direct and vicarious malpractice liability risk.[29,33]

The legal rules governing referrals to licensed medical and rehabilitation specialists probably extend to referrals to providers of CAM.[13] Physicians typically are not held liable for simply making a referral to another provider who is negligent.[20] Direct liability for referrals can occur, however, when the referral itself is negligent and the client is harmed. In CAM, for example, if a client could be managed adequately by standard care but is delayed or denied that care because of a referral to a CAM practitioner, the referring health care professional may be held liable if the client suffers harm from not receiving standard care.

Health care professionals also may have direct or vicarious liability if they refer clients to a provider who is a "known incompetent."[20] In standard medicine and rehabilitation, known incompetents are individuals who have had sanctions imposed against them or who have a significant history of malpractice claims. In CAM the condition of known incompetence may extend to practitioners who do not have the necessary credentials to perform the intervention or have been otherwise deemed incompetent by colleagues in that therapy or discipline.

Another possible situation of vicarious liability may occur with "joint treatment."[13,20] Sometimes, referring physicians and the treating practitioners and clinicians practice within the same medical group and may jointly diagnose and treat a case with a common goal. Some courts have declined to find vicarious liability in this situation, whereas others have found that participants in a group may be held liable for the negligent actions of one member.[13] It seems likely that shared liability must be an acceptable risk for health care professionals who choose to integrate CAM into their traditional practices of medicine and rehabilitation and refer clients to other health care providers and CAM practitioners. In the future, as research outcomes begin to provide evidence for the use of specific CAM interventions, such as acupuncture for postoperative nausea and vomiting, health care providers also may need to consider whether *not referring* to a CAM practitioner would violate a standard of care and be grounds for malpractice.[13]

## ETHICAL ISSUES

Ethics is grounded firmly in moral theory and refers to the process of deciding what is right or wrong. *Bioethics, biomedical ethics,* and *medical ethics* are terms commonly used to describe the ethics that deal with clients and health care.

In the practice of physical therapy and other health-related professions, the distinction between the law and ethics is blurred because often professional conduct considered to be a breach of ethics is likely also to violate the law and vice versa.[34] Ethical rules of conduct for health care providers typically are found in their respective professional association's codes of ethics. The American Physical Therapy Association (APTA), for example, has set forth ethical guidelines for the physical therapy profession in two documents. The *Code of Ethics* governs the conduct of member physical therapists and the *Standards of Ethical Conduct for the Physical Therapist Assistant* provides guidelines for ethical behavior for affiliate members.[34] These documents reflect the four foundational principles of biomedical ethics: beneficence, nonmaleficence, autonomy, and justice.

### Beneficence and Nonmaleficence

Beneficence is the obligation to act in the best interest of the client regardless of the self-interest of the health care provider. Nonmaleficence is the obligation "to do no harm" and requires that the health care provider not intentionally harm or injure a client. Nonmaleficence also applies to omissions, and the ethical duty to try and prevent harm that could be incurred by the client.[34,35] When applied to CAM, these ethical principles can be interpreted to require health care providers to be knowledgeable about the risks and benefits of CAM and to openly discuss their client's use of CAM.[35] Not surprisingly, the behaviors recommended to reduce malpractice liability risk are consistent with the ethical principles of beneficence and nonmaleficence. Clients expect a plan of care to include interventions that will improve their condition and to not include treatments or activities that will harm them or worsen their condition. A health care professional's knowledge of the best scientific evidence in terms of treatment safety and efficacy is critical for development of any client's plan of care. This situation is no different for a plan of care that includes CAM, except that scientific evidence may be difficult to obtain. Regardless, the risks and benefits based on the best available CAM research must be shared with the client so that decisions for care adhere to the principles of bioethics and science.

### Justice

The bioethical principle of justice refers to equity or fair treatment and often includes considerations of cost. Comparative justice is concerned with how health care is delivered on an individual basis and is debated every day when primary caregivers believe a client's condition warrants a particular intervention. However, sometimes the health maintenance organization (HMO) refuses to give authorization for that procedure. Distributive justice addresses the distribution of equitable health care

Derby Hospitals NHS Foundation
Trust
Library and Knowledge Service

across society.[34] Issues such as the eligibility of certain populations to receive government-funded interventions and the rationing of health care services often are raised when distributive justice is discussed. In CAM, discussions exist whether resources should be expended for CAM interventions in addition to the most commonly delivered care, thereby making fewer resources available for standard care.[35,36] Resource allocation for CAM also is debated from the perspective of relative merit, efficacy, safety, and cost-effectiveness, which may be different depending on the therapy, the client population, and the goals of treatment.

## Autonomy

*Autonomy* means self-governance. Applied as a bioethical term, respect for autonomy means respect for clients' rights to make their own decisions regarding health care and to control what tests and treatments are being done to and for them.[3,34]

Client autonomy rights are reflected in the law, which upholds clients' rights to make health care decisions, including refusal of potentially life-saving treatments. However, for clients to exercise autonomy, they must be told the truth about their health status and should be informed of the risks and benefits of treatment versus no treatment. The American Hospital Association's *Client Care Partnership*[37] and requirements that clients must provide informed consent before all medical and therapeutic procedures reflect the value placed upon client autonomy. Once again, behaviors recommended to reduce malpractice liability risk, such as full disclosure of a procedure's risks and benefits and acquisition of a client's informed consent, are consistent principles of bioethics.

Many experts support the application of these ethical principles to CAM,[35,36,38] whereas others suggest that the practice of CAM requires ethical principles that incorporate the values implicit in those practices.[26,40] The Institute of Medicine's report on CAM in the United States calls for the adherence to five ethical principles when integrating CAM into a client's plan of care. The first three principles or values are consistent with beneficence, nonmaleficence, and autonomy. The other two values call for greater consideration and a broader view of integrative care. The first, medical pluralism, is a principle that supports "a moral commitment of openness to diverse interpretations of health and healing" and a "commitment to finding innovative ways to assess efficacy."[26] The second,

public accountability, requires consideration of a wide variety of healing traditions along with fair assessment and use of health care resources.

Acceptance of all these bioethical principles may require a shift in attitude by critics and supporters of CAM and provide support for the expansion of CAM research. Skeptics of CAM may need to become more open to the assumptions of health, illness, and healing embraced by different cultures and ethnic groups and be willing to investigate CAM in ways that provide measurable and reproducible outcomes.

CAM practitioners may need to develop an appreciation for and contribute to rigorous scientific inquiry into the mechanism, safety, and efficacy of a wide array of therapies and practices so that health care providers can best serve their clients' interests through evidence-based practice. Still, many health care professionals may feel uncomfortable in situations in which they want to ack-nowledge and respect their clients' values but are challenged to incorporate these values into ethical and medically responsible advice and care. To address this concern, Adams and colleagues[40] have recommended a list of factors to be considered in analysis of the risk-benefits of CAM versus standard or conventional care (Figure 3-2).

## CULTURAL ISSUES

Culture has a powerful influence on health and illness.[11] Thought characteristics of a population that guide their world view, personal experiences, values, and customs provide the foundation for decision making during illness.[41] Some suggest that American health care providers constitute a cultural group that has been greatly influenced by the Flexner Report of 1910.[41-43] This report, which established the standards for scientific and clinical education of physicians, also encouraged medicine's use of the scientific method to study the mechanical workings of the body and disease. The report was published at a time when technological developments facilitated scientific breakthroughs in pharmacology, surgery, germ theory, and other areas, solidifying the value of science in the practice of medicine. Lost during this period was acceptance for a unitary system of mind, body, and spirit even though Western medicine had been under the auspices of organized religion until the seventeenth century, and healers were often medical and spiritual leaders.[44]

Severity and acuteness of illness

Curability with conventional treatment

Degree of invasiveness, associated toxicities, and side effects of conventional treatment

Quality of evidence of safety and efficacy of the desired CAM treatment

Degree of understanding of the risks and benefits of CAM treatment

Knowledge and voluntary acceptance of those risks by the client

Persistence of the client's intention to use CAM treatment

**Figure 3-2** Factors in risk-benefit analysis of complementary and alternative versus conventional medical treatment. Reproduced with permission from Adams KE, Cohen MH, Eisenberg DM, Jonsen AR. *Ann Intern Med* 137:661, 2002.

Today, however, the resurgence of interests in spirituality and holistic health care in the United States[23,44] and in Europe[45] challenges the primacy of scientific rationality and materialistic views[44] and suggests that people are seeking approaches to health and illness that are less secular and authoritative. Not surprisingly, many of those people have turned to CAM, which is derived from cultural beliefs and assumptions of health and illness that are radically different from traditional medicine or "biomedicine."[46] For many American-born, English-speaking, middle-class people the transition from biomedicine to CAM or integrative medicine is self-initiated and self-directed and represents a clear paradigm shift in health care. For many immigrant and refugee groups, Western biomedicine is considered "alternative medicine," so such a shift may not be so obvious or even necessary depending on their explanatory model of health and wellness. Details of a few alternative medical systems such as Ayurveda and traditional Chinese medicine can be found in Chapter 4.

An explanatory model as described by Pachter[41] is the way an episode of sickness is conceptualized and includes beliefs, behaviors related to the assumed etiology of the illness and symptoms, and the roles and expectations of the sick individual.[47] Health care providers are advised to inquire about clients' beliefs regarding the cause and treatment of their illnesses especially if the clients are from cultures whose assumptions or "truths" of health and illness may be in conflict with the assumptions or "truths" of biomedicine. This conflict is well-described by Fadiman[48] in *The Spirit Catches You and You Fall Down*, a true story about Lia, a Hmong immigrant who was brought to a county hospital

at 3 months of age with epileptic seizures. Her family was unable to communicate in English, and for many months and years the hospital staff and county workers were unable to fully and competently communicate with them. Many conflicts arose between health care and social service personnel and Lia's family because the professional caregivers did not understand the parent's beliefs regarding the etiology and meaning of the illness. In the Hmong culture, the behaviors of epilepsy were known as "*quag dab peg*" or "the spirit catches you and you fall down." From their explanatory model, Lia's parents viewed their daughter's experiences as the fleeing of her soul. "Treatment" according to the Hmong traditions should therefore include interventions by which Lia's soul could be welcomed back and restored. Both Lia's parents and her health care team wanted to provide the best care for Lia, but the conflicts that arose from each interested party not understanding or misinterpreting the other's intentions led to tragedy and harm for everyone.

In the Hmong culture the foremost traditional healer is the shaman.[49] The scope and power of the shaman, who is believed to have been "chosen" and trained by the spirits, go beyond the capacities and expertise of Western physicians.[49] Shamans work with a person's soul rather than the physical body. Their goal is to communicate with the spirit(s) causing the illness and to make peace between good and evil through ritual practices such as animal sacrifice and the burning of incense. Other traditional Hmong healers who have not been chosen by the spirits are the "Kws tshuaj" and the "Tu kws khawv koob." These healers use herbs and powerful magic words respectively to treat a variety of physical conditions such as wounds, infertility, and broken bones.

As in the Hmong culture, folk practitioners or healers of other cultures are regarded as highly valuable members of their community. These healers can be divinely chosen, elders of the community, and descendants of gifted healers, spiritual leaders, herb doctors, or practitioners of magicoreligious rituals.[11] Depending on the traditions of a culture and the acculturation of that group into the Western health care system, folk healers may provide treatments exclusive from Western biomedical care, or they may provide support for clients as they receive care from Western physicians, nurses, and therapists. In a group of Hmong immigrants, for example, Plotnikoff et al[49] found that 75% reported using a shaman, but only 2 out of 32 subjects used shamans only. A total of 25% of the subjects who sought only Western health care did so because they converted to Christianity and no longer followed traditional spiritual or religious practices. Interestingly, all 11 shamans interviewed sought Western medical care for themselves, yet only 1 of the 43 persons surveyed cited a situation in which a Western physician referred a client to a shaman.

Health care providers are encouraged to consider the possibility that their clients may be conferring with a folk healer or engaged in healing rituals or treatments while at the same time seeking Western health care. Similarly, health care providers are advised to consider the possibility that people who ordinarily follow a biomedical approach for managing health and illness may seek a complementary therapy or alternative medical approach because the practice appeals to their sense of well-being or because they have not achieved their goals with biomedicine. Regardless of the client's situation, inquiries about clients' explanatory models of health and illness and the health care practices commonly sought and used can serve many purposes. Questions about health traditions such as, "What are the things you do to maintain and protect your health?," "What do you do when you feel like you're getting a cold or have pain?," and "What are the family or folk remedies or treatments that help you when you're sick or in pain?"[9,11] suggest an interest in establishing open and honest communication. Furthermore, the answers can provide valuable information for development of plans of care that best serve clients. Survey studies by Eisenberg et al[50] and Najm et al[51] reported that 38.5% and 37.6% of CAM users do not tell their physicians about their use of CAM. Arush et al[52] found that in a mixed Western and Middle-Eastern population, 64% of parents with children who used CAM to manage symptoms associated with cancer did not inform their physicians or nurses of their use.

Encouraging clients to describe their use of folk remedies and CAM is an important first step in determination if all practices can be integrated safely into a proposed biomedical or rehabilitation plan of care. This kind of communication has the potential to address risk management, and it may facilitate a client-clinician alliance in which clients are able to participate in the development of a plan of care that is culturally appropriate, efficient, and efficacious.

## SUMMARY

The core of most legal and ethical issues in health care is centered on four basic ethical principles or values: beneficence, nonmaleficence, autonomy, and justice. These principles underpin standard or traditional medicine and CAM. The practice of CAM has not been tested thoroughly in the courts, although a few court decisions have indicated that licensed health care providers who practice CAM will be held to the same laws and rules of conduct as professionals who provide and recommend standard care.[53,54] To help manage their risk for liability, licensed and unlicensed practitioners of CAM and licensed health care professionals who integrate CAM into their clients' plans of care are encouraged to be knowledgeable about medical practice acts and the legal requirements for practicing CAM such as disclosure, training requirements, and credentials. Health care providers also are advised to seek out the best scientific literature available on a possible CAM approach and to obtain explicit informed consent from clients to assist in minimizing practitioner and client risk.

The bioethical principle of autonomy is particularly relevant in the practice of CAM, especially when cultural issues are considered. Many interventions or healing practices considered to be complementary or alternative in the United States are thought to be a part of a standard of care in other parts of the world and within different subcultures across America. Acknowledgment and respect for different views of health, illness, and health care help to encourage a positive client-practitioner alliance, one that will allow for client autonomy and likely will advance support for the integration of CAM into standard biomedical care.

## REFERENCES

1. Scott RW: *Promoting legal awareness in physical and occupational therapy*, St Louis, 1997, Mosby.
2. Swisher LL, Krueger-Brophy C: *Legal and ethical issues in physical therapy*, Philadelphia 1998, Butterworth-Heinemann.
3. Aiken TD: *Legal and ethical issues in health occupations*, Philadelphia, 2002, WB Saunders.
4. Follin SA: *Nurses legal handbook*, ed 5, Ambler, Penn, 2004, Lippincott Williams & Wilkins.
5. Guido GW: *Legal and ethical issues in nursing*, ed 3, Upper Saddle River, NJ, 2000, Prentice-Hall.
6. Jonsen AR, Siegler M, Winslade WJ: *Clinical ethics: a practical approach to ethical decisions in clinical medicine*, ed 5, Columbus, Ohio, 2002, McGraw Hill.
7. Monagle JF: *Health care ethics: critical issues for 21st century*, ed 2, Sudbury, Mass, 2005, Jones and Bartlett.
8. Bigby J, editor: *Cross-cultural medicine*, Philadelphia, 2003, American College of Physicians-American Society of Internal Medicine.
9. Spector RE: *Cultural diversity in health & illness*, ed 6, Upper Saddle River, NJ, 2003, Prentice-Hall.
10. Rundle A, Carvalho M, Robinson M, editors: *Cultural competence in health care: a practical guide*, San Francisco, 1999, Jossey-Bass.
11. Purnell LD, Paulanka BJ: *Transcultural health care: a culturally competent approach*, ed 2, Philadelphia, 2003, FA Davis.
12. Lattanzi JB, Purnell LD: *Developing cultural competence in physical therapy practice*, Philadelphia, 2005, FA Davis.
13. Cohen MH: *Beyond complementary medicine: legal and ethical perspectives on health care and human evolution*, Ann Arbor, Mich, 2000, University of Michigan Press.
14. Cohen MH: *Legal issues in alternative medicine: a guide for clinicians, hospitals, and clients.* Victoria, BC, Canada, 2003, Trafford.
15. Cohen MH: *Complementary and alternative medicine: legal boundaries and regulatory perspectives*, Baltimore, Md, 1998, Johns Hopkins University Press.
16. Cohen MH: *Legal issues in integrative medicine: a guide for clinicians, hospitals, and clients*, Chaplin, Conn, 2005, National Acupuncture Foundation.
17. Alternative Link Systems, Inc: *The state legal guide to complementary and alternative medicine and nursing*, Albany, NY, 2001, Thomson Delmar Learning.
18. National Center for Complementary and Alternative Medicine: What is CAM? Available at: *http://nccam. nih.gov/health/whatiscam/.* Accessed October 20, 2006.
19. Beck RL: An overview of state alternative healing practices law, *Altern Ther Health Med* 2:31-3, 1996.
20. Cohen MH: Legal issues in complementary and integrative medicine: a guide for the clinician, *Med Clin North Am* 86(1):185-96, 2002.
21. Thomas CL: *Taber's cyclopedic medical dictionary*, ed 17, Philadelphia, 1993, FA Davis.
22. Green JA: Collaborative physician-client planning and professional liability: opening the legal door to unconventional medicine, *Adv Mind Body Med* 5:83-100, 1999.
23. Eisenberg DM et al: Unconventional medicine in the United States. Prevalence, costs, and patterns of use, *N Engl J Med* 328:246-52, 1993.
24. Carlston M, Stuart MR, Jonas W: Alternative medicine instruction in medical schools and family practice residency programs, *Family Med* 29:559-62, 1997.
25. Scherwitz L et al: An integrative medicine clinic in a community hospital, *Am J Pub Health* 93:549-52, 2003.
26. Institute of Medicine at the National Academy of Sciences: *Complementary and alternative medicine in the United States*, Washington, DC, 2005, The National Academies Press.
27. Wong SS, Nahin RL: National Center for Complementary and Alternative Medicine perspectives for complementary and alternative medicine research in cardiovascular diseases, *Cardiol Rev* 11(2):94-8, 2003.
28. Barnes J et al: Articles on complementary medicine in the mainstream medical literature: an investigation of MEDLINE, 1966 through 1996, *Arch Intern Med* 159(15):1721-25, 1999.
29. Cohen MH, Eisenberg DM: Potential physician malpractice liability associated with complementary and integrative medical therapies, *Ann Intern Med* 136(8):596-603, 2002.
30. Acupuncture. *NIH Consensus Statement.* 15(5):1-34, 1997.
31. Ernst E, Cohen MH: Informed consent in complementary and alternative medicine, *Arch Intern Med* 161:2288-92, 2001.
32. Eisenberg DM: Advising clients who seek alternative medical therapies, *Ann Intern Med* 127:61-9, 1997.
33. Studdard DM et al: Medical malpractice implications of alternative medicine, *JAMA* 280:1610-5, 1998.
34. Scott R: *Professional ethics: a guide for rehabilitation professionals*, St Louis, 1998, Mosby.
35. McNaughton C, Eidsness LM: Ethics of alternative therapies. *S D J Med* 48(7):209-11, 1995.
36. Ernst E: The ethics of complementary medicine, *J Med Ethics* 22:197-8, 1996.
37. *The client care partnership.* Chicago, 2003, American Hospital Association.
38. Schneiderman LJ: Medical ethics and alternative medicine, *Sci Rev Altern Med* 2(1):63-6, 1998.

39. Guinn DE: Ethics and integrative medicine: moving beyond the biomedical model, *Altern Ther Health Med* 7(6):68-72, 2001.

40. Adams KE et al: Ethical considerations of complementary and alternative medical therapies in conventional medical settings, *Ann Intern Med* 37:660-4, 2002.

41. Pachter LM: Culture and clinical care: folk illness beliefs and behaviors and their implications for health care delivery, *JAMA* 271(9):690-4, 1994.

42. Nash RA: The biomedical ethics of alternative, complementary and integrative medicine, *Altern Ther Health Med* 5(5):92-5, 1999.

43. Hufford DJ: Cultural and social perspectives on alternative medicine: background and assumptions, *Altern Ther Health Med* 1(1):53-61, 1995.

44. Engebretson J: Folk healing and biomedicine. Culture clash or complementary approach? *J Holist Nurs* 12:240-50, 1994.

45. Fisher P, Ward A: Complementary medicine in Europe, *Br Med J* 309:107-10, 1994.

46. Trotter G: Culture, ritual, and errors of repudiation: some implications for the assessment of alternative medical traditions, *Altern Ther Health Med* 6(4):62-8, 2000.

47. Kleinman A, Eisenberg L, Good B: Culture, illness, and care: clinical lessons from anthropologic and cross-cultural research, *Ann Intern Med* 88:251-8, 1978.

48. Fadiman A: *The spirit catches you and you fall down,* New York, 1997, Farrar, Straus, and Giroux.

49. Plotnikoff GA et al: Hmong shamanism. Animist spiritual healing in Minnesota. *Minnesota Med* 85(6):29-34, 2002.

50. Eisenberg DM et al: Trends in alternative medicine use in the United States, 1990-1997: results of a follow-up national survey, *JAMA* 280(18):1569-75, 1998.

51. Najm W et al: Use of complementary and alternative medicine among the ethnic elderly, *Altern Ther Health Med* 9(3):50-7, 2003.

52. Arush MWB et al: Prevalence and characteristics of complementary medicine used by pediatric cancer clients in a mixed western and middle-eastern population, *J Pediatr Hematol Oncol* 28(3):141-6, 2006.

53. *Charell v Gonzales* 660 NY (Supp.II) 665,668, S.Ct., NY County, 1997.

54. *Schneider v Revici*, 817 F.2d 987, 2d Cir, 1987.

# CHAPTER 4

# Whole Medical Systems

*Judith E. Deutsch, Suzanne McDonough*

Traditional or whole medical systems are defined by the National Center for Complementary and Alternative Medicine (NCCAM) as those that "involve complete systems of theory and practice that have evolved independently from or parallel to allopathic (conventional) medicine."[1] They are practiced by individual cultures throughout the world. Examples of whole medical systems include Ayurvedic and traditional Chinese medicine (TCM) from the East, and homeopathy and naturopathy from the West. Other systems have been developed by Native American, African, Middle Eastern, Tibetan, and Central and South American cultures.[1] Because entire books are dedicated to the description and evaluation of each of the whole medical frameworks, in this chapter the coverage of these systems is brief. Introductions to selected whole medical systems, specifically, Ayurveda, TCM, Native American medicine, and naturopathy, are presented here. These whole medical systems were selected to introduce the reader to ancient classical systems in contrast with a more modern system, such as naturopathy. Selecting four systems allows the novice reader to appreciate commonalities and differences between the rationale and approaches of whole medical systems and to contrast the evidence base for each system. Further, Ayurveda and TCM serve as the basis for many individual therapies used in rehabilitation (such as yoga and tai chi) and are reported among the most frequently used therapies in the United States.[2] Homeopathy is covered in some detail in Chapter 6. Two excellent complementary and alternative medicine (CAM) books that cover all of the topics presented here in more detail are recommended for additional reading.[3,4]

Clinical decision making is influenced by health frameworks. Making clinical decisions is a shared responsibility between therapist and client. Therefore an understanding of the therapist's and client's health framework is important. The goals of the chapter are to provide enough background information on whole medical systems to aid therapists in (1) understanding specific complementary therapies described in the book (see, for example, acupuncture (Chapter 5), tai chi (Chapter 9), and qigong (Chapter 15), which are specific TCM approaches) and (2) understanding the client, who may be approaching care from a theoretical perspective different from the therapist's. Each section in the chapter is organized the same way using the following headings: Background, Foundational Principles, Examination and Diagnosis, and Therapeutic Techniques. More detail is provided in the TCM section because the literature available in MEDLINE from 1996 to June 2007 used to evaluate TCM was greater (3420 citations) than Ayurveda (596 citations), naturopathy (281), or Native American Medicine (11). This format is designed to aid the reader in comparison and contrast of the whole medical systems described in the chapter.

## AYURVEDA

### Background

Ayurveda is a whole medical system that began in India and has evolved over 5000 years.[5,6] The word *Ayurveda* is based on two Sanskrit words, *ayur,* meaning "life," and *veda,* meaning "science" or "knowledge."[6] Ayurveda originated as a spiritual tradition with the evolution into a systematic approach to health and disease.[6] Ayurvedic medi-

cine was formalized by the writing of three major and several minor books. Three books in poem form (*sutra*) are considered the most important texts on Ayurvedic medicine.[7] The oldest book, the *Charaka Samhita,* relates to internal medicine and contains a classification of diseases based on organ systems, including signs and symptoms of ill-defined conditions.[6] The definition of health is anchored in a tripod of mind, spirit, and body. The second major text, the *Susruta Samhita,* was written by the surgery school. In addition to surgery and surgical equipment is a discussion of the human anatomy, including the musculoskeletal, circulatory, and nervous systems. Eight distinct branches of medicine are delineated in the book.[6] The third text, the *Astanga Hrdayam Samhita,* also relates to internal medicine and describes human physiology in addition to therapeutic use of minerals and metals.[7] Translation of these three texts in addition to other important books forms the basis of the West's understanding of Ayurvedic practices.[6] Reportedly the Vedic texts were translated into Chinese and influenced the development of TCM in addition to other systems of medicine in Europe and the Middle East.[6]

### Foundational Principles

Ayurvedic practice connects people to a universal context. The universe was created by female and witnessed by male energy.[7] This universe is composed of five elements: space, air, fire, water, and earth. All of these elements are believed to be in every human cell.[7] Therefore people are a representation of the larger cosmos.[8]

The five elements have three active forms or energies (*doshas*): vata, pitta, and kapha (Table 4-1).[7] The energies are composed of elements found in varying amounts. Vata is composed primarily of space and air and is associated with movement. Pitta is composed primarily of fire and water and is considered the body's metabolic system, and kapha is composed primarily of earth and water and forms the body structure that holds the cells together.[7] Each of these *doshas* has a body function associated with physiological and personality characteristics in addition to a propensity for certain disease conditions (see Table 4-1). People are composed of the three *doshas* (tri-dosha) but may have a dominant *dosha.* The seven normal body constitutions are a combination of the three *doshas.* The rarest constitution (*sama*) is one in which the three *doshas* are balanced perfectly.[9]

| Table 4-1 | | Doshas and Their Relationship to Physiological Function and Disease | | | |
|---|---|---|---|---|---|
| DOSHA | ELEMENTS | PHYSIOLOGICAL FUNCTION | IN BALANCE | OUT OF BALANCE | DISEASE SUSCEPTIBILITY |
| Vata | Space<br>Air | Breathing<br>Blinking<br>Muscle, membrane, and<br>  cytoplasm<br>Movement<br>Heartbeat | Creativity<br>Flexibility | Fear<br>Anxiety | Emphysema, pneumonia<br>Arthritis<br>Flatulence, constipation<br>Tics and twitches<br>Dry skin and hair<br>Nervous system disorders<br>Mental confusion |
| Pitta | Fire<br>Water | Digestion<br>Absorption<br>Nutrition<br>Metabolism<br>Body temperature | Understanding<br>Intelligence | Anger<br>Hatred<br>Jealousy | Fevers<br>Inflammatory diseases<br>Jaundice<br>Rashes, burning<br>  sensations, ulcers |
| Kapha | Earth<br>Water | Lubricates joints<br>Moisturizes skin<br>Water-related function | Love<br>Calmness<br>Forgiveness | Attachment<br>Greed<br>Possessiveness | Influenza<br>Sinus congestion<br>Obesity<br>Diabetes<br>Headaches |

Modified from Lad V: Ayurvedic medicine. In Jonas WB, Levin JS, editors: *Essentials of complementary and alternative medicine,* Philadelphia, 1999, Lippincott, Williams, and Wilkins, pp 200-15.

## Examination and Diagnosis

In Ayurveda the anatomy and physiology of the body are organized by tissues, mental states, waste products, and channels. The physical constitution of the body is based on seven tissues: plasma, blood, fat, muscle, bone, nerve, or reproductive. The mental constitution or states are balance (*sattva*), energy (*rajas*), and inertia (*tamas*).[9] The body produces three types of waste *(malas):* feces, urine, and sweat. The body is composed of thirteen channels through which all substances circulate. Knowing one's own psychological and physiological constitution allows a person to make lifestyle decisions aimed at maintaining equilibrium to live a balanced, happy, and fulfilled life.[7] When the *doshas* are balanced, the person is in a state of health.

Disease occurs when an imbalance exists between mind, body, and consciousness.[8] This can be manifested as an imbalance in the *doshas* in addition to the accumulation of *ama.*[9] Sources of disease can be classified into three categories: external (such as trauma or lifestyle), internal (such as hereditary), or supernatural causes (such as lightning or planetary bodies).[9]

### Examination and Diagnosis

The examination process consists of interview, observation, and physical examination of the individual. Knowledge of the *doshas* is used as a basis for all aspects of examination. Interviewing includes gaining information about past actions to search for mental imbalances[9] in addition to inquiry into a person's lifestyle. The physical exam, according to Lad,[7] has eight clinical modalities. These include examination of the pulse, urine, feces, eyes, touch, general physical exam, and observation of the voice and tongue.

Tongue, pulse, and urine examinations are related to the *doshas* in addition to the condition of the body tissues. In the pulse examination, done with the ring, index, and middle fingers over the radial artery, each *dosha* has a distinct form. For example, a pulse resembling a snakelike movement under the index finger is considered a vata pulse.[9] A person has 12 different radial pulses, six on each side; three are superficial and three are deep. These pulses correspond to organs and can be used to determine their physiological condition.[8] In the tongue examination, the organ systems are mapped to a specific location in the tongue. Tongue discolorations and sensitivities correspond to specific diseases. For example, a black or brown discoloration indicates a vata tongue, whereas a white, pale tongue indicates a decrease in red blood cells and is a kapha tongue (Figure 4-1).[8]

Similarly, in the urine exam, color and odor are used to identify a *dosha* or body tissue imbalance.

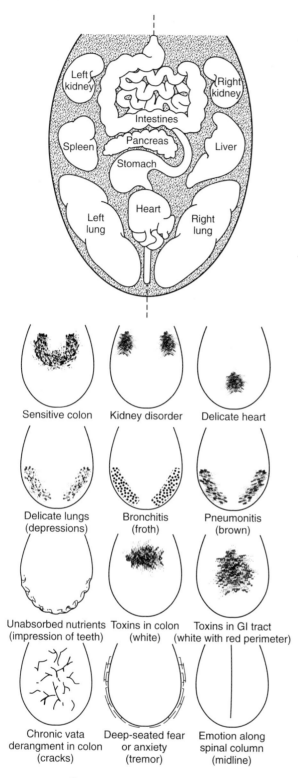

**Figure 4-1** Ayurvedic tongue exam.

For example, intense yellow, reddish, or blue urine indicates pitta.[9] The dropping of sesame oil into the urine also is used to determine the *dosha* (based on the shape of the drops as they move through the urine, again a snakelike shape is consistent with vata), in addition to the client prognosis (if the drop of sesame oil sinks to the bottom of the vessel, the disease may be very difficult to treat).[8] Finally, the odor of the urine is also diagnostic. Foul-smelling urine is an indication of accumulation of toxins, whereas sweet-smelling urine indicates a diabetic condition.[8] Many of the exam techniques used in Ayurveda persist in the physical exam even with the advent of new diagnostics.

Diseases are staged according to the balance of the *doshas*, from the least severe stage of accumulation (too much *dosha* in a particular organ system) through the provocation stage (irritation of the *dosha* in the local tissue), spread stage (*dosha* moving into other systems), deposition stage (*dosha* disrupting other organ systems), manifestation (signs and symptoms are apparent), and differentiation (tissue damage) stages.[7] Interestingly, it is not until manifestation that the cardinal signs and symptoms of the disease are evident. Therefore diagnosis of the disease at the earlier stages can be viewed as preventive, and prognosis worsens as a person moves toward the manifestation and differentiation phases of disease.

## Therapeutic Techniques

Interventions are categorized as preventive or therapeutic. Prevention includes a lifestyle that involves knowing a person's constitution and how to maintain a balance between external and internal forces and then engaging in proper nutrition, exercise (yoga), and purification. The approach to intervention in Ayurvedic medicine is to rebalance the person's *doshas* and then to identify the disease. Disease identification includes localization of the specific tissues and channels affected in addition to the staging of the disease.[9] Treatment is applied at the physical, emotional, and spiritual level.[7] The repertoire of interventions includes diet and herbs, massage, yoga, aroma, color, and music therapies.

Once disease has been identified, a person may go through two types of cleansing and restorative processes: palliation or panchakarma.[7] Each of these processes involves the use of herbs, fasting, and exposure to the correct elements and breathing to strengthen the body and eliminate the *ama,* in addition to lifestyle changes to maintain the benefits of the treatment. Panchakarma, a five-step process, is recommended when individuals have the strength to remove the extra *doshas* and toxins from the body. After preparatory steps with oil massage and sweat therapy, an individual may undergo therapeutic vomiting, purgatives and laxatives, therapeutic enemas, nasal administration of medications, and blood purification.[7] Palliation consists of toxin removal but in a more gentle manner than panchakarma; it includes herbal remedies, fasting, and sunbathing or windbathing.[7]

The use of herbs in Ayurvedic medicine is extensive. More than 2000 plant species are described in the ancient Ayurvedic texts.[10] Herbs have properties just like the *doshas*. They often can be administered as antidotes to excess *dosha*. For example, the common cold has properties of kapha, which include mucus, congestion, thickness, and lethargy. Ginger is an herb considered to have the opposite qualities and is given as an antidote.[7] Herbs also can be administered to strengthen a body tissue or restore balance in a *dosha*. Therapies involving exercise, massage, and yoga also are practiced in Ayurveda in addition to therapies that use color.

## Evidence

A MEDLINE search (performed on February 12, 2007, of references from 1950 to the present) of the key term *Ayurvedic medicine* yielded 1290 references with approximately 100 additional references when the key word *Ayurveda* was searched. No Cochrane topic reviews, three evidence-based medicine reviews,[11-13] and 70 clinical trials were found. Two reviews found support for Ayurveda in management of irritable bowel syndrome[11] and selected menopausal symptoms.[12] The evidence for the use of Ayurveda for the management of arthritis was lacking.[13]

A subset of articles dealt with the validation of the *dosha* concepts.[14-16] The authors used different approaches to validate independently the existence of the *doshas*. Support for the construct of *doshas* was found by relating them to thermodynamics[16] with use of an algorithmic heuristic approach,[15] and identification of an invariant co-enzyme that the authors proposed was a unifying construct for all organisms.[14] In each study the *dosha* identification of hundreds of subjects was compared with the independent measurement.

Many clinical trials were conducted to determine the efficacy of *plant preparations* and *Ayurvedic*

*herbs*. Applications were to varied client populations or medical conditions such as Parkinson's disease,[17,18] hepatitis,[19,20] diabetes,[21-26] asthma,[27-29] osteoarthritis,[30] insomnia,[31,32] acne,[33,34] rheumatoid arthritis,[13,35,36] obesity,[37,38] and jaundice.[39] Effects of herbs on memory,[40] cognition,[41] and decline of vision with aging[42] also were studied.

Support for Ayurveda was reported in the treatment of insomnia, diabetes, asthma, acne, and cognition. Ayurvedic herbs were found to decrease sleep latency in healthy adults,[32] whereas yoga was superior to an Ayurvedic herb for improvement of sleep in the elderly.[31] In the management of diabetes, improvements were found in the $HbA_{1c}$ levels of a subgroup of clients who took pancreas tonic[24]; and cogent db (an Ayurvedic herbal supplement), when added to allopathic medicines, improved client's blood profile without any adverse kidney effects.[25] Asthma symptoms were alleviated completely in a group of children who discontinued their allopathic medication and replaced it with an herbal supplement[27]; anti-asthmatic effects also were reported for adults in a combined clinical study with a corroborating animal model.[28] Acne preparations administered internally and externally were found to be superior to oral administration alone.[33] Finally, aspects of cognition related to memory and retention of newly learned information[41] also were reported.

Whole system or multimodality Ayurveda was studied in only two populations.[43,44] Clients with type II diabetes who were treated with Ayurveda consisting of diet, exercise, meditation, and an herb supplement were compared to a control group who had standard diabetes education classes and a follow-up with a primary care health care provider. For a subset of clients with elevated glycosylated hemoglobin, Ayurveda had better outcomes, including reduced weight, cholesterol levels, and fasting glucose, than the controls.[44] Similar findings were reported for elderly subjects with coronary heart disease (CHD) of varying risk levels. Three groups—multimodal Ayurvedic (labeled Maharishi Vedic Medicine, or MVM), modern, and usual care—were studied for 1 year. The MVM group participated in a program to promote health and decrease the risk of disease. The program included transcendental meditation, an herbal supplement high in antioxidants, Vedic diet (seasonal variation of low-fat high fruit and vegetable diet), yoga, and walking. The modern care group had modifications in their exercise and diet, and took a placebo vitamin. The usual care group did not receive interventions. On the primary outcome measure of intima-media thickness (IMT), a measure of atherosclerosis, there was a significant decrease for the high-risk CHD clients in the MMV group compared with the modern care and usual care groups. These studies are interesting because they focus on prevention of disease and present promising findings for a multimodal approach.

## TRADITIONAL CHINESE MEDICINE

### Background

The practice of TCM has a longstanding history that has evolved over many centuries. It has developed empirically in China and other parts of East Asia, and although the practice of TCM has been characterized by many schools of thought and a great deal of heterogeneity, several fundamental principles have been retained. These fundamental principles provide the framework to explain the use of medicinal herbs, acupuncture (used in conjunction with other techniques such as moxibustion and cupping), nutrition, massage, and therapeutic exercise such as qigong and tai chi.

### Foundational Principles

The first fundamental principle of TCM is based on the Taoist concept of yin and yang.[45] Yin-yang theory is based on the philosophical construct of two polar but complementary opposites (Figure 4-2).

These complementary opposites are used to explain the continuous process of natural change and describe how things function in relation to one another and to the universe. In this system of thought all things are seen as part of a whole and can be explained only by relative relationships to other entities.[46] This is demonstrated graphically in Figure 4-2, in which yin is signified by black relative to the white of yang; and yet within yin is a com-

ponent of yang, and vice versa. The curve separating yin and yang indicates that it is a gradual transition from yin to yang.

Some of the correspondences of yin and yang in nature and in the body are summarized in Table 4-2. This table demonstrates that yin-yang theory is used to describe the human body (organs, tissues, fluids) and its functions. Disease (or disharmony) in the body is caused by a relative imbalance of yin and yang, and therefore the aim of any treatment (either herbal or acupuncture) is to prevent an imbalance or rebalance of any disharmony. (See the section on the Eight Principle Patterns on p. 42.) A simple example of disharmony of yin and yang could be seen in the regulation of a client's temperature. For example, from Table 4-2 yang is hot and thus provides heat or warmth for the body, whereas yin is cold, and this cools the body. Normally if yin and yang are balanced, the body should feel neither too hot nor too cold; however, if an excess of yang exists, as could happen in an acute sports injury, then part of the body will feel hot. By contrast, if an excess of yin exists because of a longstanding chronic illness, the person will feel cold, and parts of the body will feel cold to the touch.

This balance of yin and yang is controlled by a vital force or energy called *qi* (pronounced "chee"), which circulates between the organs along channels called *meridians*[45] (see also Table 5-1, Chapter 5). Although the meridians are proposed to carry *qi* and blood through the body, they are not blood vessels but rather are an invisible network that

| Table 4-2 | Yin-Yang Correspondences in Nature and the Body | |
|---|---|---|
| | YIN | YANG |
| Nature | Night | Day |
| | Cold | Heat |
| | Stillness | Movement |
| Body structure | Internal | External |
| | Solid organs | Empty organs |
| | Ventral | Dorsal |
| Physiological function | Nutritive substances | Functional activities |
| | Storage | Movement |
| Pathological changes | Cold | Heat |
| Diagnosis | Interior | Exterior |
| | Deficiency | Excess |
| | Cold | Heat |

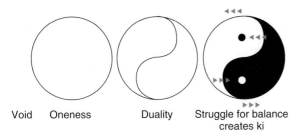

Void      Oneness          Duality       Struggle for balance creates ki

**Figure 4-2** Symbols representing yin and yang.

links all the fundamental substances and organs. Fundamental substances are described by Kaptchuk[46] and can be summarized as the following:

- Blood (does not correspond with Western concept of blood but has some of the same functions)
- Qi (five types of qi in the body)
- Jing (or essence that is the substance that underlies organic life, growth, and development). Jing has two sources: prenatal Jing, inherited from the parents, and postnatal Jing, produced from ingested food.
- Shen (spirit, considered the vitality behind qi and jing in the body)
- Fluids (sweat, saliva, gastric juices, and urine)

An interrelation exists between all these substances. For example, prenatal Jing is the root of all qi, and qi helps to transform food to postnatal Jing, which adds to the ability to grow and develop. *Qi* also moves the blood, and movement of blood is required to nourish and moisten the organs and tissues to maintain their function and overall health of the body. Through good health the production of qi can be maintained, and thus the cycle continues.

## Examination and Diagnosis

Chinese medicine is based on holistic patterns of observed phenomena gathered to form a pattern of disharmony. The client's physiological and psychological characteristics (from an Eastern perspective) and their environment are considered. Four classic methods of examination are used: visual observation (body, face, emotional state, and movement), listening and smelling (voice, breathing, smell), questioning (diet, sleep, menstruation, pain, bowel function), examination, and palpation (pulse, abdomen, meridians) (see Chapters 3 and 6[47] for more detail). The diagnostic system of TCM was developed on the basis of yin-yang polarity and the theory of the five phases (or elements).

### Five Elements

TCM beliefs are that the universe is composed of five elements, or phases: wood, fire, earth, metal, and water. A more detailed description of the five elements, or phases, can be found in Chapter 3.[47] In brief, they are used in TCM to classify functions of internal organs, tissues, and sensory organs with features of nature (Table 4-3).

As can be seen in Table 4-3, each element is linked to internal organs of the body, body tissues, emotions, colors, and climatic conditions. Each element can interact with the four other elements, and the health of the individual is dictated by the appropriate balance between all the elements.

By using the correspondences from the five phases, the practitioner can start to piece together a pattern of disharmony: for example, a very red face could indicate a fire type of person, who is more likely to suffer with problems of their heart and blood vessels, whereas a kidney typology may have a dark complexion (commonly dark circles under their eyes), complain of being cold, dislike the cold, and have problems with their bones and joints. In Chapter 5 of this text, (TCM diagnosis), these correspondences are used to help with the diagnosis of the client who is considered to be linked with the element, earth, and thus is more likely to have a disharmony of his stomach and spleen organs and be affected by dampness (either the climatic condition of damp, or eating foods that cause dampness in the system).

### Eight Principle Patterns

In TCM diagnosis, use of the Eight Principle Patterns provides a framework to describe the client's complaint in terms of yin and yang balance. TCM recognizes many patterns of disharmony. All of them can, however, be grouped according to the Eight Principle Patterns: yin/yang, hot/cold, internal/external, and excess/deficient (see Chapters 3 and 6).[47] It is difficult in this chapter to summarize TCM diagnosis using these principles without

| Table 4-3 | Correspondences of the Five Elements, or Phases | | | | | | |
|---|---|---|---|---|---|---|---|
| ELEMENTS | INTERNAL ORGAN | HOLLOW ORGAN | SENSE ORGAN | TISSUES | EMOTION | COLOR | CLIMATIC CONDITION |
| Wood | Liver (LIV) | Gallbladder (GB) | Eye | Muscle function | Anger | Green | Wind |
| Fire | Heart (HT) | Small intestine (SI) | Tongue | Blood vessels | Joy | Red | Heat |
| Earth | Spleen (SP) | Stomach (ST) | Mouth | Muscle bulk | Brooding | Yellow | Damp |
| Metal | Lung (LU) | Large intestine (LI) | Nose | Skin | Sadness | White | Dryness |
| Water | Kidney (KI) | Bladder (BL) | Ear | Bones, joints | Fear | Black | Cold |

oversimplification; however, one example of application of the Eight Principle Patterns is the following: all illness is rooted in a disturbance of qi. It can be either a deficiency (yin) or excess (yang) of qi, either in an internal organ (yin) or an external meridian (yang), and this may be associated with heat (yang) or cold (yin). As summarized in Table 4-3 exterior/hot/excess and interior/cold/deficient are classified as yang or yin criteria, respectively. A common example of an excess of qi, which is external, hot, and yang, is an acute sports tissue injury. Finally, the causes of disease in TCM are very different from Western medicine and are divided according to whether they are internal or external. Nutrition and mental/emotional stress are internal causes, whereas climatic conditions and trauma are external causes. It is therefore perfectly acceptable in TCM to diagnose a painful back as an attack of damp cold, which may be due to a damp, cold climate or getting soaked in cold water.

## Therapeutic Techniques

### Manual Acupuncture

Needles are always inserted by hand but can then be stimulated (to increase the activation of the acupuncture system) by hand or by electrical currents or moxibustion. If needles are stimulated by hand, then this is termed *manual acupuncture.*

### Electroacupuncture

In electroacupuncture (EA), needles are inserted by hand but then attached to a device that generates electrical current that cause stimulation of the needles. This can be produced with use of an ordinary TENS machine attached to the needles with wires and crocodile clips or with commercially available units specifically for EA. Regardless of the unit used, practitioners should be able to alter the frequency, intensity, and pulse duration of the electric current. Two modes of EA are used commonly: low-frequency (1 to 4 Hz), high-intensity EA and high-frequency (50 to 200 Hz), low-intensity EA.

### Moxibustion

Moxibustion describes the burning of materials, collectively called moxa, which is used to energize the patient's system. Moxa is placed directly on the skin overlying an acupuncture point or on the end of an acupuncture needle and burned. If placed on the end of an inserted acupuncture needle, the client feels a mild, comfortable heat, and it is thought that this heat can penetrate deep into the body, strengthen *qi,* and energize the system.[48] A common form of moxa is the dried herb Chinese mugwort. Because of the strong characteristic smell of and smoke produced by mugwort, some practitioners favor the use of smokeless moxa.

### Cupping

In cupping, suction is created by warming the air inside a glass jar and placing it over acupuncture points. The vacuum created is thought to promote the free flow of qi and blood in the meridians, dispel cold dampness, and reduce pain and swelling.[48]

### Chinese Herbal Medicine

Herbal medicine is central to TCM. About 500 common clinical prescriptions can rebalance a range of disharmonies in the body. Herbs rarely are used singly; they are combined normally in prescriptions containing 5 to 15 substances. As with acupuncture the practitioner prescribes these herbs to influence the flow of *qi* in the meridians and thus balance yin and yang.[47]

### Qigong

*Qigong* comprises meditation, movement exercises, self-massage, and special healing techniques to regulate internal functions of the human body. Those who practice qigong believe that through the integration of mind, body, and breathing a person can learn to promote, preserve, circulate, balance, and store qi within the body and thus maintain or improve health.[49] A more detailed description of qigong can be found in Chapter 15.

### Tai Chi

Tai chi is a form of movement that has developed into many forms from 13 basic postures. Smooth movement through these postures is believed to harmonize and balance the body's yin and the yang.[50] A more detailed description of tai chi can be found in Chapter 9.

## Scientific Basis of TCM

In this era of evidence-based medicine, the need for scientific evidence to support treatments used in clinical practice is considered paramount. However, attitudes toward the need for evaluation have been one of the greatest hindrances in evaluation of TCM. Indeed recently it has been argued that for TCM advocates, every treatment works, so evaluation is unnecessary, and for skeptics, TCM is quackery, so evaluation is pointless.[51] However, despite these standpoints, acupuncture is probably one of the most extensively researched forms of CAM, but it has been studied primarily within the framework of Western medicine. Initial studies concentrated on identifying its physiological mechanism of action in terms of analgesic effects (see Chapter 5), and more recently researchers also have started to explore the basis for some effects thought to be mediated via the autonomic nervous system, which may explain how acupuncture could affect disease states in the body.

Since the early 1990s greater efforts have been made to try to answer research questions in keeping with the TCM model of diagnosis. For example, researchers have attempted unsuccessfully to define the nature of disease in TCM.[51] This lack of success, in addition to the difference in attitudes between some TCM and Western medicine advocates for the need for research, explains in part why an abundance of research explains acupuncture used from a Western medical standpoint, but little research explains acupuncture from a TCM perspective. This can be seen clearly in Chapter 5 in which no evidence was found to support the TCM aspects of acupuncture management.

## Clinical Evidence

Over the last decade the use of CAM has increased dramatically in Australia,[52] the United States,[53] and the United Kingdom.[54] In surveys of the use of CAM, acupuncture is cited consistently among the most commonly used[1] and has been estimated to be the fourth most popular form of CAM in the United Kingdom (14%).[54] Acupuncture is used most commonly for the treatment of chronic pain, particularly musculoskeletal complaints,[55] and as such has become an integral part of physical therapy practice (e.g., United Kingdom, Ireland, Canada, New Zealand, and Sweden), recognized by the respective professional organizations. In the United States, however, acupuncture is not considered to be part of the scope of practice (American Physical Therapy Association [APTA], personal communication). This issue is discussed in more detail in the section on education and training in Chapter 5.

## Critical Reviews

The Cochrane collection of databases was searched from 1999 up to November 2006, using the key words *acupuncture, Chinese herbal medicine, tai chi,* and *qigong* to determine which critical reviews had been published.

### Acupuncture

There are 21 completed systematic reviews in the Cochrane Database of Systematic Reviews (CDSR) on the effectiveness of acupuncture for a range of areas: for example, neck disorders,[56] stroke rehabilitation,[57] shoulder pain,[58] low back pain,[59] lateral elbow pain,[60] postoperative vomiting and nausea,[61] rheumatoid arthritis,[62] Bell's palsy,[63] chronic asthma,[64] headache,[65] induction of labor,[66] and smoking cessation.[67]

The Database of Abstracts Reviews Effects (DARE) holds summaries of other relevant systematic reviews on acupuncture published in journals. On DARE there are more than 50 abstracts of quality-assessed systematic reviews and four other bibliographic reviews on acupuncture. Examples of systematic reviews are low back pain,[68-71] stroke rehabilitation,[72-74] osteoarthritis,[75,76] neck pain,[70,77] asthma,[78] headache,[79] fibromyalgia,[80] cancer-related nausea and vomiting,[81] and chronic pain.[82]

In summary, acupuncture has been shown to be safe when practiced by doctors and physiotherapists[83] and is more effective than sham acupuncture or no treatment for chronic low back pain and neck disorders.[56,59] Electroacupuncture reduces first-day vomiting after chemotherapy, but comparisons need to be made against modern antivomiting drugs.[81] Systematic reviews of acupuncture for fibromyalgia,[80] osteoarthritis,[75,76] chronic pain,[82] lateral elbow pain,[60] shoulder pain,[58] and headaches[65] indicate promising results for acupuncture. Further high-quality studies are required to confirm the effect of acupuncture for other clinical conditions: for example, stroke rehabilitation,[57,72-74] irritable bowel syndrome,[84] induction of labor,[66] smoking cessation,[67] Bell's palsy,[63] and asthma.[64,78]

### Chinese Herbal Medicine

In the CDSR, a total of 13 reviews were identified in the areas of schizophrenia,[85] irritable bowel syndrome (IBS),[86] preeclampsia,[87] influenza,[88] type 2 diabetes,[89] bronchitis,[90] acute pancreatitis,[91] chronic hepatitis,[92] atopic eczema,[93] unstable angina,[94,95] acute ischemic stroke,[96] and vascular dementia.[97] In two areas no randomized controlled trials were identified: preeclampsia and vascular dementia.[87,97] For other conditions a wealth of literature was found based in China following TCM principles, that is, using an individualized approach to treatment (e.g., IBS[86] and type 2 diabetes).[89] Although these trials showed benefits, poor study design precludes routine use in clinical practice at present. Similar conclusions were made for acute pancreatitis, bronchitis, influenza, atopic eczema, acute stroke, and unstable angina.[88,90,91,93,95,96] Although benefits were seen, especially when herbal preparations were combined with conventional treatment studies, they were too few or too weak to support their current use.

### Tai Chi

In the CDSR, tai chi has been reviewed in people with rheumatoid arthritis[98] and in prevention of falls in the elderly.[99] The evidence for tai chi was limited but positive. In Chapter 9 the evidence supporting the use of tai chi for balance and fall prevention is discussed in great detail.

### Qigong

In the CDSR there were no Cochrane reviews for qigong; however, four trials in the English were identified in Cochrane Central, which suggests benefits in chronic low back pain,[100] multiple sclerosis,[101] type 2 diabetes,[102] and cardiac rehabilitation of the elderly.[103] In Chapter 15 the evidence supporting the use of qigong to improve function for a person who is status post myocardial infarct and a triple coronary artery bypass graft procedure presenting with pain and anxiety while participating in a phase I and II cardiac rehabilitation program is described.

## NATIVE AMERICAN MEDICINE OR HEALING

### Background

Native American medicine or healing encompasses the beliefs and practices of many diverse groups. However, some commonalities have been used to describe a pan-Indian approach to health. Native American medicine is characterized by concepts and ideas rather than just remedies and treatments.[104] This approach to health has a long tradition that may date back 12,000 or even 40,000 years ago.[105] Documenting Native American healing practices is a challenge for several reasons. Many nations exist with varying practices, and more importantly the customs and traditions are shared in an oral form, and it may be considered improper

to study them at all.[105,106] However, interest and research support exist for learning more about Native American health practices. An overview of the available literature on Native American practices is summarized by Cohen.[105,106] For more detailed information about Native American practices the reader is referred to several well-written chapters in CAM books[105,107,108] and a book on American Indian medicine,[109] in addition to a web-based resource sponsored by the National Library of Medicine.[110]

### Foundational Principles or Beliefs

Core principles in Native American Medicine are wholeness and interconnectedness.[105] The connection of individuals is to themselves, their community, the environment, and spirituality.[111] Health and wellness are achieved when all of these elements are in balance. Sources of illness can be internal and external. Internal causes are generated by the individual (e.g., negative thinking). External causes are pathogenic forces that can invade the mind, body, and spirit.[106] Examples of external causes are negative thoughts by others, environmental poisons, and physical and emotional trauma, in addition to breach of taboo (e.g., the violation of cultural mores, cruel words, and abusive behavior).[106]

### Examination and Diagnosis

The process of examination and diagnosis is highly individualized, and it is partly the responsibility of the client to identify the correct healer.[112] The process of diagnosis begins with observation of the symptoms and follows with an extensive history in which the client-healer relationship is established. All aspects of the illness are explored, such as the clients' lifestyles, relationships, and impact of the disease on their families and communities. This information gives the healer a sense of the greater community's involvement with the person.[106] If the healer or medicine elder is unable to obtain the information from his exam, he can consult a diagnostic specialist, who may go into a trance to examine the body more carefully. Divination, the process of eliciting medical information from the spiritual forces, also is practiced.[106] Divination can be achieved by praying, examining dreams, or having visions or omens. The spirits can yield information about diagnosis and about prognosis and treatment.[106]

## Therapeutic Techniques

The Native American repertoire for health management includes remedies, therapeutic procedures, and hygienic practices.[113] Health management is provided by a healer, also known as a *medicine man* or a *shaman*, who has multiple roles as a healer, sorcerer, seer, educator, and priest.[104] Ritualistic procedures are practiced to address supranatural or external causes of disease[113]; these procedures include prayers, chanting, music, voice, drum, and rattle, which can be combined into ceremonies.[104,106]

A variety of herbal remedies are used as anesthetics, stimulants, astringents, cathartics and emetics, febrifuges, vermifuges, and poisons.[113] Many drugs used currently, such as morphine, taxol, and quinine, were used first in their botanical forms in Native American medicine.[108,114] Specific examples of applications in dermatology include geranium root and dogwood bark, which were used as astringents to treat thrush.[114] Used as an over-the-counter Native American remedy, echinacea presumably boosts immunity and prevents respiratory infections.[115] With the renewed enthusiasm for herbs and herbal supplements, an important reminder is that plants used for medicinal purposes can be dangerous.[108]

Consistent with a holistic and interconnected view of health, healing practices involve a network of people and spirits. As depicted in Figure 4-3 the sick person at the center is surrounded by spirits, relatives, and singers. A connection exists between people and animals, the natural, and the supernatural.[107] Efforts to integrate Native American concepts of healing, such as ceremony and counseling, in the treatment of chronic illness have been reported.[116]

### Evidence

Limited evidence can be found in the medical literature to support Native American healing practices. A search in MEDLINE (from 1996 to the present), conducted in January 2007, using the term *Native American medicine* yielded eleven articles, many of which were not research articles.

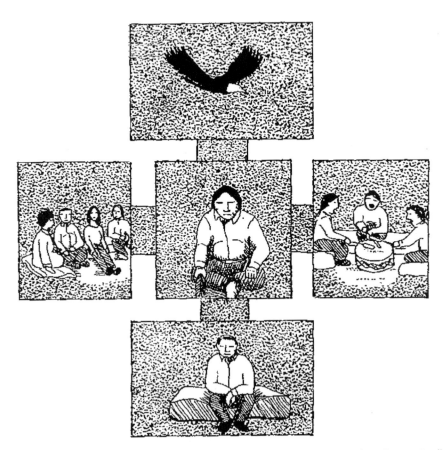

**Figure 4-3** Native American healing. Spirits, relatives, singers, and sick person in the shape of two intersecting lines. Courtesy Sinte Gleska University.

Several challenges exist to researching Native American medicine. One is the ritualistic symbolic and religious and supernatural nature of the healing approaches[114]; another is the subdivision into different healing practices by Native American groups. The state of the literature was summarized aptly by the authors of a recent review paper on use of Native American medicine in cardiology.[117] Strong testimonial support exists for its use, but scrutiny and further study are warranted.

## NATUROPATHY

### Background

Naturopathy is a whole medical system practiced in the West that was influenced by Ayurvedic medicine, TCM, and Native American medicine. The practice originated with Benedict Lust, a German who brought natural cures to the United States in the latter part of the nineteenth century. Subsequently, he acquired degrees in osteopathic, chiropractic, homeopathic, and eclectic medicine, all of which form part of naturopathy.[118] The practice took shape in the early twentieth century as American dietetic practices were integrated with homeopathy, spinal manipulation, and herbalism, in addition to mental and emotional healing.[119] The practice flourished in the United States between 1918 and 1937, when allopathic medicine was not meeting the needs of the population. It was later suppressed by the allopathic movement and resurged in the 1960s along with the interest in other complementary therapies. Laws regulating the practice of naturopathy exist in the following states: Alaska, Arizona, California, Connecticut, Hawaii, Idaho, Kansas, Maine, Montana, New Hampshire, Oregon, Utah, Vermont, Washington, and the District of Columbia.[120]

### Foundational Principles

Naturopaths view health as a continuum with optimal function at one end and death at the other.[119] Nature plays an integral role in health and possesses healing qualities. An essential tenet of naturopathy is that the body has the power to heal itself, and this process should be facilitated naturally. Murray and Pizzorno summarized seven principal concepts of naturopathy:

1. The healing power of nature
2. Identification and treatment of the cause of the disease (not just the symptoms)
3. Do no harm
4. Treat the whole person
5. The physician as a teacher
6. Prevention is the best cure
7. Establish health and wellness[119]

Naturopathy emphasizes wellness and prevention.

### Examination and Diagnosis

Examination consists of an interview and physical exam. The interview emphasizes lifestyle and nutrition and establishing the health care provider–client relationship. Conventional laboratory tests (such as radiology tests) are supplemented with techniques to assess nutritional status, toxin load, detoxification function, food intolerance, intestinal bioses, and digestive function.[119] Diagnostic tests include urine, blood, and stool analysis. Client education on health and wellness is also part of the examination.

The interview questions that guide naturopaths in making the diagnosis were summarized by Murray and Pizzorno and include the following:

- Is the person in balance with nature?
- Will healing be aimed at suppression of the disease, palliation, or a cure?
- What are the limiting factors in the person's life?
- Where is the center of the person's disease (physical, mental, or emotional)?[119]

Many other questions are raised to help determine individuals' readiness to heal themselves and change their lifestyle to prevent further illness.

### Therapeutic Techniques

Given the many influences on the development of naturopathy, it is not surprising to find that naturopathy's repertoire of therapies includes clinical nutrition, botanical medicine, homeopathy, TCM and acupuncture, hydrotherapy, manual and body-based therapies, exercise and mind-body therapies, detoxification, counseling, and lifestyle modification.[121]

Nutrition and botanical medicine are core interventions used by naturopathic doctors (NDs). NDs recommend a healthy diet based on whole foods and nutritional supplements. Controlled fasting is used therapeutically. NDs are trained as herbalists and use herbs to complement the body's natural healing process. Detoxification is performed on the liver and bowel to reduce the toxic load on the body. Also central to the NDs' repertoire of treatment are counseling and lifestyle modification. Client education to identify their own barriers and resources for health promotion are consistent with the ND approach to allowing the body to heal itself.

Healing modalities such as homeopathy, TCM, acupuncture, hydrotherapy, and physical medicine (modalities and manipulative therapies) are well described elsewhere in the book and will not be elaborated on here. NDs have to be trained in multiple modalities and approaches.

## Evidence

A MEDLINE search (from 1996 to the present) performed on February 15, 2007, using the key word and MESH term *naturopathy* yielded one Cochrane review and 220 articles, of which 9 survived the clinical trials limit. The Cochrane review was on speleotherapy for asthma.[122] Speleotherapy is the use of subterranean environments to reduce chronic obstructive pulmonary disease. The findings were not reliable, and therefore it was not possible to determine if speleotherapy reduces asthma.

The most frequently reported trials were on the use of naturopathic herbs to manage specific conditions. Preliminary positive findings were reported for reducing rheologic properties in people with systemic sclerosis who consumed a garlic preparation.[123] Two trials found support for the use of different herbal preparations for the management of otitis media.[124,125] In both trials an herb preparation was compared with antibiotic treatment of otitis media and found to be superior or comparable. One dosing study and one incidence report were found. The dose of Icelandic moss (a lichen harvested in Scandinavia) to reduce oral mucosal irritation was reported to be the lowest administered dose in the trial.[126] The incidence of phytotherapeutic drugs used by pregnant women was reported to be 96%, and it decreased to 84% for lactating women.[127]

Contained in the nine clinical trials search that survived the search limit clinical trials were two articles that grouped naturopathy with other CAMs for the management of diabetes[128] and the likelihood of reducing relapses from drug-induced headaches.[129] The number of clinical trials on naturopathy identified in this search was small. The number, however, may be an underestimation because some trials conducted by NDs may not be identified as naturopathy studies. For example, a recent trial on echinacea was conducted by individuals from a naturopathic institution but missed in the search because *naturopathy* was not a key word.[130]

A recent summit between NDs and "conventional" physicians and scientists produced a research agenda. In it the study of naturopathy for the management of diabetes in the elderly was identified as a research priority.[131] As with any of the complementary therapy approaches, constant study of the literature is necessary to be current with the evidence base.

## SUMMARY

Two of the whole medical systems briefly described in this chapter represent two of the largest systems of medicine practiced outside of the West: Ayurvedic and TCM. The other two systems originated and are practiced in the West: Native American medicine and naturopathy. The youngest system, naturopathy, clearly is influenced by the three others. Commonalities between these systems include the respect for and incorporation of nature into health; the definition of health based on balance between all relevant elements that may cause and prevent disease; prevention; a holistic view of the individual, whether in the context of nature or the community; the focus on incorporation of diet and herbs in treatment; and the goal of eliminating toxins from the body. Commonalities can be found in some of the exam and diagnosis procedures in addition to intervention techniques. Elements of spirituality are found in all of the systems except naturopathy.

The evidence to support the use of these whole medical systems varies in quantity and quality. TCM has the greatest number of studies and level of evidence to support specific aspects of the work such as acupuncture, whereas Native American medicine has the least amount of evidence and lowest quality of evidence to support it. The challenge to investigate the efficacy of an entire whole medical system was overcome by a couple of studies of comprehensive Ayurvedic interventions.

The richness of the history and the alternative approaches to diagnosis and comprehension of human physiology are academically interesting but more importantly may contribute to enhancement of Western medicine. Enhancements can be derived from a more holistic view of the client during examination and intervention in addition to a better understanding of the client's health background. This chapter was only a brief introduction to a select group of whole medical systems, and the reader is referred to the other chapters in this book and to additional references for additional information.

## REFERENCES

1. NCCAM: Whole Medical Systems: An Overview. Backgrounder, 2006. Available at: *http://nccam. nih.gov/health/backgrounds/wholemed.htm.* Accessed November 20, 2006.
2. Barnes PM et al: Complementary and alternative medicine use among adults: United States, 2002, *Advance Data* May 27, 2004, 343:1-19.
3. Jonas WB, Levin JS: *Essentials of complementary and alternative medicine*, Baltimore, 1999, Lippincott.
4. Micozzi MS: *Fundamentals of complementary and alternative medicine,* ed 3, St Louis, 2006, Saunders.
5. NCCAM: A closer look at Ayurvedic medicine, *CAM at the NIH Focus on Complementary and Alternative Medicine*, vol 12, 2005. http://nccam. nih.gov/news/newsletters/2006_winter/ayurveda. htm accessed on 2-19-2006
6. Mishra L-C, Singh BB, Dagenais S: Ayurveda: a historical perspective and principles of the traditional healthcare system in India, *Altern Ther* 7(2):36-40, 2001.
7. Lad V: Ayurvedic medicine. In Jonas WB, Levin JS, editors: *Essentials of complementary and alternative medicine,* Philadelphia, 1999, Lippincott, Williams and Wilkins, pp 200-215.
8. Lad V: An introduction to ayurveda, *Altern Ther Health Med* 1(3):57-63, 1995.
9. Zysk KG: Traditional Ayurveda. In Miccozi MS, editor: *Fundamentals of complementary and integrative medicine,* ed 3, St Louis, 2006, WB Saunders, pp 494-507.
10. Mukherjee PK, Wahile A: Integrated approaches towards drug development from ayurveda and other Indian systems of medicine, *J Ethnopharmacol* 103:25-35, 2006.
11. Liu JP et al: Herbal medicines for treatment of irritable bowel syndrome, *Cochrane Database of Systematic Reviews* 1:CD004116, 2006.
12. Kronenberg F, Fugh-Berman A: Complementary and alternative medicine for menopausal symptoms: a review of randomized, controlled trials, *Ann Intern Med* 137(10):805-13, 2002.
13. Park J, Ernst E: Ayurvedic medicine for rheumatoid arthritis: a systematic review, *Semin Arthritis Rheum* 34(5):705-13, 2005.
14. Hankey A: A test of the systems analysis underlying the scientific theory of ayurveda's tridosha, *J Altern Complement Med* 11(3):385-90, 2005.
15. Joshi RR: A biostatistical approach to ayurveda: quantifying the tridosha, *J Altern Complement Med* 10(5):879-89, 2004.
16. Hankey A: Ayurvedic physiology and etiology: Ayurvedo Amritanaam. The doshas and their functioning in terms of contemporary biology and physical chemistry, *J Altern Complement Med* 7(5):567-74, 2001.
17. Nagashayana N et al: Association of L-DOPA with recovery following ayurveda medication in Parkinson's disease, *J Neurol Sci* 176(2):124-7, 2000.
18. An alternative medicine treatment for Parkinson's disease: results of a multicenter clinical trial. HP-200 in Parkinson's Disease Study Group, *J Altern Complement Med* 1(3):249-55, 1995.
19. Katiyar CK et al: Management of chronic hepatitis B with New Livfit in end stage renal disease, *Ind J Physiol Pharmacol* 49(1):83-8, 2005.
20. Antarkar DS et al: A double-blind clinical trial of Arogya-wardhani—an ayurvedic drug—in acute viral hepatitis, *Ind J Med Res* 72:588-93, 1980.
21. Rao NK, Nammi S: Antidiabetic and renoprotective effects of the chloroform extract of terminalia chebula Retz. seeds in streptozotocin-induced diabetic rats, *BMC Complement Altern Med* 6:17, 2006.
22. Saxena A, Vikram NK: Role of selected Indian plants in management of type 2 diabetes: a review, *J Altern Complement Med* 10(2):369-78, 2004.
23. Elder C: Ayurveda for diabetes mellitus: a review of the biomedical literature, *Altern Ther Health Med* 10(1):44-50, 2004.
24. Hsia SH, Bazargan M, Davidson MB: Effect of pancreas tonic (an ayurvedic herbal supplement) in type 2 diabetes mellitus, *Metab Clin Experiment* 53(9):1166-73, 2004.
25. Shekhar KC et al: A preliminary evaluation of the efficacy and safety of cogent db (an ayurvedic drug) in the glycemic control of patients with type 2-diabetes, *J Altern Complement Med* 8(4):445-57, 2002.
26. Indian Council of Medical Research (ICMR), Collaborating Centres, New Delhi: Flexible dose open trial of Vijayasar in cases of newly-diagnosed non-insulin-dependent diabetes mellitus, *Indian J Med Res* 108:24-9, 1998. (Erratum, *Indian J Med Res* 108:253, 1998.)
27. Kumar SS, Shanmugasundaram KR: Amrita bindu—an antioxidant inducer therapy in asthma children, *J Ethnopharmacol* 90(1):105-14, 2004.
28. Sekhar AV et al: An experimental and clinical evaluation of anti-asthmatic potentialities of Devadaru compound (DC), *Indian J Physiol Pharmacol* 47(1):101-7, 2003.
29. Gupta I et al: Effects of *Boswellia serrata* gum resin in patients with bronchial asthma: Results of a

double-blind, placebo-controlled, 6-week clinical study, *Eur J Med Res* 3(11):511-4, 1998.

30. Singh BB et al: The effectiveness of commiphora mukul for osteoarthritis of the knee: an outcomes study, *Altern Ther Health Med* 9(3):74-9, 2003.

31. Manjunath NK, Telles S: Influence of yoga and ayurveda on self-rated sleep in a geriatric population, *Indian J Med Res* 121(5):683-90, 2005.

32. Farag NH, Mills PJ: A randomised-controlled trial of the effects of a traditional herbal supplement on sleep onset insomnia, *Complement Ther Med* 11(4):223-5, 2003.

33. Lalla JK et al: Clinical trials of ayurvedic formulations in the treatment of acne vulgaris, *J Ethnopharmacol* 78(1):99-102, 2001.

34. Paranjpe P, Kulkarni PH: Comparative efficacy of four Ayurvedic formulations in the treatment of acne vulgaris: a double-blind randomised placebo-controlled clinical evaluation, *J Ethnopharmacol* 49(3):127-32, 1995.

35. Thabrew MI et al: Antioxidant potential of two polyherbal preparations used in Ayurveda for the treatment of rheumatoid arthritis, *J Ethnopharmacol* 76(3):285-91, 2001.

36. Chopra A et al: Randomized double blind trial of an ayurvedic plant derived formulation for treatment of rheumatoid arthritis, *J Rheumatol* 27(6):1365-72, 2000.

37. Bhatt AD et al: Conceptual and methodologic challenges of assessing the short-term efficacy of Guggulu in obesity: data emergent from a naturalistic clinical trial, *J Postgrad Med* 41(1):5-7, 1995.

38. Paranjpe P, Patki P, Patwardhan B: Ayurvedic treatment of obesity: a randomised double-blind, placebo-controlled clinical trial, *J Ethnopharmacol* 29(1):1-11, 1990.

39. Rege N et al: Immunotherapy with *Tinospora cordifolia*: a new lead in the management of obstructive jaundice, *Indian J Gastroenterol* 12(1):5-8, 1993.

40. Joshi H, Parle M: Antiamnesic effects of *Desmodium gangeticum* in mice, Yakugaku Zasshi— *J Pharm Soc Japan* 126(9):795-804, 2006.

41. Stough C et al: The chronic effects of an extract of *Bacopa monniera* (Brahmi) on cognitive function in healthy human subjects, *Psychopharmacology* 156(4):481, 2001.

42. Gelderloos P et al: Influence of a Maharishi Ayurvedic herbal preparation on age-related visual discrimination, *Int J Psychosom* 37(1-4):25-9, 1990.

43. Fields JZ et al: Effect of a multimodality natural medicine program on carotid atherosclerosis in older subjects: a pilot trial of Maharishi Vedic Medicine, *Am J Cardiol* 89(8):952-8, 2002.

44. Elder C et al: Randomized trial of a whole-system ayurvedic protocol for type 2 diabetes, *Altern Ther Health Med* 12(5):24-30, 2006.

45. Zollman C, Vickers A: ABC of complementary medicine: users and practitioners of complementary medicine, *Br Med J* 319(7213):836-8, 1999.

46. Kaptchuk TJ: *Chinese medicine: the web that has no weaver*, London, 1993, Rider.

47. Stux G: Background and theory of traditional Chinese medicine. In Stux G, Berman B, Pomeranz B, editors: *Basics of acupuncture*, ed 5, Berlin, Germany, 2003, Springer Verlag, pp 1-6.

48. Xinnong C: *Chinese acupuncture and moxibustion*, ed 2, Beijing, China, 1999, Foreign Languages Press.

49. Londorf D, Winn M: QiGong. In Novey D, editor: *Clinicians' complete reference to complementary and alternative medicine*, St Louis, 2000, Mosby.

50. Liu Y, Morgan T: Tai chi. In Novey D, editor: *Clinicians' complete reference to complementary and alternative medicine*, St Louis, 2000, Mosby.

51. Tang J: Research priorities in traditional Chinese medicine, *Br Med J* 333:391-4, 2006.

52. MacLennan A, Wilson D, Taylor A: The escalating cost and prevalence of alternative medicine, *Prev Med* 35:166-73, 2002.

53. Eisenberg DM et al: Trends on alternative medicine use in the United States, 1990-1997, *JAMA* 280(18):1569-74, 1998.

54. Ernst E, White A: The BBC survey of complementary medicine use in the UK, *Complement Ther Med* 8:32-6, 2000.

55. Effective Health Care. Acupuncture, NHS Centre for Reviews and Dissemination Acupuncture, vol 7, 2001. Available at: http://www.york.ac.uk/inst/crd/ehc72.pdf. Accessed July 29, 2004.

56. Trinh K et al: Acupuncture for neck disorders, *Cochrane Database of Systematic Reviews* 3, 2006.

57. Wu H et al: Acupuncture for stroke rehabilitation, *Cochrane Database of Systematic Reviews* 3, 2006.

58. Green S, Buchbinder R, Hetrick S: Acupuncture for shoulder pain, *Cochrane Database of Systematic Reviews* 2, 2005.

59. Furlan A et al: Acupuncture and dry-needling for low back pain, *Cochrane Database of Systematic Reviews* 1, 2005.

60. Green S et al Acupuncture for lateral elbow pain, *Cochrane Database of Systematic Reviews* 1, 2002.

61. Lee A, Done M: Stimulation of the wrist acupuncture point P6 for preventing postoperative nausea and vomiting, *Cochrane Database of Systematic Reviews* 3, 2004.

62. Casimiro L et al: Acupuncture and electroacupuncture for the treatment of RA, *Cochrane Database of Systematic Reviews* 4, 2005.

63. He L, Zhou D, Wu B: Acupuncture for Bell's palsy, *Cochrane Database of Systematic Reviews* 1, 2004.

64. McCarney R, Brinkhaus B, Lasserson T: Acupuncture for chronic asthma, *Cochrane Database of Systematic Reviews* 3, 2003.

65. Melchart D, LiInde K, Fischer P: Acupuncture for idiopathic headache, *Cochrane Database Syst Rev Reviews* 1, 2001.

66. Smith C, Crowther C: Acupuncture for induction of labour, *Cochrane Database of Systematic Reviews* 3, 2004.

67. White A, Rampes H, Ernst E: Acupuncture for smoking cessation, *Cochrane Database of Systematic Reviews* 1, 2006.

68. Strauss A: Acupuncture and the treatment of chronic low-back pain, *Chiropractic J Aust* 29(3):112-8, 1999.

69. Ernst E, White A: Acupuncture for back pain, *Arch Intern Med* 158(20):2235-41, 1998.

70. Smith L, Oldman A, McQuay H: Teasing apart quality and validity in systematic reviews: an example from acupuncture trials in chronic neck and back pain, *Pain* 86(1-2):119-32, 2000.

71. Cherkin D, Sherman K, Deyo R: A review of the evidence for the effectiveness, safety and cost of acupuncture, massage therapy and spinal manipulation for back pain, *Ann Intern Med* 138(11):898-906, 2003.

72. Ernst E, White A: Acupuncture as an adjuvant therapy in stroke rehabilitation? *Wiener Medizinische Wochenschrift* 146(21-22):556-8, 1996.

73. Park J, Hopwood V, White A: Effectiveness of acupuncture for stroke, *J Neurol* 248(7):558-63, 2001.

74. Kai-hoi Sze F, Wong E, Or K: Does acupuncture improve motor recovery after stroke, *Stroke* 33(11):2604-19, 2002.

75. Ernst E: Acupuncture as a symptomatic treatment of osteoarthritis, *Scand J Rheumatol* 26(6):444-7, 1997.

76. Ezzo J, Hadhazy V, Birch S: Acupuncture for osteoarthritis of the knee, *Arthritis Rheum* 44(4):819-25, 2001.

77. White A, Ernst E: A systematic review of randomized controlled trials of acupuncture for neck pain, *Rheumatol* 38(2):143-7, 1999.

78. Martin J: Efficacy of acupuncture in asthma: systematic review and meta-analysis of published data from 11 randomised controlled trials, *Eur Respir J* 20(4):846-52, 2002.

79. Manias P, Tagaris G, Karageorgiou K: Acupuncture in headache, *Clin J Pain* 16(4):334-9, 2000.

80. Hadhazy V, Berman B, Ezzo J: Is acupuncture effective in the treatment of fibromyalgia? *J Fam Pract* 48(3):213-8, 1999.

81. Ezzo J et al: Acupuncture-point stimulation for chemotherapy-induced nausea or vomiting, *Cochrane Database Syst Rev* 2, 2006.

82. Ezzo J, Berman B, Hadhazy V: Is acupuncture effective for the treatment of chronic pain, *Pain* 86(3):217-25, 2000.

83. White A, Hayhoe S, Hart A: Adverse effects following acupuncture, *Br Med J* 323(3):485-6, 2001.

84. Lim B et al: Acupuncture for treatment of irritable bowel syndrome, *Cochrane Database Syst Rev* 4, 2006.

85. Rathbone J et al: Chinese herbal medicine for schizophrenia, *Cochrane Database Syst Rev* 4, 2005.

86. Liu J, Yang M, Liu X: Herbal medicines for treatment of irritable bowel syndrome, *Cochrane Database Syst Rev* 1, 2006.

87. Zhang JZ, Wu T, Liu G: Chinese herbal medicines for treatment of pre-eclampsia, *Cochrane Database Syst Rev* 2, 2006.

88. Chen X et al: Chinese medicinal herbs for influenza, *Cochrane Database Syst Rev* 1, 2005.

89. Liu J et al: Chinese herbal medicines for type 2 diabetes mellitus, *Cochrane Database Syst Rev* 3, 2002.

90. Wei J et al: Chinese medicinal herbals for acute bronchitis, *Cochrane Database Syst Rev* 3, 2005.

91. Qiong W et al: Chinese medicinal herbals for acute pancreatitis, *Cochrane Database Syst Rev* 1, 2005.

92. Liu J, McIntosh H, Lin H: Chinese medicinal herbs for chronic hepatitis B, *Cochrane Database Syst Rev* 4, 2000.

93. Zhang W et al: Chinese herbal medicine for atopic eczema, *Cochrane Database Syst Rev* 4, 2004.

94. Wu T et al: Tongxinluo capsule for unstable angina pectoris, *Cochrane Database Syst Rev* 4, 2006.

95. Wang Q et al: Puerarin injection for unstable angina pectoris, *Cochrane Database Syst Rev* 3, 2006.

96. Zeng X et al: Ginkgo biloba for acute ischemic stroke, *Cochrane Database Syst Rev* 4, 2005.

97. Jirong Y et al: Zhiling. decoction for vascular dementia, *Cochrane Database Syst Rev* 4, 2004.

98. Han A et al: Tai chi for treating rheumatoid arthritis, *Cochrane Database Syst Rev* 3, 2004.

99. Gillespie LD et al: Interventions for preventing falls in the elderly, *Cochrane Database Syst Rev* 4, 2003.

100. Berman BM, Singh BB: An outcome analysis of a mind-body intervention, *Complement Ther Med* 5(1):29-35, 1997.

101. Mills N, Allen JB, Carey-Morgan S: Does Tai Chi-QiGong help patients with multiple sclerosis? *J Bodywork Movement Ther* 4(1):39-48, 2000.

102. Tsujuichi T et al: The effect of Qi-gong relaxation exercise on the control of Type 2 diabetes mellitus: a randomized controlled trial, *Diabetes Care* 25(1):241-2, 2002.

103. Stenlund T et al: Cardiac rehabilitation for the elderly: Qi Gong and group discussions, *Eur J Cardiovac Prevent Rehabil* 12(1):5-11, 2005.

104. Vogel VJ: *Indian theories of disease and shamanistic practices:* American Indian medicine, Norman, Okla, 1970, University of Oklahoma Press, pp 13-35.

105. Cohen K: Native American medicine. In Jonas WB, Levin J, editors: *Essentials of complementary and alternative medicine,* Baltimore, 1999, Lippincott, pp 233-51.

106. Cohen KBH: Native American medicine, *Altern Ther Health Med* 4(6):45-57, 1998.

107. Voss RW, Douville V, Edwards ED: Native American healing. In Micozzi M, editor: *Fundamentals of complementary and integrative medicine*, ed 3, St Louis, 2006, Saunders.

108. Moerman D: Native American medicinal plants. In Miccozi MS, editor: *Fundamentals of complementary and integrative medicine,* ed 3, St Louis, 2006, Saunders, pp 571-7.

109. Vogel VJ: American Indian therapeutic methods: American Indian medicine, Norman, Okla, 1970, University of Oklahoma Press.

110. NLM: American Indian Health. Available at: *http://americanindianhealth.nlm.nih.gov/tradition alhealing.html.* Accessed December 28, 2006.

111. Portman TAA, Garret MT: Native American healing traditions, *J Disabil Dev Educ* 53(4):453-69, 2006.

112. Native American Medicine: Treatment Approaches. Available at: *http://www.healthandhealingny.org/ tradition_healing/native_treat.asp.* Accessed December 28, 2006.

113. Vogel VJ: American Indian therapeutic methods: American Indian medicine, Norman, Okla, 1970, University of Oklahoma Press, pp 162-266.

114. Weigand DA: Traditional Native American medicine in dermatology, *Clin Dermatol* 17(1):49-51, 1999.

115. Borchers AT et al: Inflammation and Native American medicine: the role of botanicals, *Am J Clin Nutr* 72(2):339-47, 2000.

116. Mehl-Madrona LE: Native American medicine in the treatment of chronic illness: developing an integrated program and evaluating its effectiveness, *Altern Ther Health Med* 5(1):36-44, 1999.

117. Nauman E: Native American medicine and cardiovascular disease, *Cardiol Rev* 15(1):35-41, 2007.

118. Cody G: History of naturopathic medicine. In Pizzorno JA, Murray MT, editors: *A textbook of natural medicine*, Seattle, 1996, John Bastyr College Publications.

119. Murray TM, Pizzorno JA, editors: *Naturopathic medicine*, Philadelphia, 1999, Lippincott Williams and Wilkins. Jonas WB, Levin JS, editors. *Essentials of complementary and alternative medicine.*

120. Physicians AAoN: Licensed States and Licensing Authorities. Available at: *http://www.naturopathic. org/viewbulletin.php?id=118.* Accessed May 15, 2007.

121. NCAAM: An Introduction to Naturopathy. Backgrounder Available at: *http://nccam.nih.gov/health/ naturopathy/.* Accessed May 1, 2007.

122. Beamon S et al: Speleotherapy for asthma, *Cochrane Database Syst Rev* 2:CD001741, 2001.

123. Rapp A et al: Does garlic influence rheologic properties and blood flow in progressive systemic sclerosis?, *Forschende Komplementarmedizin* 13(3): 141-6, 2006.

124. Wustrow TPU: Naturopathic therapy for acute otitis media. An alternative to the primary use of antibiotics, *HNO* 53(8):728-34, 2005.

125. Sarrell EM, Cohen HA, Kahan E: Naturopathic treatment for ear pain in children, *Pediatrics* 111(5 Pt 1):e574-9, 2003.

126. Kempe C et al: Icelandic moss lozenges in the prevention or treatment of oral mucosa irritation and dried out throat mucosa, *Laryngorhinootologie* 76(3): 186-8, 1997.

127. Gut E et al: Natural remedies during pregnancy and lactation, *Gynakologisch-Geburtshilfliche Rundschau* 44(4):233-7, 2004.

128. Garrow D, Egede LE: Association between complementary and alternative medicine use, preventive care practices, and use of conventional medical services among adults with diabetes, *Diabetes Care* 29(1):15-9, 2006.

129. Suhr B et al: Drug-induced headache: long-term results of stationary versus ambulatory withdrawal therapy, *Cephalalgia* 19(1):44-9, 1999.

130. Weber W et al: *Echinacea purpurea* for prevention of upper respiratory tract infections in children, *J Altern Complement Med* 11(6):1021-6, 2005.

131. Standish LJ, Calabrese C, Snider P: The naturopathic medical research agenda: The future and foundation of naturopathic medical science, *J Altern Complement Med* 12(3):341-5, 2006.

# CHAPTER 5

## Acupuncture

*Suzanne McDonough, Sheelagh McNeill*

### ▀ Initial Examination

***Client Report:*** Richard has had right lateral elbow pain for 4 months; it is continuing to worsen despite use of nonsteroidal antiinflammatory drugs (NSAIDs). He is currently unable to work and also has great difficulty lifting and carrying objects in his right hand. The onset of his pain was insidious.

***Client Goals:*** Reduce pain, return of full function of the arm, especially gripping objects and driving

***Employment:*** Bus driver

***Recreational Activities:*** Football referee

***General Health:*** Moderate; had shingles 12 years ago and since then suffers from headaches; also complains of left sciatica, right neck pain, and left ankle fracture, which required open reduction internal fixation

***Medications:*** NSAID

***Musculoskeletal:*** Range of motion (ROM): unable to actively extend the elbow because of pain and swelling; passive stretching of the extensor muscle group, and elbow supination and pronation (with the forearm flexed to 90 degrees) all produce pain. Swollen around lateral complex of the elbow.

***Neuromuscular:*** Force generation: unable to test right elbow extension, right wrist extension, or right grip strength because of aggravation of pain. Tests for left arm all scored 5/5 on manual muscle testing.[1]

***Function:*** Severe sharp pain, aggravated by any light pressure such as clothes touching his arm, unable to sleep on right side, sharp pain: visual analogue scale (VAS)=8 to 9 out of 10 at worst during movement; and dull throbbing pain: VAS=2 to 3 out of 10 at rest. Activities of daily living (ADL): unable to safely lift and carry heavy objects in his right hand; unable to safely drive.

### ▀ Plan of Care

The plan of care includes ice, massage, and stretches to the muscles of extensor complex of lateral elbow. The initial home exercise program given was to hold stretch for 10 seconds three to five times per session and repeat three times per day within his limits of pain. Functional activities were not commenced because of the extreme pain, and the client was told to ice and use antiinflammatory gel to control his pain at home.

### ▀ Reevaluation

After two sessions over 2 weeks little change exists: the client can tolerate only very light pressure around the right elbow. Passive stretching of the extensor muscle group, resisted finger extension of the middle digit, and elbow supination and pronation (with the forearm flexed to 90 degrees) all produce high levels of pain. Self-treatment with ice and antiinflammatory gel has little impact on his pain, and he is unable to comply with the home exercise program.

## Incorporating CAM into the Plan of Care

Physical therapy treatment has been limited by this client's inability to tolerate any level of pressure on or around his right lateral elbow. The client therefore was referred to another therapist who practices acupuncture from a TCM perspective as an alternative to the current plan of care. The therapist carries out a diagnosis from a TCM perspective and notes the following.

## TCM Examination

**Appearance:** Overweight especially around his abdomen; facial expression indicates pain, good vital energy in his eyes
**Listening:** Normal level of speech
**Presenting Tongue:** Pale, damp with slight teeth marks
**Pulses**

| RIGHT HAND | | LEFT HAND | |
|---|---|---|---|
| [1]LI deficient | LU deficient | SI deficient | HT deficient |
| ST OK | SP deficient | GB excess | LIV excess |
| TE OK | HC (KI Yang) OK | BL OK | KI (KI Yin) deficient |

**Palpation:** Extremely tender on palpation along the large intestine (LI) meridian of the right arm; also swollen. Severe pain limits movement and increases with light pressure, which suggests a yin problem.
**Meridian/Organ Involvement:** Painful along right LI meridian from LI 11 to LI 9 and also LI organ involvement (see bowel function below).
**Diet:** Majority of his food is fried fatty foods and carbohydrates; chicken, pork, and eggs aggravate his symptoms of irritable bowel syndrome (IBS).
**Fluid Intake:** Drinks at least three to four cups of tea/coffee daily.
**Bowel/Urinary Function:** Symptoms of IBS are worse than typical over last 9 months with chronic diarrhea daily (usually preceded by left-sided abdominal cramps) and intermittent constipation. Client is also complaining of abdominal distension after eating food. Increased frequency of urine at night.

**Sleep:** Suffers from nocturia and sluggishness first thing in the morning; complains of tiredness and energy dips in the afternoon; falls asleep in front of the television by 9 PM every night.
**Other Health Problems:** Complaining of dizziness and headaches that travel from back of left eye over temporal aspect of his head along the GB meridian (linked to shingles attack 12 years ago).

## TCM Diagnosis and Plan of Care

In this case study, internal organ problems and local channel problems appear to overlap.[2] In TCM, local channel problems may be explained by invasion of a single or a combination of four external pathogenic factors (cold, heat, damp, or wind), which may lead to painful obstructive syndrome or Bi syndrome.[3] In this case study, the symptoms of severe pain, which limits movement, and swelling could be explained by an invasion of cold and damp into the body.[3] This invasion alters the balance of yin and yang, upsets the circulation of qi in the channel, and causes qi and blood to stagnate. Local stagnation of qi and blood along the LI meridian (Figure 5-1) of this client's right forearm causes significant pain and swelling and lack of nourishment of the tendons and skin. This type of pain is improved by heat and aggravated by cold, which explains why the use of cryotherapy by the first physiotherapist was unhelpful.[3] Another frequent cause of lateral elbow pain, according to Ji,[4] is local trauma, which could be a likely explanation in this case study and would fit with a Western medical diagnosis of repetitive strain injury (RSI). Obviously in this case study this is linked to the client's occupation as a bus driver.

However, this client also is showing signs of disharmony in several organs, which suggests deficiency of his system and may explain why he was susceptible to an invasion of cold/damp. His reported symptoms of diarrhea/constipation

---

[1]LI, large intestine meridian, LU, lung meridian, SI, small intestine meridian, HT, heart meridian, ST, stomach meridian, SP, spleen meridian, GB, gallbladder meridian, LIV, liver meridian, TE, triple energiser meridian, HC, heart constrictor meridian, BL, bladder meridian, KI, Kidney meridian; kidney meridian is subdivided into yin (KI Yin) and yang (KI Yang) components, see also Table 5-1 and Figure 5-1).

reflect changes in large intestine function. directly linked to his local large intestine channel problem manifested in his elbow. This may be due to an underlying spleen qi deficiency, which causes collapse of the LI. The pattern of spleen qi deficiency is manifested by the symptoms of fatigue and chronic diarrhea and can be seen on his tongue (pale, damp, swollen, and tooth marked, which also may indicate yang deficiency of the kidney),[5] his body type (overweight, especially the abdomen), and his pulse. He also is showing signs of liver disharmony in his pulses and reports of dizziness and temporal headaches along the GB line. His bowel symptoms, along with abdominal bloating and cramps and his reported intolerance to some foods, are suggestive of IBS. According to Gascoigne[6] in TCM this corresponds to liver qi stagnation invading the spleen with an underlying kidney deficiency. Kidney deficiency in this case study is seen in the pulses, his sleep pattern, and tongue. A predominance of spleen qi deficiency explains the loose stools, and the abdominal distension and pain are caused by stagnation of liver qi.

## Incorporating CAM into the Plan of Care

Using a TCM approach the plan of care is extended from one that treated the local problem (channel problem in TCM) to one that treats the organ disharmonies revealed by the detailed TCM diagnosis. Local channel problems will be treated in this case by use of a combination of local (LI 10, LI 11, LI 12) and distal points (LI 4, LI 5, TE 5). (See Table 5-1 for a list of the 12 main meridians and their corresponding organs.) Several organs show signs of disharmony and are treated accordingly. Use of large intestine points may help to resolve the large intestine organ problems (e.g., diarrhea and constipation).

However, the other underlying organ deficiencies already identified in the TCM diagnosis also need to be addressed. For example, spleen qi deficiency should be addressed through a change in diet in addition to the use of specific acupuncture points to strengthen spleen function. The client should avoid dairy products, bananas, refined foods high in sugar, and raw cold food because these all can injure the spleen. In addition he should reduce consumption of fried, greasy foods and alcohol because these can damage the spleen (and liver). A reduction in tea and coffee also may be helpful and can be achieved by a switch to herbal teas and diluted apple juice. During acupuncture treatment, specific points to reinforce the function of the spleen (and kidney) could be used (B 120, ST 36, SP 6, KI 3, KI 6 with moxibustion), if required. Improvement of the flow of liver qi also would be important to address by use of either GB or LIV points (GB 40, LIV 3). In the case study, points were altered as required depending on the client's response and on reassessment during each visit. In TCM, acupuncture points may have several actions, and points to treat organ disharmony may be useful for treatment of the local problem (and vice versa). For example, LIV 3 and SP 6 aid the movement of qi and blood anywhere in the body and thus reinforce the action of local and distal points along the arm meridian.

This chapter describes the case of a 58-year-old male bus driver with lateral elbow pain, who is unable to work. The client is examined with use of a physical therapy and a traditional Chinese medicine (TCM) approach. The physical therapists, both trained as acupuncturists, consider including acupuncture, using a TCM approach in the plan of care. The decision is based on the physical therapists' training, in the United Kingdom, where PTs can use acupuncture as an adjunctive analgesic modality after a conventional physiotherapy assessment or as part of treatment after a TCM diagnosis (see Appendix 1).

In this case study the therapists use a TCM approach and acupuncture analgesia (AA). The therapists, also acupuncture researchers, thoroughly review the literature relevant to lateral elbow pain and after a discussion of the findings with the client initiate a course of acupuncture. The investigation of the literature and the therapists' clinical decision making are described in this chapter.

## INVESTIGATING THE LITERATURE

The therapist uses two strategies to investigate the literature. The first is a detailed approach in which preliminary background reading is performed on the pathophysiology of pain and acupuncture therapy, including Eastern and Western perspectives on TCM. Next comes a search of databases and evaluation of the literature with use of reviews and primary sources. The second strategy is the use of the PICO format for a focused search to answer the clinical question generated by the case.

## Preliminary Reading

A multitude of publications provide an introduction to acupuncture, many of which start with some form of historical perspective on acupuncture in East Asia,[6,7] and how it was introduced to and embraced in the Western world.[8] For example Pomeranz explains that although acupuncture was first brought to Europe in the seventeenth century, it only recently has been accepted widely because of the clash of Eastern and Western paradigms in health care.[9] Briefly, acupuncture is a form of treatment derived from TCM, which is more than 2000 years old. Although the term *TCM* is used throughout this chapter, a great deal of heterogeneity exists in the practice of acupuncture in eastern Asia, and it is not a single, historically stable therapy. For example, whereas many Chinese practitioners insert needles deep into the tissues, Japanese practitioners use shallow needle and noninsertion needling techniques.[10] Although the details of practice may vary, all traditional acupuncture is based on the Daoist concept of yin and yang[10] (see Chapter 4).

To maintain health, yin and yang energies must be balanced; otherwise imbalance will result in disharmony/disease of the human body. This balance of yin and yang is controlled by a vital force or energy called *qi* (pronounced "chee"), which circulates between the organs along channels called *meridians*.[10] The surface of the body has 12 regular meridians (Figure 5-1 and Table 5-1), and these correspond to 12 major functions or "organs" of the body. Although they have the same names (e.g., liver, kidney, heart), Chinese and Western concepts of the organs correlate only very loosely. Qi must flow in the correct strength and quality (and direction) through these meridians, which connect to interior organs, for health to be maintained.[10] To stimulate healing and alter the energetic flow of qi and thus maintain the balance of yin and yang, acupuncture needles are applied at external points along the meridians. Each acupuncture point is considered to have a defined therapeutic action (some of which have been confirmed by MRI studies[11]), and thus particular defined points are

| Table 5-1 | The 12 Main Meridians and Their Corresponding Organs | | |
|---|---|---|---|
| MERIDIAN | NO. OF POINTS | YIN/YANG | ARM/LEG |
| Lungs (LU) | 11 | Yin | Arm |
| Large intestine (LI) | 20 | Yang | Arm |
| Heart (HT) | 9 | Yin | Arm |
| Small intestine (SI) | 19 | Yang | Arm |
| Pericardium (PC) | 9 | Yin | Arm |
| Triple energizer (TE) | 23 | Yang | Arm |
| Spleen (SP) | 21 | Yin | Leg |
| Stomach (ST) | 45 | Yang | Leg |
| Kidneys (KI) | 27 | Yin | Leg |
| Bladder (BL) | 67 | Yang | Leg |
| Liver (LIV) | 14 | Yin | Leg |
| Gallbladder (GB) | 44 | Yang | Leg |

The number of acupoints for each meridian is identified; six meridians have points along the arms and six have points along the legs. Each meridian/organ is paired so that a balance of yin and yang exists. For example, LU/LI, HT/SI, PC/TE, SP/ST, KI/BL, LIV/GB are yin-yang couples.

chosen to treat a specific condition. Pain along a meridian could indicate a dysfunction of that meridian only or could reflect a dysfunction of the corresponding organ.[7] In this particular case history, Richard appears to have a dysfunction of the meridian and corresponding organ.

When acupuncture is practiced from a TCM perspective, the interpretation of how the body functions is different from Western medicine, and a complex examination of many systems is carried out to diagnose the location of an imbalance in energy (see Chapter 4).

### Western Medical Acupuncture

Many of the health professionals such as physical therapists, medical doctors, and dentists who practice acupuncture have dispensed with these TCM concepts[6] and practice "Western medical acupuncture." In Western medical acupuncture the clinician diagnoses the client from an orthodox point of view and applies acupuncture, based on the published scientific evidence, as an adjunctive technique.[12] Acupuncture points are seen to correspond to physiological and anatomical features such as peripheral nerves and muscular trigger points,[10] and the aim of treatment is to reduce pain and/or deactivate trigger points. Now a large body of scientific evidence details the mechanisms of action of acupuncture, in particular acupuncture

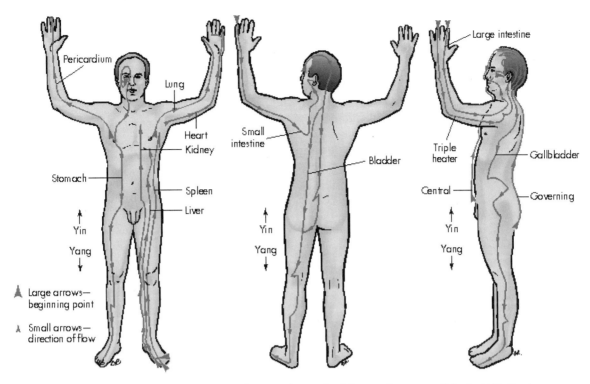

**Figure 5-1** The 12 main meridians. From Fritz S: *Fundamentals of therapeutic massage,* St Louis, 2004, Elsevier.

| Table 5-2 | **Classification of Nerve Fibers** | | | | |
|---|---|---|---|---|
| SENSATION | | SKIN | MUSCLE/JOINTS | MEAN FIBER DIAMETER (μm) | MEAN CONDUCTION VELOCITY (m/s) |
| Touch and proprioception | | A beta | Group II | 8 | 50 |
| Pinprick, cold, heavy pressure, muscle ergoreceptor | | A delta | Group III | 3 | 15 |
| Deep pain and itch | | C | Group IV | 0.5 | 1 |

Nerve fibers are classified by diameter and conduction velocity. The numerical classification typically is used for muscle afferents, whereas the alphabetical scheme is used for cutaneous nerves.

analgesia. Several sources can be found on this topic.[13-16]

A starting point is an understanding of pain control mechanisms. Additional references provide information on the neuroanatomy of the nociceptive system and neurophysiology of pain and its modulation.[17-20] To minimize confusion in reading these texts remember that nerve fibers are classified by diameter and conduction velocity. The numerical classification typically is used for muscle afferents, whereas the alphabetical scheme is used for cutaneous nerves (Table 5-2).

Scientific research suggests that acupuncture needles activate sensory afferents (variously A

delta/Group III, A beta/Group II, and C fiber/ Group IV afferents), which send impulses to the spinal cord and activate three centers (spinal cord, midbrain, and hypothalamus-pituitary) to cause analgesia through the release of endorphins and monoamines.[16] Another suggestion is that activation of ergoreceptors in the muscle, which normally signal muscle load and are activated during voluntary muscle contraction, occurs by low-frequency ture. These receptors, which are served by group III muscle afferent fibers, are proposed to play a particularly important role in the production of AA.[21]

The main mechanisms of AA are outlined in the first three points below. The secondary mechanisms of AA are outlined in points four and five. Some of these are less well understood than others, and research to elucidate mechanisms is ongoing.

1. Segmental inhibition: At the spinal cord level, pain relief is produced by blocking incoming pain messages (mainly transmitted along C fibers) through the presynaptic or/and postsynaptic release of endogenous opiates (dynorphins or enkephalins),[16] which can close the "pain gate," as described by Melzack and Wall.[22] Much of the research in this area has used electroacupuncture to investigate these mechanisms. However, manual acupuncture also can block pain in the spinal cord,[23] possibly through similar mechanisms.

2. Descending pain suppression system (DPSS): When appropriately stimulated, ascending afferents from the spinal cord excite the periaqueductal grey (PAG) in the midbrain, which releases the opioid enkephalin; this in turn activates other centers in the brainstem, for example, the medulla (the raphe nucleus) and the pons (locus ceruleus) with descending projections onto the spinal cord. These descending projections inhibit the transmission of pain by postsynaptic inhibition of A delta and C fibers at the level of the spinal cord via the synergistic effects of the neurotransmitters serotonin and norepinephrine.[16] These neurotransmitters excite inhibitory interneurons, which inhibit the pain-transmitting fibers through the release of enkephalin.

3. Hypothalamus-pituitary axis: Evidence suggests that hypothalamic nuclei have a central role in mediating the effects of AA (as well as autonomic effects) by releasing beta-endorphin, which reinforces the midbrain DPSS.[14,16] This system may be activated by vigorous physical exercise with repetitive muscle contractions or low-frequency EA, at sufficiently high intensities to cause muscle contraction. This muscle contraction excites high-threshold and low-threshold mechanoreceptors called *ergoreceptors* in muscle and other tissues, as described earlier.[14] When activated, the hypothalamus-pituitary releases beta-endorphin by two methods: either into the CSF of the brain to produce AA or into the blood via the pituitary (along with equal amounts of cortisol). The role of beta-endorphin released into the blood is unclear, although the release of cortisol may play an important antiinflammatory role in the body's tissues.

4. Peripheral effects: Electrical stimulation at intensities likely to recruit A delta fibers can reduce conduction velocity and amplitude of potentials in A delta fibers.[24] Presumably EA (at least) can block transmission through this mechanism. In addition, acupuncture has been shown to lead to the release of substances in the periphery (substance P, vasoactive intestinal polypeptide, and calcitonin gene-related peptide), which are likely to result in vasodilatation, and in increased nutrition from improved blood flow, and thus may accelerate the removal of pain-inducing substances.[15]

5. Oxytocinergic system: Acupuncture and muscle exercise release endogenous opioids and oxytocin.[14] The oxytocinergic system is activated by mild, nonpainful sensory stimulation such as a 2-Hz EA, massage, vibration, and thermal stimulation and affects beta-endorphin release,[15] which mediates AA in the hypothalamus-pituitary axis.

The choice of acupuncture points is important. Activation of acupuncture analgesia is believed to depend on several factors: the stimulation of the sensory afferents, the length of time the needles are retained, the location of the needles relative to the site of pain, and the intensity/method of stimulation.[16] First, a dull ache, numbness, or heaviness indicates that the sensory afferents have been activated as a result of insertion and stimulation of the needle, and because maximum acupuncture analgesia occurs after 20 minutes of retention, needles should be retained for at least this time period.[16,25]

Second, needles can be stimulated in two ways: by hand, termed *manual acupuncture*, or by the use of electrical current at either low or high frequencies (EA). The majority of evidence on the mechanisms of AA is based on studies of EA in laboratory animals or transcutaneous electrical nerve stimulation (TENS) on the skin overlying acupuncture points, as opposed to manual acupuncture. The reason for this is that the stimulation parameters can be controlled carefully and precisely quantified with use of EA. The centers activated in AA (using EA) depend on the method and site of stimulation (i.e., within the segment of pain or extrasegmentally). Needles placed in the same segment as the pain can produce effects through all three principal mechanism described above, whereas needles placed distally produce analgesia via the hypothalamus and brainstem only. Local segmental needling therefore gives a more intensive analgesia than distal nonsegmental needling.[16]

Early experiments were seminal: they did establish that opioids were released in response to acupuncture needle insertion and stimulation. However, much debate still exists about the influence of parameter choice (for electrical stimulation) and the types of opioids released. Two main forms of EA have been explored: low-frequency, high-intensity needling, which activates all three principal mechanisms, and high-frequency, low-intensity needling, which activates the spinal cord and brainstem only.[16] Low-frequency, high-intensity electrical stimulation produces pain relief through the release of beta-endorphin and enkephalins, whereas high-frequency currents produce analgesia via the opioid dynorphin.[26,27] However, other parameter factors such as intensity and pulse duration may influence which opioid is released in the spinal cord.[28] More research is required to explore these mechanisms in more detail.

Finally, the majority of scientific evidence for AA is based on EA in animals, and this has been extrapolated to provide evidence for AA in humans. However, other forms of evidence, such as laboratory studies and clinical studies in humans, which have explored the analgesic effects of EA and manual acupuncture, have shown conflicting results. Systematic review evidence for using EA in human laboratory studies (using acute pain models) suggests that a genuine analgesic effect exists; however, the evidence to date has not been able to show a similar clear effect for manual acupuncture.[13] Moreover, although a systematic review of the effectiveness of acupuncture (EA and manual acupuncture) for chronic pain in clients demonstrated a clear analgesic effect compared with no treatment, inconsistent results have been reported compared with placebo, sham, or other treatments.[29] Further research in humans therefore is required to establish definitively the mechanism for acupuncture-mediated analgesia.

### Typical Acupuncture Treatment

The experience of the client during the first acupuncture treatment may differ depending on whether the clinician is using Western medical or TCM acupuncture. In the Western medical approach, acupuncture is used mainly as a pain-relieving modality after an orthodox diagnosis of the client. In contrast, a more complex whole system diagnosis takes place with TCM, and the explanations for effects given to the client may be different from those given by the Western acupuncture clinician. In Western acupuncture, points are chosen within the segment of pain and extrasegmentally: however, the choice of specific points for pain relief is not considered important. In TCM, acupuncture points may have multiple functions, as described for this case study in the section on plan of care and in Table 5-6 on p. 69, and may treat the local problem by moving stagnation of qi and blood (and thus reduce pain and swelling) and treat the organ disharmony.

Regardless of the approach, a combination of points is used and a typical treatment entails the insertion of 3 to 15 needles, which are left in place for up to 30 minutes (Figure 5-2). Usually clinicians activate the needles to produce needle sensation or de qi because this is considered important from a Western and an Eastern perspective. De qi refers to a deep ache, a numbness, or a distending feeling around the point where the needle is inserted. Western medical acupuncturists interpret this as the activation of sensory afferents, which will produce AA, whereas TCM clinicians consider that the "arrival of de qi at each point" is important because it will help to open the channel, move qi, and rebalance the body's energies.

### Searching the Databases and Evaluating the Literature

The Cochrane Library and other relevant databases were searched to identify systematic reviews of treatment for lateral elbow pain. Data from these reviews were extracted in a standardized fashion (Table 5-3).[30-34] These reviews identified a range of primary studies, and only the evidence most pertinent to this case study was examined in more detail; that is, studies on laser acupuncture were excluded from more detailed analysis. Table 5-4 includes data extracted from clinical needle acupuncture according to STRICTA guidelines[35] (Table 5-4).[36-40]

### Reviews

The Cochrane Library was searched up to July 2004, using the key word *acupuncture* to determine which critical reviews had been published. Ten systematic reviews were identified (see Chapter 4 for details on these reviews). Only one was relevant to the case study in this chapter,[31] which was last updated in June 2001. This review is one of a series of reviews of interventions for lateral elbow pain in

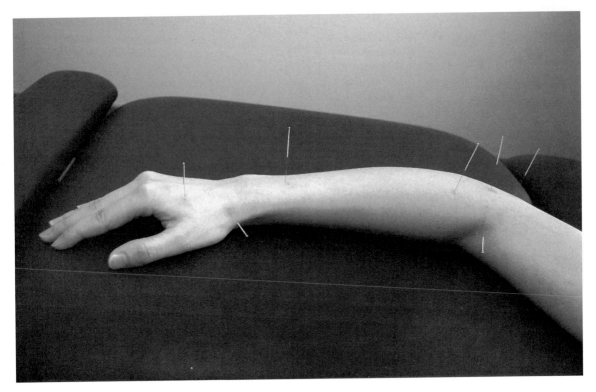

**Figure 5-2** Acupuncture needles commonly used for lateral elbow pain.

the Cochrane Library, and its objectives were to determine the effectiveness of acupuncture in the treatment of adults with lateral elbow pain with respect to pain reduction, improvement in function, grip strength, and adverse effects.

To identify any additional reviews since the last Cochrane review searches the therapist completed a search of CAM on MEDLINE/PubMed, CINAHL, AMED, and EMBASE electronic databases with use of the key words *tennis elbow* or *tendonitis* or *lateral elbow pain* or *epicondylitis* or *common extensor origin* and *acupuncture* with a limit to review articles. CAM on PubMed was searched as well as MEDLINE because this database holds additional life sciences journals, which may have revealed additional articles (Table 5-5).

In addition, *Clinical Evidence* was searched using the key word *acupuncture*. *Clinical Evidence* (published by the *British Medical Journal*) is an international source of the best available evidence for effective health care, which summarizes systematic review evidence plus any recent randomized controlled trials (RCTs). *Clinical Evidence* had seven reviews, one of which was on lateral elbow pain.[32]

Therefore four additional review articles were identified[30,32-34] and are summarized along with the

Cochrane review[31] in Table 5-3. The aims of these systematic reviews varied. Two reviews included trials using laser acupuncture and needle acupuncture,[31,32] one of laser only,[40] one of needle acupuncture only,[33] and one of needle acupuncture and laser.[34] The reviews by Smidt et al[30] and Trudel et al[34] were a subset of a more global review on the effectiveness of physiotherapy/conservative treatments for lateral epicondylitis, where laser may have been used over acupuncture points or simply over the painful area. The review by Assendelft et al[32] is an update of the Cochrane review, Green et al,[31] by some of the same authors. Two additional references comparing needle acupuncture to sham acupuncture (non acupoints 5 cm away from real points[39,41]) or electroacupuncture[40] were included. Finally, the review by Trinh et al[33] reviewed studies of needle acupuncture only. Apart from reviewing Fink et al,[39,41] Trinh et al[33] included three additional studies in comparison with Assendelft et al,[32] one unpublished article by Irnich and colleagues, one pilot study,[38] and an Italian language publication.[42]

Three out of five of these systematic reviews concluded that insufficient evidence exists to support or refute the effects of either needle or laser

| Table 5-3 | Recent Systematic Reviews on Lateral Elbow Pain | | | | |
|---|---|---|---|---|---|
| | SMIDT ET AL (2003)[30] | GREEN ET AL (2004)[31] | ASSENDELFT ET AL (2003)[32] | TRINH ET AL (2004)[33] | TRUDEL ET AL (2004)[34] |
| Search date | January 1999 | June 2001 | April 2003 | January 2004 | March 2003 |
| Inclusion criteria | (1) Lateral epicondylitis, or lateral elbow pain increased by pressure on lateral epicondyle and during resisted dorsiflexion of the wrist; (2) at least one of the treatments included a physical therapy intervention and had to be contrasted with placebo, no treatment, or another conservative treatment; (3) treatments have to be randomly allocated; (4) at least one clinically relevant outcome measure has to be mentioned; (5) follow up was at least 1 day; (6) published as a full report before July 1999; (7) all languages; (8) Quality rating ≥7/14* | (1) Adults >16 years of age; (2) lateral elbow pain for greater than 3 weeks; (3) no history of significant trauma or systematic inflammatory conditions such as arthritis; (4) studies that included other sites with separate report of lateral elbow results or >90% of clients with lateral elbow pain; (5) randomized controlled trials; (6) outcome assessor blind or not blind to allocated group; (7) all languages | (1) Adults >16 years; (2) tennis elbow, lateral elbow pain, lateral epicondylitis, rowing elbow, tendinitis common extensor origin, peritendinitis of elbow: (3) no history of significant trauma or systematic inflammatory conditions such as arthritis; (4) studies that included other sites with separate report of lateral elbow results or >90% of clients with lateral elbow pain; (5) pain for greater than 3 weeks; (6) laser or acupuncture treatments; (7) systematic reviews, RCTS, or quasi-RCTs | (1) Pain from tennis elbow, lateral epicondyle pain, lateral elbow pain, lateral epicondylitis, and description of pain originating from the common origin of the extensor tendon; (2) needle acupuncture as primary intervention; (3) random or quasi random; (4) any language; (5) original study | (1) Adults (18 years +); (2) tennis elbow; (3) randomized and quasi-randomized controlled trials; (4) physical therapy techniques, rehabilitation, complementary therapies, conservative treatment, ultrasound, acupuncture, laser, TENS, electrical stimulation, friction massage, manual therapy, mobilizations, exercise, SWD, steroid injections, exercise movement techniques; (5) English language only |
| Number of studies identified | 9/23 (laser vs. placebo for elbow pain) 1/23 laser vs. physical therapy for elbow pain | 11 | One systematic review (Green et al) Two additional RCTs | 8 | 31: 5 on acupuncture and 6 on laser |
| Number of studies excluded | 2 because of low-quality score; Lundeberg 1987 and Gudmundsen 1987 | 6 (see original article) | — | 2, one because it included medial elbow pain (Brattberg et al, 1983); second acupuncture not the primary intervention (Wang, 1997) | No detail given |

*Continued*

| Table 5-3 | Recent Systematic Reviews on Lateral Elbow Pain–cont'd | | | | |
|---|---|---|---|---|---|
| | SMIDT ET AL (2003)[30] | GREEN ET AL (2004)[31] | ASSENDELFT ET AL (2003)[32] | TRINH ET AL (2004)[33] | TRUDEL ET AL (2004)[34] |
| Number of studies evaluated | 6/7 laser vs. placebo for elbow pain 1/7 laser vs. physical therapy for elbow pain | 4/5 (one duplicate publication) 2/4 needle acupuncture vs. placebo 1/4 laser acupuncture vs. placebo 1/4 acupuncture and vitamin B12 injection vs. vitamin B12 injection alone | 3/6 RCT acupuncture vs. sham 1/6 laser acupuncture vs. placebo 1/6 acupuncture and vitamin B12 injection vs. vitamin B12 injection alone 1/6 RCT MA vs. EA | 4/6 needle acupuncture vs. placebo 2/6 needle acupuncture vs. US | 1/5 comparing two acupuncture techniques 4/5 needle acupuncture vs. placebo |
| Summary of results | Contradictory results for *laser acupuncture* vs. placebo or physical therapy | Needle acupuncture to be of short-term benefit for pain based on n=2 trials; no differences in other comparisons | As for Green et al (2004) plus needle acupuncture of short-term benefit for pain and function compared to sham acupuncture; EA of greater short-term pain relief than MA | Best evidence synthesis showed that five out of six trials indicated that needle acupuncture was more effective than a control treatment | Level 2b evidence to support the use of acupuncture to relieve pain and improve function; similarly level 2b evidence that laser was not an effective treatment |
| | Insufficient evidence to demonstrate benefit or lack of effect | Insufficient evidence to support or refute the use of acupuncture | Insufficient evidence to assess the effects of acupuncture (either laser or needle) | Strong evidence that suggests that acupuncture is effective in short-term pain relief | Weak evidence that acupuncture is effective in short-term pain relief and functional improvement |

MA, manual acupuncture; EA, electroacupuncture; US, ultrasound.
*Amsterdam-Maastricht consensus list (van der Heijden GJ, van der Windt DA, de Winer AF): Physiotherapy for clients with soft tissue disorders: a systematic review of randomized clinical trials, *Br Med J* 315:25-30, 1997.

acupuncture for lateral elbow pain.[30-32] Only the more recent systematic reviews stated that strong to weak evidence existed to suggest that needle acupuncture is effective in the short-term relief of pain[33,34] plus weak evidence for an improvement in function.[34] Trinh et al[33] based their statement on the evidence that in five of the six trials acupuncture was more effective than a control treatment (see Tables 5-3 and 5-4). Trudel et al[34] stated that at least level 2b evidence[43] exists to support the use of acupuncture in the reduction of pain and improvement in function, and at least level 2b evidence that laser therapy was ineffective in this condition. The main differences between the reviews, which may account for the differences in the interpretation of the findings, were the included trials and the authors' assessment of the methodological quality of these trials. For example, Trinh et al[33] included two additional positive trials and excluded two negative trials in comparison with Assendelft et al,[32] so on balance the majority of studies provided evidence for acupuncture. The other important difference was the interpretation of methodological quality: whereas Trinh et al[33] stated that all trials were of high quality (based on Jadad scores), Assendelft et al[32] found important problems with the methodology of some of the same studies and therefore concluded that the balance of evidence was insufficient to support the use of acupuncture. The authors in both of these reviews were unable to carry out a meta-analysis because of the lack of clinical heterogeneity. Additional high-quality studies of similar comparisons are required to establish definitively the effectiveness of acupuncture. None of the systematic reviews were able to provide any evidence to support or refute the effect of acupuncture on quality of life or return to work. The effects of acupuncture on swelling, the autonomic nervous system, and the link between pain along the LI meridian and LI organ involvement were not explored either. Two RCTs provided some evidence that acupuncture improved functional return (see Table 5-4),[37,39,41] which would be expected to affect some of the former outcomes.

### Primary Sources

Despite the usual focus on internal validity in systematic reviews, clinicians often are more concerned about the external validity of a study and whether the treatment intervention used was clinically appropriate. The development of the standards for reporting interventions in controlled trials of acupuncture (Standards for Reporting Interventions in Controlled Trials of Acupuncture, STRICTA) recommendations[35] has attempted to address this issue. The STRICTA recommendations[35] were developed specifically to enhance the conduct and reporting of trials in acupuncture and were prompted by the publication of the Consolidated Standards of Reporting Trials (CONSORT statement).[44] However, the STRICTA recommendations[35] are also a useful tool to extract information from research articles so that a judgment on clinical appropriateness of the intervention can be made.

Using the STRICTA recommendations[35] the treatment details for all the English language published articles included in the systematic reviews above (with objective outcome measures) were extracted to inform the clinical hypothesis and treatment plan for the client (see Table 5-4).

Two articles compared acupuncture with sham acupuncture. Sham in one case was superficial needle insertion of the same points for the same length of time as the real (verum) acupuncture group[37] (see Table 5-4); in the other paper it was pressure on B 113 with a penlike probe.[36] Based on these two articles a single acupuncture needle inserted in the lower limb (GB 34) for a single treatment[36] or 10 acupuncture treatments (two to three times weekly) using five acupuncture points inserted in the affected upper limb (LI 10, 11, 12,

Lu 5 and TE 5[37]; see Figure 5-2) were found to be of short-term benefit in terms of pain relief. This evidence was not considered strong evidence because both trials were small (n = 48, n = 82, respectively) and the results could not be combined in a meta-analysis. The other two articles compared acupuncture in combination with an injection of vitamin B12 versus an injection of vitamin B12 alone,[45] or laser acupuncture to placebo laser acupuncture[46]; neither study showed any differences between groups. The reviewers stated that no evidence from any of the trials was found to support the use of acupuncture for changes in grip strength, function, or adverse effects. However, Haker and Lundeberg[37] did report that verum acupuncture significantly increased pain-free grip strength and increased the amount that the client could lift pain free. In summary, the reviewers concluded that insufficient evidence exists to either support or refute the use of acupuncture (either needle or laser) in the treatment of lateral elbow pain (see Table 5-3).

The age range in the studies varied slightly, with mean ages of 47.5 years[38] versus 52 years[39] and age ranges from 52 to 70 years.[37] All studies included clients with chronic lateral elbow pain with average time since injury from 6 to 9 months.[37-39] The majority of trials, three out of five, chose segmental acupuncture points commonly used for lateral elbow pain, based on TCM theory,[37-39] whereas two trials used extrasegmental points in the lower limb.[36,40] However, despite the fact that these trials used a TCM approach, management focused only on the treatment of the local channel problem. The issue of underlying organ disharmony was not identified in any of these studies, which makes it possible to use only the evidence from these studies to inform treatment of the local elbow problem. This lack of detail on organ disharmony may be simply a reporting problem; alternatively, to standardize treatment in these trials, perhaps only local problems were addressed.

A summary of the parameters used is still helpful because they inform the treatment of an elbow problem with acupuncture. All acupoints were treated unilaterally with between one and six needles, the most commonly used local points were LI 10, LI 11, and distal points TE 5, LI 4/LI 5[37-39] in the upper limb and GB 34 in the lower limb.[36,40] LU 5 and LI 12 and local Ashi points also were used.[37-39] Needles were inserted manually to a depth of 1.25 to 2.5 cm, for 20 to 25 minutes in all of the studies except for Molsberger and Hille,[36] who retained one

## Table 5-4    STRICTA Guidelines[35]

| STRICTA | MOLSBERGER & HILLE, 1994[36] | HAKER & LUNDEBERG, 1990[37] | DAVIDSON ET AL, 2001[38] | FINK ET AL, 2002[39] | TSUI AND LEUNG, 2002[40] |
|---|---|---|---|---|---|
| Client characteristics | N=48, details on age, gender not identified | N=82, aged 25-70 years, 52 males, 32 females | N=16, mean ± SD age=47.5 (8.4) years, 6 male, 10 female | N=45, mean age=52 years; gender distribution unclear | N=20, details on age, gender not identified |
| Time since injury | ≤2 months | Median (range)=9 (1-120 months) | Mean=6.16 months | Median=9 months | Not identified |
| Outcome | Verum acupuncture significantly reduced pain (11-point box scale) compared with sham acupuncture (55.8% vs. 15%) with an increased average duration of pain relief (20.2 hours vs. 1.4 hours). | Classical deep needling of acupuncture points was significantly more effective than superficial needling for reducing pain (5 point scale), increasing pain-free grip strength, and increasing the amount that the client could lift pain free. No differences were observed between the groups at 2-month follow up. | Acupuncture significantly more effective than ultrasound at reducing pain when change scores were used; no differences found when raw data were analyzed. Possible type II error. Power analysis using a retrospective power analysis showed that n=168 (90% power, alpha=0.05) required to show changes on VAS (100-mm scale) and pain-free grip. | Acupuncture significantly reduced pain, increased function and muscle strength at 2 weeks; at 2 months only function was still significantly better than sham acupuncture. Power analysis using a five-point difference on the subjective rating of pain (0-30 scale) at start of trial indicated that n=34 subjects required for 80% power at alpha level 0.05. | Significantly greater reduction in pain (VAS; 50% EA vs. 32% with MA) and pain-free grip with EA over MA in this small study: no power analysis; possible type II error |
| Style of acupuncture | TCM | TCM | TCM | TCM | TCM |
| Rationale for treatment (e.g., syndrome patterns, segmental levels, trigger points) and individualization if used | Nonsegmental | Segmental: prescriptive use of points commonly advocated for lateral elbow pain in TCM | Segmental: prescriptive use of points commonly advocated for lateral elbow pain in TCM | Segmental: prescriptive use of points commonly advocated for lateral elbow pain in TCM | Nonsegmental points |
| Literature sources to justify rationale | Three textbooks | One textbook | One textbook | One textbook | Molsberger & Hille, 1994[36] |
| Points used (unilateral/bilateral) | GB 34 Control: Pressure on UB 13 | LI 10, 11, 12, LU5, TE 5 (unilaterally) | LI 4, 10, 11, 12, TE 5 (unilaterally) | One Ashi pt, LI 5, 10, 11 Lu 5, TE 5 (unilaterally) | GB 34, ST 38 |
| Numbers of needles inserted/points activated. | 1 | 5 | 5 | 6 | 2 |
| Depths of insertion (e.g., cun or tissue level) | 2 cm | 1.25-2.5 cm into muscle | 1.25-2.5 cm | Into muscles | 2 cm |
| Responses elicited (e.g., de qi or twitch response) | De qi | De qi, every 5 min | De qi., every 5 min | De qi | De qi |

| | | | | | |
|---|---|---|---|---|---|
| Needle stimulation (e.g., manual or electrical) | Manual | Manual | Manual | Manual | Manual or low-frequency electroacupuncture (4 Hz) at tolerable pounding sensation |
| Needle retention time | 5 minutes | 20 minutes | 20 minutes | 25 minutes | 20 minutes |
| Needle type (gauge, length, and manufacturer)/material)/acupressure material | – | Seirin B-type No. 8, 0.3 mm×30 mm, Neu Isenberg, Germany Control: Seirin B-type No. 3, 0.2 mm×15 mm | Seirin disposable needles 0.23 mm×40 mm. | Seirin B-type, 0.25×40 mm, Neu Isenberg, Germany | Disposable needles 0.22 mm×25 mm |
| Number of treatment sessions | 1 | 10 | 8 | 10 | 6 |
| Frequency of treatment | | 2-3/week | 2-3/week | 2/week | 3/week |
| Other interventions (e.g., moxibustion, cupping, herbs, exercises, lifestyle advice) | Movement of arm during verum needling only | None | 3 repetitions of forearm stretches held for 10 seconds | None | General active flexion/extension exercises of the involved arm 50 times in 5 minutes |
| Duration of relevant training | Not specified but orthopedic doctor trained in Chinese acupuncture | Not specified but in Academy of Traditional Chinese Medicine, Beijing in 1985 | Not stated | Not stated | Not stated |
| Length of clinical experience | Not stated | 5 years in acupuncture | Not stated | Physician with a sound knowledge of TCM techniques | Not stated |
| Expertise in specific condition | Not stated | Not stated | Not stated | Not stated | Not stated |
| Intended effect of control intervention and its appropriateness to research question and, if appropriate, blinding of participants (e.g., active comparison, minimally active penetrating or nonpenetrating sham, inert) | To compare the verum effects of one acupuncture treatment to placebo effects using a nonpenetrating sham | To compare the effects of classical "deep" acupuncture to elicit de qi to superficial needle insertion with no sensation of de qi | Comparative trial of acupuncture with current standard treatment for this condition (i.e., ultrasound) | Controls for effects of correct point location. Comparable penetration at non acupoints | No separate control group; control data collected for n=14/20 2 weeks before treatment. Then a comparative trial of two methods of stimulating acupuncture needles was compared with these control data. |
| Explanations given to clients of treatment and control interventions, details of control intervention (precise description, as for item 2 above, and other items if different) | Clients in both groups given the same information, both told that they were getting acupuncture treatment | Comparing two different types of acupuncture technique | Clients naive to expected differences between the two forms of treatment | Not stated | Not stated |
| Sources that justify choice of control | Published research articles | Published research articles | Published research articles | Published research article | Published review |

Data extracted from published English language needle acupuncture trials only. The second through fourth rows of this table are not part of the STRICTA guidelines but were included for completeness of reporting.

| Table 5-5 | The Number of Hits for Each Electronic Database | | | | |
|---|---|---|---|---|---|
| DATABASES | AMED 1985-2004 | CAM ON PUBMED 1966-2004 | MEDLINE 1966-2004 | CINAHL 1982-2004 | EMBASE 1980-2004 |
| Acupuncture or laser | 6,506 | 10,636 | 73,935 | 3,898 | 69,435 |
| Tennis elbow or tendonitis or lateral elbow pain or epicondylitis or common extensor origin | 219 | 120 | 1067 | 319 | 964 |
| #1 and #2 | 45 | 45 | 48 | 23 | 66 |
| Limit to review | 1 | 19 | 11 | 2 | 19 |
| Relevant articles | 0 | 4 | 0 | 1 | 2 |

The databases were searched up to week 3 in August 2004. Reviews were mainly excluded because they were not systematic reviews, did not consider treatment of lateral elbow pain, or were short reviews of individual research trials.

needle for 5 minutes only, and all studies elicited de qi. The numbers of treatments ranged from one[36] to ten[37,39] and were given two to three times per week for 2 to 5 weeks.

The details on the training of the practitioners were reported poorly, although two were trained in TCM.[36,37] Overall the size of these studies was small, ranging from 16 to 82 subjects. Only two studies carried out a power analysis.[38,39]

None of the studies made the same treatment comparisons. For example, manual acupuncture was compared with nonpenetrating sham acupuncture[36] or superficial needling[37] or low-frequency EA[40] of the same points in three studies, or comparable penetration to nonacupoints[39] or standard treatment of the painful elbow (e.g., with ultrasound).[38] The larger trials showed that manual acupuncture was significantly more effective for the treatment of lateral elbow pain,[36,37,39] improvement of arm function,[37,39] and pain-free grip.[37]

The therapist in this chapter performs a literature search that involves five databases. If she were pressed for time she could generate a PICO question and search a single database such as MEDLINE.

## CLINICAL DECISION MAKING

Richard is typical of the clients described in the trials above. He is 58 years of age and male and has chronic elbow pain; thus the results of these studies are relevant to his case.

### Generate a Clinical Hypothesis

Having considered the evidence, the therapist feels that manual acupuncture will help to reduce this

---

### PICO BOX

For people with tennis elbow or lateral elbow pain, does the use of acupuncture decrease pain and swelling and improve organ harmony and function?

P: People with tennis elbow or lateral elbow pain
I: Acupuncture
O: Pain
O: Swelling or edema
O: "Organ harmony"
O: Function:
Combining all of the terms listed in the PICO (tennis elbow or lateral elbow pain, acupuncture, pain, swelling or edema, organ harmony and function) yielded zero references. She then performs the search with each outcome term separately. Pain and function yield 18 and 3 references, respectively. When she combines pain and function, three references are identified. This result is four references less than the one she identified using the more comprehensive approach.

P = **Population** (patient/client, problem, person condition or group attribute)
I = **Intervention** (the CAM therapy or approach)
C = **Comparison** (standard care or comparison intervention)
O = **Outcomes** (the measured variables of interest)

---

client's pain in the short term and increase the functional use of the arm in the longer term. The evidence does not support or refute the use of acupuncture to reduce swelling in lateral elbow pain. However, other evidence suggests that acupuncture can stimulate the autonomic nervous system, so it seems reasonable to hypothesize this effect.[21] No evidence supports the link between function of the large intestine and pain along the LI meridian or the accompanying organ disharmony of spleen, liver, and kidney. This was despite the fact that the majority of papers stated that clients were treated according to TCM.

## Examine

Based on this information the clinician hypothesizes that acupuncture will reduce the client's pain and promote return of function of the arm so that he can return to work more quickly. However, it is not possible to use the evidence to inform the other aspects of treatment (reduction of swelling and rebalancing of organ disharmony). Before the client begins acupuncture the therapist should conduct a reexamination of the client with standardized tools for outcome measurement. To find standardized outcome measures for TCM, diagnosis and reassessment (e.g., tongue and pulse diagnosis) are difficult. Therefore this next section concentrates mainly on measures used for changes in impairment and function of the local problems, which link with a Western medical model of client care. However, some suggestions are made for quality of life and individualized outcome measures, which are more consistent with the individualized and holistic concepts of TCM.

The Vigorimeter test is considered an excellent tool for evaluation of pain threshold when gripping and in appraising the progress of treatment in lateral elbow pain.[47] This paper also showed that the most frequent pain-provoking tests were palpation of the lateral epicondyle (99.7%), resisted wrist extension (86%), and the middle finger test (84%).[47] These could be measured on a numerical rating scale, which has been shown to be best for chronic pain clients.[48] In contrast to these lateral epicondyle-specific measures, Waugh et al advocated using the Disabilities of the Arm, Shoulder, and Hand (DASH) outcome measure because it has been evaluated more extensively and its validity was comparable with joint-specific measures.[49] The DASH is a 30-item questionnaire with five response options for each item. It is scored out of 100, with a higher score indicating a greater level of disability.[50] Finally, to measure quality of life the MYMOP questionnaire (Measure Yourself Medical Outcome Profile) could be used to measure changes in the client's perception of symptoms and well-being.[51] It is considered particularly suitable for measuring the effects of complementary therapies, because it takes a client-centered approach and may address the more holistic aspects of TCM. It has been vali-

dated and found to be more sensitive to change than the SF36,[51] and qualitative evaluation has led to minor amendments, such as the addition of a question about medication use.[52]

## Intervene

The therapist explains to the client that scientific evidence suggests that acupuncture will reduce his pain and improve the function of his right arm. In addition a wealth of anecdotal evidence exists that acupuncture can address organ disharmonies, as identified by the TCM diagnosis. However none of the retrieved literature reported on this aspect, although the majority stated that they used a TCM approach to treatment.

Based on the reviewed literature, a maximum of 10 sessions of treatment, two to three times per week, will be required to produce a local treatment effect, and approximately six needles will be used in each session (based on the data extracted from 5 RCTs using the STRICTA guidelines,[35] see Table 5-4). Needles will be inserted to a depth of between 1.25 and 2.5 cm (depending on the depth of the point) within the segment of pain. The majority of needles will be inserted directly into muscular tissue (LI 12, LI 11, LI 10, LI 4), whereas other needles will be inserted into the anatomical snuff box (LI 5) or close to tendons (LU 5, TE 5). The specific action and location of these points are described in Table 5-6. In addition, tender points found on palpation (Ashi points) could also be used.[37-39] The treatment protocol used will be reviewed after reassessment at each visit. Possibly more (or fewer) needles will be used, which will depend on the assessment and whether an improvement since the last treatment occurs.

Although the insertion of the needles during each treatment should be relatively painless, the therapist will manipulate the needles to produce a dull ache, numbness, or heaviness (de qi) in the forearm. This has been shown to improve the outcome of treatment in this condition.[37] All needles will be manually stimulated every 5 minutes by the therapist to stimulate de qi and retained for at least 25 minutes. A suggested optimum time for needle retention is 25 minutes because acupuncture analgesia will have been activated fully within the first 20 minutes.[25]

Before obtaining written informed consent the therapists should identify contraindications to treatment[53,54]; state that only disposable sterile needles will be used on each occasion[54]; and explain

**Table 5-6    Location and Action of the Points Used for Elbow Pain**

| ACUPUNCTURE POINTS | ANATOMICAL LOCATION | ACTION |
|---|---|---|
| LI 4 | On the dorsum of the hand between the first and second metacarpal bones, approximately in the middle of the second metacarpal on the radial side | Distal point for elbow pain |
| LI 5 | On the radial side of the wrist, in the anatomical snuff box between the tendons of extensor pollicis longus and brevis | Distal point for elbow pain |
| LI 10 | 2 cun distal from LI 11 in a line between LI 11 and LI 5 | Local point for elbow pain |
| LI 11 | When the elbow is flexed in the depression at the lateral end of the transverse cubital crease, midway between LU 5 and the lateral epicondyle of the humerus | Local point for elbow pain |
| LI 12 | When the elbow is flexed, 1 cun above LI 11, in a line between LI 11 and LI 15 | Local point for elbow pain |
| LU 5 | In the depression on the radial side of the tendon of biceps in the cubital crease | To resolve swelling and pain in elbow |
| TE 5 | 2 cun proximal to the dorsal crease of the wrist, on the line connecting TE 4 and the tip of the olecranon, between the radius and the ulna | Distal point for elbow pain |
| Ashi | Any tender point | Local points for elbow pain |
| **ORGAN DISHARMONY** | | |
| SP 6 | Meeting point of three yin meridians of the leg, 3 cun above the tip of the medial condyle of the ankle, behind the fibula | Strengthens spleen, resolves damp, promotes liver function and smooth flow of liver qi, tonifies the kidneys, nourishes blood and yin, benefits urination, stops pain, moves blood, and eliminates stasis |
| ST 36 | 3 cun below ST 35 | Tonifies qi and blood, regulates the intestines, expels wind and damp, benefits stomach and spleen |
| LIV 3 | 1 cun in a dip between the fourth and fifth metatarsals of the foot | Promotes smooth flow of qi, calms abdominal pain, moves local stagnation of qi and blood |
| KI 3 | Level with the tip of medial condyle of the ankle in a depression between the condyle and the Achilles tendon | Tonifies the kidneys in any deficiency pattern |

the possible side effects of acupuncture (e.g., bleeding, needling pain, and aggravation of symptoms) in the context that in skilled hands, it is one of the safer forms of medical intervention.[55] Clients always should be treated in a supine position on the first occasion, with a limited number of needles retained for a maximum of 20 minutes so that the client response can be evaluated. The therapist should be aware that clients who are anxious about acupuncture treatment may experience an increase in sympathetic activity, which can be heightened by the insertion of needles and may lead to fainting in extreme cases. Practitioners must identify their approved qualifications because a considerable range of standards and levels of training for acupuncture practitioners exists, depending on geographical location and national legal requirements. The issue of training is dealt with in more detail later in the chapter.

### Evaluate

In this case, the patient received 12 treatments, and his VAS score reduced from 8/10 to 2/10 during movement and he had no pain at rest. He regained full ROM of the elbow, and his swelling completely resolved. His DASH score reduced from 78 to 53, so that he still had some functional difficulties that related to reduced grip strength, which was being addressed by the use of a home exercise program. His MYMOP score changed from 4.6 to 1, and it was notable that there was a great improvement in his feeling of well-being. He demonstrated notable improvements in his IBS symptoms by treatment 4, which suggested that organ disharmonies had been addressed. At this stage he was referred back to mainstream physical therapy to finish addressing his grip strength problems to allow him to return to work.

## Report the Outcomes

Regardless of the client's outcome, the therapist considers writing a case report to describe how and why acupuncture was incorporated into the client's plan of care. In addition the therapist should reflect on whether the initial hypothesis, based on scientific evidence, was supported by the clinical outcome.

One of the key findings of this case study was that acupuncture can be used for pain relief and return of function in lateral elbow pain and is supported by a wealth of scientific evidence. The scientific evidence only partially supported the original plan of care, that is, the local channel problem and not the organ disharmonies. Moreover, the literature did not discuss the rationale for pain relief from a TCM perspective (e.g., clearing cold from the system in addition to promoting the flow of qi and blood to remove stagnation) but based on only the scientific evidence for acupuncture analgesia. The evidence for other effects in this case study was not reported in the retrieved literature and therefore should be highlighted. For example, the reduction in swelling, which in TCM is explained by the dispersal of damp along the meridian, could have been achieved through local antiinflammatory actions[16] and/or via activation of the autonomic nervous system.[18] Although it was not possible to hypothesize, from the research literature, that the client's IBS and bowel dysfunction would be affected by acupuncture treatment, interestingly the abdominal pain, cramps, and diarrhea did resolve quickly. Whether this was a combination of dietary advice and the effects of specific acupuncture points was unclear; however, the fact that acupuncture can influence the autonomic nervous

system would suggest that the function of internal organs may be affected. Further research is required to identify the links between meridians and organs/functions as defined in TCM and the autonomic effects of acupuncture. These results could be reported in the *Journal of the Acupuncture Association of Physiotherapy; Acupuncture in Medicine Journal* (published by the British Medical Acupuncture Society), or the *International Journal of Clinical Acupuncture.*

## REFERENCES

1. Kendall FP, Kendall-McCreary E, Provance P: *Muscles: testing and function,* ed 4, Philadelphia, 1993, Lippincott, Williams & Williams.
2. Maciocia G: *The foundations of Chinese medicine. A comprehensive text for acupuncturists and herbalists.* London, 1989, Churchill Livingstone, p 307.
3. Hopwood V: *Acupuncture in physiotherapy,* ed 1, Oxford, UK, 2004, Butterworth Heinemann, pp 34-35.
4. Ji X-P: Two cases of mechanical injury. *Int J Clin Acupunct* 6(3):295-7, 1995.
5. Xinnong C: *Chinese acupuncture and moxibustion,* ed 2, Beijing, China, 1999, Foreign Languages Press, p 270.
6. Gascoigne S: *The clinical medicine guide. A holistic perspective.* Clonakilty, Co. Cork Ireland, 2001, Jigme Press, p 245.
7. Kaptchuk TJ: *Chinese medicine. The web that has no weaver,* London, 1993, Rider, p 78.
8. Birch SJ, Felt RL: *Understanding acupuncture,* London, 1999, Churchill Livingstone.
9. Pomeranz B: Introduction. In Stux G, Berman B, Pomeranz B, editors: *Basics of acupuncture,* ed 5, Berlin, Germany, 2003, Springer-Verlag, pp 1-6.
10. Zollman C, Vickers A: ABC of complementary medicine. Users and practitioners of complementary medicine, *Br Med J* 319:836-8, 1999.
11. Cho ZH et al: Functional magnetic resonance imaging of the brain in the investigation of acupuncture. In Stux G, Hammerschlag R, editors: *Clinical acupuncture: scientific basis,* Berlin, 2001, Springer-Verlag, pp 83-95.
12. Filshie J, Cummings TM: Western medical acupuncture. In Ernst E, White A, editors: *Acupuncture: a scientific appraisal,* Oxford, UK, 1999, Butterworth Heinemann, pp 31-59.
13. White A: Neurophysiology of acupuncture analgesia. In Ernst E, White A, editors: *Acupuncture: a scientific appraisal,* Oxford, 1999, Butterworth Heinemann, pp 60-92.
14. Lundeberg T, Stener-Victorin: Is there a physiological basis for the use of acupuncture in pain? In Sato A, Li P, Campbell J, editors: *Acupuncture—is there a*

*physiological basis?* Amsterdam, 2002, Elsevier, pp 3-10.

15. Stener-Victorin E et al: Alternative treatments in reproductive medicine: much ado about nothing, *Hum Reprod* 17(8):1942-6, 2002.

16. Pomeranz B, Berman B: Scientific basis of acupuncture. In Stux G, Berman B, Pomeranz B, editors: *Basics of acupuncture*, ed 5, Berlin, 2003, Springer-Verlag, pp 7-55.

17. Walsh DM: Pain and its modulation. In *TENS: clinical application and related theory*. London, 1997, Churchill Livingstone, pp 11-23.

18. Cho ZH, Wong EK, Fallon J: *Neuroacupuncture. Scientific evidence of acupuncture revealed*. Los Angeles, California, 2001, Q-puncture, Inc.; 2001, p 72.

19. Galea MP: Neuroanatamy of the nociceptive system. In Strong J, Unruh A, Wright A, Baxter GD, editors: *Pain: a textbook for physiotherapists*, London, 2001, Churchill Livingstone, pp 13-41.

20. Wright A: Neurophysiology of pain and pain modulation. In Strong J, Unruh A, Wright A, Baxter GD, editors: *Pain: a textbook for physiotherapists*, London, 2001, Churchill Livingstone, pp 207-225.

21. Andersson S, Lundeberg T: Acupuncture—from empiricism to science: functional background to acupuncture effects in pain and disease, *Med Hypotheses* 45:271-81, 1995.

22. Melzack R, Wall P: Pain mechanisms: a new theory, *Science* 150:971-9, 1965.

23. Hashimoto T, Aikawa S: Needling effects on nociceptive neurons in rat spinal cord. *Proceedings of the 7th World Congress on Pain IASP*. Seattle, 1993, p 428.

24. Ignelzi RJ, Nyquist JK: Direct effect of electrical stimulation on peripheral nerve evoked activity: Implications in pain relief, *J Neurosurg* 45:159-65, 1976.

25. Pomeranz B, Cheng R: Suppression of noxious responses in single neurons of cat spinal cord by electroacupuncture and its reversal by the opiate antagonist naloxone, *Exp Neurol* 64(2):327-41, 1979.

26. Baxter D, Barlas P: Electrophysical agents in pain management. In Strong J, Unruh A, Wright A, Baxter GD, editors: *Pain: a textbook for physiotherapists*, London, 2001, Churchill Livingstone, pp 207-25.

27. Han J-S: Acupuncture: neuropeptide release produced by electrical stimulation of different frequencies, *Trends Neurosci* 26:17-22, 2003.

28. Sluka K et al: Low frequency TENS is less effective than high frequency TENS at reducing inflammation-induced hyperalgesia in morphine-tolerant rats, *Eur J Pain* 4:185-93, 2000.

29. Ezzo J et al: Is acupuncture effective for the treatment of chronic pain: a systematic review? *Pain* 86(3):217-25, 2000.

30. Smidt N et al: Effectiveness of physiotherapy for lateral epicondylitis: a systematic review, *Ann Med* 35:51-62, 2003.

31. Green S et al: Acupuncture for lateral elbow pain, *Cochrane Database Syst Rev*, 3, 2004.

32. Assendelft W et al: Tennis elbow, *Clin Evid* 11:1633-44, 2004.

33. Trinh KV et al: Acupuncture for the alleviation of lateral epicondyle pain: a systematic review. *Rheumatology (Oxford)*. Jun 22, 2004. Available at: *http://rheumatology.oupjournals.org/cgi/reprint/keh247v1*. Accessed July 22, 2004.

34. Trudel D et al: Rehabilitation for clients with lateral epicondylitis: a systematic review, *J Hand Ther* 17: 243-66, 2004.

35. MacPherson H et al: Standards for reporting interventions in controlled trials of acupuncture: The STRICTA recommendations, *Acupunct Med* 20(1):22-5, 2002.

36. Molsberger A, Hille E: The analgesic effect of acupuncture in chronic tennis elbow pain, *Br J Rheumatol* 33:1162-5, 1994.

37. Haker E, Lundeberg T: Acupuncture treatment in epicondylalgia: a comparative study of two acupuncture techniques, *Clin J Pain* 6:221-6, 1990.

38. Davidson JH et al: The effect of acupuncture versus ultrasound on pain level, grip strength and disability in individuals with lateral epicondylitis: a pilot study. *Physiother Can* 53:195-202, 2001.

39. Fink M et al: Acupuncture in chronic epicondylitis: a randomized controlled trial, *Rheumatology* 41:205-9, 2002.

40. Tsui P, Leung MCP: Comparison of the effectiveness between manual acupuncture and electroacupuncture on clients with tennis elbow, *Acupunct Electrother Res* 27:107–17, 2002.

41. Fink M: Chronic epicondylitis: effects of real and sham acupuncture treatment: a randomised controlled client- and examiner-blinded long-term trial, *Forsch Komplementarmed Klass Naturheilkd* 9:210-5, 2002.

42. Grua D et al: L'agopunturanel trattamento dell'epicondilite laterale: valutazione dell'efficaciae confronto con ultrasuonoterapia. [Acupuncture in the treatment of lateral epicondylitis: evaluation of the effectiveness and comparison with ultrasound therapy], *G Ital Riflessot Agopunt* 11:63-9, 1999.

43. Center for Evidence Based Medicine: Levels of evidence and grades for recommendation. Available at: *http://www.cebm.net/levels_of_evidence.asp*. Accessed September 26, 2004.

44. Begg CB et al: Improving the quality of reporting of randomized controlled trials: the CONSORT statement, *JAMA* 276:637-9, 1996.

45. Wang Y: Acupuncture and injection for the treatment of tennis elbow: 30 cases, *Shanghai Acupunct J* 16:20, 1997.

46. Haker E, Lundeberg T: Laser treatment applied to acupuncture points in lateral humeral epicondylagia. A double blind study, *Pain* 40:243-7, 1990.

47. Haker E: Lateral epicondylagia. *A diagnostic and therapeutic challenge*, PhD thesis, Stockholm, Sweden, 1991, Karolinska Institute.

48. Jensen MP, Karoly P, Braver S: The measurement of clinical pain intensity: a comparison of six methods, *Pain* 27:117-26, 1986.

49. Waugh EJ et al: Factors associated with the prognosis of lateral epicondylitis after 8 weeks of physical therapy, *Arch Phys Med Rehabil* 88:308-18, 2004.

50. Beaton DE et al: Measuring the whole or parts? Validity, reliability and responsiveness of the disabilities of the arm, shoulder and hand outcome measure in different regions of the upper extremity, *J Hand Ther* 14:128-42, 2001.

51. Paterson C: Measuring outcomes in primary care: a client generated measure, MYMOP, compared to the SF36 health survey, *Br Med J* 312(7037):1016-20, 1996.

52. Paterson C, Britten N: In pursuit of patient-centered outcomes: a qualitative evaluation of the "Measure Yourself Outcome Profile," *J Health Serv Res Policy* 5(1):27-36, 2000.

53. Hopwood V: Safe practice, needle techniques and types of needles. In Hopwood V, Lovesey M, Mokone S, editors: *Acupuncture and related techniques in physical therapy,* London, 1997, Churchill Livingstone, pp 61-8.

54. WHO: Guidelines on basic training and safety in acupuncture 1999. Available at: *http://www.who.int/medicines/library/trm/acupuncture/who-edm-trm-99-1/who-edm-trm-99-1en.shtml.* Accessed April 1, 2004.

55. White A, Hayhoe S, Hart A, Ernst E: Survey of adverse events following acupuncture (SAFA): a prospective study of 32,000 consultations. *Acupunct Med* 19(2):84, 2001.

56. Dawson V: Membership director's report, *J Acupunct Assoc Physiother,* July 2004, p 9.

57. Chartered Society of Physiotherapy's guide to physiotherapy and complementary health. Available at: *http://www.csp.org.uk/physiotherapy/complementary.cfm.* Accessed August 4, 2004.

58. Acupuncture Association of Chartered Physiotherapists. Available at: *http://www.aacp.uk.com/.* Accessed August 4, 2004.

59. National Center for Complementary and Alternative Medicine: Research report on acupuncture, 2002. Available at: *http://nccam.nih.gov/health/acupuncture/.* Accessed July 22, 2004.

60. White House Commission on Complementary and Alternative Medicine Policy: Interim progress report: White House Commission on Complementary and Alternative Medicine Policy. Washington, DC, 2001, The Commission.

## ADDITIONAL RESOURCES

Accreditation Commission for Acupuncture and Oriental Medicine (ACAOM): *http://www.acaom.org/*

International Acupuncture Association of Physical Therapists IAAPT: *http://wcpt.org/subgroups/wcptsubgroups/iaapt/index.php*

# APPENDIX 1

# Education, Training, and Regulation of Acupuncture within the Physical Therapy Profession

The World Health Organization (WHO) published guidelines on basic acupuncture training and safety in 1999.[54] These guidelines cover the basic requirements for training physicians, non-physician acupuncturists, and other health personnel and include a core syllabus to assist national health authorities in setting standards and establishing official examinations. The guidelines address four categories of personnel (Table 5-7).

Acupuncturists who do not have a background in conventional health care train for 3 to 4 years full time as recommended by WHO.[54] Medical physicians and other health professionals who wish to practice acupuncture from a TCM perspective require fewer hours of training if they want to incorporate acupuncture as an adjunctive treatment into their clinical practice because they already have conventional medical training.

These guidelines make no specific statement with respect to the training requirements for physical therapists, and as stated in the introduction of this chapter this varies from country to country. An overview of those guidelines follows.

## International

The International Association of Acupuncture in Physical Therapy (IAAPT) is a subgroup of the World Congress of Physical Therapy (WCPT). The IAAPT aims to promote standards of safe acupuncture practice and sharing of information on education, training, and research between individual and group members. Currently in eight core member countries (United Kingdom, New Zealand, Sweden, Argentina, Ireland, Hong Kong, Australia, and Canada) acupuncture is considered within the scope of practice for physiotherapists. Until recently no agreed minimum training requirement existed between these countries; however, in 2003 a minimum of 80 hours of training for physiotherapists was decided by consensus at a meeting of the IAAPT at the World Congress of Physical

Therapy in Spain. This level of training aims to ensure that physical therapists can use acupuncture to treat painful conditions in a safe and effective manner. This practice should be supported by the scientific evidence underpinning the mechanisms of action of acupuncture, especially AA, and the clinical evidence of its effectiveness in certain conditions.

## United Kingdom

Physiotherapists are one of the key groups of statutory health professionals, alongside medical doctors, for whom acupuncture has become a core skill for the management of painful conditions. As such it is taught at undergraduate and postgraduate levels. In the United Kingdom more than 2800 physical therapists practice acupuncture but rarely specialize in it. Rather the majority offer treatment for musculoskeletal and other painful conditions within the National Health Service (NHS) or private practice.[56] Currently four universities provide acupuncture for pain relief as an optional module at the physiotherapy undergraduate level (Birmingham, Coventry, Nottingham, and Southampton). Coventry University, Keele University, and the University of Ulster all provide graduate-level acupuncture training for qualified physiotherapists. The Acupuncture Association of Chartered Physiotherapists (AACP) approves these courses, and many others, which take place outside the university sector. The AACP is a special interest group, recognized and accredited by the Chartered Society of Physiotherapy, and plays an important role in monitoring training and maintaining standards of acupuncture practice by physiotherapists.[57,58]

Members of the CSP can become members of the AACP once they have gained an approved level of acupuncture training. Currently two levels of membership exist: accredited and advanced. Accredited membership requires 80 hours of cer-

| Table 5-7 | Basic Training in Acupuncture[50] | |
|---|---|---|
| CATEGORY OF PERSONNEL | LEVEL OF TRAINING | HOURS OF TRAINING |
| Licensed acupuncturists | Full course of training | 2500 |
| Qualified physicians | Full course of training | 1500 |
| Qualified physicians | Limited training in acupuncture as a technique in their clinical work | Not less than 200 hours |
| Other health personnel | Limited training in acupuncture for use in primary health care | Varies according to application |

tificated training, whereas advanced membership requires more than 200 hours of training, evidenced by an acupuncture portfolio. To maintain membership in the AACP, evidence of 10 hours continuing professional development (CPD) is required every 2 years. Currently the AACP has 2813 members, either working in the National Health Service (NHS) or in private practice.[56] Indeed they are the largest group of health professionals providing acupuncture for pain relief within the NHS. All members of the AACP are approved to provide acupuncture for pain relief, although advanced members may use acupuncture in a broader remit because many of them are TCM trained. The AACP is affiliated with the British Medical Acupuncture Association (BMAS), which also promotes the use of acupuncture as a therapy after orthodox medical diagnosis.

### United States

According to the American Physical Therapy Association (APTA) acupuncture is not within the scope of practice for physical therapists and is not in the *Guide to Physical Therapist Practice*, developed by the APTA. However, acupuncture increasingly is being used to complement conventional therapies in the United States, but mostly by medical doctors in conventional health care.[59] This may be explained by the fact that in some states medical doctors do not require any additional training to use acupuncture in their practice. About 40 states have established training standards for acupuncture certification, but states have varied requirements for obtaining a license to practice acupuncture.[60] To practice acupuncture, physical therapists would need to contact each state agency responsible for acupuncture licensing to establish the training

requirements. Most states that license acupuncture or TCM practitioners use standards set by the Accreditation Commission for Acupuncture and Oriental Medicine (ACAOM). The ACAOM, the only national accrediting agency recognized by the U.S. Department of Education, accredits professional programs in the acupuncture and Oriental medicine professions.

### SUMMARY

In this chapter the case of a 58-year-old male who initially presented to physiotherapy with severe right lateral elbow pain is presented. A therapist uses both a physical therapy and TCM approach to expand examination and intervention and identifies the local (channel) problem and organ disharmony of three yin organs (spleen, kidney, and liver), which have affected the balance of yin and yang and Richard's overall health. Only the highest quality scientific literature on acupuncture, as it related to this case, was reviewed and evaluated. This highlighted the difficulty in identifying scientific evidence that is methodologically rigorous and clinically relevant to a client who is being treated with a TCM approach to acupuncture.

The therapist determined that strong evidence supports the use of acupuncture for the local channel problem (based on acupuncture analgesia). However, no evidence supports or refutes the use of acupuncture to address swelling or organ disharmony. The use of acupuncture may be supported for these latter symptoms based on the known analgesic and autonomic nervous system effects of acupuncture. The therapist, who is from the United Kingdom, applies the acupuncture treatment herself based on a TCM approach (and in the chapter explains the regulation of acupuncture in the United States and the United Kingdom). The client has decreases in pain and return to function, which are comparable with those reported in the cited literature in this chapter. Changes in gastrointestinal function related to the relevant acupuncture points and a decrease in swelling also resulted, which are not reported in the literature. The therapist proposes to report her findings as a case study.

# CHAPTER 6

## Arnica

### Lori Zucker

---

## CASE

Samantha is a 48-year-old interior decorator. She is the mother of two teenage children. Samantha fell at home on a marble floor, badly spraining her ankle and bruising her elbow. She was discharged from the emergency room with negative x-rays, a pair of crutches to be used as needed, and scripts for pain and antiinflammatory medications.

### ■ Initial Examination

***Past Medical History:*** Samantha's medical history includes a bout of mononucleosis in her late teens, colitis, anaphylactic shock secondary to antiinflammatory medications, and severe abuse during childhood.

***Client Report:*** Client complains of pain (5/10) in her right ankle radiating into her foot and up her leg. She also complains of pain (6/10) in her right upper extremity primarily around her elbow. She reports that she is limited in most of her household, social, and work-related activities since the slip and fall. She is also limited in her yoga practice.

***Client Goals:*** (1) Decrease muscle pain and soreness; (2) Walk pain free without an assistive device; (3) Decrease swelling; (4) Return to work; (5) Pain-free use of her right arm; (6) Return to her active yoga practice

***Employment:*** As an interior decorator, Samantha makes her own schedule with her clients, which allows her to be available to her two teenage children. Work-related activities require her to drive, walk around clients' homes and showrooms, and carry or move moderately heavy furniture. She also has several hours of paperwork, primarily on the computer, related to her business or her household finances.

***Recreational Activities:*** Samantha enjoys yoga, painting, knitting, reading, and visiting museums.

***General Health:*** Samantha reports that she has been generally healthy much of her adult life. Her history of abuse includes use of electrical impulses. As such, therapeutic electrical stimulation is not an available treatment option. Client is reluctant to try ultrasound, although she may be willing to try it if absolutely necessary.

***Medications:*** Antidepressants, vitamins

***Musculoskeletal:*** Strength in the right upper extremity is limited by client's complaints of pain. Client is able to move against gravity at all joints, but added resistance is not indicated at this time.

***Neuromuscular:*** Posture is unremarkable. Strength in the left upper extremity is WNL throughout.

| LOWER EXTREMITY | ROM MEASUREMENTS |
| --- | --- |
| Dorsiflexion | Limited to neutral secondary to pain |
| Eversion | Not measured secondary to pain |
| Inversion | Not measured secondary to pain |
| Plantar flexion | +20 degrees with complaints of pain |
| Knee flexion/extension | WNL |
| Hip mobility | WNL |
| Upper extremity | ROM measurements |
| Elbow flexion | 0-100 degrees |
| Elbow extension | −15 degrees, painful and limited at end range |
| Shoulder mobility | WFL throughout |
| Wrist mobility | WFL throughout |

*WNL*, Within normal limits; *WFL*, within functional limits; *ROM*, range of motion.

**Palpation:** Client has right upper quarter muscle spasms, swelling around the elbow, and soreness of the forearm musculature. Palpation around the right ankle elicits a painful reaction.

**Function:** Client is ambulating with a single crutch for partial weight bearing on the right ankle. Bilateral crutches may have been more appropriate given the severity of the sprain, but the client's right elbow bruise precludes her from bearing weight through the right arm. Client is limited in household ADL and many of her work-related and recreational activities.

## Plan of Care

The initial plan was for the client to receive physical therapy three times a week for 3 weeks. At home, the client was advised to rest, ice her ankle and elbow, use a light compressive garment, and elevate her leg. In the clinic, interventions included the following:

1. Active and active assistive range of motion at the ankle and elbow
2. Gentle soft tissue mobilization of the right foot, ankle, lower leg, and arm to decrease swelling and muscle soreness
3. Gait training to facilitate proper heel-toe pattern
4. Balance training
5. Light resistive exercises when tolerated by the client. Client taught home exercises as appropriate at each physical therapy visit

## Incorporating CAM into the Plan of Care

The client has inquired about the use of arnica to decrease muscle soreness. The therapist reviews the literature to decide if arnica should be included in the plan of care.

This case is used to illustrate the clinical decision-making process of whether to include a homeopathic remedy in the plan of care. The client's goal is to "get back to normal." During the initial physical therapy visit, the client inquires if arnica may help with management of her muscle soreness. The client explains that she is exploring the use of homeopathic remedies given her past medical history of colitis and anaphylactic shock after a dose of antiinflammatory medication. The therapist will make recommendations after examination of the client and a review of the evidence to support the use of arnica for this particular client.

## INVESTIGATING THE LITERATURE

To respond to the client's inquiry about homeopathic arnica, the therapist needs to become more familiar with the practice of homeopathic medicine and the specific literature on arnica for relief of

muscle soreness. While the use of arnica is being investigated, the client's treatment would remain the same. The therapist may not always have time to do such an extensive search. Instead she may use a targeted PICO approach.

### Preliminary Reading

The therapist uses a resource available on the Internet and two books[2,3] to gain some general knowledge about homeopathy. She then reads about arnica.

#### Homeopathy

The word *homeopathy*, derived from the Greek words *homoios*, meaning "like" or "similar," and *pathos*, meaning "suffering," was first used by Dr. Samuel Hahnemann in 1796 to explain his idea of "letting likes be treated with likes."[1] Hahnemann, the founder of homeopathic medicine, was trained as an allopathic physician in Europe in the late 1700s. His experiences led him to believe that treating illness by trying to suppress symptoms was not the optimal approach. He began to believe that if a specific substance caused illness in a person, that same substance given in extremely dilute preparations could effect a cure. Hahnemann called this concept the *Law of Similars*. He began to explore these specific substances through a process called *provings*.[2] Provings followed a systematic administration of a given substance to healthy individuals. During the proving period, all signs and symptoms, including changes in temperature, intellectual acuity, alertness, body irritation, pain, and emotional state, were recorded daily. Hahnemann then organized the information in order of importance.[1] In 1810 Hahnemann published *The Organon*, a reference book that described his beliefs in the Law of Similars and identified many of the homeopathic remedies still used today.[3]

The American Institute of Homeopathy was founded in 1844 and by the turn of the century, the United States had approximately 22 homeopathic medical schools and 15,000 practitioners. American interest in homeopathy dwindled through the early 1900s so much that the last homeopathic hospital closed in 1938, although the practice continued to thrive in European countries.[2] Today, clinicians interested in becoming homeopathic physicians are trained in schools of homeopathy outside the traditional medical establishment.

Approximately 3000 documented remedies exist in the homeopathic literature. They are derived from plants, minerals, animals, and pathogenic substances. Today, remedies are made much as they were in Hahnemann's time. A mother tincture is prepared by maceration of the fresh substance in alcohol. This suspension is aged for a defined period of time before the suspension is filtered by compression, which yields a concentrated "mother tincture." The mother tincture then is used to make remedies in various potencies. Common potencies available to the public are 6×, 6C, 30C, and 200C.[2] To make a 6C preparation, one drop of the mother tincture would be diluted into 100 drops of solvent. Then one drop of the new solution would be further diluted into 100 drops of solvent. This procedure would occur six times to produce a 6C remedy or 30 times to make a 30C remedy. In homeopathy, the most dilute remedies are considered the most potent. Thus a 6× dosage, which actually has the most of the original "mother tincture," is considered less potent than the more dilute 200C preparation.[4]

The practice of homeopathy relies heavily on individual treatment of symptoms and dosing according to individual needs. Unlike an allopathic approach, which may vary dosages of a particular medicine by weight or age, dosages of homeopathic remedies most often are determined through an interview. During the interview process, the practitioner evaluates many different factors, including physical concerns, emotional or psychological concerns, dietary and sleeping patterns, and habits.[2] Table 6-1 provides a brief summary of homeopathic remedies, their sources, and their uses.[3]

### Table 6-1    Summary of Homeopathic Remedies

| HOMEOPATHIC REMEDY | SOURCE | USE |
| --- | --- | --- |
| Arsenicum album | Arsenopyrite | Digestive disorders, deep-seated insecurity |
| Calcium carbonicum | Oyster shell | Joint and bone pain, body odor |
| Ignatia | St. Ignatius beans | Bereavement, insomnia, acute grief |
| Phosphorus | Phosphorus | Circulation problems, excessive bleeding, anxiety and fear |
| Pulsatilla | Meadow anemone | Runny nose, loose cough, greenish/yellow phlegm, depression |
| Sepia | Cuttlefish | Gynecological problems, PMS, menopausal symptoms |
| Nux vomica | Poison nut, Quaker buttons | Overindulgence in foods, alcohol, coffee |
| *Rhus toxicodendron* | Poison ivy or poison oak | Skin complaints with burning, itchy, red, or swollen scaly skin (shingles, chicken pox), also used for osteoarthritis, musculoskeletal problems, and sciatica |
| *Ruta graveolens* | Herb-of-grace or rue | Periosteal bruising and deep achy pain of rheumatism, tendon injuries, sciatica, and eye strain |
| Magnesium phosphorus | Magnesium phosphate | Neuralgic pain, constricting feeling, headaches, toothaches, and colic |

In the United States, the FDA regulates the production of all homeopathic remedies. Given that the remedies contain infinitesimal amounts of active ingredient, the FDA considers them safe and without risk of side effects or toxicity. Many substances used to make homeopathic remedies also are used in herbal preparations. Herbal medicines are not FDA regulated at this time, and although they bear similar names to those of the homeopathic remedies, an herbal preparation may have side effects and may cause toxicity.

## Arnica

*Arnica montana*, a yellow flowering plant found native to northwest America, Mexico, Siberia, and parts of Europe, is also known as *leopard's bane, mountain tobacco*, or *wolfsbane* (Figure 6-1). The use of arnica as a healing herb first was recognized in the sixteenth century.[3] Hahnemann published his findings of arnica in 1805 through the process of proving as mentioned above. It has been used as a homeopathic remedy since that time. For homeopathic purposes, it is used primarily to treat the inflammation caused by muscle injuries such as sprains, strains, and blunt trauma.

The Commission E, Germany's regulatory agency for herbs, has approved herbal arnica only for topical use because it can be toxic if ingested orally. The FDA considers homeopathic arnica safe for oral and topical use.[5,6]

Arnica can be purchased over the counter in pill or cream form in most health food stores, pharmacies, and specialty grocery stores, and over the Internet. A typical 30C vial of arnica purchased in a health food store costs approximately $6.00 (Figure 6-2). An arnica gel or ointment costs approximately $10.00.

### Searching the Databases

Once a basic understanding of homeopathy, remedies, and arnica has been established, the therapist must look at the specific literature to evaluate the use of arnica for muscle soreness. Several important databases must be included in a search of the lit-

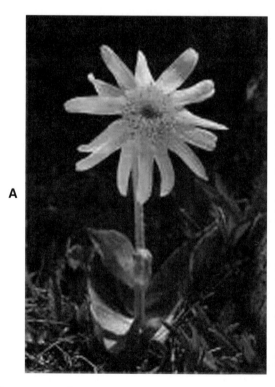
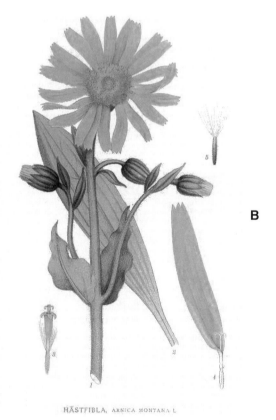

HÄSTFIBLA, ARNICA MONTANA L.

**Figure 6-1** Arnica flower. (From *http://www.herbmed.org/Herbs/Herb92.htm* and *http://caliban.mpizkoeln.mpg.de/~stueber/lindman/22.jpg.*)

erature for homeopathic studies. PubMed and MEDLINE are often the first databases searched because they are the most traditional places to find critical literature on medical issues. The Cochrane database of reviews ensures that the therapist will find meta-analyses or systematic reviews if they exist on a specific subject. For CAM-related issues, CINAHL is often another good database to search because it includes journals that do not appear in

MEDLINE searches. Specifically for homeopathy, it is important to search the British Homeopathic Library database. The British Homeopathic Library has an extensive database of international journals reporting or tracking the practice of homeopathy (Box 6-1). This database is available through the Internet. It is housed at Glasgow Homeopathic Hospital and often is referred to as the *Glasgow Homeopathic Library.*

Using a search term of *arnica* alone gleans articles on the herbal use of arnica, the botanical properties of arnica, and many references that do not help the therapist assess the client's request to use arnica to relieve muscle soreness. Combining the search terms to *arnica* and *pain* and *arnica* and *muscle soreness* narrows the literature search to more appropriate references. Search results are summarized in Table 6-2.

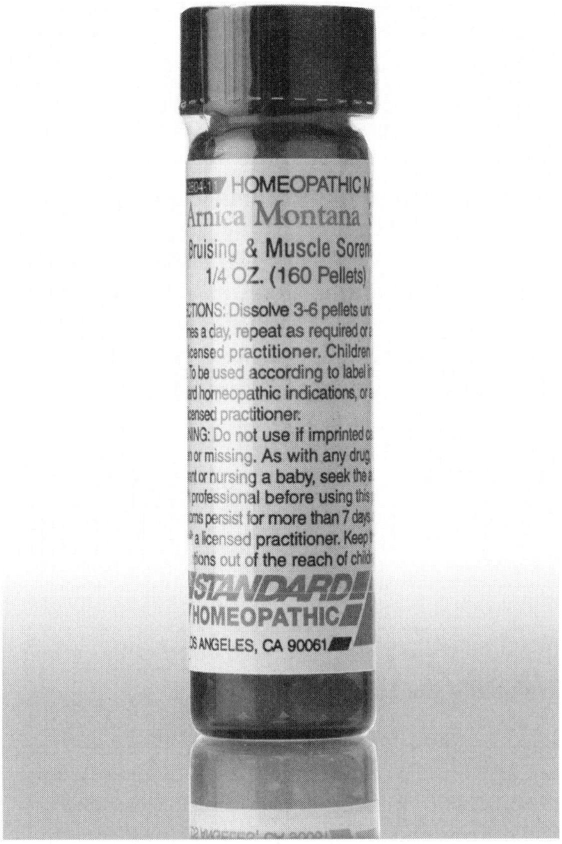

**Figure 6-2** Arnica vial. Copyright 2007, Standard Homeopathic Company/Hyland's, Inc.

---

**Box 6-1    Home Page of British Homeopathic Library**

The British Homeopathic Library is a library and information service dedicated to the research and practice of homeopathy.

They supply comprehensive library services, including the following:

- A database of more than 25,000 article and book references on homeopathy, **free** to search from this website (*http:hominform.soutron.com*).
- Hom-Inform, an individualized search and query service available to anyone and a document supply service available to members only.
- Borrowing access to our substantial collection of books and audiotapes, to Members and Associates of the Faculty of Homeopathy and to Affiliate Members of the library.

The British Homeopathic Library is affiliated with Ad Hom, the Academic Departments of Homeopathy at Glasgow Homeopathic Hospital. Their website address is *http://www.adhom.com.*

---

**Table 6-2    Literature Search Results**

|  | PUBMED | MEDLINE | CINAHL | COCHRANE EBM REVIEWS | GLASGOW HOMEOPATHIC LIBRARY |
|---|---|---|---|---|---|
| Arnica | 169 | 67 | 7 | 10 | 114 |
| Arnica and pain | 14 | 14 | 14 | 13 | 0 |
| Arnica and muscles | 4 | 2 | 1 | 2 | 0 |

Based on the hierarchy of evidence, meta-analyses are considered to be at the top. Thus the most expedient place to look first would be at the Cochrane reviews for any meta-analyses on homeopathy and arnica. *The Lancet* published a 1997 meta-analysis specifically looking at 89 placebo-controlled clinical trials of homeopathy.[7] The pooled data across these trials favored homeopathy over placebos, but the results were not specific to any one remedy. The therapist now has some information that homeopathy may be a more useful tool than just a placebo, and it is time to focus on arnica literature.

The most commonly cited review of arnica is that of Ernst and Pittler published in the Archives of Surgery.[8] This systematic review identified that arnica was used for postoperative ileus, after dental work, after acute stroke, and for symptoms of delayed onset muscle soreness. The authors conclude that arnica is no better than a placebo and that the efficacy of arnica use is in doubt. This review, however, only peripherally addresses the concerns of the client because it includes studies of arnica use in many different situations. The therapist could not necessarily make a clinical recommendation regarding arnica use for muscle soreness based on Ernst and Pittler's systematic review. As such, the therapist would look toward individual clinical trials that more closely resemble the client's concerns.

The database searches identify five articles that deal more specifically with muscle soreness. Three articles evaluate the use of arnica to relieve muscle soreness after running and two articles evaluate the use of arnica to relieve the pain of delayed onset muscle soreness after a stepping protocol.[9-13] The therapist may decide that muscle soreness after running is more similar to the client's complaints of muscle soreness after crutch walking and choose to review those three articles.

Tveiten's randomized, double-blind, placebo-controlled trial was done on a relatively small sample size of only 46 experienced marathon runners.[10] The placebo group included 22 runners and the arnica group 24 runners. A dosage of arnica 30C was used twice a day for 5 days and visual analog scales were used to assess muscle soreness on those days in the morning and evening. Tveiten reported a significant 10% difference between the arnica and placebo group's mean visual analog scale (VAS) score for muscle soreness immediately after running a marathon. Tveiten also reported that the arnica group ran the marathon 9 minutes faster than the placebo group. This result was not statistically significant but it is potentially clinically meaningful particularly when combined with the finding that the arnica group reported less soreness immediately after running the marathon.

Vickers' randomized, double-blind, placebo-controlled trial used the same dosages of arnica in a much larger study of runners.[11] This study had a sample size of 400 runners: 200 in the arnica group and 200 in the placebo group. Rather than look only at marathon runners, Vickers chose to look at people running in races varying from 1-mile fun runs to full marathons. Volunteers for the study anticipated being sore after running. The only significant finding in this study was a change in VAS score 2 days after running. Interestingly, the placebo group demonstrated a lower score than the arnica group.

The third study of this group evaluated muscle soreness in novice runners after a 3.5-mile race.[9] Out of 141 runners total, 44 subjects in an arnica group used a 1× arnica ointment, 46 subjects in an arnica group used a 6C arnica ointment, and 51 used a placebo. Schmidt used only descriptive data of median, mode, and percent variability on a 10-point scale of muscle soreness. The data suggest that both groups who used arnica ointments had less muscle soreness than the group using a placebo ointment. Schmidt's trial, although seemingly positive for the use of arnica, is the least rigorous in study design of the three chosen.

## Evaluating the Literature

Making a decision whether to support the client's use of arnica for muscle soreness is the next step in the process. The therapist is now more educated on the history and philosophy behind homeopathic medicine. On a more global approach, a study supports the idea that homeopathy is not just a placebo effect but a generalized systematic review does not support the efficacy of arnica.[7,8] A review of the specific trials of arnica for muscle soreness after running provides only mixed results. The most positive trial is the least rigorous.[9] The trial that has some meaningful results that may be applicable to the client has a small sample size.[10] And the most rigorous of the three trials does not support the use of arnica to reduce muscle soreness after running, but the length of the races varies dramatically.[11] The therapist decides that given the state of the literature at this point in time, it is not possible to provide the client with a definitive answer.

In the absence of time the therapist may opt to do a PICO-based search and read the articles exclusively targeted for her case. The PICO approach is summarized in the PICO Box.

---

### PICO BOX

For persons with ankle sprains or muscle soreness, does the use of arnica decrease pain and swelling?

P: Persons with ankle sprains
P: Persons with muscle soreness
I: Arnica
C: Comparison (none)
O: Pain
O: Inflammation

A search of MEDLINE from 1966 forward using the terms *ankle sprain* (injuries), *arnica, pain,* and *inflammation* does not yield any references. A search of the same database using *muscle soreness, arnica,* and *pain* yielded two references that the therapist already had found.[10,11] Findings from these two citations showed conflicting support for the use of arnica for muscle soreness (induced by marathon running). The therapist then chose to look at the terms separately. Using this approach she found references for arnica and inflammation that dealt with cellular[14] and animal preclinical work,[15] arnica and musculoskeletal pain reduction that was osteoarthritis (OA) of the knee,[16] postsurgical carpal tunnel pain,[17] and arnica used preventively to decrease pain and bruising associated with hand surgery.[18] Findings were conflicting, supportive for arnica for the OA and carpal tunnel study but not for the prevention of surgical pain and inflammation.

For a topic such as arnica it may be necessary to search more than one database to get useful information. The therapist chooses CINAHL to repeat her PICO search using the terms *muscle soreness, arnica,* and *pain* and finds 11 citations, three of which she identified in her original search.[10,12,13] Additional articles were not supportive of arnica on exercise-induced arnica[19] or amelioration of soft tissues.[20]

In the studies no adverse effects were reported for the use of arnica. The challenge, of course, in application of it to this case is that all the studies are about muscle-induced soreness using exercise, which is not the mechanism for soreness experienced by the client.

P = **Population** (patient/client, problem, person condition or group attribute)
I = **Intervention** (the CAM therapy or approach)
C = **Comparison** (standard care or comparison intervention)
O = **Outcomes** (the measured variables of interest)

---

## CLINICAL DECISION MAKING

The therapist chooses to share the information learned on the history and philosophy of homeopathy and the strengths and weaknesses of the current literature.

### Generate a Clinical Hypothesis

If the cost of taking arnica is not prohibitive to the client and the client is motivated to try this homeopathic remedy, the therapist supports the client in adding homeopathic arnica to her treatment. The therapist generates a clinical hypothesis that homeopathic arnica will reduce the muscle soreness experienced after injury.

### Intervene and Evaluate the Outcome

Before Samantha takes arnica, the therapist evaluates Samantha's muscle soreness using a VAS much like that used in the studies by Tveiten and Vickers.[10,11] The client's physical therapy treatments would remain unchanged, with the only addition being that of the arnica.

The therapist and the client must agree on the dosage and potency of arnica to be used. The dosing in homeopathy is determined on an individual basis. However, use of a 30C dose may be appropriate to mimic the published clinical trials. Alternatively, the client could consult with a homeopath on specific dosages or simply follow the directions on the vial. The dosages and the potency must be recorded and held constant. The therapist decides to reevaluate both measures after 2 weeks.

After 2 weeks of physical therapy with the addition of arnica, the client reported less pain and irritation on a VAS. She was able to progress from crutch walking to ambulation with only an Aircast ankle support. ROM at the ankle improved such that client was able to move through full ROM actively. Strengthening exercises were initiated for the right ankle and elbow. Pain, as measured on a standard pain scale, decreased by 50% and edema measurements improved. As such, therapy was scheduled for two times a week thereafter. The client's home exercise program was updated accordingly.

### Report the Outcome

Regardless of the results of this 2-week trial the therapist considers writing a case report and presenting the findings of this particular intervention as a poster presentation. This would allow her to communicate the information she learned with other therapists. Therefore she targets a physical therapy conference as a venue for the poster. This decision is based on the evaluation of the literature in homeopathy, which has a few studies on arnica and muscle soreness, but nothing on this specific application. A case study or poster presentation, which provides outcomes that are easily measured and reproducible, would enhance the available literature on the topic of homeopathic arnica for muscle soreness.

## SUMMARY

In this chapter the clinical decision-making process is applied to answer the question of whether arnica should be added to the plan of care for an individual who could not tolerate traditional medications. The client's complaints involved muscle soreness and bruising after a slip and fall that interfered with function After investigating and evaluating the literature, the therapist decides that the quality of the literature is fair and that she cannot endorse the use of arnica; however, she does not believe it will harm the client. She chooses to educate the client on what she has learned and gives the client the option of deciding after consulting with the physician. As the client does take arnica, the therapist generates a clinical hypothesis about the potential outcome and examines the client specifically to try to capture any of the changes. These include using a VAS score for pain, tracking the number of days the client has relief, monitoring ambulation status, and measuring strength and ROM. The client demonstrates decreases in pain, improved ROM, improved strength, and gradual improvements in ambulation. The therapist chooses to report her findings in a poster format to summarize the available literature on arnica and discuss with other therapists how they may have managed this case.

## REFERENCES

1. Fischbacher E: The medical science of homeopathy. Available at: *http://www.arnica.com/homeo/homeopath2.html.* Accessed May 23, 2004.
2. Weiner M: *The complete book of homeopathy,* Garden City Park, NY, 1989, Avery.
3. Lockie A, Geddes N: *Complete guide to homeopathy,* New York, 2000, Doring Kindersley.
4. Tedesco P, Cicchetti J: Like cures like: homeopathy, *Am J Nurs* 101:43-9, 2001.
5. Blumenthal M, editor: *The complete German Commission E. monographs: therapeutic guide to herbal medicines,* Austin, Tex, 1998, American Botanical Council.
6. Fetrow C, Avila J: *Complementary and alternative medicines,* Springhouse, Penn, 1999, Springhouse.
7. Linde K, Clausius N, Ramirez G: Are the clinical effects of homeopathy placebo effects? A meta-analysis of placebo controlled trials, *Lancet* 250:834-43, 2004.
8. Ernst E, Pittler MH: Efficacy of homeopathic arnica: a systematic review of placebo-controlled clinical trials, *Arch Surg* 133:1187-90, 1998.
9. Schmidt C: A double-blind, placebo-controlled trial: *Arnica montana* applied topically to subcutaneous mechanical injuries, *J Am Inst Homeopath* 312:71-2, 1996.
10. Tveiten D et al: Effects of homeopathic remedy arnica D30 on marathon runners: a randomized, double-blind study during the 1995 Oslo marathon, *Complement Ther Med* 6:71-4, 1998.
11. Vickers AJ et al: Homeopathic arnica 30X is ineffective for muscle soreness after long distance running: a randomized, double-blind, placebo controlled trial, *Clin J Pain* 14:227-31, 1998.
12. Jawara N et al: Homeopathic arnica and *rhus toxicodendron* for delayed onset muscle soreness, *Br Homeopath J* 86:10-5, 1997.
13. Tuten C, McClung J: Reducing muscle soreness, *Altern Complement Ther* 5:369-72, 1999.
14. dos Santos MD et al: Analgesic activity of dicaffeoylquinic acids from roots of *Lychnophora ericoides* (Arnica da serra), *J Ethnopharmacol* 96:545-9, 2005.
15. Macedo SB, Ferreira LR, Perazzo FF, Carvalho JC: Anti-inflammatory activity of *Arnica montana* 6cH: preclinical study in animals, *Homeopath J Faculty Homeopathy* 93:84-7, 2004.
16. Knuesel O, Weber M, Suter A: *Arnica montana* gel in osteoarthritis of the knee: an open, multicenter clinical trial, *Adv Ther* 19:209-18, 2002.
17. Jeffrey SL, Belcher HJ: Use of arnica to relieve pain after carpal-tunnel release surgery, *Altern Ther Health Med* 8:66-8, 2002.
18. Stevinson C et al: Homeopathic arnica for prevention of pain and bruising: randomized placebo-controlled trial in hand surgery, *J Royal Soc Med* 96:60-5, 2003.

19. Plezbert JA, Burke JR: Effects of the homeopathic remedy arnica on attenuating symptoms of exercise-induced muscle soreness, *J Chiropract Med* 4:52-61, 2005.

20. Bauer CM, Weight L, Lambert MI: The use of arnica for the treatment of soft-tissue damage, *S African J Physiother* 58:34-40, 2002.

# CHAPTER 7

## Overview of Mind-Body Therapies

*Susan Gould Fogerite, Gary L. Goldberg*

Mind-body therapies reflect a view that, rather than being isolated physical constructs whose health is determined solely by genetic coding, wear and tear, and the presence or absence of foreign pathogens, human beings are a complex blend of the mental and physical. This view holds that mental processes and the state of the mind can affect the biochemical, immunological, and physical status of the body.[1-9]

Cognitive and behavioral therapy, group and social support, meditation, imagery, and hypnosis are tools of mind-body therapies that use the power of the mind to lead the body into better health. Relaxation, biofeedback, tai chi, and elements of the traditional sciences of yoga and qigong are believed to harness the body's resources to bring balance and healing to the mind.

In mind-body-spirit practice, the mind-body dyad is expanded to include the dynamic of the spirit.[2,4,9-12] The world's religions and wisdom traditions have long taught the importance of the spiritual component in the human experience. Now methods of modern clinical research are being applied to elucidate the effects of belief, ritual, and prayer on health, recovery, and the experiences of illness and death.[11,13-17]

Complementary and alternative medicine (CAM) also has been called "the New Medicine." A recent review by J. Gordon and D. Murray Edwards entitled, "MindBodySpirit Medicine" discusses aspects of the "New Medicine," particularly as defined in the model developed at the Center for Mind-Body Medicine in Washington, DC.[8] These authors list seven concepts that underlie this approach:

1. The *uniqueness* of all human beings and the need for individually tailored care
2. A *holistic* view of the integrated nature of body, mind, spirit, and the social context in which individuals function
3. *Healing partnerships* between the individual and health care professionals
4. *Self-care* for health maintenance in addition to disease intervention
5. Respect and use of *other healing systems*, especially in collaboration with practitioners and clients from these traditions
6. Use of *group support* to alleviate a sense of isolation, to foster community, and to provide coping strategies
7. Seeing *illness as a journey* or challenge that can lead to transformation of many aspects of a person's beliefs and life activities

The practices categorized as mind-body medicine, which are reviewed in this chapter, incorporate these seven principles. They can be used to promote wellness, personal empowerment, and transformation and to serve as therapeutic interventions in disease states.

The National Center for Complementary and Alternative medicine (NCCAM) of the National Institutes of Health (NIH) lists mind-body medicine as one of the five major areas of CAM.[18] This is a convenient and useful categorization. However, other groupings are possible, and overlap exists between practices and perspectives among these groups. In many clinical trials two or more CAM practices, and mind-body therapies in particular, have been used together. These practices also have been reviewed together regarding their effectiveness for various clinical outcomes and disease states. This orientation toward specific disease states reflects the specialization of the practice of modern Western medicine and the typical design of clinical trials.

An excellent and detailed review of mind-body medicine by Astin et al, published in 2003, took this approach.[3] That review supported the biopsychosocial model and found significant data for efficacy of mind-body therapies for a number of important diseases.[3] Of particular interest to rehabilitative therapy clinicians was evidence for the effectiveness of multimodal mind-body therapies (MBTs), including stress management, psychological, educational, and psychosocial support for osteoarthritis and rheumatoid arthritis, cancer, chronic and low back pain, coronary heart disease, chronic obstructive pulmonary disease, tinnitus, and diabetes, in addition to use before and during surgery.[3] Biofeedback for postsurgical recovery, in addition to migraine and chronic headaches, also was found to be effective, whereas limited evidence for the effectiveness of MBTs for fibromyalgia existed at the time that Astin's 2003 review was written.[3] A separate review by Astin, published in 2004, of MBTs for the management of pain reinforced and updated the findings of the earlier review discussed above.[19] Yoga, tai chi, qigong, and spirituality were not included in either review. Luskin et al's "A Review of Mind/Body Therapies in the Treatment of Musculoskeletal Disorders with Implications for the Elderly," although published earlier, also is recommended highly for its breadth (including yoga, tai chi, and qigong), clarity, and focus on a topic of high interest to physical therapists.[20]

This book is organized into overview chapters on the major categories of CAM practices and individual chapters with case studies on selected CAM practices. This overview chapter on mind-body therapy includes yoga (Chapter 8) and tai chi (Chapter 9), which are covered in more depth in chapters within this section of the book. Qigong is explained and reviewed Chapter 15 and in the overview in the section on energy therapies (Chapter 13).

## BRIEF HISTORY OF MIND-BODY MEDICINE

Throughout most of history people have believed in the importance of the mind, spirit, and environment in health and healing. This belief and practices that have incorporated it have been maintained to the present day in many locations and cultures.[2,4,18,21] However, in much of the Western world, and more recently in the East, the growth of science and some philosophical trends led to a separation of mind and body, in addition to a diminution of the role of spirit in health.[2,6,18,21] The discoveries of Copernicus, Galileo, and Newton brought about a more mechanistic view of the universe. In the 1800s, the philosopher Rene Descartes separated a transcendent and nonmaterial mind from the material and mechanical operations of the body.[18] The telescope, the microscope, biochemistry, and molecular biology have revealed microcosms and macrocosms of seemingly endless physical complexity. Western civilization's rational, scientific, mechanistic worldview has helped to bring about enormous technological and material advances. In general, the practice of Western medicine has reflected this view and depended upon technology to support and advance its practice. In particular, the discovery of microbial pathogens, a greater understanding of disease pathogenesis, the development of successful surgery, and antibiotics, have led to a disease-based model of health and medical intervention.

Despite the impressive achievements medicine has made in the past century, this biomedical model has narrowed human perspective over time. Many people have come to view all illness as primarily a malfunction of mechanical parts and to regard physicians and other health practitioners as technicians responsible for their repair. They have lost sight of the importance of psychological, social, economic, and environmental influences on health and illness and of the extraordinary power of the mind to affect the body. A trend that has contributed to this lack of a holistic view has been the specialization of education and the paucity of intellectual discourse between the fields and practitioners of medicine, basic research, philosophy, and psychology.

As our understanding increases, this purely mechanistic model and the division of mind and body begin to look more like a product of a particular period and viewpoint, rather than a complete vision of reality.[1,2,4-6] Modern science's view is coming more into alignment with earlier, even ancient, understandings of the unity of body and mind.[1,2,5,22,23] This is reflected in the frequent use of a hyphen between the words *mind* and *body* or even fusing them together as mindbody or bodymind. Indeed, the nature of consciousness and the rela-

tionship of mind to brain and body are areas of active scientific investigation and philosophical debate.[3,10,18,24] A major focus of biomedical research over the coming decade will be to determine the efficacy of mind-body practices, to optimize protocols, and to further elucidate their mechanisms of action.[3,18]

## THE BIOLOGICAL BASIS OF MIND-BODY THERAPIES

In the last 30 years scientists have begun to explore the complex interconnections between mind and body. Much evidence exists for the powerful impact that the mind has on our physical health and the influence of the body's condition upon our mental state.[1,2,25-32]

### Correlation of Condition, Mood, and Health

Biomedical research has begun to elucidate the important roles that stress, depression, and anxiety play in causing illness, exacerbating symptoms, and delaying or blocking recovery. Of equal importance is the correlation of positive emotions and thoughts with health and the ability to use the mind and body to heal and to maintain health.[1,2,25-33]

Many studies have shown that people who live with poverty, long-term loneliness, or job dissatisfaction or those who suffer from prejudice or the sudden loss of a loved one are far more vulnerable to illness and death than those who are fulfilled in their social and interpersonal experiences. Idler, Kasl, and Lemke have found that mood, attitude, and belief can affect virtually every chronic illness.[34] Fear and cynicism, in addition to a sense of hopelessness and helplessness, can have a detrimental effect on health. On the other hand, courage, good humor, a sense of control, and hopefulness can be beneficial. Optimistic people are less likely to become ill and, when they do become ill, tend to have a better chance of recovery, to live longer, and to suffer less. The authors of this study indicated that the opinion of an individual's health status may be the best predictor of well-being and future health.[34]

A clinical study published in 1991 had a strong impact on perceptions and research in this field.[28] This study showed that people with higher levels of perceived stress and more stressful events in the previous year were more susceptible to illness when experimentally infected with a cold virus.[28] This observation was corroborated and expanded in a later study involving experimental exposure to an upper respiratory virus.[35] This clinical trial showed that individuals with more stress and negative moods developed more severe illness than those with more positive moods and less stress.[35] Science has now been able to at least partially explain these results by confirming that emotional fluctuations and emotional status directly influence the probability that the human organism will get sick or be well.[33]

## The Nervous System and the Stress Response

To begin to understand how it is possible for the mind to affect the health of the body, we can look at the structure and function of the nervous system. The nervous system is composed of the peripheral nervous system (PNS), 31 pairs of spinal nerves, and 12 pairs of cranial nerves, which branch off from the central nervous system (CNS), the spinal cord, and the brain. The PNS has been categorized as comprising the voluntary or somatic system involved in muscle sensing and movement and the involuntary or autonomic system enervating muscles, tissues, and glands responsible for maintaining homeostasis and not requiring conscious control. However, a high degree of control over the "involuntary" nervous system can be obtained, as demonstrated by yogic adepts and more recently through the effectiveness of biofeedback.

The autonomic nervous system is divided further into sympathetic and parasympathetic systems, having complementary or opposing actions. The "flight or fight response," first described by Cannon in the 1920s, is associated with adrenal and sympathetic nervous system activation.[36] This response prepares the body to deal with a threat by running or fighting. It shuts down activities temporarily not needed, including digestive and reproductive systems, and some immune functions. Blood is shunted away from the interior critical organs and toward the muscles and brain. Blood pressure rises as heart and breathing rate increase. The brain and senses become hyperaware, and sensitivity to pain is decreased.

## Pathways of Stress and Relaxation

Two major pathways are used to bring about the stress response and recovery from it. They are the sympathetic-adrenal-medullary (SAM) axis and the hypothalamic-pituitary-adrenal cortex (HPA) axis.[37-39] In the HPA axis, signals of emotional stress

or physical threats are received and interpreted in the emotional or limbic system of the brain. These stress signals are communicated to the hypothalamus, which secretes corticotrophin-releasing hormone (CRH), which causes the pituitary to secrete adrenocorticotropic hormone (ACTH). ACTH circulating in the blood causes the adrenal cortex to release the major stress hormone, cortisol. Cortisol has the immediate effects of mobilizing energy stores, inhibiting immune and inflammatory responses, and increasing sensitivity to other stress hormones. The SAM axis comprises the direct effects of autonomic sympathetic nervous system activation. These include secretion of epinephrine by the adrenal medulla and increases in blood levels of various stress hormones and peptides, including norepinephrine, renin, calcitonin, substance P, neuropeptide Y, thyroxine, parathyroid hormone, and insulin.

Although this response is necessary and helpful in acutely dangerous situations, it is important that this state passes and is followed by a return to a less excited state. Biochemical feedback pathways, conscious mental control, and the parasympathetic nervous system are responsible for returning the body-mind to a state of calmer homeostasis.

Chronic stress, associated with long-term sympathetic activation in response to the challenges of daily life, or a failure to recover from traumatic events, causes physical and chemical states within the body that promote or lead to illness. Hans Selye's work was seminal in the early definition and description of the response to stress and its negative impacts on health.[40] A condition of excessive sympathetic tone contributes to many of the chronic diseases from which modern man suffers.[37,41] Chronically cold hands can be indicative of this state, because of the decreased peripheral blood flow that is part of this response. Indeed, learning to increase hand temperature is one of the major techniques used in biofeedback to promote a calmer state and reduce migraine headaches (see the section on biofeedback in this chapter for related references).

Samuel Mann has proposed that emotions that are not perceived at a conscious level may be playing an important role in hypertension and other pathological conditions believed to involve the mind-body connection.[42] This hypothesis would be consistent with the large placebo effects seen in hypertension trials and with the lack of consistently strong correlations between hypertension and self-reported stress. If this is the case, mind-body therapies may be appropriate and effective and should be considered, even when the client does not have a significant awareness of stress or recollection of traumatic events.[42]

## Psychoneuroimmunology and the Mind-Body Connection

Psychoneuroimmunology (PNI) is the study of the connections and communication between the psychological, neurological, endocrine, and immune systems.[32,43-47] Within the context of this short space, it is not possible to describe thoroughly or review this burgeoning field of science, or to do justice to the many researchers who have made important contributions. The reader is instead referred to a few review articles and other references within this chapter as an overview and introduction. Dr. Candice Pert, a pioneer and leader in the field of PNI and former Chief of the Section on Brain Biochemistry of the Clinical Neuroscience Branch at the National Institute of Mental Health, has written a book on alternative medicine and a review article on PNI that provide a good overview and history of psychoneuroimmunology.[48,49] A recent article by Dr. Ronald Glaser gives a personal history of the field, with an emphasis on his collaborative work with Dr. Janice Kiecolt-Glaser and others in their research group, which has moved the field forward significantly.[44]

The discovery of naturally occurring peptides or neuropeptides (messenger molecules made up of amino acids), which could cause alterations of mood, pain, and pleasure, revolutionized thinking about the nature of emotions and physical sensations. Among the first of these substances identified were *endorphins*, which is shorthand for endogenous morphine, meaning "the brain's own morphine." When endorphins are released, they produce pleasurable responses, similar to those associated with opiates.

The most amazing aspect of these discoveries was that these endorphins and other chemicals like them were found not just in the brain, but in the immune system, the endocrine system, and throughout the body. Likewise, these peptides were seen to affect the functioning of all systems of the body, including the immune system. The communication between these systems is extensive and constant and uses neurotransmitters, neuropeptides, hormones, and cytokines as messengers.[45,50,51] Many examples of the connections and communi-

cation between the immune system and the nervous system (NS) exist, including the following[41]:

- Innervation of primary and secondary lymphoid organs
- Temporal and quantitative correspondence in immune and neural hormonal activation
- Lesions in specific areas of the brain producing consistent correlating immune defects
- Receptors for neurotransmitters and cytokines on NS and immune cells
- Production of cytokines by the NS and neuropeptides and hormones by immune cells
- Inhibition of the immune system by stress
- Effects on immune system by NS stimulatory or inhibitory substances (e.g., alcohol, nicotine, drugs of abuse)
- NS pathologies associated with immunological responses or imbalances

Virtually any cytokine, hormone, neuropeptide, or neurotransmitter could be used as an example of the communication within these systems. Corticotropin-releasing hormone (CRH), for instance, plays a critical role in coordinating physiological and behavioral responses to stress and has also been implicated strongly in mediation of immunological sequelae.[52] Another possible mediator of mind-body connections is the hormone insulin-like growth factor (IGF-1).[53] High levels of IGF-1 have been correlated with certain cancers and with depression. Depression has been associated independently with higher risks of cancer. The pineal gland and the secretion of melatonin also have been hypothesized to play a role in depression and cancer progression.[54] Research in PNI has progressed to the level of studying the modulation of gene expression. A fascinating article by Ernest Lawrence Rossi, Ph.D., outlines some of the research in this area on differential expression of mRNA splicing variants of acetylcholinesterase (AChE) in response to stress.[37] He hypothesizes the existence of temporal and biochemical connections between gene expression changes, cognitive-behavioral changes, insight, creativity, brain remodeling, and variations in performance throughout the day.[37] The connections and communications between the immune, neurological, and endocrine system are extensive. Future research will continue to define and refine the details and mechanisms of action.

## Placebo and "Nonspecific" Effects

Another area of active investigation is in what has been called the "physiology of expectancy." This is at least partially responsible for what is widely known as the "placebo effect." Dr. Henry Beecher first coined this term during World War II. He observed that saline injections, given when morphine was unavailable, could control a substantial amount of pain if the soldiers believed they were getting the drug. His later work demonstrated that belief accounted for a large percentage (as much as 35%) of the response to any medical treatment.[55] Current brain and psychological research seeks to understand the basis of placebo and other cognitive modulation of the perception of pain.[56,57] Factors contributing to "nonspecific" or placebo effects include the client's expectations that the therapy will work, the client's degree of suggestibility, and a desire to please the health practitioners dispensing the treatment.[58] A subset of effects that are not specific to a particular drug or treatment includes the positive effect of interacting with a person who listens to the client's problems, who cares about whether the client will get well, and who dispenses reassurance, information, and suggestions for how to get better. These factors play a role in conventional and alternative medicine and contribute to positive outcomes in both.[59] The observation that people in the control arms of clinical trials get better as a result of the time in contact with study personnel and attention paid to them has been termed the *Hawthorne effect*. Considerations of placebo and Hawthorne effect play a significant role in the design of clinical trials and interpretation of their results. The design and development of appropriate controls and clinical trial design for complementary and alternative medicine practices, particularly in mind-body therapies, has proved challenging and is still evolving.

Many mind-body interventions are being shown to affect the status of the psycho-neural-endocrine-immune network. Although many of the basic interactions are understood, still much work must be done to define the detailed mechanisms of action of these therapies.

## Use of Mind-Body Therapies in the United States

CAM use by the American public is significant and has grown rapidly over the past few decades.[18,60-63] A 1990 National Survey published in 1993 by Eisenberg et al brought public, government, and medical community attention to the popularity and high out-of-pocket costs of CAM.[64] This survey reported that about a third of the U.S. adult population had used one or more complementary therapies in the last year, with visits to alternative medicine practitioners estimated at 427 million.[64]

A follow-up survey in 1997 documented a 25% increase over the 1990 statistics in CAM usage, to 42% of those surveyed, with the largest increases in herbal medicine, massage, high-dose vitamins, self-help groups, folk remedies, homeopathy, and energy healing.[65] Visits to CAM practitioners increased 47%, topping visits to primary care physicians. Projected out-of-pocket expenditures for CAM and for all U.S. physician services were similar, conservatively estimated at $27 billion.[65] A review of these data by Wolsko et al looked specifically at use of mind-body therapies, documenting their extensive use and application to a variety of chronic diseases in particular.[62]

Tindle et al. compared results of that 1997 survey to the 2002 Alternative Health/Complementary and Alternative Medicine Supplement to the National Health Information Survey (NHIS).[66] The prevalence of CAM use remained stable during this time period at more than one third of the U.S. population, or a projected 72 million adults, using at least one CAM modality (not including prayer) in the previous year.[66] Multiple therapy use was common, as more than 40% of those using CAM had used more than one CAM modality during this time period. Mind-body therapies continued to be among the most popular relaxation techniques (defined in this survey as including meditation, guided imagery, deep breathing, and progressive relaxation), used by 14.2%, or a projected 28 million adults. These came in second only to herbal medicine usage, which was 18.6% or 38 million.[66] Yoga had the second largest increase in usage, from 3.7% of adults in 1997, up to 5.1% or 10.4 million adults in 2002.[66] Tai chi (1.2%, 3.4 million), hypnosis (0.2%, 505,000), and biofeedback (0.1%, 278,000) round out the mind-body therapies covered in this chapter that were specifically assessed in this comparison. This article did not include a comparison of statistics on cognitive-behavioral therapy, group therapy, or prayer. The 2002 National Health Survey reported that when prayer was included as a CAM practice, the number responding positively to use in the last year increased to 62% of the U.S. adult population.[66]

According to a number of surveys, CAM usage varies somewhat with sociodemographic determinants, with the highest associations of use occurring with white, female, higher education, and higher socioeconomic status.[62,66-71] However, although interesting differences among patterns of use exist, utilization by all major ethnic, racial, age, and socioeconomic groups, in addition to both genders, is high.[62,66-69,71-73]

These and other surveys have found that the use of CAM is significantly underreported to health practitioners.[62,64,65,68-70,74-76] Nonjudgmental elicitation of information on CAM use from clients is important.[77] This can prove invaluable in determination of a course of treatment involving CAM, in addition to identification of practices that may interfere or be synergistic. Current or former CAM practices may have contributed positively or negatively to a client's present condition.

Partially in response to widespread public use and support in Congress, the NIH has steadily increased funding for CAM research and has instituted the National Center for Complementary and Alternative Medicine.[18] Other NIH divisions, especially the National Cancer Institute, also are financing ongoing research into the efficacy of various mind-body modalities in achieving recovery and maintaining health.[78] See the NIH CRISP database for titles and abstracts of funded studies.

Mainstream medicine is moving more and more in the direction of integrating mind-body practices into treatment plans.[60,79,80] Prestigious medical centers throughout the country are opening centers of integrative medicine that include mind-body techniques.[79] The Consortium of Academic Health Centers for Integrative Medicine (CAHCIM) is an organization that currently includes 36 highly esteemed North American academic medical centers. Its "mission is to help transform medicine and health care through rigorous scientific studies, new models of clinical care, and innovative educational programs that integrate biomedicine, the complexity of human beings, the intrinsic nature of healing and the rich diversity of therapeutic systems."[81] Although significant research supports the efficacy of mind-body therapies, they still are underutilized by the public and underprescribed by the medical community. Although a trend toward greater reimbursement for CAM practices and mind-body therapies exists, this remains an area in which expansion is still needed.[18,82]

CAM modalities, and mind-body therapies in particular, often are used for specific diseases, syndromes, and symptoms. Many review and research articles on conditions of interest to the rehabilitative practitioner include, but are not limited to, rheumatologic disorders,[27,83] pain,[19,84-86] anxiety and depression,[87] physical disabilities,[88,89] cancer and palliative care,[71,72,90-98] diabetes,[99] and

cardiovascular diseases.[100] Much of the use and highest utility of mind-body therapies is for the management and amelioration of chronic diseases and symptoms. Major mind-body practices and some of the research done on their applications in health and disease are reviewed below. An exhaustive review of these broad topics is not possible within the space of a book chapter. The goal here is to introduce and give an overview of the history, general components, and biomedical research. Recent or classic work that may be of particular interest and use in rehabilitation also has been highlighted.

## YOGA

Yoga is an ancient practical science that leads to the purification and the integration of mind, body, and spirit.[101-110] The goal of yoga is self-knowledge and ultimately self-realization (enlightenment).[102,103,105,109] Yoga comes from the Sanskrit root word *yug*, which means "yoke" or "to bind together." It also means "unity," which refers to a unity of principles, aspects, and energies, or the union of the individual self with the supreme universal self.[107,108,110,111]

A number of paths of yoga exist, such as bhakti (love, devotion), jnana (knowledge), karma (action, selfless service), kundalini (primal force), mantra (sound), tantra (expanded consciousness), and raja (the royal path, or path of enlightenment). These paths are not mutually exclusive, and a person may practice some combination of paths at any one time. However, the choice of path is influenced by a person's tendencies and state of development.[101,104,106,110]

Raja yoga, the eight-limbed path, is a systematic practice to obtain enlightenment. Through the practice of raja yoga, an individual obtains mastery over the physical, mental, and spiritual aspects and is led to full realization of the self. It is also referred to as a ladder with eight rungs (Box 7-1).[103,110,111]

The physical yoga that comprises the postures and some breathing practices with which we are most familiar in the United States today is an aspect of hatha yoga. The word *hatha*, in its grossest form, means "force."[103] It is a gentle forcing, for breaking habits. It also is composed of "ha," for Sun (active), and "tha," for moon (passive). The practice integrates and balances the opposite forces within us.[102-104] This concept of the balance of opposites associated with an optimal state of health and well-being was arrived at intuitively and through centu-

| Box 7-1 | The Eight Rungs of Raja Yoga |
|---------|------------------------------|
| Yamas | Restraints (nonviolence, nonlying, nonstealing, continence or control of the senses, nonpossessiveness) |
| Niyamas | Observances (cleanliness, evenmindedness, or contentment; practices perfecting the body and senses; study of the self and scriptures; surrender to the ultimate reality) |
| Asanas | Postures and cleansings |
| Pranayama | Energy regulation through the breath |
| Pratyahara | Sense withdrawal |
| Dharana | Concentration |
| Dhyana | Meditation |
| Samadhi | Absorption, enlightenment |

ries of observation and practice. This view has direct corollaries in modern science's understanding of biochemical, immunological, and psychological health and the mind-body connection.

Many styles of hatha yoga are practiced in the United States. The reader is referred to Chapter 8 for a list and discussion of some of the major schools. These include, but are not limited to Ashtanga (power), Jivamukti, Bikram (hot), and some Vinyasa practices. These practices are oriented more toward fitness, are quite challenging, and are not recommended for beginners or the significantly ill. Iyengar yoga is a strong and popular tradition that emphasizes perfection of postures and the use of props. It can be good for the medical client but may be too rigid or focused on perfection. It would be important to know the teacher or studio before recommending this as a therapeutic option. Some other schools include Anahata, Ananda, Anusara, Himalayan, Integral, Kripalu, Phoenix Rising, Svaroopa, Sivananda, Vinyasakrama, and Viniyoga. These have an emphasis on healing and enlightenment. They are gentle and use an integrated approach (mind, body, spirit). They are mainly individualized and appropriate for medical clients. Integrative yoga therapy is designed specifically for medical and mainstream wellness settings.

## Brief History of Yoga

The origins of yoga many thousands of years ago are obscure.[110] It is a practical science developed over thousands of years through revelation in higher states of consciousness, meditation, observation, and experimentation in the cave monasteries of the Himalayas.[102-104] It was handed down directly from teacher to student, known only to a select few. The Sage Patanjali codified yoga science about two thousand years ago in the "Yoga Sutras."[102,104] Sutras (Sanskrit for "threads," related to the word *suture*) are brief statements with deep meaning. These short aphorisms facilitated the oral transmission of this knowledge. Personal practice, study with a bona fide teacher, and reading a commentary on the sutras are recommended to get the most benefit and understanding of this knowledge. The translations and commentaries written by Swami Veda Bharati have received critical acclaim and are recommended highly.[102,104] The knowledge and practice of yoga have spread throughout the world in the last 100 years, directly from teachers and from ancient and modern writings. Recently, television, videos, the Internet, and a tremendous increase in the number of yoga studios and teachers have contributed to its accessibility.

Yoga is important for health care practitioners and clients because it is one of the most popular CAM practices in the world today.[66,112,113] Millions of people are exploring yoga as therapy for a wide array of health problems.[112] A growing body of research on its effectiveness in cardiovascular, neuroendocrine, musculoskeletal, immunological, mental, and behavioral diseases[114-116] exists.

## Review of Yoga Scientific Literature

Medical intervention and research have focused mainly on pranayama (breathing practices), asana (postures), and dhyana (meditation), or integrated interventions involving two or all three types of practices.

### Pranayama

Pranayama comes from the Sanskrit *prana*, which means "breath, energy, or life force," and *yama*, which means "pause, regulation, or expansion."[103,110,117] It often is translated as "breathing practices," but it refers more broadly to regulation of the breath, or control or expansion of the life force.[117] Relatively few clinical studies of only breathing practices have been performed. However, a long history exists of practice and belief in effectiveness.[104,106,117,118] Positive effects on lung function and blood oxygenation may seem likely, and clinical trial evidence exists for effectiveness in asthma,[119,120] in chronic bronchitis,[121] and in decreasing concentrations of circulating free radicals.[122] Improvements in cardiac function[123] and enhanced grip strength[124] have been seen with specific pranayama practices. Bhastrika (bellows breathing) resulted in faster reaction times in healthy young men immediately after practice.[125]

Sudharshan kriya yoga (rhythmic hyperventilation at different rates) significantly improved various symptoms of clinical depression with no negative side effects (although outcomes were somewhat inferior to electroconvulsive therapy).[126] Changes in brain activity with various pranayama practices also have been shown.[127,128] Pranayama is often part of hatha yoga and meditative practices, which have demonstrated efficacy in a variety of clinical medical and psychological conditions. More well-designed research in pranayama practices is needed to fully characterize and take advantage of their considerable potential for health promotion and for treatment of disease.

### Asana

Asanas are postures that promote physical well-being that are performed with a state of mental awareness.[101-104,106,129] Mental and breath awareness are attributes that distinguish yoga asanas from simple exercise.[103] Research studies on hatha yoga have shown positive effects on a wide variety of diseases, disorders, and symptoms, many of which are likely to be encountered in the practice of physical therapy and rehabilitation (see below and Chapter 8).[130-132] Physical benefits of hatha yoga practice include increased strength, flexibility, energy, and improved posture, in addition to improved functioning of the digestive, immune, and neuroendocrine systems. Although the evidence is significant and growing, still a strong need exists for more well-designed clinical trials. Many of the studies referred to in this section on "asana" practice are integrated practices that include pranayama, meditation, and even yoga philosophy components.

A number of trials have provided evidence for yoga's efficacy in improvement of function, psychological parameters, and decreasing asthma symptoms or medication use.[119,120,133-136] A recent trial of a 4-week Iyengar intervention compared with a stretching class, however, showed no statistical difference between the yoga group and the controls.[137] Further controlled studies are needed to determine optimal types, content, and duration of interventions, in addition to their effectiveness. It also may be desirable to have a standard care control arm in clinical studies. Many mind-body interventions represent significant improvements over standard care but may not be statistically different from similar or alternative controls. Qualitative and semi-quantitative research also can improve the sensitivity of the research and pick up changes that may be missed with only physical parameters or validated quantitative analytical assessment tools.

Many studies, particularly in India, have demonstrated positive effects of yoga on cardiovascular and cardiopulmonary diseases (including hypertension), in addition to improvement of respiratory capacity and cardiorespiratory performance in elderly and healthy young populations.[138-151] Another common health problem investigated for potential treatment with yoga is type 2 diabetes, in which clinical trials have shown improvements in blood glucose control, pulmonary function, and nerve conductance.[152-154] Positive preliminary results have been achieved with irritable bowel syndrome (IBS),[155] urologic disorders,[156] drug addiction,[157] and insomnia.[158,159]

Improvements in various brain and psychological functions, including anxiety,[160,161] perceived stress,[162] depression,[163] intellectual performance,[162] subjective well-being,[164] relaxation,[165] obsessive compulsive disorder,[166] attention deficit hyperactivity disorder,[167,168] and seizure disorders such as epilepsy,[169-171] have been obtained in yoga clinical studies. Yoga practices have been seen to improve pregnancy outcomes (including delivery and birth weight) in a number of randomized controlled trials.[172-174]

Cancer clients and survivors are another group likely to benefit from yoga interventions, based on outcomes from a number of clinical trials and a review published in 2005 by Bower et al.[175-177] Experimental support exists for the feasibility and efficacy of yoga interventions for cancer, with modest improvements seen in sleep quality, mood, stress, cancer-related distress, cancer-related symptoms, and overall quality of life.[176]

Positive results with neuromuscular diseases, (including multiple sclerosis),[178] musculoskeletal disorders (including arthritis),[20,149,179,180] pain (including low back pain),[181-184] and carpal tunnel syndrome[185-187] have been achieved. See Chapter 8 for an in-depth discussion of the research and results for low back pain, stress, and carpal tunnel syndrome.

A small pilot study in clients suffering from the weakness and fatigue of postpolio syndrome showed improvements after a 5-day retreat and 12 weeks of home practice with a video prepared specifically for this trial.[115] Although the numbers in this study were small and no control group was used, the results were encouraging for a client population in whom a lack of deterioration is generally viewed as positive.[115]

### Dhyana-Meditation

Meditation is the use of specific techniques for resting the mind and attaining a state of consciousness that is different from waking, dreaming, and sleeping (Figure 7-1).[188,189] This fourth state is known as *turiya*. It is alert, clear, relaxed, and inwardly focused.[188,189] Meditation is not thinking hard, contemplating, daydreaming, or fantasizing. Another definition is "making the mind to flow as an even stream," or "the unbroken even flow of the mind on a single cognition."[102,109] A large number of studies and clinical trials on meditation have been completed or are in progress. Early on in the U.S. research, Herbert Benson, MD, coined the term "relaxation response." He and co-workers described a variety of changes that occurred in meditation, including decreased metabolic rate, temperature, heart rate, lower blood pressure and oxygen consumption, stress hormone reduction, and brain wave changes.[190] More recent work has also demonstrated transient and long-term brain changes.[191-194]

Mindfulness-based stress reduction (MBSR), developed by Jon Kabat-Zinn, PhD, is a program based on Buddhist meditation practices, along with some hatha yoga.[195,196] Numerous clinical studies have been completed and are in progress using this system, which was originally developed for

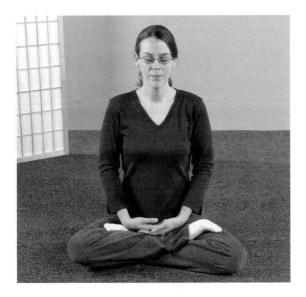

**Figure 7-1** A woman performing a sitting mediation.

clients with chronic pain.[196,197] At the University of Massachusetts Medical Center, Kabat-Zinn found that 72% of clients with chronic pain conditions achieved at least a 33% reduction in pain after participating in an 8-week period of mindful meditation, whereas 61% of the clients achieved at least a 50% reduction.[198] Dr. Kabat-Zinn was also first author on an interesting study that showed increased rates of lesion healing in psoriasis clients when an audiotape with MBSR guidance (and some guided imagery) was played during ultraviolet phototherapy (UVB) or photochemotherapy (PUVA), compared with clients who did not have the tape.[197]

Systematic MBSR programs currently are used in many medical settings. A systematic review of clinical studies of MBSR for cancer, published in 2005, reported numerous positive outcomes including psychology, sleep, and symptomatology.[199] Individual clinical trials with improved outcomes in a variety of parameters also have been published for breast and prostate cancer,[200] with qigong for fibromyalgia,[86] for physical symptoms, psychological parameters, and spiritual experiences,[25] and on stress hormones, physical functioning, and submaximal exercise responses.[201]

An ongoing dialogue between scientists and practitioners of Buddhism has been fostered by the Mind and Life Institute through conferences and research. Mind and Life board member Richard Davidson, MD, has been focusing primarily on brain function and physiological studies with Buddhist monks with years of meditation practice.[202] In addition, a recent collaborative study with Kabat-Zinn, with subjects who had not previously meditated, showed an increase in antibody titer to flu vaccine after a short introductory meditation course and practice, compared with a control group who did not meditate.[196]

Transcendental meditation (TM) probably has been studied in the largest number of clinical trials.[203-215] Robert Schneider, MD, has been a leading researcher on the effects of TM, particularly in hypertension and cardiovascular disease.[207,209,211-215] Improvements in cardiovascular parameters, blood chemistries, and blood pressure, and decreases in negative outcomes such as myocardial infarctions, hospitalizations, and even mortality, have been seen with shorter and long-term practice of TM.[207,209,211-215]

Various other meditative practices also have been studied, although much need and opportunity still exists to explore different modalities and interventions. Some examples include kundalini yoga meditation techniques for specific psychiatric problems[216] and cancer,[98] and Tibetan yoga meditation for cancer.[177]

## Yoga Summary

Significant clinical evidence exists to support the effectiveness of integrated yoga practices, in addition to individual breathing, meditation, and physical asana practices for improvement of medical conditions. Positive effects on cardiovascular, cardiopulmonary, and musculoskeletal diseases; addiction; migraine; pain; pregnancy and delivery; the immune system; cancer; infectious diseases; anxiety; insomnia; stress; depression; ADHD; and seizure disorders have been demonstrated. Many groups and individuals have been and are continuing to push this exciting area of research forward throughout the world, including India. More high-quality research is needed to determine optimal interventions, extent of efficacy, client variables, and mechanisms of action.

## TAI CHI

Tai chi is a physical practice involving flowing movements coordinated with breath and performed with mental awareness.[217,218] Properly performed, tai chi becomes a moving meditation.[218] It is a conditioning exercise designed to promote health, balance, strength, breathing, relaxation, and concentration. The balance it promotes does not just refer to an ability to stay on your feet but balance of the energy or chi (qi) of the body. The belief is that the vital forces within the body need to be balanced and flowing for a condition of health. Disease is thought to be the result of blockages or imbalances in the energy. In tai chi, the physical balance is shifted constantly from side to side, forward and back, and even on to one leg at a time. Coordinated arm movements also are varied in direction. Much of the time is spent with bent knees and a low center of gravity.[218] Tai chi is extremely popular in China, particularly among older people, because of its benefits supporting health and longevity.[219] It has gained increasing popularity in the United States, where it has been studied and promoted primarily in older populations as an intervention for decreasing falls and fear of falling and for cardiovascular benefits.[219-222] (See Chapter 9.)

## Brief History of Tai Chi

Tai chi (other spellings include t'ai chi ch'uan, tai qi quan, and tai chi chun) has its roots in ancient Chinese martial arts. The practice prepares and conditions the individual for fighting, and the movements and stances themselves actually are used in defense and attack. Five major schools of tai chi have evolved, which are named after the families who originated them. These styles have differences and similarities.[217] The school used most often for elderly people and for health promotion in the West is Yang, because of its gentle flowing movements. There is a Yang long form and short form.[218] Variations on these forms have been developed for use in older and frail populations and have been used in clinical trials.

The practice of tai chi is intimately connected with the Taoist Chinese philosophy that describes the material universe as being composed of pairs of opposites, yin and yang, feminine and masculine, passive and active, dark and light. This reality is depicted in the yin-yang symbol: a circle with swirling black and white sections. A small circle of the opposite color resides within the widest part of each side, representing the seed of the opposite existing within either of the extremes. The understanding is that although things appear to be opposites, they are in fact inseparable aspects of the same reality, and the underlying reality is unity.

Many parallels exist between the beliefs and practices of tai chi, qigong, and yoga. Yoga, originating several thousand years ago, predates tai chi, which has been practiced for several hundred years.[218] Trade and the travels of scholars, sages, and warriors throughout what is now India, the Himalayas, Tibet, China, Korea, and Japan spread philosophy, medicine, and the arts of war. This knowledge and these practices have come to the West and have become subjects of interest to the public and medical science in recent decades.

## Review of Tai Chi Scientific Literature

The major health applications investigated for the use of tai chi are to improve balance, prevent falls, and lower fear of falling in the elderly (see Chapter 9). The evidence for its effectiveness in these application consists of one large multisite trial and numerous smaller ones.[223-236] Various physical parameters have been assessed to attempt to determine the physical changes that accompany the positive outcomes of reduced falling, including isokinetic knee extensor length, postural sway, muscle action patterns, multidirectional reach, and center of pressure trajectory.[237,238]

Tai chi also has been shown to result in improvements in cardiovascular parameters, including high blood pressure.[239-241] The weight-bearing, gentle movement of tai chi may be predicted to produce positive effects on bone and joint health. Indeed, preliminary evidence exists for prevention of bone mineral loss in early post-menopausal women[242] and increased functional mobility and satisfaction with health status, with decreased tension, for people with lower extremity osteoarthritis.[243]

Immune system improvements also have been seen. Varicella zoster is the virus that causes chicken pox upon first infection and causes shingles later in life when virus-specific cell-mediated immunity wanes. A 50% increase in varicella zoster–specific cell-mediated immunity and improvements in health functioning were seen in healthy functioning older adults after 1 week of tai chi classes.[244] Breast cancer clients exhibited increased health-related quality of life and self-esteem after participating in a 12-week course of tai chi chuan, as compared with a psychosocial support group, although a larger trial is needed to assess statistical significance.[245]

Neuromuscular and neurological diseases and function are also potential targets for tai chi, with improved general functioning poststroke being achieved in one clinical trial.[246] Preliminary qualitative research indicates a potential positive role for tai chi classes for persons with Parkinson's disease and their support partners.[247] In addition, modulation of autonomic nervous system activity has been observed.[248]

Another significant problem in older adults that tai chi may help with is nighttime sleep disturbance and daytime sleepiness.[167] General physical functioning in older adults also can be improved with tai chi training.[227,249]

## Tai Chi Summary

Strong evidence exists for tai chi improving balance and reducing falls and fear of falling in older, community-dwelling populations. Less evidence exists for more elderly people in nursing and long-term care residences. Positive effects on blood pressure, strength, flexibility, and quality of life in middle-aged and older populations also have been shown. Preliminary evidence exists for improvements in neuromuscular, neurological, and immunological functioning, although the number of trials and subjects is not large. Certainly enough encouraging evidence exists to support the need for additional trials to further define optimal tai chi interventions and their efficacy for a wide variety of applications, in addition to support for general healthy functioning.

## GUIDED IMAGERY

Guided imagery is a mind-body therapy that uses the imagination to evoke images involving several or all of the senses.[3,20,250,251] It can be considered a kind of focused, purposeful daydreaming.[250,252] These images that may contain components that can be seen, heard, felt, smelled, or tasted can be used to heal the mind and body or to improve performance.[250,252,253] Imagery is a natural way the nervous system stores, accesses, and processes information. This makes it especially effective for maintaining the dialogue between mind and body, which is the source of its power in the healing process. A relaxed state of mind and body, receptive to suggestion, is an important component for guided imagery, which is a form of hypnosis.[250,251,254] Music also is used often in conjunction with the verbal cues of guided imagery, because of its emotionally evocative properties, its right brain connection, and its ability to help induce and maintain the relaxed state supportive of optimal effectiveness.

Imagery has three main characteristics that lend it great value in medicine and healing:

- It directly affects physiology.
- Through the mental processes of association and synthesis, it provides insight and perspective into health.
- It has an intimate relationship with emotions, which are often at the root of many common health conditions.

## Brief History of Guided Imagery

Guided imagery probably has been practiced by people on themselves, and by parents for children, for millennia. The use of a pleasant daydream or story to distract or soothe, or rewriting unpleasant memories or nightmares to help with fears, seems to be a natural human response. The induction of a trancelike state, with a guided journey evoking the senses and emotions, is also a powerful technique used in Shamanism and other traditional healing modes probably since the dawn of time.[255] Greek tragedy also contains the same elements, which were used to bring about an emotional catharsis and healing. In more modern times, imagery has been an element in hypnosis, biofeedback, and autogenic training.[20] In the last decade or so it has been used as a stand-alone treatment and investigated as such.[256]

## Review of Guided Imagery Scientific Literature

Research in guided imagery has demonstrated that in a relaxed state of mind, people possess a remarkable range of self-regulatory capacities. According to Martin L. Rossman, MD, co-founder of the Academy for Guided Imagery, imagery seems to arise from unconscious processes, body processes, and memories and perception from the cerebral cortex.[257] Some imagery having to do with smell or feelings may arise from older, more primitive brain centers. Wherever its origin, imagery is believed to have its effect by sending messages from the higher centers of the brain through to the lower centers that regulate most of a person's physiological functions, such as breathing, heart rate, blood flow and pressure, digestion, immunity, and temperature, in addition to waking and sleeping rhythms, hunger, thirst, and sexual function.

Recent research with PET scans (a test involving radioactive material that is used to examine brain tissue) indicates what parts of the brain are active when a person is performing certain tasks. The PET scans seem to indicate that the optic cortex, the same part of the brain activated when a person is seeing, is activated when a person visualizes. Similarly, when people imagine hearing things, the auditory cortex is active, and when they imagine feeling sensations, the sensory cortex is active. Therefore it appears that the cortex can create these imaginary realities and in the absence of conflicting information, the lower centers of the nervous system respond to this information. This is one reason why health care professionals using guided imagery attempt to recruit as many senses as they can in creating an image. Comprehensive sensory recruitment increases the subjective reality of the image and probably increases the amount of information sent through the lower brain centers and autonomic nervous system, which makes it more likely to elicit the desired response.

Beyond simple relaxation, imagery can have specific effects in relief of numerous common symptoms and improvement of health in disease states. Imagery often is used for relief of pain. Clinical studies have shown reduction in pain from joint replacement,[258] osteoarthritis,[259] headaches, neck, back, and experimentally delivered, or medical procedural pain.[260-262] Particularly interesting to the field of physical therapy is the evidence that guided imagery can also accelerate healing and minimize discomfort from all sorts of acute injuries, including sprains, strains, and broken bones. In addition, because it can be used to enhance performance, it can have use in recovery of function subsequent to stroke, surgery, or traumatic injury.[263-267] Use of imagery to produce relaxation and improve motor performance is presented in a case in Chapter 2.

Cardiovascular disease and rehabilitation,[268] including high blood pressure; benign arrhythmias (heartbeat irregularities); stress-related gastrointestinal symptoms, including IBS and recurrent abdominal pain of childhood;[269] functional urinary complaints; and reproductive irregularities including premenstrual syndrome, irregular menstruation, dysmenorrhea (painful menstruation), and even excessive uterine bleeding, are all applications in which at least some support exists for the use of guided imagery.

Given the information in the section on PNI above, it makes sense that guided imagery can affect immune system function. Consequently, a great deal of interest exists among researchers of mind-body therapies for applying it to a broad spectrum of autoimmune diseases, including rheumatoid arthritis, ulcerative colitis, and systemic lupus erythematosus. Clinical evidence also exists for positive effects on the symptoms of the common cold, flu, other infections, and acute and chronic allergies, including hay fever and asthma.[270,271]

Finally, a great number of people with cancer have used imagery as part of their recovery process. Imagery, as a tool in cancer therapy, was pioneered by radiation oncologist O. Carl Simonton. He used imagery as a means to reinforce traditional medical treatments and suggested that his clients imagine their cancer cells as "anything soft that can be broken down, like hamburger meat, or fish eggs," and their warrior white cells as "aggressive and eager for battle."[272] Simonton's program was successful in helping clients to tolerate treatment and in some cases show remarkable improvements in their condition. In addition to cellular imagery focused on fighting cancer cells, guided imagery has been used successfully in many other cancer applications, including reducing pain, anxiety, and the effects of chemotherapy, such as nausea and fatigue and improving quality of life.[273,275,276]

Eye movement desensitization and reprogramming (EMDR) is a technique that involves having clients imagine a stressful or traumatic situation or memory while rapidly moving a finger in front of their eyes.[277] It is a type of imagery or exposure therapy. Although it has been considered controversial, it has been and is being used extensively with positive outcomes, particularly in posttraumatic stress disorder (PTSD). In addition to EMDR, standard guided imagery has been effective in a number of studies for treatment for PTSD.[252]

## Imagery Summary

Guided imagery is thought to be effective because of the mind-body connection, the "reality" of sensory images, the power and abilities of the altered state, and the feeling of being in control that the individual has in practicing it. One of the most attractive aspects of guided imagery as a mind-body modality is that it readily adapts itself to client education and self-care. It provides a formal methodology for increasing personal empowerment and self-control. Furthermore, it appears to offer significant and effective therapeutic benefits after only a few weeks or months of therapy.

## HYPNOSIS

Hypnosis generally can be described as an artificially induced state characterized by a heightened receptivity to suggestion. This state is attained by first relaxing the body then shifting attention away from the external environment toward a narrow range of objects or ideas as suggested by the hypnotherapist or by oneself in self-hypnosis. Absorption, dissociation, and suggestibility are three important components of the hypnotic trance state.[278]

It has been said that all hypnosis is self-hypnosis. The hypnotherapist is just a facilitator. Without a willing client no hypnosis can occur. The client enters hypnosis in a natural way, of his or her own accord, simply by following the suggestions of the hypnotherapist. Regardless of what procedure is used, the main concern during hypnosis is to quiet the client's conscious mind and to make the unconscious mind more accessible. Because the unconscious mind is less critical, suggestions have a better chance of being effective than they would if given during a normal waking state.

In the *superficial* hypnotic state, the client accepts suggestions but does not necessarily carry them out. Clients who reach the deep, or *somnambulistic*, state benefit most from hypnotherapy. In this state posthypnotic suggestions (suggestions that take effect after the client awakens from the trance)

to relieve pain are most successful. According to the World Health Organization, 90% of the general population can be hypnotized, with 20% to 30% having a high enough susceptibility to enter the somnambulistic state, which makes them highly receptive to treatment.[279] A review article by Barber, published in 2000, noted that individuals who are strongly prone to fantasy, able to compartmentalize unwanted memories or emotions, or highly cooperative are highly responsive to hypnotherapy.[280]

Conditions essential to successful hypnotherapy:
1. Rapport between hypnotist and subject
2. A comfortable environment, free of distraction
3. Willingness and desire by the subject to be hypnotized

Factors affecting the hypnosis:
1. The socialization of the subject
2. The effectiveness of the induction
3. The unique talents of the hypnotist
4. The power or depth of meaning of the suggestions.[280]

A hypnotherapy session usually lasts from 1 hour to 90 minutes. The number of sessions required to produce results varies according to each individual and according to the nature of the issue being addressed. However, 6 to 12 sessions, 1 per week, is about the average for many applications.

## Brief History of Hypnosis

For thousands of years the power of suggestion has played a major role in healing in cultures as varied as ancient Greece, Persia, and India. Hypnotherapy uses the power of suggestion and trancelike states to access the deepest levels of the mind to effect positive changes in a person's behavior and to treat a range of health conditions.

Hypnosis became popular for a variety of medical conditions in the late 1700s.[281] In 1955 the British Medical Association approved the use of hypnotherapy as a valid medical treatment. The American Medical Association followed suit in 1958, and its Council on Scientific Affairs continues to encourage more research on the subject of hypnotherapy. At the same time, the American Society of Clinical Hypnosis, a professional organization of physicians, psychologists, and dentists, has grown from 20 members in 1957 to more than 4300. Approximately 15,000 doctors now combine hypnotherapy with traditional treatments, and recent studies show that 94% of clients benefit from hypnotherapy, even if the only benefit is relaxation.[282] A 2005 review by Stewart found much benefit for a wide variety of medical conditions and recommended further study and greater use.[281]

Over the past 2 decades, hypnotherapy has become used more widely as a method for treatment of many medical conditions. Because of the fact that hypnotherapy induces a deep state of relaxation, increases tolerance to adverse stimuli, eases anxiety, and reinforces positive imagery, it has been adapted to maximize the mind's ability to heal. Recent studies demonstrate the ability of hypnotherapy, especially immune system targeted intervention, to have positive effects on immune status and health.[283,284]

## Review of the Hypnosis Scientific Literature

Hypnotherapy has therapeutic applications for psychological and physical disorders. A skilled hypnotherapist can facilitate profound changes in respiration and relaxation on the part of the client to create positive shifts in behavior and in health. A physiological shift can be observed in the hypnotic state, as can greater control of autonomic nervous system functions formerly considered to be beyond an individual's ability to control. Stress reduction is a common occurrence, as is a lowering of blood pressure. These changes are similar to and overlap with the "relaxation response." The underlying mechanisms for the effectiveness of hypnotherapy and its concomitant changes in perception, biochemistry, and physiology are a topic of investigation that includes functional brain mapping, protein chemistry, and gene expression.[285-287] This research may provide answers central to an understanding of the mind-body connection.

Research has demonstrated that a person's body chemistry actually changes during hypnosis. Scores of well-documented studies prove this fact. In one, a girl was unable to hold her hand in a bucket of ice water for more than 30 seconds. Testing showed that the blood cortisol levels were high, which indicates that she was undergoing severe stress. Under hypnosis, she was able to keep the same hand in ice water for 30 minutes while no rise in blood cortisol levels occurred.[288] This type of finding and the ability to reduce pain in a wide variety of situations (see below) appear to be due to interruptions or reprocessing of pain messages in the cortex of the brain, particularly the anterior cingulate cortex, although the exact mechanisms are not understood fully at present.[285,286,289]

Hypnotherapy has been employed successfully to control pain.[57,290,291] Some examples of applications include burns,[292] headaches, facial neuralgia, sciatica, osteoarthritis, rheumatoid arthritis, multiple sclerosis,[293] whiplash, menstrual pain, upper limb repetitive strain injuries,[294] and tennis elbow. A 2005 review article by Cuellar discusses the use and efficacy of hypnotherapy for pain in older adults.[295] Various mind body therapies, including hypnosis, are recommended in the treatment of pain in children.[296,297] A recent trial that trained children in self-hypnosis reduced distress and duration of an invasive medical procedure.[298] The reader is referred to a recent (2006) review of psychological interventions for pain management by Osborne et al, which is geared specifically toward rehabilitative medicine applications and practitioners.[299]

Labor and delivery pain is another application for hypnotherapy, with reductions in need for medication and less perceived pain reported.[300,301] However, a 2004 review (with different criteria) concluded that insufficient evidence existed for the efficacy of any alternative therapies (including hypnotherapy) for labor pain, except for intracutaneous sterile water injections.[302] A broad review of non-pharmacological treatments for labor and delivery pain found widespread satisfaction among users of all methods, promising results for hypnotherapy, and a need for more well-controlled studies to determine efficacy of many interventions.[303]

A 2002 review article by Oakley et al concluded that hypnotic imagery is helpful as an adjunctive therapy to standard movement therapies for phantom limb pain. The interventions reviewed contained elements of hypnosis and guided imagery.[304] Long-term pain relief benefits of hypnotherapy have been demonstrated. One comprehensive study of 178 clients suffering from chronic pain between 1981 and 1983 reported that 78% remained pain free after 6 months; 47% after 1 year; 44% after 2 years; and 36.5% after 3 years after a hypnotherapy intervention.[305]

Hypnotherapy has been used instead of, or with, reduced anesthesia, in a variety of surgical procedures, including hysterectomies, hernias, breast biopsies, hemorrhoidectomies, and Cesarean sections, and for the treatment of second-degree and third-degree burns.[56,306,307] A variety of alternative therapies can be helpful in decreasing pain, and suffering, and improving outcomes in surgery.[308] Dentists have been successful in using hypnotherapy for tooth extractions when clients were allergic to all Novocain-type drugs.

Psychotherapists have been employing hypnotherapy successfully to treat an array of anxiety disorders such as generalized anxiety disorder, simple phobias, and posttraumatic stress disorder, although more controlled studies are needed to define efficacy.[309,310-312] Like guided imagery, hypnosis may be coupled with EMDR[313] and may be effective particularly for treatment of posttraumatic stress.[314] The efficacy of hypnotherapy as compared with psychoanalysis and behavior therapy was pointed out in another study.[315] After 600 sessions of psychoanalysis, 38% of the clients reported recovery from their conditions; those receiving behavior therapy improved in 72% of all cases after 22 sessions, whereas hypnotherapy produced a 93% success rate after only six sessions.

Physical ailments with strong emotional components, such as IBS, are amenable to treatment with hypnosis.[316,317] A review by Tan, published in 2005, concludes that strong evidence exists for hypnosis improving colonic and noncolonic symptoms of IBS and that hypnosis meets the criteria for the highest level of acceptance of the American Psychological Association.[318] Improvements in hot flashes, mood, anxiety, and sleep have been seen with hypnosis for breast cancer survivors.[319] Nocturnal enuresis (bedwetting) is another condition in which some evidence exists for efficacy, although larger, well-designed trials are needed.[320] Evidence of efficacy exists also for asthma, particularly in children.[135,321] A recent review of complementary therapies for weight reduction noted a lack of large, well-designed trials and indicated some evidence for effectiveness of hypnotherapy.[322] A 2005 Cochrane review of psychological interventions for nonulcer dyspepsia reported one randomized control trial of hypnotherapy, which showed improvement of symptoms at treatment completion and at 1 year follow-up.[323]

Hypnotherapy often is applied to help people to give up unwanted habits such as cigarette smoking. A Cochrane systematic review published in 2000, using strict criteria for trial design and lack of smoking for 6 months, showed variable results and no strong effect for hypnosis over no treatment.[324] Another, more recent review concluded that hypnosis can play a significant role in supporting smoking cessation,[325] whereas another classified it as possibly efficacious.[326]

## Hypnosis Summary

Hypnosis is still far from being fully understood; however, it has achieved increasing professional acceptance and use. More basic and clinical research is needed to understand its mechanisms of action. Large, well-designed trials are necessary to further determine the effectiveness of hypnosis for the many medical and psychological applications for which it is being used and to promote its greater application, where it can be of the most help.

## COGNITIVE-BEHAVIORAL AND GROUP THERAPY

Cognitive-behavioral therapy (CBT), which uses the mind-body connection and was formerly considered complementary medicine, has now come to be considered more of a mainstream conventional therapy. CBT combines two kinds of psychotherapy: cognitive therapy and behavior therapy. Using behavior therapy, a person weakens the connections between difficult situations and his habitual reactions to them. Self-damaging and self-defeating behavior in addition to rage, fear, and depression are some of the reactions that a person can have to these situations. Employing cognitive therapy, a person learns that certain thinking patterns are causing the symptoms that he or she is experiencing. These patterns lead to a distorted image of a person's life, which causes inappropriate anxiety, anger, and depression. As Aaron Beck describes it, CBT teaches people how to answer themselves when the way that they are talking to themselves is dysfunctional.[327]

The therapist takes an active role in solving a client's problems, rather than taking the traditional passive role that other therapies require. A precise history and evaluation of the present situation are necessary to give the therapist a clear picture of the client's needs and problems.

A concrete treatment plan is developed that is structured, flexible, and clearly explained to the client. CBT often is compared with coaching and tutoring. The client and the therapist set treatment goals and decide upon strategies to be employed. The CBT session is structured and focused. Homework projects are assigned regularly. The purpose of these assignments is to reinforce and expand the work done in the therapist's office. Prepared materials related to the presenting problem often are given to the client to read at home. All of this is geared to be solution oriented and to expedite change.

CBT focuses on the present and the future. Past experiences may explain a person's difficulties but do not add anything to present-day solutions. Therefore clients are encouraged to stay focused on the here and now and limit an exploration into their histories.

The cognitive aspect of CBT works on transforming a client's attention, thoughts, ideas, attitudes, beliefs, assumptions, and mental imagery in a more rational and healthy direction. The behavioral aspect of CBT leads a client to act in a positive, productive manner by using rational judgment.

Some applications for CBT include depression and mood swings; shyness and social anxiety; panic attacks and phobias; obsessions and compulsions; posttraumatic stress symptoms; chronic anxiety or worry; eating disorders; insomnia and other sleep problems; difficulty establishing and staying in relationships; marital problems; job, career, and school difficulties; stress; low self-esteem; substance abuse; and anger management.[328]

Strategies used in CBT include challenging irrational beliefs, relaxation training, self-monitoring, cognitive rehearsal, thought stopping, communication skills training, assertiveness skills training, social skills training, bibliotherapy, and homework assignments.

### Brief History of Cognitive-Behavioral Therapy

In the 1950s and 1960s Aaron Beck and Albert Ellis, both former psychoanalysts, and both considered founders of the cognitive-behavioral school, became disenchanted with the practice of psychoanalysis. They believed that relying on unconscious processes, the need for long-term treatment, and extensive historical exploration limited this approach. It also was found that classical behavioral therapy was limited to behavioral problems or to behavioral aspects of problems that were behavioral and cognitive in their presentation. Cognitive methods were needed to bridge this divide. Clinical research also was pointing to the relevance of cognition in mental disorders and personal problems. Evidence was mounting that people do not simply respond to aspects of their environment, they also employ self-regulation and self-control.[328]

### Review of Cognitive-Behavioral Therapy Scientific Literature

The field of CBT is broad and longstanding, and detailed review in this chapter is impossible. The reader again is referred to review articles for more references and in-depth discussion of various applications. A recent review of meta-analyses for cognitive-behavioral interventions found evidence for efficacy in a large number of psychological and physical health applications.[329]

Pain management has been a significant and effective application for cognitive and behavioral therapy,[253,330] including acute pain in children.[331]

Surgical outcomes can be improved, as seen when a cognitive-behavioral tape was played repeatedly during and immediately after bariatric surgery. Clients in the group listening to the tape performed better in the postsurgical recovery program and were released an average of 1.6 days earlier than the control group.[332]

Clinical trials and case studies indicate that cognitive-behavioral therapy is helpful in treatment of posttraumatic stress disorder (PTSD) in children and adolescents.[309,312] A review of PTSD after single-incident trauma in children found that CBT studies tended to be better designed than other interventions, and improvements were noted after treatment. However, the review also demonstrated that this field needs more rigorous trials to determine efficacy and optimize interventions for different PTSD populations.[333]

A randomized controlled trial with adult civilian trauma survivors showed CBT better than supportive counseling, and CBT plus hypnosis better than CBT alone.[334] As may be predicted from PNI and the mind-body connection, cognitive-behavioral interventions can affect the immune system. A 10-week CBT program with HIV-infected men resulted in lowered stress hormones, positive changes in immune cell populations and function, and improved psychological status.[50]

### Group Therapy and Other Psychotherapy

Group therapy or support is used as a component in many psychological and medical treatments. A seminal study involving women with metastatic breast cancer showed almost a doubling of survival time for women who were participants in group therapy.[335] A systematic review of psychological interventions for cancer by Newell, Sanson-Fisher, and Savolainen was published in 2002, which made recommendations for future research.[97] Astin et al performed a meta-analysis of trials with psychological interventions for rheumatoid arthritis, which found significant pooled effect sizes for a number of parameters, including pain, functionality, and coping.[27] In a study performed in a methadone maintenance clinic, hatha yoga and psychodynamic group therapy were found to be equally effective at reduction of drug use and criminal behavior.[157]

Transpersonal psychology blends modern psychology with the knowledge of the world's religions or wisdom traditions. It holds that people are biopsychospiritual beings and that the main business of being a human is spiritual evolution. In this context, frameworks that describe human development in terms of progression through well-described stages linked by transformative experiences have been postulated. The perspectives of human nature as biopsychospiritual and life as a transformative journey are common elements of the individual human experience. The reader also is referred to a review entitled "Transformative Practices for Integrating Mind-Body-Spirit" by Frederick Luskin for a more detailed description of the field of transpersonal psychology and its applications.[10]

### Group and Cognitive-Behavioral Therapy Summary

The extensive and ongoing research in group therapy and CBT supports their efficacy for many diseases and disorders and further strengthens the evidence of the mind-body connection and its importance in heath and disease. As with the other mind-body therapies, further research will be beneficial.

## BIOFEEDBACK

Biofeedback generally uses sensing devices to monitor subtle biological processes or states and provide some sort of "feedback" that indicates the current and changing status of that process or state (Figure 7-2). It has been described by John Basmajian, a pioneer in electromyogram (EMG) biofeedback, as "the technique of using equipment to reveal internal physiological events in the form of visual and auditory signals in order to teach the person to manipulate these otherwise involuntary and unfelt events by manipulating the displayed signals."[336]

A variety of measurements and instruments are used in biofeedback. Skin temperature (ST), which is influenced by blood flow beneath the skin, is one such measurement. In the flight-or-fight response, blood flow to the periphery is reduced. By learning to warm the hand, individuals can reverse this effect and bring themselves into a calmer biological state. The galvanic skin response (GSR) measures the electrical conductivity of the skin. If a person becomes even slightly more stressed, sweat is produced and the skin conductivity increases. Depolarization of the muscle sheath, which usually leads to muscle tension, is measured with an EMG. EMG has been used extensively in rehabilitation (see below for discussion and references). An electroencephalogram (EEG) is used to measure brain wave activity. Very complex systems that monitor the frequencies of brain waves being produced in various parts of the brain have been developed for research and therapeutic applications.

Heart rate and heart rate variability also have been the subject of intensive diagnostic and biofeedback research in recent years. The regulation of heart rate may be used as an example of how biofeedback is done. First, the person is connected to a computer or monitor by means of electrodes or a small sensor that the finger can be placed into. The computer may be programmed to transmit one blinking light or one audible beep (or both) per heartbeat. Techniques such as meditation, breathing, relaxation, and visualization may be used to achieve a slower heart rate. With practice, the person is able to alter the rate of the flashes and beeps (and heart rate) at will. As the person learns to tune in to aspects of their physiological state, they are able to modulate these processes without the assistance of the feedback from the computer. This self-regulation has been compared with taking tennis lessons. If an individual stops taking lessons but continues to play, he or she will continue to improve. As with most learned behaviors, more practice results in higher-level skills.

### Brief History of Biofeedback

Biofeedback was first developed in the 1960s, grew rapidly in the 1970s, and the number of articles

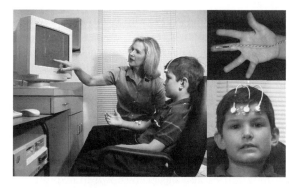

**Figure 7-2** A child used biofeedback to affect skin temperature and promote relaxation.

published peaked in the 1980s.[337] EMG instrumentation grew out of the studies of neuromuscular and spinal cord functions. It began with a classic paper in 1929 by Adrian and Bronk, which showed that the electrical responses in individual muscles provided an accurate reflection of the actual functional activity of the muscles. Applications of EMG to neuromuscular reeducation and stroke rehabilitation were developed in the 1960s and have remained important uses of this technology to this day.[337,338]

The use of biofeedback in treatment of migraines was found accidentally in the late 1970s, when researchers at the Menninger Clinic were employing biofeedback to help a woman to relax.[339] While undergoing a series of relaxation exercises, the researchers found that the woman's hand temperature suddenly increased 10 degrees. She reported that at the same time a severe headache she was experiencing totally disappeared. The researchers then used this technology to teach clients to alleviate migraines, while at the same time lowering the medications that they were taking to ease their symptoms.[338] This thermal biofeedback is still one of the most effective therapeutic modalities for the treatment of migraines.[81,340,341]

In the 1960s correlations between electroencephalographic (EEG) waves of certain frequencies, particular states of consciousness, and the ability to modulate these frequencies were reported.[190,191] Measurement of brain waves by EEG and the use of neurofeedback have been areas of active research and clinical application since that time.

For most of the time that biofeedback has been used for diagnostics or therapeutics, equipment has been expensive to purchase and complicated to use. People could obtain the benefits of biofeedback only under the care of trained professionals. Indeed, this is still the case and necessary for most applications, particularly for rehabilitation, in which the practitioner plays a crucial role in designing the intervention, placing sensors, setting and adjusting parameters, and providing human feedback.[338] Recently, however, the development of small sensors with digital readouts and sensors that can interface with affordable computer programs available to the public is broadening the base of use of biofeedback.[342,343]

## Review of Biofeedback Scientific Literature

The Association of Applied Pyschophysiology and Biofeedback is an international organization of professionals and other individuals interested in research, education, and use of biofeedback.[344] The reader is referred to this organization's website for additional background information and references on biofeedback research.[344]

One of the most common uses for biofeedback training is the treatment of stress and stress-related disorders. The evidence supporting the use of biofeedback for headaches, particularly EMG for tension headache and thermal biofeedback for migraine, is strong.[340,341,345-347] Biofeedback often is used with some combination of relaxation, imagery, hypnosis, education, or CBT for many applications, including headache and other pain disorders.[340,346-350] A review by McNeely of physical therapies for temporomandibular joint disorders (TMJ) concluded that evidence exists for the effectiveness of postural exercises, manual therapy plus active exercise, muscular awareness relaxation therapy, biofeedback training, and low-level laser therapy treatment, but that most studies were of poor methodological quality.[351]

Biofeedback training has a vast range of applications for health and prevention, particularly in which psychological factors play a role. Sleep disorders, hyperactivity in children, and other disorders respond well to biofeedback training. One more recent advance in biofeedback training is the use of neurofeedback, with people suffering from conditions caused by an unhealthy pattern of brain waves.[352-354] Biofeedback has been used extensively to test and alter states of arousal and brain waves. The practitioner helps the client to increase the appropriate brain frequency to achieve optimal performance. Neurofeedback has been shown to be helpful for people suffering from attention deficit disorder (ADD) and attention deficit hyperactivity disorder (ADHD).[354-356] Improvement in performance for individuals with learning disabilities also has been achieved. It also has shown promise in helping people who suffer from various addictions.

Dysfunctions that stem from inadequate control over the muscles or muscle groups, such as incontinence, postural problems, back pain, and even loss of control because of brain or nerve damage, have shown improvement when clients undergo biofeedback training. The evidence supporting the use of biofeedback for treatment of urinary or fecal incontinence is strong.[357-360]

Biofeedback also has been shown to help other problems such as heart dysfunctions, gastrointestinal disorders (acidity, ulcers, IBS), difficulty swallowing, esophageal dysfunction, tinnitus, twitching of the eyelids, fatigue, and cerebral palsy.[361]

The use of biofeedback to retrain muscles after physical trauma or stroke is well known to physical therapists and is integrated into standard practice. It has been said that all learning involves feedback. Biofeedback (EMG) can be used to help the client identify which muscles are involved and what actions are required, in addition to when, and to what degree, these actions are being achieved. It is also a means of nonbiased feedback that clients know is not being given just to make them feel better. For the therapist, it can aid in diagnosis, targeting, or clarification for the client and monitoring of progress. Understanding of the principles involved, limitations of the instruments, proper placement of electrodes, setting of parameters, and personal monitoring and verbal feedback are important skills and activities of the physical therapist employing biofeedback.[338] The utility of biofeedback in physical therapy is widely accepted, and clinical evidence supports this.[362-364] However, a 2004 review by Van Peppen et al found little evidence for its efficacy in improvement of functional outcomes after stroke.[365]

The latest developments in biofeedback concern the self-regulation of bodily functions that, until now, were considered inaccessible. If therapists are able to help people to have moment-to-moment feedback of the levels of chemicals in the bloodstream and give feedback that enables them to influence their hormone levels (such as insulin), then individuals may have the ability to profoundly influence their health.

### Biofeedback Summary

Strong clinical evidence exists for biofeedback's efficacy for a wide variety of psychological and physical ailments. Future research should increase the understanding of mechanisms and optimize interventions.

## SPIRITUALITY AND PRAYER

Spirituality may take many forms but may be considered to be a belief in something that helps give meaning to existence. It may be a way of thinking, feeling, and being that brings comfort in the face of the challenges and losses in life and appreciation for life's gifts. It may or may not be associated with some formal religion. Prayer most often is thought of as directed heartfelt thoughts or words, which

may be accompanied by ritual actions. It may seek a specific outcome or may be offered as worship. Meditation also can be considered a form of prayer and has been referred to as "centering prayer" in some contemporary Christian traditions.

### Brief History of Spirituality and Prayer

Some argue that spirituality is an intrinsic human quality. Although the presence and strength vary in individuals, and even at different times within a person's life, it is found across all cultures and throughout the course of history. For as far back as artifacts and art of prehistoric cultures exist is evidence of ritual and probable belief in the "supernatural." The cave drawings of ancient civilizations in the European continent could be seen as a form of prayer to enhance the outcome of hunting expeditions. Fertility goddesses and praying statues of the ancient Near East, the huge and elaborate temples and tombs of Egypt, artwork, artifacts and temples of the Americas and the Indian subcontinent, in addition to the practice in China of burying replicas of soldiers and horses with the ruler, give voice to the complex and powerful beliefs of the people of those times and places.

It only has been fairly recently that man's spiritual beliefs and prayer have been examined in the context of clinical trials to attempt to determine their effects on health in other than anecdotal reports. The major types of studies have been for intercessory prayer or "third person" praying for someone else, at a distance, or in personal contact. Other studies look at personal spirituality and prayer and look at correlation with various outcomes of health and well-being (Figure 7-3).

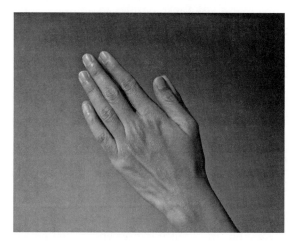

**Figure 7-3** A traditional hand position during prayer.

## Review of the Spirituality and Prayer Scientific Literature

Scientific studies on intercessory prayer and distance healing have yielded mixed results. A review by Astin, Harkness, and Ernst in 2000 of randomized trials of "distant healing" showed a positive trend.[366] However, most major, well-controlled trials since that time have been negative. Further research is needed to determine the true efficacy of prayer in improvement of the health of clients.

In one study, distance healing was performed on 40 clients with advanced AIDS. Numerous religions and spiritual traditions were represented by the participating healers. After 6 months, researchers discovered that clients who had been the subjects of distance healing had shown statistically significant improvements in their health. These clients had acquired fewer new AIDS-defining illnesses and lower illness severity. They also had significantly fewer doctor visits and hospitalizations; when hospitalized, the length of their stay was significantly shorter. In addition, clients who had received distance healing showed significantly improved mood. This study showed that distance healing had a statistically significant positive impact on the health of clients with advanced AIDS.[367]

Intercessory prayer is a popular method of distance healing. Its effectiveness is controversial; many studies have found that it has a significant positive impact on clients, but many others have found no difference between the health of clients receiving intercessory prayer and of those who are not. One study found that clients who unknowingly received remote, intercessory prayer after being admitted to a coronary care unit generally had lower CCU course scores. This shows that intercessory prayer may have a positive effect on a client's health.[368] Another study on prayer's effect on cardiovascular disease found no that it had no significant effect on the health of clients recently discharged from a coronary care unit. Five people prayed for the health of each client randomly chosen to receive intercessory prayer. At the end of the study, no significant difference was found between the progression of cardiovascular disease in clients who had received intercessory prayer and those who had not.[369] In another study, remote intercessory prayer was associated with shorter hospital stays and shorter fever durations in clients with bloodstream infections.[370] Yet another study found no significant improvements in the health of children with psychiatric conditions after they received intercessory prayer.[371]

Intercessory prayer also has been used to increase the likelihood of successful in vitro fertilization–embryo transfer (IVF-ET). Women undergoing this procedure in Seoul, South Korea, were not informed that prayer groups in the United States, Australia, and Canada were praying for them. Women who received intercessory prayer had a 50% rate of pregnancy (the control group's rate was 26%) and an implantation rate of 16.3% (instead of the control group's 8%). This study showed a statistically significant increase in the success rate of IVF-ET when it is accompanied by intercessory prayer.[372]

Effectiveness between remote and direct-contact intercessory prayer may differ. The previously discussed studies studied the effects of remote prayer on unsuspecting subjects. Research has been done on the effects of direct-contact prayer as well. In one study, clients suffering from class II or III rheumatoid arthritis received a 3-day treatment that included 6 hours of direct-contact prayer. Some of these clients were randomly selected to receive additional prayer performed by people in distant locations. After 1 year, clients who had received intercessory prayer from a person in close proximity showed significant improvement in the severity of their arthritis. Clients who received long-distance prayer showed no significant additional improvement.[373]

The benefits of intercessory prayer may derive from a client's belief in its effectiveness. A study of clients undergoing hemodialysis found neither intercessory prayer nor positive visualization to be effective treatments. Clients who expected to receive prayers did report feeling significantly better than clients expecting to be the subjects of positive visualizations, but no physical changes were attributed to either method of complementary therapy.[374]

Directed prayer asks for a specific outcome to occur; nondirected prayer asks for the generalized improvement of a situation without specifying the way in which such improvement should occur. One study measured the difference between directed and nondirected prayer when used for healing. The volunteers who prayed and those who were prayed for took five tests that scored them on 11 measures of objective well-being. After 12 weeks of either directed or nondirected prayer, all participants retook the test. Those who had been prayed for improved significantly on all measures of well-being and all who had prayed improved on all but one measure. Those who had prayed had significantly higher scores than those for whom someone had prayed. The more time a participant had spent praying, the more his or her scores increased on the objective tests. This study suggests that praying may have benefits for all participants of intercessory prayer. Improvement on some of the objective measures was associated positively with the subject's belief in the effectiveness of prayer and the subject's belief that someone was praying for him or her.[375]

Other studies also have hinted that a client's belief in prayer can affect the effectiveness of intercessory prayer. One study used prayer directed at solving a specific problem each participant mentioned at the beginning of the study. No significant effect on the resolution of each subject's problem was found, but concern about the problem was reduced in participants in the prayer group. Those who had been prayed for and believed in prayer had better physical functioning, whereas those in the control group who did not believe in prayer had better mental health.[376]

Research has been conducted to determine whether intercessory prayer is an effective complement to standard treatments for alcohol abuse. The relevant study assigned 40 clients in a public substance abuse treatment center into two groups; one received prayer from outside volunteers, whereas the other did not. No differences in alcohol consumption were found between the two groups; in fact, participants in the study did not reduce their drinking as soon as clients at the same treatment facility who were not involved in the study. Surprisingly, clients who had a friend or family member praying for them in addition to the volunteers in the study were drinking significantly more after 6 months of treatment than clients who did not have any extra people praying for them. Although intercessory prayer was found to have no positive impact on clients undergoing treatment for alcohol abuse, prayer performed by the clients was associated with less drinking after a few months.[377]

The recently released results of the largest study of prayer completed conclude that distant intercessory prayer was not effective in reduction of complications after heart surgery.[378] The study involved 1802 bypass clients from six hospitals who were assigned randomly to one of three groups. Group 1 received intercessory prayer after being told they may or may not receive it. Group 2 did not receive intercessory prayers after being told they may or may not receive it. Group 3 were told they would be receiving intercessory prayer and did receive it. The study of the therapeutic effects of intercessory prayer, or STEP, is the sixth study to find that inter-

cessory prayer has no real effect on the well-being of clients. An unexpected finding was that the group of heart clients who knew they were receiving prayers from strangers did not do as well as those who did not know. Perhaps having been selected to receive prayer may have caused more worry about their health and potential outcomes. Some individuals may not have been comfortable with the idea of strangers praying for them. Given these and other unresolved issues, investigators said that possibly intercessory prayer may not be amenable to randomized control methodology and that a large-scale study like this may not be replicated.

Although intercessory prayer has a mixed record of effectiveness, personal spirituality generally is associated with greater well-being. One study found that clients leaving drug abuse treatment who regularly attended religious services had fewer drug problems after treatment ended.[379] Although the sense of community fostered by religious services also may have decreased a subject's likelihood of relapse, personal religious faith is also a likely factor in deterrence of continued drug abuse. Intercessory prayer did not assist the recovery of alcohol abusers, but personal faith may aid recovering drug addiction.

Clients with strong religious backgrounds often benefit from treatment that incorporates their beliefs. In a study of clients with strong personal faith and depression or anxiety disorders, psychotherapy that incorporated religious beliefs caused a significantly faster initial response to treatment.[380] Religious belief also influences treatment preferences of clients with advanced lung or colon cancer. Those who believe in divine intervention and cite spirituality as a major strategy for coping with cancer were more likely to want hospitalization, CPR, and mechanical ventilation to sustain life.[381] Health providers must take religious belief into account in the treatment of clients, especially elderly clients. A study of clients over age 60 admitted to a hospital found that more than one half (53.4%) of the clients attended weekly religious services, 85% reported holding intrinsic religious attitudes, and 40% claimed that religious faith was their most important method for coping with ill health. Strong religious faith was associated with African Americans and individuals with lower levels of education and greater life stressors.[382] If incorporating spirituality with standard treatment is shown to significantly help the recovery of religious clients, these statistics show that many people would benefit.

Psychological stress is associated with the presence and severity of symptoms in clients with fibromyalgia. A study of women with fibromyalgia found that those reporting low levels of intrinsic spirituality had a less regular cortisol rhythm. Clients with greater spirituality had high cortisol levels in the morning and low levels in the evening, whereas those with low spirituality had less variation in cortisol levels. Spirituality therefore is correlated positively with more normal patterns in this marker of stress in women with fibromyalgia.[383] A study of women with metastatic breast cancer also found that spirituality may affect the immune system. Women who reported greater spirituality had more circulating white blood cells and a greater number of lymphocytes, including helper and cytotoxic T-cells.[384]

## Spirituality and Prayer Summary

The results of studies to determine the efficacy of intercessory prayer for improvement of health are mixed. Some feel that certain methodological challenges make it impossible to perform definitive randomized clinical trials on intercessory prayer. Others propose that this is not a subject amenable to clinical trials because the effect of prayer is not a replicable commodity. However, strong and consistent evidence exists for personal spirituality and prayer having positive health correlations.

## DISCUSSION AND CONCLUSIONS

Much of modern theoretical and experimental physics has strong overlap in its understanding of the nature of reality with ancient views arrived at intuitively in higher states of conciousness.[385,386] The view of the universe as composed of opposites with underlying unity, and the need for balance between these opposites, is congruent with the emerging understanding of the mind-body and its physical, biochemical, and psychological makeup.

This is an exciting time of exploration and transition in medicine throughout the world. It will be interesting to see to what degree the tools and methods of modern biological and psychological science will elucidate and be informed by knowledge from the ancient sources. Mind-body (and mind-body-spirit) research should continue to provide new insights and improved methodologies for years to come. Hopefully, what will emerge will be a synergistic melding of the best of ancient traditional practices with modern scientific tools, understanding, and proof, which will benefit the earth and all of its inhabitants.

## ACKNOWLEDGMENTS

Dr. Gould Fogerite wishes to thank Ms. Julia Fogerite for excellent assistance with research and writing of the section on prayer and spirituality and Dr. Rene David Alkalay for general critical review and helpful suggestions for the yoga and biofeedback sections. She also is grateful to Ms. Marie K. Saimbert for help with literature searches to Dr. Peter Kurzynski for sharing meditation research and references, and to Dr. Adam Perlman and Dr. Judith Deutsch for patience and support during the lengthy process of researching and writing this chapter.

## ADDITIONAL RESOURCES
### Journal Articles
#### Mind-Body Medicine
Astin JA: Mind-body therapies for the management of pain, *Clin J Pain* 20(1):27-32, 2004.

Astin JA et al: Mind-body medicine: state of the science, implications for practice, *J Am Board Fam Pract* 16(2):131-47, 2003.

Barrows KA, Jacobs BP: Mind-body medicine. An introduction and review of the literature, *Med Clin North Am* 86:11-31, 2002.

Gordon JS, Edwards DM: MindBodySpirit Medicine, *Semin Oncol Nurs* 21(3):154-8, 2005.

Luskin FM et al: A review of mind/body therapies in the treatment of musculoskeletal disorders with implications for the elderly, *Altern Ther Health Med* 6(2):46-56, 2000.

Pert CB, Dreher HE, Ruff MR: The psychosomatic network: foundations of mind-body medicine, *Altern Ther Health Med* 4(4):30-41, 1998.

#### Yoga
Bijlani RL: Influence of yoga on brain and behaviour: facts and speculations, *Ind J Physiol Pharmacol* 48(1):1-5, 2004.

Garfinkle M, Schumacher HR: Yoga, *Rheum Dis Clin North Am* (1):125-32, 2000.

Khalsa SBS: Yoga as a therapeutic intervention: a bibliometric analysis of published research studies, *Ind J Physiol Pharmacol* 48(3):269-85, 2004.

Raub JA: Psychophysiologic effects of Hatha Yoga on musculoskeletal and cardiopulmonary function: a literature review, *J Altern Complement Med* 8(6):797-812, 2002.

Sovik R: The science of breathing—the yogic view, *Progr Brain Res* 122:491-505, 2000.

#### Meditation
Krisanaprakornkit T et al: Meditation therapy for anxiety disorders, *Cochrane Database Syst Rev* (1): CD004998, 2006.

Smith JE et al: Mindfulness-based stress reduction as supportive therapy in cancer care: systematic review, *J Advanc Nurs* 52(3):315-27, 2005.

### Tai Chi

Adler PA, Roberts BL: The use of Tai Chi to improve health in older adults, *Orthop Nurs* 25(2):122-6, 2006.

Gillespie LD et al: Interventions for preventing falls in elderly people, *Cochrane Database System Rev* (4): CD000340, 2003.

### Guided Imagery

Gruzelier JH: A review of the impact of hypnosis, relaxation, guided imagery and individual differences on aspects of immunity and health, *Stress* 5(2):147-63, 2002.

Liu KP et al: Mental imagery for promoting relearning for people after stroke: a randomized controlled trial, *Arch Phys Med Rehabil* 85(9):1403-8, 2004.

### Hypnosis

Barber TX: A deeper understanding of hypnosis: its secrets, its nature, its essence, *Am J Clin Hypnosis* 42(3-4):208-72, 2000.

Stewart JH: Hypnosis in contemporary medicine, *Mayo Clin Proc* 80(4):511-24, 2005.

### Cognitive-Behavioral Therapies

Beck AT: The current state of cognitive therapy: a 40-year retrospective, *Arch Gen Psychiatr* 62(9):953-9, 2005.

Butler AC et al: The empirical status of cognitive-behavioral therapy: a review of meta-analyses, *Clin Psychol Rev* 26(1):17-31, 2006.

Adams N, Poole H, Richardson C: Psychological approaches to chronic pain management: part 1, *J Clin Nurs* 15(3):290-300, 2006.

### Biofeedback

Haythornthwaite JA, Benrud-Larson LM: Psychological assessment and treatment of clients with neuropathic pain, *Curr Pain Headache Rep* 5(2):124-9, 2001.

McNeely ML, Armijo Olivo S, Magee DJ: A systematic review of the effectiveness of physical therapy interventions for temporomandibular disorders, *Phys Ther* 86(5):710-25, 2006.

Penzien DB, Rains JC, Andrasik F: Behavioral management of recurrent headache: three decades of experience and empiricism, *Appl Psychophysiol Biofeedback* 27(2):163-81, 2002.

Van Peppen RPS et al: The impact of physical therapy on functional outcomes after stroke: what's the evidence? *Clin Rehabil* 18(8):833-62, 2004.

### Spirituality and Prayer

Astin JA, Harkness E, Ernst E: The efficacy of "distant healing": a systematic review of randomized trials, *Ann Intern Med* 132(11):903-10, 2000.

Dusek JA et al: Healing prayer outcomes studies: consensus recommendations, *Altern Ther Health Med* 9(3 suppl):A44-53, 2003.

Seeman TE, Dubin LF, Seeman M: Religiosity/ spirituality and health. A critical review of the evidence for biological pathways, *Am Psychol* 58(1):53-63, 2003.

### Selected Books
### Mind-Body Medicine

Dossey L: *Healing beyond the body: medicine and the infinite reach of the mind,* Boston, 2001, Shambhala.

Liebowitz R et al, editors: *The Duke University encyclopedia of the new medicine,* New York, 2006, Rodale.

Ornish D: *Dr. Dean Ornish's program for reversing heart disease,* New York, 1990, Random House.

Rakel D, editor: *Integrative medicine,* ed 2, Philadelphia, 2007, Saunders Elsevier.

### Yoga

Anderson S, Sovik R: *Yoga, mastering the basics,* Honesdale, Penn, 2000, Himalayan Institute Press.

Arya U: *Philosophy of Hatha yoga,* ed 2, Honesdale, Penn, 1998, Himalayan Institute of Yoga Science and Philosophy of the USA.

Arya U: *Yoga sutras of Patanjali with exposition of Vyasa, translation and commentary,* vol I, Honesdale, Penn, 1986, Himalayan Institute of Yoga Science and Philosophy of the USA.

Coulter H: *Anatomy of Hatha yoga: a manual for students, teachers, and practitioners,* Honesdale, Penn, 2001, Body and Breath.

Rama S, Ballentine R, editors: *Joints and gland exercises,* Honesdale, Penn, 1996, Himalayan Institute Press.

Rama S, Ballentine R, Hynes A: *Science of breath,* Honesdale, Penn, 1998, Himalayan Institute Press.

Ramaswami S: *Yoga for the three stages of life: developing your practice as an art form, a physical therapy, and a guiding philosophy,* Rochester, Vt, 2000, Inner Traditions International.

Veda S: *Yoga sutras of Patanjali with exposition of Vyasa, translation and commentary,* vol II, Delhi, 2001, Motilal Banaridass Publishers.

### Meditation

Arya U: *Superconscious meditation,* Honesdale, Penn, 1978, Himalayan Institute of Yoga Science and Philosophy of the USA.

Benson H: *The relaxation response,* New York, 1993, Outlet Books.

Chernin D: *How to meditate using chakras, mantras and breath,* Ann Arbor, Mich, 2002, Think Publishing.

Goleman D: *The meditative mind,* Los Angeles, 1988, Jeremy P Tarcher.

Kabat-Zinn J: *Full catastrophe living: using the wisdom of your body and mind to face stress, pain, and illness,* New York, 1991, Delta (Dell Publishing).

Keating T: *Foundations for centering prayer and the Christian contemplative life: open mind, open heart, invitation to love, mystery of Christ*, New York, 2002, The Continuum International Publishing Group.

Murphy M, Donovan S: *The physical and psychological effects of meditation. a review of contemporary research and a comprehensive bibliography, 1931-1996*, Sausalito, Calif, 1999, Institute of Noetic Sciences.*

Rama S: *Meditation and its practice*, Honesdale, Penn, 1998, Himalayan Institute Press.

Rama S et al: *Meditation in Christianity*, Honesdale, Penn, 1989, Himalayan Institute of Yoga Science and Philosophy of the USA.

### Tai Chi

Liao W: *The essence of tai chi*, Boston, 1995, Shambhala Publications.

See Chapter 9 for additional references.

### Guided Imagery

Borysenko J: *Minding the body, mending the mind*, Reading, Mass, 1988, Bantam.

Bresler D: *Free yourself from pain*, Topanga, Calif, 1992, The Bresler Center.

Naparstek B: *Survivors of trauma and how they heal*, New York, 2004, Bantam Books.

### Hypnosis

Elman D: *Hypnotherapy*, Glendale, Calif, 1984, Westwood Publishing Company.

Rhue J, Lynn S, Kirsch I: *Handbook of clinical hypnosis*, Washington, DC, 1993, American Psychological Association.

Tinterow M: *Hypnosis, acupuncture, and pain*, Wichita, Kan, 1989, Bio-Communication Press.

### Cognitive-Behavioral Therapies

Banks S: *The enlightened gardener*, Edmonton, Calif, 2001, Lone Pine Publishing.

Burns D: *Feeling good: the new mood therapy*, New York, 1999, Harper Collins, 1999.

Ellis A: *Overcoming destructive beliefs, feelings and behaviors: new directions for rational emotive behavior therapy*, Amherst, NY, 2001, Prometheus Books.

Linehan M, Miller A, Rathus J: *Dialectical behavior therapy with suicidal adolescents*, New York, 2007, Guilford Press.

### Biofeedback

Basmajian J: Introduction: principles and background. In Basmajian J, editor: *Biofeedback: principles and practice for clinicians*, Baltimore, 1989, Williams and Wilkins.

Danskin D, Crow M: *Biofeedback: an introduction and guide*, Palo Alto, Calif, 1981, Mayfield Publishing.

Murphy M: *The future of the body: explorations into the further evolution of the human species*, Los Angeles, 1992, Jeremy Tarcher.

Yucha C, Gilbert C: *Evidence based practice in biofeedback & neurofeedback*, Wheat Ridge, Colo, 2004, AAPB.

### Spirituality and Prayer

Dossey L: *Healing words: the power of prayer and the practice of medicine*, New York, 1993, Harper Collins.

Hanh TN: *The energy of prayer: how to deepen your spiritual practice*, Berkeley, Calif, 2006, Parallax Press.

Keating T: *Foundations for centering prayer and the Christian contemplative life: open mind, open heart, invitation to love, mystery of Christ*, New York, 2002, The Continuum International Publishing Group.

Ross M: *The fire of your life*, London, 2007, Seabury Books.

### Selected Websites
### Mind-Body Medicine

*National Center for Complementary and Alternative Medicine, National Institutes of Health: http://nccam.nih.gov*

Benson-Henry Institute for Mind Body Medicine: http://www.mbmi.org

### Yoga and Meditation

*Bindu. Gateway to the Himalayan Yoga Tradition:http://www.bindu.org*

*Integrative Yoga Therapy: http://www.iytyogatherapy.com*

*Swami Veda Bharati's World Wide Mission http://www.swamiveda.org*

*Traditional Yoga and Meditation of the Himalayan Masters:http://www.swamij.com/self-realization-himalayan-tradition-htm*

### Tai Chi

*International TaiChi Chuan Association: http://www.itcca.org*

*Tai Chi and Qigong Links: http://www.mtsu.edu/~jpurcell/Taichi/tc-links.htm*

### Guided Imagery

*Eupsychia Institute: http:// www.eupsychia.com*
*Guided Imagery Inc.:*
*Health Journeys. Resources for Mind, Body, Spirit: http://www.healthjourneys.com*
*http:// www.guidedimageryinc.com*

### Hypnosis

Hypnosis Motivation Institute: http://www.hypnosis.edu

*This bibliography and an update to September 2002 are available on the IONS website (*http://www.ions.org*).

**Derby Hospitals NHS Foundation Trust**
**Library and Knowledge Service**

Mayo Clinic. Hypnosis: Altered State of Consciousness: http://www.mayoclinic.com/health/hypnosis/SA00084

*The Milton H. Erickson Foundation http://www.erickson-foundation.org*

### Cognitive-Behavioral Therapies

*National Association of Cognitive-Behavioral Therapists: http://www.nacbt.org*

*PsychNet-UK. Cognitive Behavioral Therapy: http://www.psychnet-uk.com/psychotherapy/psychotherapy_cognitive_behavioural_therapyhtm*

### Biofeedback

*Applied Psychophysiology & Biofeedback: http://www.aapb.org*

*Biocybernaut Institute The Gold Standard in Neurobiofeedback: http://www.biocybernaut.com*

*The Institute of Noetic Sciences: http://www.ions.org*

### Spirituality and Prayer

Association for Transpersonal Psychology http://www.atpweb.org

John Templeton Foundation: http://www.templeton.org

## REFERENCES

1. Benjamin SA et al: Alternative medicine, part two: mind-body medicine: expanding the health model, *Patient Care* 31(14):126-8, 1997.
2. Astin JA, Forys K: Psychosocial determinants of health and illness: integrating mind, body, and spirit, *Adv Mind Body Med* 20(4):14-21, 2004.
3. Astin JA et al: Mind-body medicine: state of the science, implications for practice, *J Am Board Fam Pract* 16(2):131-47, 2003.
4. Gilbert MD: Weaving medicine back together: mind-body medicine in the twenty-first century, *J Altern Complement Med* 9(4):563-70, 2003.
5. Gordon JS: Mind body medicine, *Total Health* 26(6):54-6, 2004.
6. Riley D: The mind/body continuum, *Altern Ther Health Med* 6(2):34, 2000.
7. McDowell B: Mind/body medicine: from the relaxation response to mindfulness, *Altern Complement Ther* 1(2):80-7, 1995.
8. Gordon JS, Edwards DM: MindBodySpirit Medicine, *Semin Oncol Nurs* 21(3):154-8, 2005.
9. Tataryn DJ: Paradigms of health and disease: a framework for classifying and understanding complementary and alternative medicine, *J Altern Complement Med* 8(6):877-92, 2002.
10. Luskin F: Transformative practices for integrating mind-body-spirit . . . *J Altern Complement Med* 10(suppl1):S-15-23, 2004.
11. Bolletino RC: A model of spirituality for psychotherapy and other fields of mind-body medicine, *Adv Mind Body Med* 17(2):90-101, 104-7, 2001.
12. Ben-Arye E et al: Is a biopsychosocial-spiritual approach relevant to cancer treatment? A study of patients and oncology staff members on issues of complementary medicine and spirituality, *Support Care Cancer* 14(2):147-52, 2006.
13. Dusek JA et al: Healing prayer outcomes studies: consensus recommendations, *Altern Ther Health Med* 9(suppl 3):A44-53, 2003.
14. Miller WR, Thoresen CE: Spirituality, religion, and health: an emerging research field, *Am Psychologist* 58(1):24-35, 2003.
15. Powell LH, Shahabi L, Thoresen CE: Religion and spirituality. Linkages to physical health, *Am Psychol* 58(1):36-52, 2003.
16. Seeman TE, Dubin LF, Seeman M: Religiosity/spirituality and health. A critical review of the evidence for biological pathways, *Am Psychologist* 58(1):53-63, 2003.
17. Sloan RP, Bagiella E, Powell T: Religion, spirituality, and medicine, *Lancet* 353(9153):664-7, 1999.
18. Rossiter T: The effectiveness of neurofeedback and stimulant drugs in treating AD/HD: Part I. Review of methodological issues, *Appl Psychophysiol Biofeedback* 29(2):95-112, 2004.
19. Astin JA: Mind-body therapies for the management of pain, *Clin J Pain* 20(1):27-32, 2004.
20. Luskin FM et al: A review of mind/body therapies in the treatment of musculoskeletal disorders with implications for the elderly, *Altern Ther Health Med* 6(2):46-56, 2000.
21. Chan C, Ho PSY, Chow E: A body-mind-spirit model in health: an Eastern approach, *Social Work Health Care* 34(3/4):261-82, 2001.
22. Martin JB: Keynote address: historical and professional perspectives of complementary and alternative medicine with a particular emphasis on rediscovering and embracing complementary and alternative medicine in contemporary Western society. Papers from the Symposium on Scientific Integration of Western Medicine and Complementary, Alternative-Mind, Body Medicine, Seoul, Korea. *J Altern Complement Med* 7(suppl 1):S11-8, 2001.
23. Hassed CS: Bringing holism into mainstream biomedical education, *J Altern Complement Med* 10(2):405-7, 2004.
24. Doggett AM: ADHD and drug therapy: is it still a valid treatment? *J Child Health Care* 8(1):69-81, 2004.
25. Astin JA: Stress reduction through mindfulness meditation. Effects on psychological symptomatology, sense of control, and spiritual experiences, *Psychother Psychosomat* 66(2):97-106, 1997.
26. Astin JA et al: Sense of control and adjustment to breast cancer: the importance of balancing control coping styles, *Behav Med* 25(3):101-9, 1999.

27. Astin JA et al: Psychological interventions for rheumatoid arthritis: a meta-analysis of randomized controlled trials, *Arthr Rheum* 47(3):291-302, 2002.

28. Cohen S, Tyrrell D, Smith A: Psychological stress and susceptibility to the common cold, *N Engl J Med* 325:606-12, 1991.

29. Jacobs GD The physiology of mind-body interactions: the stress response and the relaxation response. Papers from the Symposium on Scientific Integration of Western Medicine and Complementary, Alternative-Mind, Body Medicine, Seoul, Korea [corrected], *J Altern Complement Med* 7(suppl 1):S83-92, 2001. (Erratum, *J Altern Complement Med* 2002 8[2]:219, 2002.)

30. Rossi EL: Psychosocial genomics: gene expression, neurogenesis, and human experience in mind-body medicine, *Adv Mind-Body Med* 18(2):22-30, 2002.

31. Bauer-Wu SM: Psychoneuroimmunology. Part II: mind-body interventions, *Clin J Oncol Nurs* 6(4):243-6, 2002.

32. Kiecolt-Glaser JK et al: Psychoneuroimmunology: psychological influences on immune function and health, *J Consult Clin Psychol* 70(3):537-47, 2002.

33. Kiecolt-Glaser JK et al: Emotions, morbidity, and mortality: new perspectives from psychoneuroimmunology, *Ann Rev Psychol* 53:83-107, 2002.

34. Idler EL, Kasl SV, Lemke JH: Self evaluated health and mortality among the elderly in New Haven, CT, and Washington Counties, IO, 1982-1986, *Am J Epidemiol* 131(1):91-103, 1990.

35. Cohen S: Emotional style and susceptibility to the common cold, *Psychosomat Med* 65(4):652-7, 2003.

36. Cannon WB: *The wisdom of the body, 1932,* New York.

37. Rossi EL: Stress-induced alternative gene splicing in mind-body medicine, *Adv Mind-Body Med* 20(2):12-9, 2004.

38. Bauer-Wu SM: Psychoneuroimmunology. Part I: physiology, *Clin J Oncol Nurs* 6(3):167-70, 2002.

39. Cardinali DP, Cutrera RA, Esquifino AI: Psychoimmune neuroendocrine integrative mechanisms revisited, *Biol Signal Recept* 9(5):215-30, 2000.

40. Selye H: *The stress of life,* New York, 1956, McGraw-Hill.

41. Friedman EM, Irwin MR: Modulation of immune cell function by the autonomic nervous system, *Pharmacol Therapeut* 74(1):27-38, 1997.

42. Mann SJ: The mind/body link in essential hypertension: time for a new paradigm, *Altern Ther Health Med* 6(2):39-45, 2000.

43. Ader R: On the development of psychoneuroimmunology, *Eur J Pharmacol* 405(1-3):167-76, 2000.

44. Glaser R: Stress-associated immune dysregulation and its importance for human health: a personal history of psychoneuroimmunology, *Brain Behav Immun* 19(1):3-11, 2005.

45. Kaplin A, Bartner S: Reciprocal communication between the nervous and immune systems: crosstalk, back-talk and motivational speeches, *Int Rev Psychiatry* 17(6):439-41, 2005.

46. Kerr D et al: The immune system and neuropsychiatric diseases, *Int Rev Psychiatry* 17(6):443-9, 2005.

47. Antoni MH: Psychoneuroendocrinology and psychoneuroimmunology of cancer: plausible mechanisms worth pursuing? *Brain Behav Immun* 17(suppl 1):S84-91, 2003.

48. Pert C: *Alternative medicine: the definitive guide,* New York, 1995, The Burton Goldberg Group, Future Medicine Publishing.

49. Pert CB, Dreher HE, Ruff MR: The psychosomatic network: foundations of mind-body medicine, *Altern Ther Health Med* 4(4):30-41, 1998.

50. Antoni MH: Stress management effects on psychological, endocrinological, and immune functioning in men with HIV infection: empirical support for a psychoneuroimmunological model, *Stress* 6(3):173-88, 2003.

51. Fleshner M, Laudenslager ML: Psychoneuroimmunology: then and now, *Behav Cogn Neurosci Rev* 3(2):114-30, 2004.

52. Friedman EM, Irwin MR: A role for CRH and the sympathetic nervous system in stress-induced immunosuppression, *Ann N Y Acad Sci* 771:396-418, 1995.

53. Moyad MA, Pienta KJ: Mind-body effect: insulin-like growth factor-1; clinical depression; and breast, prostate, and other cancer risk-an unmeasured and masked mediator of potential significance? *Urology* 59(4 suppl 1):4-8, 2002.

54. Callaghan BD: Does the pineal gland have a role in the psychological mechanisms involved in the progression of cancer? *Med Hypotheses* 59(3):302-11, 2002.

55. Beecher H: *Measurement of subjective responses,* New York, 1959, Oxford University Press.

56. Kupers R, Faymonville M-E, Laureys S: The cognitive modulation of pain: hypnosis- and placebo-induced analgesia, *Prog Brain Res* 150:251-69, 2005.

57. Rainville P, Bushnell MC, Duncan GH: Representation of acute and persistent pain in the human CNS: potential implications for chemical intolerance, *Ann N Y Acad Sci* 933:130-41, 2001.

58. De Pascalis V, Chiaradia C, Carotenuto E: The contribution of suggestibility and expectation to placebo analgesia phenomenon in an experimental setting, *Pain* 96(3):393-402, 2002.

59. Schweizer E, Rickels K: Placebo response in generalized anxiety: its effect on the outcome of clinical trials, *J Clin Psychiatry* 58(suppl 11):30-8, 1997.

60. Astin JA et al: A review of the incorporation of complementary and alternative medicine by mainstream physicians, *Arch Intern Med* 158(21):2303-10, 1998.

61. Astin JA: Why patients use alternative medicine: results of a national study, *JAMA* 279(19):1548-53, 1998.

62. Wolsko PM et al: Use of mind-body medical therapies, *J Gen Intern Med* 19(1):43-50, 2004.

63. Astin JA et al: Complementary and alternative medicine use among elderly persons: one-year analysis of a Blue Shield Medicare supplement, *J Gerontol A Biol Sci Med Sci* 55(1):M4-9, 2000.

64. Eisenberg DM et al: Unconventional medicine in the United States: Prevalence, costs, and patterns of use, *N Engl J Med* 328:246-52, 1993.

65. Eisenberg DM et al: Trends in alternative medicine use in the United States, 1990-1997: results of a follow-up national survey, *JAMA* 280(18):1569-75, 1998.

66. Tindle HA et al: Trends in use of complementary and alternative medicine by US adults: 1997-2002, *Altern Ther Health Med* 11(1):42-9, 2005.

67. Graham RE et al: Use of complementary and alternative medical therapies among racial and ethnic minority adults: results from the 2002 National Health Interview Survey, *J Nat Med Assoc* 97(4):535-45, 2005.

68. Conboy L et al: Sociodemographic determinants of the utilization of specific types of complementary and alternative medicine: an analysis based on a nationally representative survey sample, *J Altern Complement Med* 11(6):977-94, 2005.

69. Fairfield KM et al: Patterns of use, expenditures, and perceived efficacy of complementary and alternative therapies in HIV-infected patients, *Arch Intern Med* 158(20):2257-64, 1998.

70. Ashikaga T et al: Use of complimentary and alternative medicine by breast cancer patients: prevalence, patterns and communication with physicians, *Support Care Cancer* 10(7):542-8, 2002.

71. Lee MM et al: Alternative therapies used by women with breast cancer in four ethnic populations, *J Nat Cancer Inst* 92(1):42-7, 2000.

72. Adler SR: Complementary and alternative medicine use among women with breast cancer, *Med Anthropol Q* 13(2):214-22, 1999.

73. Owens B, Dirksen SR: Review and critique of the literature of complementary and alternative therapy use among Hispanic/Latino women with breast cancer, *Clin J Oncol Nurs* 8(2):151-6, 2004.

74. Diehl DL, Eisenberg D: Complementary and alternative medicine (CAM): epidemiology and implications for research, *Progr Brain Res* 122:445-55, 2000.

75. Eisenberg DM: The Institute of Medicine report on complementary and alternative medicine in the United States: personal reflections on its content and implications, *Altern Ther Health Med* 11(3):10-5, 2005.

76. Adler SR, Fosket JR: Disclosing complementary and alternative medicine use in the medical encounter: a qualitative study in women with breast cancer, *J Fam Pract* 48(6):453-8, 1999.

77. Perlman AI, Eisenberg DM, Panush RS: Talking with patients about alternative and complementary medicine, *Rheum Dis Clin North Am* 25(4):815-22, 1999.

78. Kaptchuk T, Eisenberg D, Komaroff A: Research. Finding out what works, *Newsweek,* Dec 2, 2002, p 73.

79. Cohen MH et al: Emerging credentialing practices, malpractice liability policies, and guidelines governing complementary and alternative medical practices and dietary supplement recommendations: a descriptive study of 19 integrative health care centers in the United States. (Erratum, *Arch Intern Med* 11;165(7):730, 2005. Note: Kemper, Kathi J [added]; Boyer, Edward W [added]]. *Arch Intern Med.* Feb 14 2005;165(3):289-295.

80. Cohen MH et al: Policies pertaining to complementary and alternative medical therapies in a random sample of 39 academic health centers, *Altern Ther Health Med* 11(1):36-40, 2005.

81. Allen KD: Using biofeedback to make childhood headaches less of a pain, *Ped Ann* 33(4):241-5, 2004.

82. Pelletier KR, Astin JA, Haskell WL: Current trends in the integration and reimbursement of complementary and alternative medicine by managed care organizations (MCOs) and insurance providers: 1998 update and cohort analysis, *Am J Health Promotion* 14(2):125-33, 1999.

83. Eisenberg D: Alternative medical therapies for rheumatologic disorders, *Arthritis Care Res* 9(1):1-4, 1996.

84. Cherkin D, Sherman K, Eisenberg D: Back pain: beyond the backache, *Newsweek,* Dec 2, 2002, p 56.

85. Wolsko PM et al: Patterns and perceptions of care for treatment of back and neck pain: results of a national survey, *Spine,* Feb 1, 2003, pp 292-297.

86. Astin JA et al: The efficacy of mindfulness meditation plus qigong movement therapy in the treatment of fibromyalgia: a randomized controlled trial, *J Rheumatol* 30(10):2257-62, 2003.

87. Kessler RC et al: The use of complementary and alternative therapies to treat anxiety and depression in the United States, *Am J Psychiatr* 158(2):289-94, 2001.

88. Krauss HH et al: Use of alternative treatments for emotional dysphoria by individuals with physically disabling conditions, *Percept Mot Skills* 85(3 Pt 2):1450, 1997.

89. Krauss HH et al: Alternative health care: its use by individuals with physical disabilities, *Arch Phys Med Rehabil* 79(11):1440-7, 1998.

90. Ernst E, Filshie J, Hardy J: Evidence-based complementary medicine for palliative cancer care: does it make sense? *Palliat Med* 17(8):704-7, 2003.

91. Weiger W, Eisenberg D: Cancer. Easing the treatment, *Newsweek,* Dec 2, 2002, p 49.

92. Ashby MA et al: Psychosocial support, treatment of metastatic disease and palliative care, *Med J Aust* 164(1):43-9, 1996.

93. Elkins G et al: Can hypnosis reduce hot flashes in breast cancer survivors? A literature review, *Am J Clin Hypn* 47(1):29-42, 2004.

94. Ernst E: Complementary therapies in palliative cancer care, *Cancer* 91(11):2181-5, 2001.

95. Monti DA, Yang J: Complementary medicine in chronic cancer care, *Semin Oncol* 32(2):225-31, 2005.

96. Nahleh Z, Tabbara IA: Complementary and alternative medicine in breast cancer patients, *Palliat Support Care* 1(3):267-73, 2003.

97. Newell SA, Sanson-Fisher RW, Savolainen NJ: Systematic review of psychological therapies for cancer patients: overview and recommendations for future research, *J Nat Cancer Inst* 94(8):558-84, 2002.

98. Shannahoff-Khalsa DS: Patient perspectives: Kundalini yoga meditation techniques for psycho-oncology and as potential therapies for cancer, *Integr Cancer Ther* 4(1):87-100, 2005.

99. Yeh GY et al: Use of complementary and alternative medicine among persons with diabetes mellitus: results of a national survey, *Am J Public Health* 92(10):1648-52, 2002.

100. Yeh GY et al: Effects of tai chi mind-body movement therapy on functional status and exercise capacity in patients with chronic heart failure: a randomized controlled trial, *Am J Med* 117(8):541-8, 2004.

101. Anderson S, Sovik R: *Yoga: mastering the basics,* Honesdale, Penn, 2000, Himalayan Institute Press.

102. Arya U: *Yoga-sutras of Patajali with the exposition of Vyasa, a translation and commentary,* vol 1, Honesdale, Penn, 1986, The Himalayan Institute of Yoga Science and Philosophy of the USA.

103. Arya U: *Philosophy of Hatha yoga,* ed 2, Honesdale, Penn, 1998, The Himalayan Institute of Yoga Science and Philosophy of the USA.

104. Arya U: *Yoga sutras of Patanjali with the exposition of Vyasa,* vol 2, Delhi, 2001, Sadhana-Pada. Motilal Banaridass Publishers.

105. Frawley D: *Yoga and Ayerveda: self-healing and self-realization,* Twin Lakes, Wis, 1999, Lotus Press.

106. Muktibodhananda S: *Hatha yoga Pradipika,* Mungar, Bihar, 2003, Yoga Publications Trust.

107. Rama S: *Path of fire and light,* vol 1, Honesdale, Penn., 1996, The Himalayan Institute Press.

108. Rama S: *Path of fire and light,* vol 2, Honesdale, Penn., 1996, The Himalayan Institute Press.

109. Rama S: *Perennial psychology of the Bhagavad Gita,* Honesdale, Penn, 1996, Himalayan Institute Press.

110. Rama S: *The Royal path: practical lessons on yoga,* ed 3, Honesdale, Penn, 1998, Himalayan Institute Press.

111. Ramaswami S: *Yoga for the three stages of life: developing your practice as an art form, a physical therapy, and a guiding philosophy,* Rochester, Vt, 2000, Inner Traditions International.

112. Saper RB et al: Prevalence and patterns of adult yoga use in the United States: results of a national survey, *Altern Ther Health Med* 10(2):44-9, 2004.

113. Tindle HA et al: Factors associated with the use of mind body therapies among United States adults with musculoskeletal pain, *Complement Ther Med* 13(3):155-64, 2005.

114. Riley D: Hatha yoga and the treatment of illness, *Altern Ther Health Med* 10(2):20-1, 2004.

115. DeMayo W et al: Hatha yoga and meditation in patients with post-polio syndrome, *Altern Ther Health Med* 10(2):24-5, 2004.

116. Holloway RG et al: Pramipexole vs levodopa as initial treatment for Parkinson disease: a 4-year randomized controlled trial, *Arch Neurol* 61(7):1044-53, 2004. (Erratum, *Arch Neurol* 62(3):430, 2005.)

117. Rama S, Ballantine R, Hymes A: *Science of breath: a practical guide,* Honesdale, Penn, 1998, Himalayan Institute Press.

118. Sovik R: The science of breathing—the yogic view, *Progr Brain Res* 122:491-505, 2000.

119. Vedanthan PK et al: Clinical study of yoga techniques in university students with asthma: a controlled study, *Allergy Asthma Proc* 19(1):3-9, 1998.

120. Khanam AA et al: Study of pulmonary and autonomic functions of asthma patients after yoga training, *Ind J Physiol Pharmacol* 40(4):318-24, 1996.

121. Behera D: Yoga therapy in chronic bronchitis, *J Assoc Physicians India* 46(2):207-8, 1998.

122. Bhattacharya S, Pandey US, Verma NS: Improvement in oxidative status with yogic breathing in young healthy males, *Ind J Physiol Pharmacol* 46(3):349-54, 2002.

123. Udupa K et al: Effect of pranayam training on cardiac function in normal young volunteers, *Ind J Physiol Pharmacol* 47(1):27-33, 2003.

124. Raghuraj P et al: Pranayama increases grip strength without lateralized effects, *Ind J Physiol Pharmacol* 41(2):129-33, 1997.

125. Bhavanani AB et al: Acute effect of Mukh bhastrika (a yogic bellows type breathing) on reaction time, *Ind J Physiol Pharmacol* 47(3):297-300, 2003.

126. Janakiramaiah N et al: Antidepressant efficacy of Sudarshan Kriya Yoga (SKY) in melancholia: a randomized comparison with electroconvulsive

therapy (ECT) and imipramine, *J Affect Dis* 57(1-3):255-9, 2000.

127. Raghuraj P, Telles S: Right uninostril yoga breathing influences ipsilateral components of middle latency auditory evoked potentials, *Neurol Sci* 25(5):274-80, 2004.

128. Naveen KV et al: Yoga breathing through a particular nostril increases spatial memory scores without lateralized effects, *Psychol Rep* 81(2):555-61, 1997.

129. Alkalay RD, Gelberman RJ: *Kabbalah in motion*, New York, 2003, Genesis.

130. Telles S, Naveen KV: Yoga for rehabilitation: an overview, *Ind J Med Sci* 51(4):123-7, 1997.

131. Khalsa SBS: Yoga as a therapeutic intervention: a bibliometric analysis of published research studies, *Ind J Physiol Pharmacol* 48(3):269-85, 2004.

132. Riley D: Hatha yoga and the treatment of illness, *Altern Ther Health Med* 10(2):20-1, 2004.

133. Manocha R et al: Sahaja yoga in the management of moderate to severe asthma: a randomised controlled trial, *Thorax* 57(2):110-5, 2002.

134. Ram FSF, Holloway EA, Jones PW: Breathing retraining for asthma, *Respir Med* 97(5):501-7, 2003.

135. Lehrer P et al: Psychological aspects of asthma, *J Consult Clin Psychol* 70(3):691-711, 2002.

136. Lewith GT, Watkins AD: Unconventional therapies in asthma: an overview, *Allergy* 51(11):761-9, 1996.

137. Sabina AB et al: Yoga intervention for adults with mild-to-moderate asthma: a pilot study, *Ann Allergy Asthma Immunol* 94(5):543-8, 2005.

138. Yogendra J et al: Beneficial effects of yoga lifestyle on reversibility of ischaemic heart disease: caring heart project of International Board of Yoga, *J Assoc Physicians India* 52:283-9, 2004.

139. Bowman AJ et al: Effects of aerobic exercise training and yoga on the baroreflex in healthy elderly persons, *Eur J Clin Invest* 27(5):443-9, 1997.

140. McCaffrey R et al: The effects of yoga on hypertensive persons in Thailand, *Holist Nurs Pract* 19(4):173-80, 2005.

141. Manchanda SC et al: Retardation of coronary atherosclerosis with yoga lifestyle intervention, *J Assoc Physicians India* 48(7):687-94, 2004.

142. Mahajan AS, Reddy KS, Sachdeva U: Lipid profile of coronary risk subjects following yogic lifestyle intervention, *Indian Heart J* 51(1):37-40, 1999.

143. Harinath K et al: Effects of Hatha yoga and Omkar meditation on cardiorespiratory performance, psychologic profile, and melatonin secretion, *J Altern Compl Med* 10(2):261-8, 2004.

144. Damodaran A et al: Therapeutic potential of yoga practices in modifying cardiovascular risk profile in middle aged men and women, *J Assoc Physicians India* 50(5):633-40, 2002.

145. Pandya DP, Vyas VH, Vyas SH: Mind-body therapy in the management and prevention of coronary disease, *Compr Ther* 25(5):283-93, 1999.

146. Mamtani R, Mamtani R: Ayurveda and yoga in cardiovascular diseases, *Cardiol Rev* 13(3):155-62, 2005.

147. Manchanda SC, Narang R: Yoga and coronary artery disease, *Indian Heart J* 50(2):227-8, 1998.

148. Innes KE, Bourguignon C, Taylor AG: Risk indices associated with the insulin resistance syndrome, cardiovascular disease, and possible protection with yoga: a systematic review, *J Am Board Fam Pract* 18(6):491-519, 2005.

149. Raub JA: Psychophysiologic effects of Hatha Yoga on musculoskeletal and cardiopulmonary function: a literature review, *J Altern Complement Med* 8(6):797-812, 2002.

150. Jayasinghe SR: Yoga in cardiac health (a review), *Eur J Cardiovasc Prevent Rehabil* 11(5):369-75, 2004.

151. Murugesan R, Govindarajulu N, Bera TK: Effect of selected yogic practices on the management of hypertension, *Indian J Physiol Pharmacol* 44(2):207-10, 2000.

152. Malhotra V et al: Study of yoga asanas in assessment of pulmonary function in NIDDM patients, *Indian J Physiol Pharmacol* 46(3):313-20, 2002.

153. Elder C: Ayurveda for diabetes mellitus: a review of the biomedical literature, *Altern Ther Health Med* 10(1):44-50, 2004.

154. Malhotra V et al: Effect of Yoga asanas on nerve conduction in type 2 diabetes, *Indian J Physiol Pharmacol* 46(3):298-306, 2002.

155. Taneja I et al: Yogic versus conventional treatment in diarrhea-predominant irritable bowel syndrome: a randomized control study, *Appl Psychophysiol Biofeedback* 29(1):19-33, 2004.

156. Ripoll E, Mahowald D: Hatha Yoga therapy management of urologic disorders, *World J Urol* 20(5):306-9, 2002.

157. Shaffer HJ, LaSalvia TA, Stein JP: Comparing Hatha yoga with dynamic group psychotherapy for enhancing methadone maintenance treatment: a randomized clinical trial, *Altern Ther Health Med* 3(4):57-66, 1997.

158. Manjunath NK, Telles S: Influence of Yoga and Ayurveda on self-rated sleep in a geriatric population, *Indian J Med Res* 121(5):683-90, 2005.

159. Khalsa SBS: Treatment of chronic insomnia with yoga: a preliminary study with sleep-wake diaries, *Appl Psychophysiol Biofeedback* 29(4):269-78, 2004.

160. Krisanaprakornkit T et al: Meditation therapy for anxiety disorders, *Cochrane Database Syst Rev* 1: CD004998, 2006.

161. Kirkwood G et al: Yoga for anxiety: a systematic review of the research evidence, *Br J Sports Med* 39(12):884-91, 2005.

162. Malathi A, Damodaran A: Stress due to exams in medical students—role of yoga, *Indian J Physiol Pharmacol* 43(2):218-24, 1999.

163. Woolery A et al: A yoga intervention for young adults with elevated symptoms of depression, *Altern Ther Health Med* 10(2):60-3, 2004.

164. Malathi A et al: Effect of yogic practices on subjective well being, *Indian J Physiol Pharmacol* 44(2):202-6, 2000.

165. Ghoncheh S, Smith JC: Progressive muscle relaxation, yoga stretching, and ABC relaxation theory, *J Clin Psychol* 60(1):131-6, 2004.

166. Kochan LD, Qureshi AI, Fallon BA: Therapeutic approaches to the treatment of refractory obsessive-compulsive disorder, *Curr Psychiatr Rep* 2(4):327-34, 2000.

167. Jensen PS, Kenny DT: The effects of yoga on the attention and behavior of boys with attention-deficit/hyperactivity disorder (ADHD), *J Atten Disord* 7(4):205-16, 2004.

168. Rojas NL, Chan E: Old and new controversies in the alternative treatment of attention-deficit hyperactivity disorder, *Ment Retard Dev Disabil Res Rev* 11(2):116-30, 2005.

169. Ramaratnam S, Sridharan K: Yoga for epilepsy [update in Cochrane Database Syst Rev. 2000;(3): CD001524; PMID: 10908505], *Cochrane Database Syst Rev* 2:CD001524, 2000.

170. Marson A, Ramaratnam S: Epilepsy, *Clin Evidence* 9:1403-20, 2003. [update in *Clin Evid.* 2003 Dec;(10):1508-26; PMID: 15555158][update of *Clin Evid.* 2002 Jun;(7):1153-68; PMID: 12230734]

171. Bijlani RL: Influence of yoga on brain and behaviour: facts and speculations, *Indian J Physiol Pharmacol* 48(1):1-5, 2004.

172. Narendran S et al: Efficacy of yoga on pregnancy outcome, *J Altern Complement Med* 11(2):237-44, 2005.

173. Fields N: Float like a butterfly . . . yoga and birth, *Pract Midwife* 8(1):22-5, 2005.

174. Berk B: Yoga for moms. Building core stability before, during and after pregnancy, *Midwifery Today Int Midwife* 59:27-9, 2001.

175. Coker KH: Meditation and prostate cancer: integrating a mind/body intervention with traditional therapies, *Semin Urologic Oncol* 17(2):111-8, 1999.

176. Bower JE et al: Yoga for cancer patients and survivors, *Cancer Control* 12(3):165-71, 2005.

177. Cohen L et al: Psychological adjustment and sleep quality in a randomized trial of the effects of a Tibetan yoga intervention in patients with lymphoma, *Cancer* 100(10):2253-60, 2004.

178. Oken BS et al: Randomized controlled trial of yoga and exercise in multiple sclerosis, *Neurology* 62(11):2058-64, 2004.

179. Kolasinski SL et al: Iyengar yoga for treating symptoms of osteoarthritis of the knees: a pilot study, *J Altern Complement Med* 11(4):689-93, 2005.

180. Dash M, Telles S: Improvement in hand grip strength in normal volunteers and rheumatoid arthritis patients following yoga training, *Indian J Physiol Pharmacol* 45(3):355-60, 2001.

181. Nelson C et al: The influence of hostility and family history of cardiovascular disease on autonomic activation in response to controllable versus noncontrollable stress, anger imagery induction, and relaxation imagery, *J Behav Med* 28(3):213-21, 2005.

182. Jacobs BP et al: Feasibility of conducting a clinical trial on Hatha yoga for chronic low back pain: methodological lessons, *Altern Ther Health Med* 10(2):80-3, 2004. (Erratum, *Altern Ther Health Med* 10(3)48, 2004.)

183. Galantino ML et al: The impact of modified Hatha yoga on chronic low back pain: a pilot study, *Altern Ther Health Med* 10(2):56-9, 2004.

184. Graves N et al: Clinical inquiries. Does yoga speed healing for patients with low back pain? *J Fam Pract* 53(8):661-2, 2004.

185. Michlovitz SL: Conservative interventions for carpal tunnel syndrome, *J Orthop Sports Phys Ther* 34(10):589-600, 2004.

186. Muller M et al: Effectiveness of hand therapy interventions in primary management of carpal tunnel syndrome: a systematic review, *J Hand Ther* 17(2):210-28, 2004.

187. O'Connor D, Marshall S, Massy-Westropp N: Nonsurgical treatment (other than steroid injection) for carpal tunnel syndrome, *Cochrane Database Syst Rev* 1:CD003219, 2003.

188. Rama S: *Meditation and its practice*, ed 2, Honesdale, Penn, 1998, Himalayan Institute Press.

189. Veda Bharati S: *Superconscious meditation*, Honesdale, Penn, 1978, The Himalayan Institute of Yoga Science and Philosophy of the USA.

190. Benson H: *The relaxation response,* 1993, New York Outlet Books.

191. Lazar SW et al: Functional brain mapping of the relaxation response and meditation, *Neuroreport* 11(7):1581-5, 2000.

192. Lazar SW et al: Meditation experience is associated with increased cortical thickness, *Neuroreport* 16(17):1893-7, 2005.

193. Peng CK et al: Heart rate dynamics during three forms of meditation, *Internat J Cardiol* 95(1):19-27, 2004.

194. Peng CK et al: Exaggerated heart rate oscillations during two meditation techniques, *Internat J Cardiol* 70(2):101-7, 1999.

195. Gazella, A. Jon Kabat-Zinn: Bringing mindfulness to medicine, *Altern Ther Health Med* 11(3):56-64, 2005.

196. Davidson RJ et al: Alterations in brain and immune function produced by mindfulness meditation, *Psychosomat Med* 65(4):564-70, 2003.

197. Kabat-Zinn J et al: Influence of a mindfulness meditation-based stress reduction intervention on rates of skin clearing in patients with moderate to severe psoriasis undergoing phototherapy (UVB) and photochemotherapy (PUVA), *Psychosomat Med* 60(5):625-32, 1998.

198. Kabat-Zinn J: *Full catastrophe living: using the wisdom of your body and mind to face stress, pain and illness*, New York, 1990, Dell Publishing.

199. Smith JE et al: Mindfulness-based stress reduction as supportive therapy in cancer care: systematic review, *J Adv Nurs* 52(3):315-27, 2005.

200. Carlson LE et al: Mindfulness-based stress reduction in relation to quality of life, mood, symptoms of stress and levels of cortisol, dehydroepiandrosterone sulfate (DHEAS) and melatonin in breast and prostate cancer outpatients, *Psychoneuroendocrinology* 29(4):448-74, 2004.

201. Robert McComb JJ et al: A pilot study to examine the effects of a mindfulness-based stress-reduction and relaxation program on levels of stress hormones, physical functioning, and submaximal exercise responses, *J Altern Complement Med* 10(5):819-27, 2004.

202. Lutz A et al: Long-term meditators self-induce high-amplitude gamma synchrony during mental practice, *Proc Natl Acad Sci USA* 101(46):16369-73, 2004.

203. Alexander CN et al: Trial of stress reduction for hypertension in older African Americans. II. Sex and risk subgroup analysis, *Hypertension* 28(2):228-37, 1996.

204. Barnes V et al: Stress, stress reduction, and hypertension in African Americans: an updated review, *J Nat Med Assoc* 89(7):464-76, 1997.

205. Castillo-Richmond A et al: Effects of stress reduction on carotid atherosclerosis in hypertensive African Americans, *Stroke* 31(3):568-73, 2000.

206. MacLean CR et al: Effects of the transcendental meditation program on adaptive mechanisms: changes in hormone levels and responses to stress after 4 months of practice, *Psychoneuroendocrinology* 22(4):277-95, 1997.

207. Schneider RH et al: Long-term effects of stress reduction on mortality in persons > or =55 years of age with systemic hypertension, *Am J Cardiol* 95(9):1060-4, 2005.

208. Schneider RH et al: Behavioral treatment of hypertensive heart disease in African Americans: rationale and design of a randomized controlled trial, *Behav Med* 27(2):83-95, 2001.

209. Schneider RH, Nidich SI, Salerno JW: The Transcendental Meditation program: reducing the risk of heart disease and mortality and improving quality of life in African Americans, *Ethnicity Dis* 11(1):159-60, 2001.

210. Schneider RH et al: Lower lipid peroxide levels in practitioners of the Transcendental Meditation program, *Psychosomat Med* 60(1):38-41, 1998.

211. Walton KG et al: Lowering cortisol and CVD risk in postmenopausal women: a pilot study using the Transcendental Meditation program, *Ann N Y Acad Sci* 1032:211-5, 2004.

212. Walton KG et al: Psychosocial stress and cardiovascular disease part 2: effectiveness of the Transcendental Meditation program in treatment and prevention, *Behav Med* 28(3):106-23, 2002.

213. Walton KG et al: Psychosocial stress and cardiovascular disease part 3: clinical and policy implications of research on the transcendental meditation program, *Behav Med* 30(4):173-83, 2005.

214. Wenneberg SR et al: A controlled study of the effects of the Transcendental Meditation program on cardiovascular reactivity and ambulatory blood pressure, *Int J Neurosci* 89(1-2):15-28, 1997.

215. Zamarra JW et al: Usefulness of the transcendental meditation program in the treatment of patients with coronary artery disease, *Am J Cardiol* 77(10):867-70, 1996.

216. Shannahoff-Khalsa DS: An introduction to Kundalini yoga meditation techniques that are specific for the treatment of psychiatric disorders, *J Altern Complement Med* 10(1):91-101, 2004.

217. Liao W: *The essence of tai chi*, Boston, 1995, Shambala Publications.

218. *Tai chi for health: yang long form with Terence Dunn*, Healing Arts.

219. Adler PA, Roberts BL: The use of Tai Chi to improve health in older adults, *Orthop Nurs* 25(2):122-6, 2006.

220. Arthur HM, Patterson C, Stone JA: The role of complementary and alternative therapies in cardiac rehabilitation: a systematic evaluation, *Eur J Cardiovasc Prevent Rehabil* 13(1):3-9, 2006.

221. Fontana JA et al: T'ai chi chih as an intervention for heart failure, *Nurs Clin North Am* 35(4):1031-46, 2000.

222. Gillespie LD et al: Interventions for preventing falls in elderly people, [update of Cochrane Database Syst Rev. 2001;(3):CD000340; PMID: 11686957] *Cochrane Database Syst Rev* 4:CD000340, 2003.

223. Li F et al: Tai chi and fall reductions in older adults: a randomized controlled trial, *J Gerontol A Biol Sci Med Sci* 60(2):187-94, 2005.

224. Wolf SL et al: The effect of Tai chi quan and computerized balance training on postural stability in older subjects. Atlanta FICSIT Group. Frailty and Injuries: Cooperative Studies on Intervention Techniques, *Phys Ther* 77(4):371-81, 1997.

225. Wolf SL et al: Reducing frailty and falls in older persons: an investigation of Tai Chi and computerized balance training. Atlanta FICSIT Group. Frailty and Injuries: Cooperative Studies of Intervention Techniques, *J Am Geriatr Soc* 44(5):489-97, 1996.

226. Li F et al: Tai chi: improving functional balance and predicting subsequent falls in older persons, *Med Sci Sports Exerc* 36(12):2046-52, 2004.

227. Li F et al: An evaluation of the effects of Tai Chi exercise on physical function among older persons: a randomized contolled trial, *Ann Behav Med* 23(2):139-46, 2001.

228. Sattin RW et al: Reduction in fear of falling through intense tai chi exercise training in older, transitionally frail adults, *J Am Geriatr Soc* 53(7):1168-78, 2005.

229. Song R et al: Effects of tai chi exercise on pain, balance, muscle strength, and perceived difficulties in physical functioning in older women with osteoarthritis: a randomized clinical trial, *J Rheumatol* 30(9):2039-44, 2003.

230. Taggart HM: Effects of Tai Chi exercise on balance, functional mobility, and fear of falling among older women, *Appl Nurs Res* 15(4):235-42, 2002.

231. Tsang WWN, Hui-Chan CWY: Effects of tai chi on joint proprioception and stability limits in elderly subjects, *Med Sci Sports Exerc* 35(12):1962-71, 2003.

232. Tsang WWN, Hui-Chan CWY: Effects of exercise on joint sense and balance in elderly men: tai chi versus golf, *Med Sci Sports Exerc* 36(4):658-67, 2004.

233. Tsang WWN, Hui-Chan CWY: Effect of 4- and 8-wk intensive Tai Chi Training on balance control in the elderly, *Med Sci Sports Exerc* 36(4):648-57, 2004.

234. Wolf SL et al: Intense tai chi exercise training and fall occurrences in older, transitionally frail adults: a randomized, controlled trial, *J Am Geriatr Soc* 51(12):1693-701, 2003.

235. Wolf SL et al: A study design to investigate the effect of intense tai chi in reducing falls among older adults transitioning to frailty, *Control Clin Trials* 22(6):689-704, 2001.

236. Wolfson L et al: Balance and strength training in older adults: intervention gains and Tai Chi maintenance, *J Am Geriatr Soc* 44(5):498-506, 1996.

237. Christou EA, Yang Y, Rosengren KS: Taiji training improves knee extensor strength and force control in older adults, *J Gerontol A Biol Sci Med Sci* 58(8):763-6, 2003.

238. Wu G et al: Improvement of isokinetic knee extensor strength and reduction of postural sway in the elderly from long-term tai chi exercise, *Arch Phys Med Rehabil* 83(10):1364-69, 2002.

239. Young DR et al: The effects of aerobic exercise and t'ai chi on blood pressure in older people: results of a randomized trial, *J Am Geriatr Soc* 47(3):277-84, 1999.

240. Hong Y, Li JX, Robinson PD: Balance control, flexibility, and cardiorespiratory fitness among older tai chi practitioners, *Br J Sports Med* 34(1):29-34, 2000.

241. Channer KS et al: Changes in haemodynamic parameters following tai chi chuan and aerobic exercise in patients recovering from acute myocardial infarction, *Postgrad Med J* 72(848):349-51, 1996.

242. Chan K et al: A randomized, prospective study of the effects of tai chi chuan exercise on bone mineral density in postmenopausal women, *Arch Phys Med Rehabil* 85(5):717-22, 2004.

243. Hartman CA et al: Effects of t'ai chi training on function and quality of life indicators in older adults with osteoarthritis, *J Am Geriatr Soc* 48(12): 1553-9, 2000.

244. Irwin MR et al: Effects of a behavioral intervention, tai chi chih, on varicella-zoster virus specific immunity and health functioning in older adults, *Psychosomat Med* 65(5):824-30, 2003.

245. Mustian KM et al: Tai chi chuan, health-related quality of life and self-esteem: a randomized trial with breast cancer survivors, *Supportive Care Cancer* 12(12):871-6, 2004.

246. Hart J et al: Tai Chi Chuan practice in community-dwelling persons after stroke, *Int J Rehabil Res* 27(4):303-4, 2004.

247. Klein PJ, Rivers L: Taiji for individuals with Parkinson disease and their support partners: a program evaluation, *J Neurol Phys Ther* 30(1):22-7, 2006.

248. Lu W-A, Kuo C-D: The effect of tai chi chuan on the autonomic nervous modulation in older persons, *Med Sci Sports Exerc* 35(12):1972-6, 2003.

249. Li JX, Hong Y, Chan KM: Tai chi: physiological characteristics and beneficial effects on health, *Br J Sports Med* 35(3):148-56, 2001.

250. Naperstek B: Health Journeys: Resources for Mind, Body and Spirit. Available at: *http://www.healthjourneys.com.* Accessed April 13, 2007.

251. Tusek DL, Cwynar RE: Strategies for implementing a guided imagery program to enhance patient experience, *AACN Clin Issues* 11(1):68-76, 2000.

252. Naperstek B: *Invisible heroes: survivors of trauma and how they heal,* New York, 2004, Bantam Books.

253. Adams N, Poole H, Richardson C: Psychological approaches to chronic pain management: part 1, *J Clin Nurs* 15(3):290-300, 2006.

254. Tusek DL: Guided imagery: a powerful tool to decrease length of stay, pain, anxiety, and narcotic consumption, *J Invasive Cardiol* 11(4):265-7, 1999.

255. Acherberg J: *Imagery in healing: shamanism in modern medicine*, Boston, 1985, Shambala.

256. Naperstek B: *Staying well with guided imagery*, New York, 1994, Warner Books.

257. Simonton C, Carl S, Creighton J: *Getting well again*, Los Angeles, 1978, Jeremy P Tarcher.

258. Antall GF, Kresevic D: The use of guided imagery to manage pain in an elderly orthopaedic population, *Orthop Nurs* 23(5):335-40, 2004.

259. Baird CL, Sands L: A pilot study of the effectiveness of guided imagery with progressive muscle relaxation to reduce chronic pain and mobility difficulties of osteoarthritis, *Pain Manag Nurs* 5(3):97-104, 2004.

260. Huth MM, Broome ME, Good M: Imagery reduces children's post-operative pain, *Pain* 110(1-2):439-48, 2004.

261. Broome ME, Rehwaldt M, Fogg L: Relationships between cognitive behavioral techniques, temperament, observed distress, and pain reports in children and adolescents during lumbar puncture, *J Ped Nurs* 13(1):48-54, 1998.

262. Borckardt JJ et al: The computer-assisted cognitive/imagery system for use in the management of pain, *Pain Res Manag* 9(3):157-62, 2004.

263. Pellino TA et al: Use of nonpharmacologic interventions for pain and anxiety after total hip and total knee arthroplasty, *Orthop Nurs* 24(3):182-90, 2005.

264. Liu KP et al: Mental imagery for promoting relearning for people after stroke: a randomized controlled trial, *Arch Phys Med Rehabil* 85(9):1403-8, 2004.

265. Callow N, Hardy L: The relationship between the use of kinaesthetic imagery and different visual imagery perspectives, *J Sports Sci* 22(2):167-77, 2004.

266. Boschker MS, Bakker FC, Rietberg MB: Retroactive interference effects of mentally imagined movement speed, *J Sports Sci* 18(8):593-603, 2000.

267. Malouin F et al: Training mobility tasks after stroke with combined mental and physical practice: a feasibility study, *Neurorehabil Neural Repair* 18(2):66-75, 2004.

268. Collins JA, Rice VH: Effects of relaxation intervention in phase II cardiac rehabilitation: replication and extension, *Heart Lung* 26(1):31-44, 1997.

269. Ball TM et al: A pilot study of the use of guided imagery for the treatment of recurrent abdominal pain in children, *Clin Ped* 42(6):527-32, 2003.

270. Hewson-Bower B, Drummond PD: Psychological treatment for recurrent symptoms of colds and flu in children, *J Psychosomat Res* 51(1):369-77, 2001.

271. Castes M et al: Immunological changes associated with clinical improvement of asthmatic children subjected to psychosocial intervention, *Brain Behav Immun* 13(1):1-13, 1999.

272. Simonton OC, Simonton SM: Belief symptoms and management of the emotional aspects of malignancy, *J Transpersonal Psychol* 7:29-47, 1974.

273. Richardson MA et al: Coping, life attitudes, and immune responses to imagery and group support after breast cancer treatment, *Altern Ther Health Med* 3(5):62-70, 1997.

274. Burns DS: The effect of the bonny method of guided imagery and music on the mood and life quality of cancer patients, *J Music Ther* 38(1):51-65, 2001.

275. Baider L et al: Psychological intervention in cancer patients: a randomized study, *Gen Hosp Psychiatr* 23(5):272-7, 2001.

276. Moye LA et al: Research methodology in psychoneuroimmunology: rationale and design of the IMAGES-P clinical trial, *Altern Ther Health Med* 1(2):34-9, 1995.

277. Cusack K, Spates CR: The cognitive dismantling of Eye Movement Desensitization and Reprocessing (EMDR) treatment of Posttraumatic Stress Disorder (PTSD), *J Anxiety Disord* 13(1-2):87-99, 1999.

278. Spiegel D, Moore R: Imagery and hypnosis in the treatment of cancer patients, *Oncology (Huntington)* 11(8):1179-89, 1997.

279. Bannerman R, Burton J, Wen Chieh C, editors: *Traditional medicine and health care coverage. Chapter 13: Hypnosis.* Geneva, Switzerland, 1983, World Health Organization.

280. Barber TX: A deeper understanding of hypnosis: its secrets, its nature, its essence, *Am J Clin Hypnosis* 42(3-4):208-72, 2000.

281. Stewart JH: Hypnosis in contemporary medicine, *Mayo Clin Proc* 80(4):511-24, 2005.

282. Findlay S, Podolsky O, Silberner J: Wonder cures from the fringe, *US News and World Report* 3(13):68-74, 1991.

283. Gruzelier JH: A review of the impact of hypnosis, relaxation, guided imagery and individual differences on aspects of immunity and health, *Stress* 5(2):147-63, 2002.

284. Gruzelier J et al: Cellular and humoral immunity, mood and exam stress: the influences of self-hypnosis and personality predictors, *Int J Psychophysiol* 42(1):55-71, 2001.

285. Rossi EL: In search of a deep psychobiology of hypnosis: visionary hypotheses for a new millennium, *Am J Clin Hypn* 42(3-4):178-207, 2000.

286. Raz A: Attention and hypnosis: neural substrates and genetic associations of two converging processes, *Int J Clin Exper Hypn* 53(3):237-58, 2005.

287. Vermetten E, Douglas Bremner J: Functional brain imaging and the induction of traumatic recall: a cross-correlational review between neuroimaging and hypnosis, *Int J Clin Exper Hypn* 52(3):280-312, 2004.

288. Olsen KG: Hypnosis and hypnotherapy, *The ency-clopedia of alternative health care,* New York, 1990, Pocket Books.

289. Faymonville ME et al: Neural mechanisms of anti-nociceptive effects of hypnosis, *Anesthesiology* 92(5):1257-67, 2000.

290. Holroyd J: Hypnosis treatment of clinical pain: understanding why hypnosis is useful, *Int J Clin Exper Hypn* 44(1):33-51, 1996.

291. Patterson DR, Jensen MP: Hypnosis and clinical pain, *Psychol Bull* 129(4):495-521, 2003.

292. Patterson DR et al: Optimizing control of pain from severe burns: a literature review, *Am J Clin Hypn* 47(1):43-54, 2004.

293. Dane JR: Hypnosis for pain and neuromuscular rehabilitation with multiple sclerosis: case summary, literature review, and analysis of outcomes, *Int J Clin Exper Hypn* 44(3):208-31, 1996.

294. Karjalainen KA et al: Biopsychosocial rehabilitation for repetitive-strain injuries among working-age adults, *Scand J Work Environ Health* 26(5):373-81, 2000.

295. Cuellar NG: Hypnosis for pain management in the older adult, *Pain Manag Nurs* 6(3):105-11, 2005.

296. Kemper KJ: Complementary and alternative medicine for children: does it work? *Arch Dis Child* 84(1):6-9, 2001.

297. Gerik SM: Pain management in children: develop-mental considerations and mind-body therapies, *South Med J* 98(3):295-302, 2005.

298. Butler LD et al: Hypnosis reduces distress and dura-tion of an invasive medical procedure for children, *Pediatrics* 115(1):77-85, 2005.

299. Osborne TL, Raichle KA, Jensen MP: Psychologic interventions for chronic pain, *Phys Med Rehabil Clin North Am* 17(2):415-33, 2006.

300. Cyna AM, McAuliffe GL, Andrew MI: Hypnosis for pain relief in labour and childbirth: a systematic review, *Br J Anaesthesia* 93(4):505-11, 2004.

301. Eappen S, Robbins D: Nonpharmacological means of pain relief for labor and delivery, *Int Anesthesiol Clin* 40(4):103-14, 2002.

302. Huntley AL, Coon JT, Ernst E: Complementary and alternative medicine for labor pain: a systematic review, *Am J Obstetr Gynecol* 191(1):36-44, 2004.

303. Simkin P, Bolding A: Update on nonpharmacologic approaches to relieve labor pain and prevent suffer-ing, *J Midwifery Womens Health* 49(6):489-504, 2004.

304. Oakley DA, Whitman LG, Halligan PW: Hypnotic imagery as a treatment for phantom limb pain: two case reports and a review, *Clin Rehabil* 16(4):368-77, 2002.

305. Tinterow MM: Hypnotherapy for chronic pain, *Kansas Med* 88 (no 6):190-2, 204, 1987.

306. Tinterow MM: The use of hypnotic anesthesia for major surgical procedures, *Am Surgeon* 26:732-7, 1960.

307. Hernandez A Jr, Tatarunis AM: The use of pre-, intra-, and posthypnotic suggestion in anesthesia and surgery, *CRNA* 11(4):167-72, 2000.

308. Petry JJ: Surgery and complementary therapies: a review, *Altern Ther Health Med* 6(5):64-74, 2000.

309. Diseth TH, Christie HJ: Trauma-related disso-ciative (conversion) disorders in children and adolescents—an overview of assessment tools and treatment principles, *Nord J Psychiatry* 59(4):278-92, 2005.

310. Cardena E: Hypnosis in the treatment of trauma: a promising, but not fully supported, efficacious intervention, *Int J Clin Exp Hypn* 48(2):225-38, 2000.

311. Beere DB, Simon MJ, Welch K: Recommendations and illustrations for combining hypnosis and EMDR in the treatment of psychological trauma, *Am J Clin Hypn* 43(3-4):217-31, 2001.

312. Robertson M, Humphreys L, Ray R: Psychological treatments for posttraumatic stress disorder: Rec-ommendations for the clinician based on a review of the literature, *J Psychiatr Pract* 10(2):106-18, 2004.

313. Bjick S: Accessing the power in the patient with hypnosis and EMDR. Eye Movement Desensitiza-tion and Reprocessing, *Am J Clin Hypn* 43(3-4):203-16, 2001.

314. Hollander HE, Bender SS: ECEM (eye closure eye movements): integrating aspects of EMDR with hypnosis for treatment of trauma, *Am J Clin Hypn* 43(3-4):187-202, 2001.

315. Barrios AA: Hypnotherapy: a reappraisal, *Psycho-therapy: theory, research, and practice* 7(1):2-7, 1970.

316. Gonsalkorale WM, Whorwell PJ: Hypnotherapy in the treatment of irritable bowel syndrome, *Eur J Gastroenterol Hepatol* 17(1):15-20, 2005.

317. Camilleri M: Review article: clinical evidence to support current therapies of irritable bowel syn-drome, *Aliment Pharmacol Ther* 13(suppl 2):48-53, 1999.

318. Tan G, Hammond DC, Joseph G: Hypnosis and irritable bowel syndrome: a review of efficacy and mechanism of action, *Am J Clin Hypn* 47(3):161-78, 2005.

319. Elkins G et al: Can hypnosis reduce hot flashes in breast cancer survivors? A literature review, *Am J Clin Hypn* 47(1):29-42, 2004.

320. Glazener CMA, Evans JHC, Cheuk DKL: Comple-mentary and miscellaneous interventions for noc-turnal enuresis in children, *Cochrane Database Syst Rev* 2:CD005230, 2005.

321. Hackman RM, Stern JS, Gershwin ME: Hypnosis and asthma: a critical review, *J Asthma* 37(1):1-15, 2000.

322. Pittler MH, Ernst E: Complementary therapies for reducing body weight: a systematic review, *Int J Obesity* 29(9):1030-8, 2005.

323. Soo S et al: A systematic review of psychological therapies for nonulcer dyspepsia, *Am J Gastroenterol* 99(9):1817-22, 2004.

324. Abbot NC et al: Hypnotherapy for smoking cessation, *Cochrane Database Syst Rev* 2:CD001008, 2000.

325. Covino NA, Bottari M: Hypnosis, behavioral theory, and smoking cessation, *J Dent Ed* 65(4):340-7, 2001.

326. Green JP, Lynn SJ: Hypnosis and suggestion-based approaches to smoking cessation: An examination of the evidence, *Int J Clin Exper Hypn* 48(2):195-224, 2000.

327. Beck AT: The past and future of cognitive therapy, *J Psychother Pract Res* 6:276-84, 1997.

328. Beck AT: The current state of cognitive therapy: a 40-year retrospective, *Arch Gen Psychiatry* 62(9):953-9, 2005.

329. Butler AC et al: The empirical status of cognitive-behavioral therapy: a review of meta-analyses, *Clin Psychol Rev* 26(1):17-31, 2006.

330. Tan SY, Leucht CA: Cognitive-behavioral therapy for clinical pain control: a 15-year update and its relationship to hypnosis, *Int J Clin Exper Hypn* 45(4):396-416, 1997.

331. Chen E, Joseph MH, Zeltzer LK: Behavioral and cognitive interventions in the treatment of pain in children, *Ped Clin North Am* 47(3):513-25, 2000.

332. Cowan GS Jr et al: Assessment of the effects of a taped cognitive behavior message on postoperative complications (therapeutic suggestions under anesthesia), *Obes Surg* 11(5):589-93, 2001.

333. Adler-Nevo G, Manassis K: Psychosocial treatment of pediatric posttraumatic stress disorder: the neglected field of single-incident trauma, *Depress Anxiety* 22(4):177-89, 2005.

334. Bryant RA et al: The additive benefit of hypnosis and cognitive-behavioral therapy in treating acute stress disorder, *J Consult Clin Psychol* 73(2):334-40, 2005.

335. Spiegel D, Bloom J, Kraemer HC: Effect of psychosocial treatment on survival of patients with metastatic breast cancer, *Lancet* 2:888-91, 1989.

336. Basmajian JV: Introduction: principles and background. In Basmajian J, editor: *Biofeedback: principles and practice for clinicians*, Baltimore, 1989, Williams and Wilkins, p 1.

337. Andrasik F: Twenty-five years of progress: twenty-five more? *Biofeedback Self Regul* 19:311, 1994.

338. Fagerson TL, Krebs DE: Biofeedback. In O'Sullivan SB, Schmitz TJ, editors: *Physical rehabilitation: assessment and treatment*, Philadelphia, 2001, FA Davis.

339. Fahrion SL: Autogenic biofeedback treatment for migraine, *Res Clin Stud Headache* 47-71, 1978.

340. Andrasik F: Behavioral treatment of migraine: current status and future directions, *Expert Rev Neurother* 4(3):403-13, 2004.

341. Biondi DM: Noninvasive treatments for headache, *Expert Rev Neurother* 5(3):355-62, 2005.

342. Institute of HeartMath: Decoding the Intelligence of the Heart. Available at: *http://www.heartmath.org*. Accessed April 13, 2007.

343. The Journey to Wild Devine. Available at: *http://www.wilddevine.com*. Accessed April 13, 2007.

344. Association for Applied Psychophysiology and Biofeedback. Available at: *http://www.aapb.org*. Accessed April 13, 2007.

345. Gobel H : Non pharmaceutical treatments for migraine, *Rev Neurol* 161(6-7):685-6, 2005.

346. Powers SW, Andrasik F: Biobehavioral treatment, disability, and psychological effects of pediatric headache, *Ped Ann* 34(6):461-5, 2005.

347. Penzien DB, Rains JC, Andrasik F: Behavioral management of recurrent headache: three decades of experience and empiricism, *Appl Psychophysiol Biofeedback* 27(2):163-81, 2002.

348. Neblett R, Mayer TG, Gatchel RJ: Theory and rationale for surface EMG-assisted stretching as an adjunct to chronic musculoskeletal pain rehabilitation, *Appl Psychophysiol Biofeedback* 28(2):139-46, 2003.

349. Medlicott MS, Harris SR: A systematic review of the effectiveness of exercise, manual therapy, electrotherapy, relaxation training, and biofeedback in the management of temporomandibular disorder, *Phys Ther* 86(7):955-73, 2006.

350. Haythornthwaite JA, Benrud-Larson LM: Psychological assessment and treatment of patients with neuropathic pain, *Curr Pain Headache Rep* 5(2):124-9, 2001.

351. McNeely ML et al: A systematic review of the effectiveness of physical therapy interventions for temporomandibular disorders, *Phys Ther* 86(5):710-25, 2006.

352. Walker JE, Kozlowski GP: Neurofeedback treatment of epilepsy, *Child Adolesc Psychiatr Clin North Am* 14(1):163-76, 2005.

353. Gruzelier J, Egner T: Critical validation studies of neurofeedback, *Child Adolesc Psychiatr Clin North Am* 14(1):83-104, 2005.

354. Butnik SM: Neurofeedback in adolescents and adults with attention deficit hyperactivity disorder, *J Clin Psychol* 61(5):621-5, 2005.

355. Holtmann M, Stadler C: Electroencephalographic biofeedback for the treatment of attention-deficit hyperactivity disorder in childhood and adolescence, *Exp Rev Neurother* 6(4):533-40, 2006.

356. Fox DJ, Tharp DF, Fox LC: Neurofeedback: an alternative and efficacious treatment for attention deficit hyperactivity disorder, *Appl Psychophysiol Biofeedback* 30(4):365-73, 2005.

357. Bliss DZ et al: Directions for future nursing research on fecal incontinence, *Nurs Res* 53(6 suppl):S15-21, 2004.

358. Aslan AR, Kogan BA: Conservative management in neurogenic bladder dysfunction, *Curr Opin Urol* 12(6):473-7, 2002.

359. Andrews CN, Bharucha AE: The etiology, assessment, and treatment of fecal incontinence, *Nat Clin Pract Gastroenterol Hepatol* 2(11):516-25, 2005.

360. Anders K: Recent developments in stress urinary incontinence in women, *Nurs Stand* 20(35):48-54, 2006.

361. Leahy A, Epstein O: Non-pharmacological treatments in the irritable bowel syndrome, *World J Gastroenterol* 7(3):313-6, 2001.

362. Glazer HI: Biofeedback vs electrophysiology, *Rehab Manag* 18(9):32-4, 2005.

363. Gibson K et al: The effectiveness of rehabilitation for nonoperative management of shoulder instability: a systematic review, *J Hand Ther* 17(2):229-42, 2004.

364. Geurts ACH et al: A review of standing balance recovery from stroke, *Gait Posture* 22(3):267-81, 2005.

365. Van Peppen RPS et al: The impact of physical therapy on functional outcomes after stroke: what's the evidence? *Clin Rehabil* 8(8):833-62, 2004.

366. Astin JA, Harkness E, Ernst E: The efficacy of "distant healing": a systematic review of randomized trials, *Ann Intern Med* 132(11):903-10, 2000.

367. Sicher F et al: A randomized double-blind study of the effect of distant healing in a population with advanced AIDS: report of a small scale study, *Western J Med* 169(6):356-63, 1998.

368. Harris WS et al: A randomized, controlled trial of the effects of remote, intercessory prayer on outcomes in patients admitted to the coronary care unit, *Arch Intern Med* 159(19):2273-8, 1999. [(Erratum, *Arch Intern Med* 26;160(12):1878, 2000].

369. Aviles JM et al: Intercessory prayer and cardiovascular disease progression in a coronary care unit population: a randomized controlled trial, *Mayo Clin Proc* 76(12):1192-8, 2001.

370. Leibovici L: Effects of remote, retroactive intercessory prayer on outcomes in patients with bloodstream infection: randomized controlled trial, *Br Med J* 323(7327):1450-1, 2001.

371. Mathai J, Bourne A: Pilot study investigating the effect of intercessory prayer in the treatment of child psychiatric disorders, *Australas Psychiatry* 12(4):386-9, 2004.

372. Cha KY, Wirth DP: Does prayer influence the success of in vitro fertilization-embryo transfer? Report of a masked, randomized trial, *J Reprod Med* 46(9):781-7, 2001. (Erratum, *J Reprod Med* 49(10):100A, 2004. Note: Lobo, RA [removed])

373. Matthews DA, Marlowe SM, MacNutt FS: Effects of intercessory prayer on patients with rheumatoid arthritis, *South Med J* 93(12):1177-86, 2000.

374. Matthews WJ, Conti JM, Sireci SG: The effects of intercessory prayer, positive visualization, and expectancy on the well-being of kidney dialysis patients, *Altern Ther Health Med* 7(5):42-52, 2001.

375. O'Laoire S: An experimental study of the effects of distant, intercessory prayer on self-esteem, anxiety, and depression, *Altern Ther Health Med* 3(6):38-53, 1997.

376. Palmer RF, Katerndahl D, Morgan-Kidd J: A randomized trial of the effects of remote intercessory prayer: Interactions with personal beliefs on problem-specific outcomes and functional status, *J Altern Complement Med* 10(3):438-48, 2004.

377. Walker SR et al: Intercessory prayer in the treatment of alcohol abuse and dependence: a pilot investigation, *Altern Ther Health Med* 3(6):79-86, 1997.

378. Dusek J et al: Study of the therapeutic effects of intercessory prayer (STEP): study design and research methods, *Am Heart J* 143(4):577-84, 2002.

379. Brown BS et al: Factors associated with treatment outcomes in an aftercare population, *Am J Addict* 13(5):447-60, 2004.

380. Razali SM et al: Religious-sociocultural psychotherapy in patients with anxiety and depression, *Aust N Z J Psychiatry* 32(6):867-72, 1998.

381. True G et al: Treatment preferences and advance care planning at end of life: the role of ethnicity and spiritual coping in cancer patients, *Ann Behav Med* 30(2):174-9, 2005.

382. Koenig HG: Religious attitudes and practices of hospitalized medically ill older adults, *Int J Geriatr Psychiatry* 13(4):213-24, 1998.

383. Dedert EA et al: Religiosity may help preserve the cortisol rhythm in women with stress-related illness, *Int J Psychiatry Med* 34(1):61-77, 2004. (Erratum, *Int J Psychiatry Med* 34(3):287, 2004.)

384. Sephton SE et al: Spiritual expression and immune status in women with metastatic breast cancer: an exploratory study, *Breast J* 7(5):345-53, 2001.

385. Zukov G: *The dancing Wu Li masters,* New York, 1979, William Morrow and Company.

386. Capra F: *The tao of physics, an exploration of the parallels between modern physics and Eastern mysticism,* Boston, 1999, Shambhala Publications.

# CHAPTER 8

# Yoga

*Mary Lou Galantino, John Musser*

Harrison is a 27-year-old graduate student with past medical history of chronic LBP for 2 years, who presents with a 3-month complaint of bilateral pain in wrists. He currently is undergoing work-up for CTS. He describes pain in wrists upon waking, which lasts for up to an hour. Pain recurs throughout the day, especially after a long duration of computer work. Pain currently is ranked 7/10 bilaterally. It radiates proximally and distally from the wrists with tingling but no numbness. He received physical therapy for his LBP 2 years ago with only fair results. He wants to know if adding a specific daily exercise program or receiving another course of physical therapy will help to reduce his wrist pain and possibly his back pain.

## Initial Examination

**Client Report:** He was referred to physical therapy by his physician to manage upper extremity pain and reassessment of LBP. He currently is scheduled for a nerve conduction velocity (NCV) study and an electromyogram (EMG) next week. He had a recent follow-up x-ray and MRI of his lumbosacral spine (LS) concerning his LBP. He is active and exercises on a regular basis. He thought that he would be able to "work out" his pain, but this resulted only in symptoms worsening.

**Diagnostic Tests:** X-ray LS: grade II L4-L5 anterior spondylolisthesis; MRI: L4-L5 anterior herniated nucleus pulposus (HNP) 50%

**Client Goals:** To decrease pain so that he can better tolerate a regular exercise program and daily activities

**Employment:** Client is a graduate student with no outside employment.

**Recreational Activities:** Strength training, skiing, hiking, camping

**General Health:** Good

**Medications:** None

**Musculoskeletal:** ROM: Trunk limited in full extension and flexion, bilateral upper and lower extremities within normal limits (WNL) except for bilateral wrists: −5 degrees of extension. Posture: Client presents with forward head and shoulders. Cervical ROM: Restricted in side-bending and rotation at end-range bilaterally.

**Neuromuscular:** Force generation: Trunk: 4/5; bilateral extremities 5/5 throughout. Sensation: Decreased at C6-C7 dermatomes, R>L. Tests for CTS: +Tinel's sign and Phalen tests bilaterally. Neural tension tests: +C5-C7 nerve root involvement

**Function:** Pain: LBP 4/10 in the seated position; 6/10 after moderate physical activity, including ambulation for >0.5 hour, repetitive forward flexion and extension. CTS pain: 7/10 on the right and 6/10 on the left

**Outcome Measurements:** SF 36=30 (below the standard norm); Oswestry Low Back Pain Disability Questionnaire (ODI) Score=38%, which indicates moderate disability.[1,2] Life Stress Inventory=225 implies about a 50% chance of a major health challenge in the next 2 years.[3] The use of these measures guides the therapist in Harrison's perceived stress and disability as it relates to plans for intervention.

## Plan of Care

Harrison attended five physical therapy sessions over the course of a month for manual therapy, including soft tissue techniques, mobilization of the spine, and instructions for an exercise program with a focus on core stabilization to improve spinal flexibility and postural dynamics. He has continued this exercise program with moderate compliance. He also incorporated proper ergonomic setup in his workspace and was given wrist splints for his CTS pain, which he wears nightly. He was able to make improvements in trunk ROM and flexibility but was not pleased with the duration of pain relief from therapy. He wanted to be able to increase his daily activities.

## Reevaluation

A reexamination demonstrated an improvement in trunk ROM and flexibility by 30% overall. He reported improvement in LBP 3/10 in sedentary situations and 4/5 with ambulation. CTS symptoms moderately improved to 4/10. He still was unable to remain significantly pain free for extended periods of time. Transcutaneous electrical nerve stimulation (TENS) was tried as an intervention to assist in the management of his pain, but he found it too cumbersome to use on a regular basis and it was discontinued. Follow-up diagnostic tests (NCV and EMG) did reveal mild CTS. The ODI score upon reevaluation is 30%, still with moderate disability.

## Incorporating CAM into the Plan of Care

The therapist, familiar with yoga, suggests that the client consider trying yoga therapeutics to manage his overall stress and pain and to resolve symptoms of CTS and LBP. Although stress management techniques were recommended throughout the PT course of treatment, little carryover into daily activities occurred. Relaxation and breathing are major components of yoga, and Harrison agreed to try this as an adjunct to his rehabilitation program. The choice of the yoga practitioner was important in this plan of care because he or she needed to be equipped to address specific needs of various impairments and disabilities presenting in a session. Harrison was referred to a yoga practitioner well known to the physical therapist. The practitioner had personal experiences with LBP and had a keen sense of adaptations necessary to progress the therapeutic process of this client and others in her classes.

The therapist had developed a plan of care that included TENS, manual therapy, soft tissue mobilization, and an exercise regimen that focused on flexibility exercises and strengthening the thoracolumbar region and abdominals. The client also was given instructions for establishment of the best ergonomic setup for his work environment. Although the client's impairments of ROM, strength, pain, and endurance were improving, the client was still not able to attain long-term pain management. His general stress level could potentiate persistent pain and disability. To evaluate the appropriateness of recommending yoga for Harrison, the therapist needs to become familiar with the effect of yoga on his condition. By evaluating the evidence supporting its use in clients diagnosed with LBP or CTS, the therapist is able to safely recommend yoga as an intervention in addition to his rehabilitation program.

## INVESTIGATING THE LITERATURE

The therapist uses two strategies to investigate the literature. The first is a detailed approach in which preliminary background reading is performed on the management of LBP and CTS with yoga. This is followed by a search of databases and evaluation of the evidence with use of reviews and primary sources for LBP and CTS and yoga. The second is the use of the PICO format for a focused search to answer the clinical questions generated by the case.

In this case two PICOs are generated to address CTS and LBP separately.

## Preliminary Reading: Yoga

This client is not alone in his quest to explore yoga as a potential therapy. Millions of people in the United States, whether by their own curiosity or by the recommendation of their doctors, physical therapists, and others, are exploring yoga as a therapy for a broad spectrum of medical conditions.[4] In fact, a recent survey of the use of CAM in American adults demonstrated that of those who used yoga specifically as a CAM therapy, 21% did so because it was recommended by a conventional medical professional, 31% did so because conventional therapies would not help, and 59% thought it would be an interesting therapy to explore.[5] For centuries yoga has been practiced as a therapeutic modality in traditional Indian medicine.[4] Yoga is now one of the most common mind-body therapies used in Western complementary medicine.[6] It uniquely brings about physical and mental benefits and involves inexpensive self-care–based activities, which makes yoga appealing as a cost-effective alternative to conventional treatments.[7,8] Yoga therapy is an emerging field and is the first attempt to integrate the traditional yogic practice with Western medicine.[9] Before they recommend yoga therapeutically, therapists first must understand the traditional practice of yoga.

### Overview of Yoga

Yoga is complex. Its long and rich history extends back 5000 years to ancient India. Therefore to explore the totality of yoga within this chapter is impossible. Additional resources are provided at the end of this chapter in Appendix 1 for further exploration of yoga's history, philosophy, and practice. More information on yoga can be found in Chapter 7.

Yoga, in the traditional sense, is a spiritual way of life that extends well beyond the complicated poses and breath work. The traditional practice of yoga is actually a rigorous spiritual discipline composed of a vast array of physical and mental exercises, in addition to philosophical, moral, and even nutritional practices, all aimed at self-transformation by union of the mind, body, and spirit. As such, yoga truly embodies a holistic approach to life and health. It takes even the most dedicated a life-time to master. For the most part, however, since its introduction to the West in the late 1880s, yoga has undergone a metamorphosis into a more physically based "fitness yoga." Many purists, however, still see this Westernized yoga form as an opportunity for exploring the deeper side of yoga and the spiritual aspects of life.[9]

Yoga is complex even to define. The word *yoga* has several translations and comes from the root "yug" (to join), or "yoke" (to bind together). Essentially, yoga describes a method of discipline or means of uniting the body to the mind. The National Center for Complementary and Alternative Medicine (NCCAM) classifies yoga as a mind-body therapy, defining it as "yoga—this combination of breathing exercises, physical postures, and meditation, practiced for over 5000 years, calms the nervous system and balances body, mind, and spirit. It is thought to prevent specific diseases and maladies by keeping the energy meridians open and life energy flowing."[5] Yoga, like other mind-body therapies, is centered on development and/or enhancement of physical, psychological, and spiritual health.[10] Yoga's belief system that strongly claims mind, body, and spirit are interwoven is manifested and realized through the dedicated practice of yoga.[9]

### Yoga Practice

What is commonly referred to as "yoga" in the West is actually Hatha yoga, one of dozens of types of Hindu yoga practiced around the world today. Hatha yoga is the "yoga of activity," with a higher focus on physical postures, deep breathing exercises, and meditation in contrast to other forms of yoga, which may focus more on ethics, meditation, or diet. Because it is one of the types of yoga one can experience, its tangibility has made it the most popular form of yoga practiced in the West and the most practical therapeutically. All styles of yoga, however, are said to lead down the same path, that being toward spiritual enlightenment through self-transformation.[9]

The traditional path of Hatha yoga is said to involve eight components, or limbs, to attain a person's full potential and live a purposeful life.[9] These components are a prescription for self-discipline, and they direct attention towards one's body, mind, and overall health. These eight paths include (1) moral precepts, (2) personal behavior concepts, (3) physical postures (most familiar to

Westerners), (4) conscious regulation of the breath, (5) focus of the senses inward, (6) concentration, (7) meditation, and (8) ecstasy. Each path is meant to lead to the next. Although to mention these paths of the traditional Hatha practice is important, the focus for this client should center on the more physical and mental aspects for which Hatha yoga is known and that the client would most likely encounter. Several elements in Hatha yoga exist, which include physical postures (asanas), breathwork (pranayama), withdrawal (pratayahara), concentration (dharana), and meditation (dhyana).

The physical postures, called *asanas,* are designed to purify, cleanse, and gain mastery over the physical body to allow the body to prepare for meditation or stillness.[11] In the yogic view, a strong, flexible, and conditioned body is necessary as a foundation for the higher spiritual pursuits. Although not typically considered an aerobic exercise, these yogic postures are meant to help the client develop strength, flexibility, and endurance in muscles and improve circulation and alignment in spine.[9]

More than 200 actual asanas exist, each with its own purpose, which creates a system designed to seek out every muscle, joint, and ligament and exercise it.[9] Within a pose, certain muscles are meant to be flexed, others stretched, which enables relaxation and improved flexibility. Procedures exist for entering, holding, and emerging from each pose, along with specific sequences of poses. Movements are typically slow and coordinated with controlled breathing so that full inhalation is achieved upon entering the pose. The pose and breath are held briefly and then released simultaneously so that the starting point is reached at full exhalation. Every pose has a counterpose to balance its effects.

Typically every practice uses a variety of poses; most involve the muscles of the back and abdomen (Figure 8-1). Standing poses are designed for centering and alignment (Figure 8-2). Seated poses are designed to be more calming than the standing poses (Figure 8-3). Forward bends, with flexion in the hips, rather than the spine, can be done seated, standing (Figure 8-4), supine, twisting, balancing, or inverted. Balancing postures are designed to develop the body's coordination and strength (see Figure 8-2). Twisting poses help activate the spine, internal organs, and muscles (Figure 8-5). Backbends are meant to strengthen the extensor muscles, stretch the flexor muscles, and stimulate the entire nervous system (Figure 8-6). Inversion postures are said to strengthen the cardiovascular system and

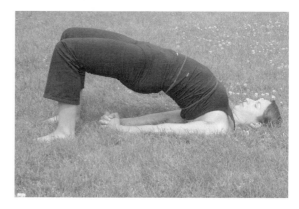

**Figure 8-1** Bridge posture illustrating the use of the back and abdomen. Reproduced with permission of Joel Stern.

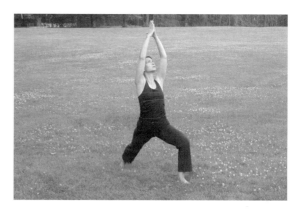

**Figure 8-2** Standing pose for alignment and balance. Reproduced with permission of Joel Stern.

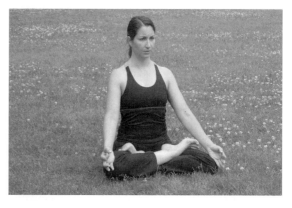

**Figure 8-3** Seated pose for meditation and stillness: lotus. Reproduced with permission of Joel Stern.

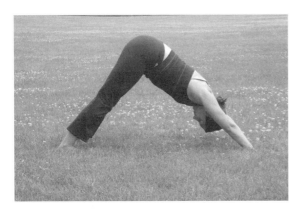

**Figure 8-4** Forward bending at the hips: downward dog. Reproduced with permission of Joel Stern.

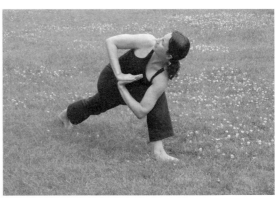

**Figure 8-5** Twisting posture. Reproduced with permission of Joel Stern.

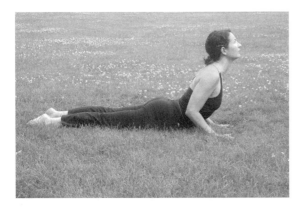

**Figure 8-6** Extensor posture: cobra. Reproduced with permission of Joel Stern.

obviously reverse the effects of gravity (see Figure 8-4).

Many various styles of Hatha yoga exist, each approaching the asana practice in a particular way (Table 8-1). Some use faster, flowing asana movements, such as Ashtanga, whereas others, such as Iyengar, use poses held for longer durations with attention to detail. Iyengar is one of the most popular styles in the West and uses props to accommodate special needs of the yoga instructor Viniyoga is another popular form, which allows poses to be customized to the individual; thus it is good for students with physical limitations.

Generally associated with the asanas is breath control, a practice called "pranayama," which also can be used as an isolated practice. The pranayamic breath is meant to be deep, rhythmic breathing through the nose during inhalation and exhalation. Pranayama is designed to gain conscious control of one of the most basic and largely unconscious bodily functions and allows realization of the connection between the breath, mind, and emotions.[9] In the yogic view, if the breath is calm and controlled, so can be the mind.[4]

Two other limbs of the yogic practice, pratyahara (withdrawal of the senses) and dharana (concentration), are important skills that increase attention and awareness. Practicing these two paths is said to place a person in "the zone" and helps bring awareness to positioning and posture. These are also important practices that allow people to sense and understand the limitations of their bodies.[9] These practices allow someone to draw attention inward, learn to recognize habitual thought patterns, and become aware of the body and its rhythms. The practice of meditation, or dhyana, results in uninterrupted concentration aimed at quieting the mind and body. It commonly is used as a practice apart from the other yogic practices.[9]

## Searching Databases and Evaluating the Evidence: Yoga

### Critical Reviews

The therapist explores the depth of scientific literature on yoga and assesses the evidence of its therapeutic application for the diagnoses relevant to the client. The therapist searches the Cochrane Collection Evidence-Based Medicine databases for any

| Table 8-1 | Different Schools of Hatha Yoga Commonly Practiced in the United States | |
|---|---|---|
| SCHOOL | FOCUS | DESCRIPTION |
| **Iyengar** | **Detail** | Technical yoga, an intense focus on the subtleties of each posture; great for beginning students |
| | | Strong focus on precise muscular and skeletal alignment; emphasizes therapeutic properties of the poses |
| | | Poses (especially standing postures) are typically held much longer than in other schools of yoga to focus on alignment |
| | | Use of props (belts, chairs, blocks, and blankets) to accommodate special needs such as injuries or structural imbalances. |
| **Ashtanga/Power Yoga** | **Fitness** | Athletic; fast paced and non-stop; not recommended for beginning students |
| | | At the core is linking the breath with each movement thoughout the practice |
| | | Power Yoga is a derivative, using a more creative sequences of postures |
| **Jivamukti** | **Fitness** | Athletic; highly meditative but physically challenging form of yoga |
| | | Combines an Ashtanga background with a variety of ancient and modern spiritual teachings |
| | | Uses chanting, meditation, reading, music, and affirmations |
| **Bikram/Hot Yoga** | **Healing** | Athletic; practiced in a room heated to 100+ degrees, thus "hot" yoga |
| | | Sauna-like effect helps move the toxins out of your body |
| **Kripalu** | **Healing** | Therapeutic; gentle and spiritually focused; Great for beginning students |
| | | Incorporates inner focus and meditation within the yoga poses; focus on alignment, breath, and the presence of consciousness |
| | | Holding of the postures to the level of tolerance and beyond |
| | | Deepens concentration and focus of internal thoughts and emotions |
| **Integrative Yoga Therapy** | **Healing** | Designed specifically for medical and mainstream wellness settings including hospitals and rehabilitation centers |
| | | Gentle postures, guided imagery, and breathing techniques for treating specific health issues |
| | | Emphasizes the healing process in detail by addressing all levels of the patient: physical, emotional, and spiritual |
| **Phoenix Rising Yoga Therapy** | **Healing** | Combination of classical yoga and elements of contemporary client-centered and mind-body psychology |
| | | Facilitates a power release of physical tensions and emotional blocks |
| | | Assisted yoga postures, guided breathing, and nondirective dialogue |
| | | Focused on experiencing the connection of the physical and emotional self |
| **Viniyoga** | **Healing** | Therapeutic; repetitious movements in and out of a posture |
| | | Individualistic; poses are synchronized with the breath in sequences determined by the needs of the practitioner |
| | | Highly adaptable, thus good for students with physical injuries or limitations |
| **Svaroopa** | **Healing** | Consciousness-oriented, emphasizing the development of transcendent inner experience, called svaroopa |
| | | Promotes healing and transformation; teaches different ways of doing familiar poses |
| | | Emphasizes the opening of the spine by beginning at the tailbone and progressing through each spinal area |
| **Ananda** | **Enlightenment** | Tool for spiritual growth while releasing unwanted tensions |
| | | Uses silent affirmations while holding a pose as a technique for aligning body, energy, and mind |
| | | Series of gentle poses designed to move energy upward to the brain, preparing the body for meditation. |

| Table 8-1 | Different Schools of Hatha Yoga Commonly Practiced in the United States—cont'd | | |
|-----------|--------|-------------|
| SCHOOL | FOCUS | DESCRIPTION |
| **Integral** | **Enlightenment** | Aimed at helping people integrate yoga's teachings into their everyday work and relationships |
| | | Incorporates guided relaxation, breathing practices, sound vibration (repetition of mantra or chant), and silent meditation |
| **Kundalini** | **Enlightenment** | Dynamic; esoteric; energizing; aimed at invoking dormant spiritual energy at the base of the spine |
| | | Incorporates breath-work, movement, postures, chanting, and meditating on mantras. |
| **Sivananda** | **Enlightenment** | Traditional approach; can become very advanced |
| | | Ridgid class structure of poses, breath-work, mediation, and relaxation. |
| | | Emphasizes 12 basic postures to increase strength and flexibility of the spine |
| | | Focus on proper pose, breathing, relaxation, and diet (vegetarian), and positive thinking and meditation |

critical reviews published on existing and definitive controlled trials using yoga. With the keyword *yoga*, a search in the Database of Abstracts of Reviews of Effects (DARE) results in only four critical reviews. However, none of these results are relevant for the client: two were for yoga and asthma, one for yoga and hypertension.

Another search using the same keyword, *yoga*, this time in the Cochrane Database of Systematic Reviews, yields 14 systematic reviews, although only one is relevant to this client. This review, "Nonsurgical Treatment (Other Than Steroid Injection) For Carpal Tunnel Syndrome,"[12] critiqued the work of Garfinkel et al.[13] This systematic review indicates that the current evidence demonstrates significant short-term benefit from yoga on symptoms of pain related to CTS and that more trials are needed to compare treatments and ascertain the duration of benefit.

The high prevalence of chronic LBP but the lack of any critical reviews on yoga's definitive application as an intervention indicates that more rigorous research is necessary to develop a stronger body of evidence for such a treatment. Likewise, given only one existing critical review for yoga's definitive effect on CTS furthers the notion that more research still needs to be undertaken on yoga's therapeutic applications.

### Primary Sources

Because only one single critical review of yoga therapy exists for CTS and no such reviews for yoga in treatment of LBP, it is necessary to search other databases to assess whatever other evidence exists. A review of the literature on the evidence of yoga as a management tool is conducted first.

Relevant studies are identified using several databases: PubMed (searched January 1960 to July 15, 2004), CAM on PubMed (searched January 1960 to July 15, 2004), Medline (searched January 1966 to July 15, 2004), CINAHL (searched January 1983 to July 2004), and PsycInfo (searched January 1960 to July 15, 2004). Non-English papers are excluded when no translation was available. The restriction to English-only studies may create some bias. Some would argue, however, that this bias should be balanced out because a recent assessment reported that non-English papers are likely of low quality and could introduce bias themselves.[14]

The yoga literature from its native India also was researched. Although currently approximately 45 Indian medical journals are indexed in MEDLINE, the Indian MEDLARS Center's IndMED database also is searched (January 1985 to July 2004) because it contains additional Indian journals. Numbers of studies identified from the search are included in Tables 8-2 and 8-3. It was decided ahead of time to not discuss these potential studies largely because of their full-text inaccessibility. In addition, surprisingly no articles of much significance or relevance to the client are found.

Using various keywords, each database was searched, and when possible, searches are limited to *clinical trial, randomized controlled trial (RCT), review, and meta-analysis* (see Tables 8-2 and 8-3).

**Table 8-2    Results of Literature Search: Part 1**

| DATABASE | PUBLICATION TYPE | LBP* | LBP + THERAPY | CTS† | CTS + THERAPY | YOGA | YOGA + PAIN | YOGA + LBP | YOGA + CTS | YOGA + MSK |
|---|---|---|---|---|---|---|---|---|---|---|
| PubMed | Clinical trial | 990 | 842 | 250 | 187 | 84 | 5 | 3 | 1 | 2 |
| | RCT | 609 | 557 | 121 | 113 | 52 | 5 | 3 | 1 | 1 |
| | Review | 1300 | 977 | 570 | 370 | 80 | 14 | 2 | 4 | 7 |
| | Meta-analysis | 44 | 34 | 12 | 10 | 2 | 0 | 0 | 1 | 0 |
| CAM | Clinical trial | 210 | 205 | 14 | 14 | 85 | 5 | 2 | 1 | 2 |
| | RCT | 162 | 158 | 10 | 10 | 52 | 5 | 2 | 1 | 1 |
| | Review | 174 | 158 | 25 | 23 | 85 | 14 | 2 | 4 | 7 |
| | Meta-analysis | 13 | 13 | 10 | 2 | 2 | 0 | 0 | 1 | 0 |
| MEDLINE | Clinical trial | 719 | 206 | 227 | 23 | 73 | 5 | 2 | 1 | 1 |
| | RCT | 434 | 153 | 112 | 14 | 41 | 5 | 2 | 1 | 1 |
| | Review | 897 | 227 | 429 | 57 | 54 | 12 | 2 | 4 | 5 |
| | Meta-analysis | 38 | 9 | 13 | 2 | 1 | 0 | 0 | 1 | 0 |
| CINAHL* | Clinical trial | 144 | 44 | 24 | 3 | 2 | 0 | 0 | 1 | 0 |
| | RCT | – | – | – | – | – | – | – | – | – |
| | Review | 253 | 44 | 39 | 0 | 12 | 5 | 1 | 0 | 1 |
| | Meta-analysis | – | – | – | – | – | – | – | – | – |
| PsycINFO | Clinical trial | 16 | 11 | 1 | 0 | 0 | 0 | 0 | 0 | 0 |
| | RCT | 0 | 0 | 0 | 0 | 0 | 0 | 0 | 0 | 0 |
| | Review | 42 | 11 | 1 | 0 | 23 | 3 | 0 | 1 | 3 |
| | Meta-analysis | 4 | 1 | 0 | 0 | 0 | 0 | 0 | 0 | 0 |
| IndMED† | All | 4 | 1 | 0 | 0 | 62 | 1 | 0 | 0 | 0 |

*LBP*, low back pain; *CTS*, carpal tunnel syndrome; *MSK*, musculoskeletal; *RCT*, randomized controlled trial.
*CINAHL does not allow limited searches of RCTs or meta-analyses.
†IndMED does not allow limited searches.

**Table 8-3    Results of Literature Search: Part 2**

| DATABASE | PUBLICATION TYPE | YOGA + COPING | YOGA + STRESS | YOGA + ANXIETY |
|---|---|---|---|---|
| PubMed | Clinical trial | 6 | 15 | 10 |
| | RCT | 4 | 9 | 8 |
| | Review | 3 | 20 | 7 |
| | Meta-analysis | 0 | 0 | 0 |
| CAM | Clinical trial | 6 | 15 | 10 |
| | RCT | 4 | 9 | 8 |
| | Review | 3 | 20 | 7 |
| | Meta-analysis | 0 | 0 | 0 |
| MEDLINE | Clinical trial | 3 | 15 | 10 |
| | RCT | 1 | 9 | 8 |
| | Review | 2 | 16 | 6 |
| | Meta-analysis | 0 | 0 | 0 |
| CINAHL* | Clinical trial | 0 | 0 | 0 |
| | RCT | – | – | – |
| | Review | 0 | 2 | 1 |
| | Meta-analysis | – | – | – |
| PsycINFO | Clinical trial | 0 | 0 | 0 |
| | RCT | 0 | 0 | 0 |
| | Review | 1 | 6 | 1 |
| | Meta-analysis | 0 | 0 | 0 |
| IndMED† | All | 3 | 11 | 4 |

*RCT*, randomized controlled trial.
*CINAHL does not allow limited searches of RCTs or meta-analyses.
†IndMED does not allow limited searches.

The PsycInfo and IndMED databases do not have the option of searching with limitations, and CINAHL does not limit to RCTs or meta-analyses. The therapist is interested in determining the depth of research about the conditions and treatment the client faces, so keywords *carpal tunnel syndrome* and *low back pain* are searched separately. Adding *therapy* to these two searches further refines the field and shows many review articles on these two subjects. A quick search using *yoga* yielded a number of studies, but a cursory review yields studies investigating yoga for asthma, epilepsy, diabetes, multiple sclerosis, stress management, psychotherapy, and more. Combining *yoga* with the additional keywords *pain* or *low back pain* or *carpal tunnel syndrome*, or even *musculoskeletal*, actually results in few studies. The small number of studies on yoga and CTS, and yoga and LBP is surprising, especially considering that yoga has long been touted to be a great therapy for musculoskeletal conditions. Obviously, much work still needs to be done to scientifically demonstrate the potential preventative and therapeutic role of yoga on the neuromusculoskeletal system.

Last, because stress has been shown to be one of the factors leading to musculoskeletal disorders such as LBP and CTS,[15] the therapist also decides to investigate the literature for studies concerning yoga's role in managing stress. The therapist used the keyword *yoga* paired with *stress, anxiety,* or *coping* (see Table 8-3). As expected, a large body of evidence investigates yoga's role in management of stress, anxiety, and coping skills. Addressing stress and improving coping strategies are important parts of any rehabilitative care.

### Searching Databases and Evaluating the Evidence: Management of Carpal Tunnel Syndrome and Yoga

In addition to reviewing the literature on yoga the therapist researches the management of diagnoses of CTS and LBP. She would like to learn about modalities used for these diagnoses and gain perspectives on nonpharmacological approaches to the management of pain.

CTS of mild to moderate severity often can be treated effectively in a primary care environment. Articles have suggested that workplace task modification and wrist splints can reduce or defer referral to the hospital for surgical decompression. Nerve and tendon gliding exercises also may be of benefit.[16] Treatments have included surgery, physical therapy, drug therapy, chiropractic treatment, biobehavioral interventions, and occupational rehabilitation. One 12-year systematic review of outcomes of these interventions on symptoms, medical status, function, return to work, psychological well-being, and client satisfaction was completed.[17] Limited evidence indicates that (1) steroid injections and oral use of vitamin B6 were associated with pain reduction; (2) in comparison with splinting, ROM exercises appeared to be associated with less pain and fewer days to return to work; (3) cognitive-behavior therapy yielded reductions in pain, anxiety, and depression; and (4) multidisciplinary occupational rehabilitation was associated with a higher percentage of chronic cases returning to work than usual care.[17]

Another study examined conservative treatment options for relief of the symptoms of CTS.[18] Their findings showed that diuretics, pyridoxine, nonsteroidal antiinflammatory drugs (NSAIDs), yoga, and laser acupuncture seem to be ineffective in providing short-term symptom relief[18] and that steroid injections seem to be effective (limited evidence).[12] Conflicting evidence exists for the efficacy of ultrasound and oral steroids.[19] Recent systematic reviews demonstrated that NSAIDs, pyridoxine, and diuretics are no more effective than placebo in relief of the symptoms of CTS.[18,20] Conservative treatment options also have included splinting the wrist in a neutral position and ultrasound therapy.[19] However, for providing long-term relief from symptoms, limited evidence exists that ultrasound is effective and that splinting is less effective than surgery.[19] One systematic review determined that all studies using splinting had serious methodological flaws.[17]

Nonsurgical treatment for CTS frequently is offered to those with mild to moderate symptoms. The effectiveness and duration of benefit from nonsurgical treatment for CTS remain unknown. An extensive search strategy was employed to evaluate the effectiveness of nonsurgical treatment for CTS versus a placebo or other nonsurgical, control interventions to improve clinical outcome.[21] The primary outcome measure was improvement in clinical symptoms after at least 3 months after the end of treatment. Current evidence shows significant short-term benefit from oral steroids, splinting, ultrasound, yoga, and carpal bone mobilization. Other nonsurgical treatments do not produce significant benefit.[21]

Conclusions from these studies are preliminary because of the small number of well-controlled studies, variability in duration of symptoms and disability, and the broad range of reported outcome measures. Although several opinions exist regarding effective treatment, little scientific support exists for the range of options currently used in practice. Despite the emerging evidence of the multivariate nature of CTS, the majority of outcome studies have focused on single interventions directed at individual etiological factors or symptoms and functional limitations secondary to CTS.[17]

The literature is sparse on studies that examine the effect of yoga on CTS. Only one RCT assesses yoga as a therapy for CTS to date. This study by Garfinkel et al[13] compared the use of yoga (Iyengar yoga) with the use of splinting. They used 11 yoga postures designed for strengthening, stretching, and balancing each joint in the upper body and held for 30 seconds, along with relaxation poses. After 8 weeks they showed that a yoga-based regimen was more effective than wrist splinting or no treatment in strengthening hand grip and relieving some symptoms (pain) and signs (Phalen's sign) of CTS. Although improvement occurred in motor and sensory nerve conduction tests for both groups, the difference between them was not statistically significant.

This lone study by Garfinkel et al[13] has been reviewed many times. A systematic review of the literature in 2002 showed yoga to be ineffective in providing short-term symptom relief (varying levels of evidence) for CTS.[19] Current review of this evidence, however, determined that a significant short-term benefit from yoga exists.[21,22] Another 2004 systematic review finds yoga "possibly effective" and recommends it as a first-line management in selected cases.[18]

In conclusion, still little is known about the efficacy of most conservative treatment options for CTS. To establish stronger evidence, more high-quality trials are needed.[19] Based on the literature review, a recommendation to include yoga as part of Harrison's CTS therapeutic regimen is taken judiciously. The use of yoga specifically for CTS incorporates cervical and thoracic mobility that may have direct impact on posture and overall reduction in symptoms of CTS. Further research regarding the nature of specific poses is also important for future recommendations. Additional research is required to clarify the relative efficacy of different mind-body therapies, factors (such as specific client characteristics) that may predict more or less successful outcomes, and mechanisms of action.

## Searching Databases and Evaluating the Evidence: Lower Back Pain and Yoga

LBP is a significant public health problem and one of the most commonly reported reasons for the use of complementary therapies. Although many potential therapies for LBP exist, currently few treatments with clearly demonstrated efficacy are known, once the pain becomes chronic. Recent research suggests a need for a more active approach with a move away from long-term rest toward progressive activity and exercise.[23,24]

Although many studies regarding the effectiveness of interventions for the treatment of LBP have been performed, a recent review of back pain studies revealed few therapies for which the trials have a high methodological quality.[25] Two areas with good evidence are the use of NSAIDs and muscle relaxants, which are effective for acute LBP.[25,26,27] The studies of manipulation, back schools, and exercise for LBP have had mixed results but suggest some efficacy.[26,28,29] Assendelft et al examined the literature to resolve the discrepancies related to use of spinal manipulative therapy and to update previous estimates of effectiveness by comparison of spinal manipulative therapy with other therapies and then incorporation of data from recent high-quality RCTs into an analysis.[30] They found that no evidence exists that spinal manipulative therapy is superior to other standard treatments for clients with acute or chronic LBP. In addition, no one treatment has been shown to be effective for all clients.[23,31] Activity-related studies that evaluate specific treatments, including back exercises and alterations in activities of daily living (ADL), have not documented long-term pain relief in many clients.[32,33] Among the studies that explore various types of exercise for LBP, even fewer examine nontraditional interventions such as tai chi and yoga.

A multidimensional approach to the understanding of pain that incorporates biopsychosocial factors has gained acceptance, emphasizing the importance of psychological factors in the realm of pain research and practice.[34,35] From a biopsychosocial perspective, chronic pain includes all three dimensions (biological, psychological, and social), which can be equally important determinants of the person's experience.[34] Interventions such as yoga that treat more than one aspect of LBP are an important group to investigate.

One small pilot study looked at the effects of a 6-week modified Hatha yoga program on 22 clients with LBP.[36] Although potentially important trends in functional measurement scores showed improved balance and flexibility and decreased disability and depression, the small sample size limited detection of significant changes. Preliminary data from a study by Williams et al indicated that the majority of self-referred persons with mild chronic LBP will comply with and report improvement on medical and functional pain-related outcomes from Iyengar yoga therapy.[37] Subjects with nonspecific chronic LBP compared 16 weeks of Iyengar yoga therapy to an educational control group. Analyses of medical and functional outcomes revealed significant reductions in pain intensity (64%), functional disability (77%), and pain medication usage (88%) in the yoga group at the post-treatment and 3-month follow-up assessments. This is important because the follow-up in physical therapy treatments is also necessary to determine effectiveness of rehabilitation interventions.

An RCT study by Sherman et al (2005) determined whether yoga is more effective than conventional therapeutic exercise or a self-care book for clients with chronic LBP. Subjects underwent 12-week sessions of yoga or conventional therapeutic exercise classes or a self-care book. Back-related function in the yoga group was superior to the book and exercise groups at 12 weeks and persisted at 26 weeks. Yoga was more effective than a self-care book to improve function and reduce chronic LBP, and the benefits persisted for at least several months.[38]

Physical therapy in conjunction with individualized exercise regimens of flexion or extension exercises that concentrate on strengthening and/or lengthening back muscles has been recommended to many clients with LBP.[39] However, because physicians may choose a course of exercises for a client based on a general concept of strengthening muscles as the goal of exercise, they do not individualize the client's regimen to the underlying abnormality in the musculoskeletal structures of the lumbosacral spine. Consequently, the maximum benefit of therapy may not be achieved.[39] Yoga therapy is beneficial in this respect because it is aspires to tailor specific postures to the individual's condition and often combines flexion and extension postures in each session.

Good general fitness has been associated with decreased incidence of back injuries and decreased duration of incapacity with a back injury.[40] The lack of endurance of back muscles plays a role in the cause and/or perpetuation of back pain.[41-43] A return of full muscle strength, joint movement, and endurance is necessary for a complete recovery of func-

tion.[39] Compared with a focus on strengthening an isolated area, strengthening and lengthening the paraspinous, psoas, and hamstring muscles to achieve normal physiological balance of the lumbosacral spine and its supporting structures result in improved outcomes of pain occurrence.[44]

In general, three types of exercise treatments exist: (1) mobility and strengthening exercises, (2) lumbar isometric flexion exercises, and (3) hyperextension exercises.

Data that demonstrate the greater efficacy of one type over another are either conflicting[45,46] or not available. Flexion exercises are known to open intervertebral foramina and facet joints, to stretch hip flexors and back extensors, to strengthen abdominal and gluteal muscles, and to mobilize the posterior fixation of the lumbosacral articulation[47,48] Extension exercises are known to improve motor strength and endurance and mobility, strengthen back extensors, or promote a shift of nuclear material to a normal position.[39] People with strong paraspinous extensors have less postural fatigue and pain, greater capacity to lift weights and to withstand axial compression, and better overall physical fitness. Existing evidence demonstrates the effects of extension exercises on strengthening lumbar extensor muscles.[49,50]

The physical postures in the asana practice of yoga have been shown to use stretching and improve muscular strength and flexibility.[51] Therefore the three studies that address the benefits of yoga present a case for its use within the rehabilitation process. Furthermore, one study[38] followed these chronic LBP clients through 26 weeks, clearly a timeframe not afforded by physical therapists in the present health care system. It does seem highly likely that various yogic postures would be potentially beneficial to treat chronic LBP. This is especially poignant considering that yoga involves flexion and extension exercises and improves flexibility.

To date, two clinical trials on the benefits of yoga use optimal clinical research methodology, whereas others lack adequate control groups. However, regular yoga practice has been shown to benefit pain management, muscle strength, and motor control in uncontrolled studies.[52,53] Because yoga can be conducted in a group setting, it is a relatively inexpensive form of physical conditioning that may prove to be a cost-effective treatment of musculoskeletal disorders. The reported benefits in nonspecific musculoskeletal syndromes have been sufficiently large with almost no serious side effects, to warrant further studies.[10] Clearly, more studies are required to determine the effects of yoga on acute and chronic LBP. Larger randomized sample sizes, group and individualized formats, and longer follow-up are needed. Control groups should involve group and nongroup settings, to detect any benefit that may be derived from group support. No reports of harm from yoga in LBP therapy were reported in the few studies found.

## Searching Databases and Evaluating the Literature: Stress and Yoga

Because the therapist suspects that stress is aggravating the client's pain complaints she searches the literature on yoga and stress. Stress has been shown to be one of the factors leading to musculoskeletal disorders such as back pain, CTS, shoulder or neck tension, eye strain, or headaches.[15]Although emerging evidence during the past several decades suggests that psychosocial factors can directly influence directly physiological function and health outcomes, medicine had failed to move beyond the biomedical model, in part because of lack of exposure to the evidence base supporting the biopsychosocial model.[54] Drawing principally from systematic reviews and meta-analyses, considerable evidence exists of efficacy for several mind-body therapies in the treatment of coronary artery disease, headaches, insomnia, incontinence, chronic LBP, disease-related and treatment-related symptoms of cancer, and improvement of postsurgical outcomes. Moderate evidence of efficacy for mind-body therapies exists in the areas of hypertension and arthritis. Now considerable evidence exists that an array of mind-body therapies can be used as effective adjuncts to conventional medical treatment for a number of common clinical conditions.[54]

Clients who practice Hatha yoga say it is valuable for prevention and management of stress-related chronic health problems, including LBP. In a survey of 3000 people receiving yoga for health ailments (1142 [38%] with back pain), 98% claimed that yoga benefited them.[55]

Yoga may reduce stress and relieve muscular tension or pain. The use of yoga in pain management includes beneficial effects on self-awareness, relaxation, approaches that use relaxation, breathing, increased self-understanding and self-acceptance, changed context of pain, increased control, lifestyle improvements, and group and social support.[53] Practicing yoga at the workplace teaches employees to use relaxation techniques to reduce stress and risks of injury on the job. Yoga at

the workplace may be a convenient and practical outlet that improves work performance by relief of tension and job stress.[15]

The therapist in this chapter performs many detailed searches. If she were pressed for time, she could generate two PICO questions—one for LBP and one for CTS. Her search could be conducted on one database.

---

### PICO BOX

For clients with LBP does the use of yoga decrease pain, stress, and disability and improve quality of life?

P: People with LBP
I: Yoga
O: Pain
O: Stress
O: Disability
O: Quality of life

A search performed in MEDLINE on July 6, 2006, combining all of the terms yielded zero references. Searches performed with each of the outcome measures separately yielded 18 for pain and 4 each for disability and quality of life. There were four overlapping references between pain, disability, and quality of life. The therapist had identified these four references in her comprehensive searching approach.

---

### PICO BOX

For clients with CTS, does the use of yoga decrease pain and stress and improve quality of life?

P: People with LBP
I: Yoga
C: Comparison (none)
O: Pain
O: Stress
O: Quality of life

A search performed in MEDLINE on July 6, 2006, combining all of the terms yields zero references. Searches performed with each of the outcome measures separately yielded 5 for pain, 1 for stress, and 0 for quality of life. The reference for stress overlapped with that of pain. Therefore a set of five references is found relating to the PICO.

P = **Population** (patient/client, problem, person condition or group attribute)
I = **Intervention** (the CAM therapy or approach)
C = **Comparison** (standard care or comparison intervention)
O = **Outcomes** (the measured variables of interest)

## CLINICAL DECISION MAKING

Integrating the findings from the CTS, LBP, stress, and yoga searches, the therapist concludes that some direct evidence supports the use of yoga for management of CTS, LBP, and stress. She feels that Harrison will benefit from a multidimensional approach to manage the conditions, which she feels are interrelated.

### Generate a Clinical Hypothesis

Yoga as a multidimensional practice incorporates breathing techniques, relaxation, and meditation along with the poses to effect greater body awareness.

Having decided to recommend yoga as an intervention, the therapist must generate a clinical hypothesis. In this case, the therapist hypothesizes that yoga will address the CTS and LBP, thereby allowing the client to increase his daily activities.

### Examine

Before Harrison begins yoga, the therapist should conduct a reexamination that includes three standardized tools. Because concerns exist regarding global pain perceptions, the Medical Outcomes Study Pain Measure (MOS) would capture severity in terms of the intensity, frequency, and duration of pain and record the impact of pain on behavior and moods.[56] This instrument offers a brief measure suitable when the goal is to assess the impact of pain on daily living, rather than to provide a detailed assessment of the nature of pain. Alternatively, the SF-36, commonly used in rehabilitation settings, is a general health survey that captures quality of life perceptions by the client. The SF-36 contains a score that represents the psychological well-being and general health perception of the respondent. This composite score is norm-based (mean=50, SD=10), with lower scores representing poorer health. The SF-36 provides the benefits of a general functional health status measure and additionally appears to provide a screening tool for depressive symptoms.[57] Depression is a common co-morbidity for clients with complaints of chronic LBP yet often goes undiagnosed in clinical practice. Depressed clients who are not identified do not receive a referral or recommendation for treatments that may help ease their total illness burden. Relative to the total outcomes of spine care this may increase costs, decrease overall functional outcomes, and limit client satisfaction.[56] Although a specific and reliable survey to detect depression could be employed, an additional survey would unnecessarily increase responder and analyst burdens if the general health status survey could be used instead.

The Oswestry Low Back Pain Disability (OLBPD) questionnaire should be used as a disease-specific instrument. The first section rates intensity of pain and the remaining nine cover the disabling effect on typical daily activities.[36,58] When self-administered, the OLBPD takes less than 5 minutes to complete and 1 minute to score. The British Medical Research Council and the journal *Spine* have recommended that the Oswestry questionnaire be used as a standard measurement for assessing back pain. Finally, the Life Stress Inventory can be used to derive a sense of major changes in a client's life and can be used as a predictor of potential future health concerns.[3]

### Intervene and Evaluate

The physical therapist explains the state of the literature to Harrison so that he is able to ask questions and participate in the decision about how to add yoga to his plan of care. The therapist refers Harrison to a yoga instructor who offers beginner classes that focus on asanas, which promote relaxation and spinal alignment. The instructor, who has been teaching yoga for 15 years, also has personal experience with LBP and has the reputation of integrating opposing and restorative postures into every session and progressing students toward improving their spinal mobility cautiously. The physical therapist and yoga instructor discuss the combination of postures specific to the published literature in which CTS and LBP postures have been tested (Table 8-4). The therapist has referred several clients to this yoga instructor and enjoys a collegial relationship in which frequent communication occurs regarding the clients' status and recommendations for progression of the various poses. She receives written permission from Harrison to contact the instructor for progress reports on the yoga sessions.

The recommendation to a specific yoga instructor is essential because currently no national requirements exist regarding the subject matter of a yoga class or the method of instruction.[9] Although several yoga groups, such as Yoga Alliance and the Yoga Research and Education Center (YREC), have

| Table 8-4 | Yoga Postures |
|---|---|

Specific Yoga Postures Tested and Published in the CTS and LBP Literature and Utilized by the PT and Yoga Instructor for this Case Presentation

| YOGA POSTURE | AREA OF EMPHASIS |
|---|---|
| Introductory breathing exercises | Improve diaphragm expansion; increase body awareness; improve focus |
| Knee to chest variations (supine) | Increases low back flexibility |
| Modified spinal twists (supine) | Improves low back flexibility with upper body maintained flat on the floor/mat |
| Butterfly position (sitting) | Improves hip ROM; maintaining proper sitting posture |
| Kneeling (lateral pose) | Increases core stability with increase in thoracolumbar lateral flexion |
| Standing mountain pose (tadasana) | Increases body awareness and proprioception in standing; active pose despite static stance |
| Warrior pose (standing) | Upper body extended, while lunge position is maintained; increases core stability and elongation of spinal muscles |
| 90 degree forward bend to the wall | Improves hamstring and low back extensibility |
| Downward facing dog pose with use of a chair—until subject is able to gradually reach the floor | Gradual increase of posterior LE muscles with UE focus in extension and stability |
| Arms extended overhead with fingers locked in prayer pose | Lateral elongation of trunk muscles |
| Hands joined in prayer behind the back | Improves ROM of anterior shoulder girdle, rib cage, and wrist extensors |
| Standing lateral pose | Arms overhead improves ROM of entire UE and trunk |
| Deep relaxation | Fosters parasympathetic nervous system to decrease stress |
| Breathing and body awareness | Improved physiology of breathing; greater awareness of body in all dimensions |

*LE*, Lower extremity; *UE*, upper extremity.

established their own professional standards and instructor certification, certification requirements at the state or national level do not exist. A new student should become familiar with the instructor's approach, personality, and level of training. Some yoga instructors at health clubs are actually fitness instructors with only a few days of training in yogic postures.[9]

Harrison attends classes, which usually last 60 to 90 minutes and cost $10 to $15 per session. In this yoga style, props such as chairs, belts, blankets, or blocks are used with the poses. Although ultimately the practice is self-discipline, easily practiced in any space at home and in the office, it typically is practiced with an instructor who demonstrates the pose and gives individual guidance and adjustments to the students.

Because the client experiences his symptoms primarily at his work station, the therapist evaluates the ergonomics of the station and makes recommendations to improve the client's biomechanics at work and instructs him to monitor his symptoms and take more frequent rests. The therapist works with the client and the yoga instructor to select a few asanas that can be practiced safely in his work environment to promote improved posture and relaxation.

## Report the Outcomes

After subsequent physical therapy and yoga experiences, the client is reexamined to evaluate the outcome of the inclusion of yoga in his plan of care. His LBP improved from a 3/10 to a 1/10 but most importantly the time interval between the onset of symptoms increased from 30 minutes to 2 hours. His wrist pain decreased from a 4/10 to a 2/10 for a 2-hour interval. ROM increased by 75%.

Outcome Measurements: SF, 36=50 (achieved standard norm); Oswestry Low Back Pain Disability Questionnaire (ODI) Score=15% which indicates minimal disability. Life Stress Inventory=155, a considerable reduction in future health challenges in the next 2 years.

At this point the client reports that management of his symptoms every 2 hours is workable; however, he would like to increase that interval to at least 4 hours. His compliance, he reports, is better than with the therapeutic exercise because he enjoys the yoga class. He reports that he feels he is more efficient at work.

The therapist is pleased with the results and would like to communicate them to a physical therapy audience. Several randomized trials exist regarding the management of this client's conditions separately, but none address the combined diagnosis with the ergonomic modifications. She chooses to submit an abstract to the combined sections meeting of the APTA to present these findings in a case report to the orthopedic session. At the time of presentation she will determine if this article would be suitable for publication in the *Journal of Orthopedic and Sports Physical Therapy*.

## SUMMARY

The case of an individual with pain symptoms and limitations in his work ability resulting from LBP and CTS was described. The individual received some benefit from physical therapy intervention but was not complying with his home exercise program and had residual symptoms. Alternative forms of exercise should be considered when the issue of adherence is observed. The therapist reviewed the literature for evidence supporting the management of LBP and CTS using yoga. She finds evidence to support the use of yoga for each condition independently. After discussing the evidence with the client, they proceed to incorporate yoga into the plan of care. Appropriate recommendations by the physical therapist and yoga practitioner are important for successful outcomes. The benefits Harrison receives in terms of decreased pain and increased time without pain are reported at a professional meeting.

## REFERENCES

1. Fairbank JC et al: The Oswestry low back pain disability questionnaire, *Physiotherapy* 66:271-3, 1980.
2. Fritz JM, Irrgang JJ: A comparison of a modified Oswestry low back pain disability questionnaire and the Quebec back pain disability scale, *Physical Ther* 81:776-88, 2001.
3. Holmes T, Rahe R: Homes-Rahe social readjustment rating scale, *J Psychosomatic Res* 11(2):213-8, 1967.
4. Farrell SJ, Ross AD, Sehgal KV: Eastern movement therapies, *Phys Med Rehabil Clin North Am* 10:617-29, 1999.
5. Barnes PM et al: Complementary and alternative medicine use among adults: United States, 2002. *Adv Data* 27(343):1-19, 2004. In Advance Data from Vital and Health Statistics, Hyattsville, Maryland,
6. Wolsko PM et al: Use of mind–body medical therapies: results of a national survey, *J Gen Intern Med* 19:43-50, 2004.
7. Sobel DS: Mind matters, money matters: the cost-effectiveness of mind-body medicine, *JAMA* 284:1705, 2000.
8. Sobel D: The cost-effectiveness of mind-body medicine interventions, *Prog Brain Res* 122:393-412, 2000.
9. Feuerstein G: *The deeper dimension of yoga: theory and practice*, Boston, 2003, Shambhala.
10. Luskin FM et al: A review of mind/body therapies in the treatment of musculoskeletal disorders with implications for the elderly, *Altern Ther Health Med* 6:46-56, 2000.
11. Garfinkel M, Schumacher HR Jr: Yoga, *Rheum Dis Clin North Am* 26:125-32, 2000.
12. O'Connor D, Marshall S, Massy-Westropp N: Nonsurgical treatment (other than steroid injection) for carpal tunnel syndrome, *Cochrane Database of Systematic Reviews* 2, 2005.
13. Garfinkel MS et al: Yoga-based intervention for carpal tunnel syndrome: a randomized trial, *JAMA* 280(18):1601-3, 1998.
14. Egger M et al: How important are comprehensive literature searches and the assessment of trial quality in systematic reviews? Empirical study, *Health Technol Assess* 7:68, 2003.
15. Gura ST: Yoga for stress reduction and injury prevention at work, *Work* 19:3-7, 2002.
16. Burke FD et al: Primary care management of carpal tunnel syndrome, *Postgrad Med J* 79:433-7, 2003.
17. Feuerstein M et al: Clinical management of carpal tunnel syndrome: a 12-year review of outcomes, *Am J Ind Med* 35:232-45, 1999.
18. Goodyear-Smith F, Arroll B: What can family physicians offer patients with carpal tunnel syndrome other than surgery? A systematic review of nonsurgical management, *Ann Fam Med* 2:267-73, 2004.
19. Gerritsen AA et al: Conservative treatment options for carpal tunnel syndrome: a systematic review of randomised controlled trials, *J Neurol* 249:272-80, 2002.

20. Viera AJ: Management of carpal tunnel syndrome, *Am Fam Physician* 68:265-72, 2003.

21. O'Connor D, Marshall S, Massy-Westropp N: Non-surgical treatment (other than steroid injection) for carpal tunnel syndrome, *Cochrane Database of Systematic Reviews.* CD003219, 2004.

22. Muller M et al: Effectiveness of hand therapy interventions in primary management of carpal tunnel syndrome: a systematic review, *J Hand Ther* 17:210-28, 2004.

23. Deyo RA et al: A controlled-trial of transcutaneous electrical nerve stimulation (TENS) and exercise for chronic low back pain, *N Engl J Med* 322:1627-34, 1990.

24. Evans C et al: A randomized controlled trial of flexion exercises, education, and bed rest for patients with acute low back pain, *Physiother Can* 39:96-101, 1987.

25. EBM Reviews-ACP, Journal Club. Review: NSAIDS and muscle relaxants reduce acute low back pain; manipulation, back schools, and exercise reduce chronic low back pain, *ACP J Club* 128:65, 1998.

26. Malanga GA, Nadler SF: Non-operative treatment of low back pain, *Mayo Clin Proc* 74:135-48, 1999.

27. Koes BW et al: Efficacy of non-steroidal anti-inflammatory drugs for low back pain: a systematic review of randomised clinical trials, *Ann Rheum Dis* 56:214-23, 1997.

28. Shekelle PG et al: Spinal manipulation for low-back pain, *Ann Intern Med* 117:590-8, 1992.

29. Hurwitz EL et al: A randomized trial of medical care with and without physical therapy and chiropractic care with and without physical modalities for patients with low back pain: 6-month follow-up outcomes from the UCLA low back pain study, *Spine* 27:2193-2204, 2002.

30. Assendelft WJ et al: Spinal manipulative therapy for low back pain. A meta-analysis of effectiveness relative to other therapies, *Ann Intern Med* 138:871-81, 2003.

31. Mannion AF, Muntener EA: A randomized clinical trial of three active therapies for chronic low back pain, *Spine* 24:2435-48, 1999.

32. Frost H et al: Randomized controlled trial for evaluation of fitness programme for patients with chronic low back pain, *Br Med J* 310:151-9, 1995.

33. Spelman MR: Back pain: how health education affects patient compliance with treatment, *Occupational Health Nurs* 32:649-51, 1984.

34. Jacobson L, Marino AJ: General considerations of chronic pain. In Loeser JD, editor: *Bonica's management of pain*, ed 3, Philadelphia, 2001, Lippincott Williams & Wilkins.

35. Linton SJ: A review of psychological risk factors in back and neck pain, *Spine* 25:1148-56, 2000.

36. Galantino ML et al: The impact of modified Hatha yoga on chronic low back pain: a pilot study, *Altern Ther Health Med* 10:56-9, 2004.

37. Williams KA et al: Effect of iyengar yoga therapy for chronic low back pain, *Pain* 115(1-2):107-17, 2005.

38. Sherman KJ: Comparing yoga, exercise, and a self-care book for chronic low back pain: a randomized, controlled trial, *Ann Intern Med* 143(12):849-56, 2005.

39. Borenstein DG, Wiesel SW, Boden SD: Medical therapy. In Borenstein DG, Wiesel SW, Boden SD, editors: *Low back and neck pain: comprehensive diagnosis and management,* ed 3, Philadelphia, 2004, Elsevier, pp 785-93.

40. Cady L et al: Strength and fitness and subsequent back injuries in firefighters, *J Occup Med* 21:269-72, 1979.

41. De Vries H: EMG fatigue nerve in postural muscles: a possible etiology for idiopathic low back pain, *Am J Phys Med* 47:175, 1968.

42. Magora A: Investigation of the relation between low back pain and occupation: IV. history and symptoms, *Scand J Rehabil Med Medica* 81-8, 1974.

43. Poulsen E: Back muscle strength and weight limits in lifting, *Spine* 6:73-5, 1981.

44. Nachemson A: The possible importance of the psoas muscle for stabilization of the lumbar spine, *Acta Othop Scand* 39:47-7, 1968.

45. Davies JE GR, Tester L: The value of exercise in the treatment of low back pain, *Rheum Rehabil* 18:243-7, 1979.

46. Kendall P, Jenkins J: Exercise for backache: a double-blind controlled trial, *Physiotherapy* 54:154, 1968a.

47. Williams P: Lesions of the lumbosacral spine. *J Bone Joint Surg* 19:343, 1937a.

48. Williams P: Lesions of the lumbosacral spine. *J Bone Joint Surg* 19:690, 1937b.

49. Pollock M et al: Effect of resistance training on lumbar extension strength, *Am J Sports Med* 17:624-9, 1989.

50. Pauley J: EMG analysis of certain movements and exercise: some deep muscles of the back, *Anat Rec* 155:223, 1966.

51. Tran MD et al: Effects of hatha yoga practice on the health-related aspects of physical fitness, *Prev Cardiol* 4:165-70, 2001.

52. Taylor MJ, Majundmar M: Incorporating yoga therapeutics into orthopaedic physical therapy. In Galantino ML, editor: *Orthopaedic physical therapy clinics of North America,* Philadelphia, 2000, WB Saunders, 341-352.

53. Nespor K: Pain management and yoga, *Int J Psychosom* 38:76-81, 1991.

54. Astin JA et al: Mind-body medicine: state of the science, implications for practice, *J Am Board Fam Pract* 16:131-47, 2003.

55. Burton Goldberg Group: *Alternative medicine: the definitive guide,* Puyallup, Wa, 1993, Future Medicine Publications.

56. Sherbourne CD: Pain measures. In Stewart AL, Ware JEJ, editors: *Measuring functioning and well-being: the medical outcomes study approach,* Durham, NC, 1992, Duke University Press, pp 220-34.

57. Walsh TL et al: Screening for depressive symptoms in patients with chronic spinal pain using the SF-36 Health Survey, *Spine J* 6(3):316-20, 2006.

58. Statford PW et al: Assessing change over time in patients with low back pain, *Phys Ther* 74:528-33, 1994.

# APPENDIX 1

## Additional Literature on Yoga

Beyond the reviews presented in this paper, numerous additional papers are published in peer-reviewed scientific journals not mentioned in this chapter. A quick search using PubMed or MEDLINE allows exploration of these reports, clinical trials, and additional reviews of yoga as a therapeutic tool. Countless books also are available on the philosophy, history, and practice of yoga, in addition to its medical use as a mind-body therapy. A list of suggested literature and other relevant resources follows.

### SUGGESTED BOOKS

Feuerstein G: *The deeper dimension of yoga: theory and practice*, Boston, 2003, Shambhala.

Feuerstein G: *The yoga tradition: its history, literature, philosophy, and practice*, Prescott, Ariz, 1998, Hohm Press.

Geeta S: *Yoga: a gem for women*, Spokane, Wash, 1990, Timeless Books.

Lasater J: *Relax and renew*, Berkeley, Calif, 1995, Rodmell Press.

Schatz M: *Back care basics*, Berkeley, Calif, 1992, Rodmell Press.

### BIBLIOGRAPHY OF YOGA LITERATURE

Touch Research Institutes Yoga bibliographies with abstracts (all of these citations but not all of the abstracts are contained in the IAYT bibliographies above): *http://www.miami.edu/touch-research/Yoga.html*

### SUGGESTED RESOURCES ON CONDUCTING YOGA RESEARCH

Black K: Yoga under the microscope: can claims of yoga's health benefits stand up to scientific scrutiny?

These three researchers think so, *Yoga J* :88-93, 130-134, 2001.

Nahin RL, Strauss SE: Research into complementary and alternative medicine: problems and potential, *Br Med J* 322:161-4, 2001.

Young J: Doing research: a tutorial for Yoga teachers, *Int J Yoga Ther* 11:23-3, 2001.

Organizations Conducting and/or Compiling Yoga Research Central Council for Research in Yoga & Naturopathy. Run by the Government of India, Ministry of Health and Family Welfare. Address: 61-65, Institutional Area, Pankha Road, Opp. D block, Janakpuri, New Delhi 110058, India, phone: 5534717, 5557602, 5543725, fax: 5613269.

International Association of Yoga Therapists. P.O. Box 2513, Prescott, AZ 86302, phone: 928-541-0004, fax: 928-541-0182.

National Center for Complementary and Alternative Medicine, National Institutes of Health. Bethesda, Maryland 20892.

Yoga Biomedical Trust. 60 Great Ormond Street, London, England WC 1N 3HR, phone: 0-171-419-7195, fax: 0-171-419-7196.

The Yoga Institute. Shri Yogendra Marg, Prabhat Colony, Santacruz (E), Mumbai (Bombay) 400055—India, phone: 6110506/6122185. For a brief history of the Institute, see the December 1999 issue of the Institute's newsletter *Yoga and Total Health*, pp 5-13.

Yoga Research Foundation. 6111 SW 74th Avenue, Miami, FL 33143, phone: 305-666-2006, fax: 305-666-4443.

Yoga Research Society. 341 Fitzwater Street, Philadelphia, PA 19147, phone: 215-592-9642, fax: 215-247-8054.

# CHAPTER 9

## Tai Chi

*Patricia Quinn McGinnis*

---

### CASE

A 70-year-old woman named Rose is screened at a senior health and fitness fair through a local community center. She expresses interest in participating in a program of tai chi because she has heard about its health benefits for older adults. The community center runs various workshops focused on health promotion and wellness, and prevention of falls is one of the topics. Based on the results of a balance screening, she is seen for further examination by a physical therapist (PT) to develop a health promotion and wellness program for her.

#### ■ Initial Examination

**Client Report:** The client reports that she is able to walk independently in the community, although she sometimes has difficulty on uneven sidewalks or terrain. She reports that she slipped on a throw rug and fell recently when she got up to go to the bathroom in the middle of the night. Fortunately she did not sustain any injuries, but she was shaken up by the incident because one of her friends recently fell, broke her hip, and was admitted to a nursing home.

**Client Goals:** Improve her balance and sense of confidence performing daily activities

**Medications:** Tarka IV 240 mg and Hydrochorot 12.5 mg for hypertension; a daily multivitamin with calcium

**Musculoskeletal:** ROM: grossly within normal limits (WNL) except for end-range tightness for

ankle dorsiflexion. Posture: in standing mild thoracic kyphosis and forward head posture

**Neuromuscular:** Hip extensors are 3+/5 and knee extensors are 4/5 bilaterally; all others are grossly WNL

**Integumentary:** Intact

**Cardiovascular and Pulmonary:** Vital signs at rest: heart rate (HR) 88; blood pressure (BP) 126/82

**Function:** Until recently Rose reports that each morning she took her dog for a walk of approximately 1 mile without difficulty. The pace was slow but steady because of her pet's arthritis. However, she discontinued her daily exercise after having to put her dog to sleep. She is a retired elementary school teacher and enjoys spending time with family and friends who live in the area.

**Living Environment:** She lives alone in a ranch style home with two steps to enter; she is able to negotiate most stairs in the community but prefers to use a railing.

**Balance Screening Measures:** Balance screening measures conducted as part of the community fitness screening day activities: forward reach 7 inches; lateral reach 4 inches; backward lean 3 inches

Timed Up and Go (TUG): 11 seconds; TUG Manual: 14 seconds

Berg Balance Scale: 52/56 total score. She received 4/4 on the first 11 items of the test. On item #12 alternate stool step, she scored 3 of 4 (completed 8 steps in >20 seconds); item #13 tandem stance scored 3 of 4 (placed feet in semi-tandem position); item #14 one-limb stance scored 2 of 4 (one leg standing time, or OLST > 3 seconds)

Self-perception: indicates fear of falling*

### Evaluation

Rose is in good health and until recently was fairly active, exercising regularly. She does have a history of falling, which could possibly be an isolated incident resulting from an environmental hazard. A difference at least 4.5 seconds for the TUG vs. TUG Manual score is associated with a greater likelihood of falls.[1] This client has only a 3-second difference on the dual task. For many older adults, polypharmacy is a risk factor for falls, but this is not an issue for Rose.

However, some of her other scores on the balance tests signal that she may be at risk for falls. Newton[2] reported the following average values for community-dwelling older adults: forward reach 9 inches, lateral reach 6 to 7 inches, backward lean $4\frac{1}{2}$ to 5 inches. This client's reach scores are all below reported averages. In addition, a forward reach of less than 10 inches has been associated with an increased likelihood of falls.[3] Likewise, the Berg Balance score, a reliable measure of balance during performance of functional tasks, is predictive of fall risk in community-dwelling older adults.[4] Shumway-Cook et al[6] reported that for Berg scores between 56 and 54, each one-point drop was associated with a 3% to 4% increase in fall risk. For Berg scores between 54 and 46, however, each one-point change in score was associated with a 6% to 8% increase in fall risk. In addition, the strongest predictor of

falls was the combination of Berg score and a self-report of imbalance. Finally, her self-perception and fear of falling alone is a risk factor.

The decreased LE strength and decreased ankle range of motion may be factors that contribute to an inability to generate an effective recovery strategy in response to a loss of balance. Given the above findings, Rose appears to fall under the Neuromuscular Practice Pattern 5A: Primary Prevention/Risk Reduction for Loss of Balance and Falling, according to the *Guide to Physical Therapist Practice*.[5]

### Plan of Care

The therapist includes the following elements in the plan of care aimed at health promotion and wellness for Rose. Client-related instruction includes safety awareness education and home environment modification: for example, installing a night light in bathroom, removing throw rugs from the home, keeping walkways free of clutter, and installing grab rails in the bathroom. The therapist also recommends that she carry a pocket flashlight if going to dim lighting situations such as restaurants, movie theaters, or auditoriums for her grandchild's school activities.

Interventions include the following: home program of therapeutic exercise consisting of ankle stretching; exercises with elastic bands for hip extension while standing at the kitchen counter and knee extension in sitting for strengthening; also heel and toe raises while standing at the kitchen counter for support. The therapist is interested in recommending tai chi as an adjunct to her plan of care because she feels it will address the balance issues for this particular client.

Tai chi has been practiced in China for centuries as a means to enhance health, fitness, and longevity for people of all ages.[6,7] This chapter addresses the use of tai chi as a mind-body intervention. In particular it focuses on the use of tai chi as an adjunct to wellness and fall prevention for a community-dwelling older adult. A variety of age-related changes in the neuromuscular system may put older adults at risk for falls. The potential impact of tai chi on these changes is presented.

### INVESTIGATING THE LITERATURE

The therapist has read a few articles in the literature related to falls in the elderly and use of tai chi as a mechanism to improve balance. Given the results of the initial examination and the client's interest in tai chi, the therapist decides to investigate the available information and evidence. The therapist uses two strategies to investigate the literature. The first is a detailed approach in which preliminary background reading is performed on tai chi and balance. This is followed by a search of the databases and evaluation of the literature with use of review articles and primary sources of research related to tai chi and balance. The second is the use of the PICO format for a focused search to answer the clinical questions generated by the case.

## Preliminary Reading

Tai chi has its origins in Chinese martial arts, and numerous books exist in the popular media on the topic. The majority of books provide background information regarding the origin, philosophy, and potential benefits of tai chi. Most provide photos or diagrams of the various movement patterns, or forms, of tai chi. For example, Chaline's[8] presentation of the 24-step simplified tai chi includes pictures of the step-by-movements for each individual form, in addition to photos of the complete sequence. A few examples of books that may be particularly helpful to the health professional interested in learning more about tai chi or in providing resources to clients seeking to promote health and wellness are: Chaline's *Tai Chi for Body Mind and Spirit*,[8] Hooton's *Tai Chi for Beginners*,[9] Carradine's *Tai Chi Workout*,[10] Liao's *The Essence of T'ai Chi*,[11] Yu's *Tai Chi Mind and Body*,[12] and Yu and Johnson's *Tai Chi Fundamentals: Health Care Professionals and Instructors* (see Chapter 7).[13]

### Philosophy and History of Tai Chi

Tai chi's underlying philosophy is based in Taoism and is described in the following quotation: "Tai chi is infused with the spirit of the Tao—the Way. Life is a never-ending journey—a process in which we must always seek to balance the opposite forces of yin and yang to find fulfillment and happiness"[8] (p. 7). One of the basic principles underlying tai chi exercise is the Chinese concept of qi (or chi), which is a life force or energy that flows through the body. If an imbalance or blockage of qi exists, then injury or illness results. Tai chi also is based on the theory of yin and yang, or the theory of opposites.[8,10,11] The yin and yang symbol represents the balance between opposites. Yin, the negative power, represents yielding, whereas yang, the positive power, represents action. These two powers oppose yet complement each other. Other examples of complementary opposites include masculine/feminine, light/dark, and hard/soft (see Chapter 4).[6]

In China, tai chi has been used to enhance health, fitness, and longevity for people of all ages.[6,7]

It is characterized by a series of movements, or forms, linked together in smooth continuous motions, with an emphasis on weight shifting and posture control. The combination of mental concentration on movements and diaphragmatic breathing promotes harmony between mind and body. Breathing, meditation, and movement combine to facilitate the smooth flow of qi throughout the body. Tai chi often is called "meditation in motion."[8,10]

Several styles of tai chi exist, with five main schools each named after their respective founding family: Chen, Yang, Sun, Wu (Jian Qian), and Wu (He Qin). Some use more of a martial arts style. Yang style, with its relaxed and evenly paced movements, often is considered the most gentle and suitable style for older adults.[1] Yang style and its variations have been used in the majority of medical and behavioral research on tai chi. Within Yang style are long and short versions with 24, 48, 88, and 108 forms. The simplified 24-step form is one of the most widely practiced styles today (Figure 9-1).[6,8]

### Overview Articles

In addition to the information available in the popular media, the therapist reads several articles from the professional literature that provide an overview of tai chi, in addition to general background information about history, philosophy, and a summary of the available literature.[6,7,14-16] One article in particular provided useful information in the choice of the type of intervention to use for this client.[6]

Also in the literature were a number of summary or overview articles related to reduction of falls or postural instability in the elderly. Many of these mentioned the tai chi literature or recommended inclusion of tai chi as one intervention to achieve these aims. For example, Skelton and Dinan[16] provided a summary of the literature plus a detailed description of a protocol that included tai chi as one element of a multidimensional program designed to reduce postural instability in older adults. Given this general background information, the therapist decides to search the professional literature for more details.

## Searching the Databases

An initial search of MEDLINE using the term *tai chi* reveals 143 journal articles, 29 items in the books/AV category, and 159 items in the consumer

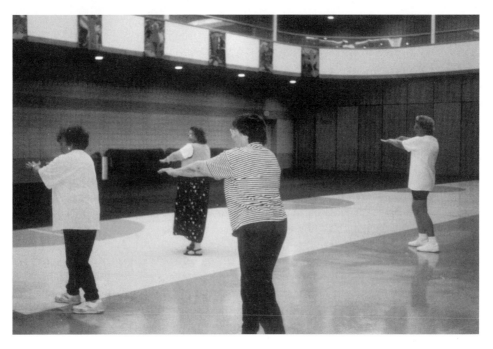

**Figure 9-1** Tai chi promotes health and fitness for people of all ages. Participants practice "white crane opens wings."

| Table 9-1 | Literature Search Results | | |
|---|---|---|---|
| DATABASE | TAI CHI | TAI CHI AND BALANCE | SYSTEMATIC REVIEW ARTICLES |
| Health Source: Nursing/Academic Edition | 203 | 19 | 1 |
| PubMed | 140 | 44 | 7 |
| CINAHL | 93 | 18 | 1 |
| MEDLINE | 143 | 50 | 7 |
| PsycInfo | 43 | 4 | 0 |

health category. Because of the widespread availability of resources about tai chi, the therapist decides to limit searches to full-text, English, and journal articles only and searched the following databases: CINAHL, PubMed, MEDLINE, and PsycInfo (Table 9-1). Because of the interest in tai chi among nursing and other health professionals, the therapist also searches HealthSource: Nursing/Academic Edition. Using the key word *tai chi* generated a combined total of 622 citations; however, because of considerable overlap of PubMed and MEDLINE, use of only the number of citations from MEDLINE yielded a more accurate representation of a combined total of 482 citations. A scan

of titles reveals that the literature reports use of tai chi for a variety of purposes, including health promotion, improving balance, reducing stress, enhancing emotional well-being, and cardiovascular effects. For example, in MEDLINE she finds 26 articles related to tai chi and cardiovascular system effects, 50 related to balance and falls, five related to effects on osteoporosis and/or menopause, and nine related to a variety of other disorders such as cancer, fibromyalgia, substance abuse, sleep disorders, dementia, head injury, and multiple sclerosis. So the therapist decides to narrow the search to address her primary interests by using the key words *tai chi and balance*.

PubMed has 44 articles for the combined terms of *tai chi* and *balance*. Of these, all but one also are listed in MEDLINE. MEDLINE has 50 citations for the combined search terms, seven not found in PubMed. Of these seven, the therapist omits three that are invited commentaries or descriptions of pilot study designs.

From PsycInfo the therapist selects three of the four titles for the combined search terms of *tai chi* and *balance*, only one of which is not found in other databases. After a visual scan of 43 titles for the search term of *tai chi*, three additional titles are selected, thus yielding a total of four citations unique to this database.

From CINAHL she scans 18 titles from combined search terms of *tai chi* and *balance*, selecting seven articles of interest, and omitting newsletters from various health-related organizations. After she reviews these selected titles, she omits two additional citations for similar reasons. Finally, omitting duplications from the other databases yields two citations of interest unique to CINAHL.

From Health Source: Nursing/Academic Edition the majority of citations are non–peer-reviewed journals or from the popular press (e.g., *Consumer Reports on Health*). Of the 19 citations for tai chi and balance, four are selected for review, all of which overlapped with CINAHL, so the therapist finds no additional contributions from this database.

After eliminating duplicates among databases, the therapist's search totals 54 articles, including seven systematic reviews,[17-23] five summary or overview articles, 20 primary sources, and a variety of clinical reports related to the areas of interest. Of the primary studies, seven were randomized controlled trials (RCTs), four were intervention studies, and nine were cross-sectional studies.

## EVALUATING THE LITERATURE

Evidence supports beneficial effects of tai chi on cardiac, respiratory, and musculoskeletal function; postural control; and the reduction of falls in the elderly.[19,22] The most relevant findings from the review of the literature are presented in the following sections.

### Community-Dwelling Older Adults

#### Prevention of Falls

Approximately 30% of adults age 65 and older fall each year.[23] Falls may have serious consequences, including fractures and other injuries, which in turn may have a significant impact on morbidity and mortality. As a result, a great deal of information in peer-reviewed literature investigates prevention of falls in older adults. This includes three systematic reviews of the literature that investigate the effectiveness of various interventions in reduction of the number of falls in community-dwelling older adults.[17,18,20] Among interventions determined "likely to be beneficial" were a 15-week tai chi group exercise intervention and a program of muscle strengthening and balance retraining that was prescribed by a health professional.[17,18,20,24] The

support for tai chi was based on the evidence from one randomized clinical trial[25] with 200 participants (risk ratio of 0.51, 95% confidence interval 0.36-0.73). This was a grade B recommendation,[20] which means that strong evidence was found from at least one level II randomized trial with an adequate sample size.

In addition, four systematic reviews focused specifically on the effectiveness of tai chi.[19,21-23] All agreed that evidence exists to support the ability of tai chi to reduce falls in community-dwelling older adults. However, their findings were somewhat less favorable than the conclusions of the previously mentioned reviews[17,18] in the Cochrane Database of Systematic Reviews (see Chapter 2). This was due to concerns that the impact of tai chi on falls was based on the results of only one study. Wu[23] and Verhagen et al[21] acknowledged that the findings of the study by Wolf et al[25] were significant. However, they concluded that limited evidence exists that tai chi was effective to reduce falls in the elderly.

The hallmark study cited in each of these systematic reviews was part of the Frailty and Injuries: Cooperative Studies of Intervention Techniques (FICSIT) studies, which were a preplanned, multicenter trial of various interventions to reduce frailty and falls in older adults. As part of this larger investigation, Wolf et al[25] conducted a trial with 200 subjects randomly assigned to one of three groups for a 15-week intervention: tai chi exercise, computerized balance training, or an education control group. Participants were community-dwelling older adults over age 70 (mean 76.2). The tai chi group met twice a week and practiced 10 "forms" drawn from the original 108-form Yang style tai chi. The tai chi group experienced fewer falls than other groups (56 in tai chi group, 76 in computer training, 77 in control) and reduced their risk of multiple falls by 47.5%.[25]

In summary, two systematic reviews consider that tai chi is likely to be beneficial in reduction of falls, based on the results of one well-designed RCT. The five remaining systematic reviews acknowledge the importance of the results of this single study but caution that additional evidence from RCTs is needed to strengthen the support for tai chi. Because these systematic reviews were published, an additional RCT by Li et al[26] found that a 6-month, three-times-per-week program of tai chi significantly reduced the frequency and risk of falls in older adults. As of yet, the mechanism of the benefits is not well understood.

### Reduced Fear of Falling

In addition to the impact on actual number of falls, participation in tai chi also appears to reduce the fear of falling among older adults.[26-28] In a later study by Wolf et al[27] tai chi participants reported reduced frequency of fear of falling (56% to 31%) after a 15-week program. Based on these results, the systematic review by Wu concluded that some evidence supports a positive effect of tai chi on prevention of falls in addition to the reduction of the fear of falling.[23]

In 2001 Li et al[29] examined whether a 6-month program of tai chi improved self-reported physical function as measured by the Short Form General Health Survey (SF-20). The researchers randomly assigned 94 physically inactive community-dwelling adults (mean age 72.8) to a tai chi or waiting list control group. The 24-form Yang style tai chi exercise took place twice a week. Results indicated significant improvements in all aspects of physical function for tai chi participants versus the control group. Participation in tai chi was associated with reduced self-report of physical function limitations. In a separate publication with the same subjects,[30] older adults in the tai chi group reported increased self-efficacy, with the amount of change in self-efficacy associated with higher levels of attendance at the sessions. In addition, participation in tai chi led to an increased self-report of physical activity and self-efficacy among older adults.

### Improved Balance Performance on Computerized Tests

Yan[31] also reported that an 8-week program of tai chi resulted in greater improvements in dynamic balance control of 28 nursing home village residents when compared with 10 residents who participated in a walking or jogging program. Dynamic balance control was measured on a stabilometer platform. Although the results appear promising, they must be viewed with caution because participants were permitted to self-select in which type of exercise program they would participate. The authors suggested that the movement experience of performing tai chi enhanced balance control; more efficient use of proprioceptive feedback to determine their center of mass and maintain stable position contributed to improved dynamic balance control.

Tsang and Hui-Chan[32] examined the effect of an intensive tai chi training program that consisted of 90-minute sessions six times per week for 8 weeks.

Elderly participants in tai chi (n=24) demonstrated improved balance control during dynamic posturography testing versus the education control group (n=27). In addition, the improvements were maintained at follow-up testing 4 weeks post intervention. The researchers noted that after week 4, the balance performance in the experimental group was comparable to that of experienced tai chi practitioners, which led to their conclusion that as little as 4 weeks of intensive tai chi practice resulted in improved balance in elderly subjects. Once again, the results must be viewed with caution because whether groups were selected by participants or randomly assigned is unclear.

A follow-up investigation of a 72-person subset of the original 200 participants in the FICSIT trial who were less active[27] revealed that computerized balance training resulted in reduced postural sway during computerized post-tests, but participation in tai chi did not. Instead, older adults who participated in tai chi responded to dynamic perturbations with more sway during the post-tests. The authors suggested that this response indicated better balance control because participants were able to move more easily toward their limits of stability on the computerized tests. This was supported by the finding that the tai chi group reported less fear of falling after the 15-week intervention than individuals who participated in computerized balance training.

### Improved Balance Performance on Clinical Tests

One of the challenges in determination of the effect of tai chi on balance improvement is that a wide variety of measures have been used, from computerized measures to a host of clinical tests. Wu[23] published a systematic review in 2002 that specifically examined the effect of tai chi on improvement of balance and prevention of falls in older adults. This article was a particularly helpful resource given the therapist's area of interest for this particular client. The author noted that one of the challenges in drawing strong conclusions from the literature was due to the wide variation in the type and duration of tai chi intervention, in addition to variation in measures of balance. For example, tai chi practice improved the ability to stand on one leg in some studies, whereas in others it did not change significantly.[23]

Also reported in the literature were measures such as tandem walking, the Romberg test, the number of losses of balance, and gait speed. Various tests of normal walking have not shown significant changes in gait speed after participation in tai chi.[23,27] A more sensitive measure such as tandem walking may be needed to detect walking-related changes. One study by Tse and Bailey[33] did demonstrate a significant difference in performance on tandem walking by tai chi practitioners, but the results were based on a cross-sectional study design.

Tai chi was found to improve balance and functional mobility, as measured by the Berg and TUG, in older women.[28] This particular study used a within-subjects design, in which each participant served as his or her own control during a 3-month "usual activity" period before participation in the 3-month twice-weekly tai chi sessions. In another intervention study, participation in tai chi significantly improved dynamic balance, with a mean increase of 7.2 cm on the functional reach test.[34]

Taken as a group, participation in tai chi improves performance on selected computerized and clinical balance measures,[22,23] although the majority of support comes from nonrandomized studies.

## Frail or Institutionalized Older Adults

### Prevention of Falls

Although clear evidence exists of the benefits of tai chi in community-dwelling older adults, the results are less conclusive for older adults who are more frail or reside in long-term care facilities. Nowalk et al[35] examined the differences in fall rates for 110 residents of long-term care facilities who were assigned randomly to an exercise group, tai chi group, or control group. No significant difference existed in the number of falls among the groups over 2 years. The authors noted that their participants were older (mean age 84.7), more frail, and more impaired cognitively than subjects in previous studies. These factors, combined with low adherence rates, contributed to the results. Wolf et al[36] also implemented tai chi for 286 older adults considered to be transitionally frail. The intervention was conducted twice a week, initially for 60-minute sessions, which increased to 90-minute sessions over 48 weeks. The authors noted that it took about 3 months for participants to progress from dependence on assistive devices during standing, to being able to perform tai chi movements without support. At the conclusion of the study, fewer tai chi participants experienced at least one fall (47.6%) than participants in the wellness edu-

cation control group (60.3%), although the risk ratio of falling was not statistically different from the control group. The authors concluded that this finding was clinically important, although not statistically significant, and recommended further study with this "at risk" population.

In summary, the evidence from RCTs shows that tai chi can reduce the rate of falls among community-dwelling older adults, but the results are inconclusive for older adults who are frail or reside in long-term care facilities.

## Benefits of Long-Term Practice of Tai Chi

### Enhanced Strength

Several studies (n=9) have examined the existing differences between a cohort of tai chi practitioners and nonpractitioners on a variety of factors such as strength, postural sway, and performance on clinical or computerized balance tests. Wu et al[37] investigated differences in lower extremity strength between individuals in Beijing, China, who had practiced tai chi for minimum of 3 years and individuals who were physically active but had not practiced tai chi. The tai chi group had significantly higher knee extensor strength on isokinetic testing and less center of pressure excursion during quiet stance. The authors concluded that long-term tai chi practice maintained eccentric strength of LE postural muscles, presumed to be beneficial for maintaining good postural stability.

### Enhanced Postural Control and Balance Performance

Tse and Bailey[33] compared performance on clinical measures of balance for tai chi practitioners versus sedentary older adults drawn from the Chinese community in Boston. They found that tai chi practitioners had significantly better postural control than the sedentary nonpractitioners for OLST and tandem walking. In a similar manner, Hakim et al[38] compared performance on balance-related measures for a convenience sample of 94 older adults, recruited from local senior centers, YMCA, or tai chi Chuan classes. Older adults participating in either tai chi or structured exercise groups demonstrated greater balance and confidence than sedentary well-elderly persons. In addition, the tai chi group performed significantly better than both groups for reaching in three directions (multi-directional reach test), which indicates greater limits of stability.

Tai chi practitioners also exhibit better performance on computerized balance tests versus nonpractitioners. Although the two groups performed similarly on simpler static tests,[39,40] older adults who practiced tai chi demonstrated greater postural stability than healthy active older adults on the more challenging sensory organization testing conditions, such as conditions with altered visual and proprioceptive input. In addition they demonstrated significantly better performance on dynamic balance tests.[39] The authors concluded that tai chi maintained postural control ability in older adults and therefore should be recommended as an exercise to prevent falls in the elderly. Tsang and Hui-Chan[40] compared 21 elderly tai chi practitioners with 21 healthy controls matched for age, gender, and physical activity level. During limits of stability testing for dynamic balance, tai chi practitioners initiated voluntary weight shifting more quickly and could lean further with a smoother trajectory to targets. In addition, the standing balance performance of tai chi practitioners on computerized dynamic posturography was comparable to that of young adults under reduced or conflicting sensory input conditions.[41]

### Enhanced Proprioceptive Awareness

Long-term practice of tai chi also enhances proprioceptive awareness for older adults, compared with sedentary older adults, in addition to those who participate in other forms of exercise. Tsang and Hui-Chan[40] noted that elderly tai chi practitioners demonstrated greater accuracy on a knee joint repositioning test when compared with healthy elderly adults matched for age, gender, and physical activity level. Although regular physical activity has been found to minimize the age-related physiological decline of older adults, the authors found that tai chi practitioners demonstrated better ankle and knee joint proprioception than sedentary older adults, in addition to better ankle joint proprioception than long-term swimmers and runners.[42] Similarly, experienced tai chi practitioners and golfers had greater limits of stability and better knee joint proprioception than elderly control subjects. Of particular interest was that their performance was similar to the young adults despite the expected age-associated decline in these areas.[43] Because age-associated decline in proprioception may influence postural control and be associated with a increased risk of falls, the ability of tai chi to maintain or enhance proprioception of ankle and knee joints

may be particularly beneficial in maintaining balance control in older adults.[42]

Two potential mechanisms have been offered to explain these findings[40] based on the current literature. First, repeated practice may have increased cortical representation of knee joints and improved joint position sense. The authors pointed to previous research in monkeys in which training and experience modified internal representation of cortical maps of the body surface. The second proposed mechanism was that repeated motor skill practice increased muscle spindle output, resulting in increased strength of synaptic connections in the central nervous system. Although these proposed explanations appear plausible, further study is needed to determine the mechanisms underlying the effects of tai chi practice.

Xu and colleagues[13,44] explored neuromuscular reaction time through EMG studies as a possible mechanism for the benefits of long-term tai chi practice. They reported that older adults who had engaged in long-term practice of tai chi or jogging exhibited faster muscle reaction times to an unexpected ankle perturbation when compared with sedentary older adults. More rapid muscle response may assist older adults in generating postural corrections needed to avoid a fall.

In summary, several studies have examined existing differences between tai chi practitioners and nonpractitioners and found that tai chi practitioners demonstrated enhanced performance on measures of lower extremity strength and proprioceptive awareness, in addition to enhanced postural control on various clinical and computerized balance tests. In some cases the comparison group was sedentary older adults, but in other studies the comparison group participated in other forms of exercise. Although the evidence supporting these findings is based on cross-sectional studies, many that use a sample of convenience, they indicate encouraging trends. A number of the authors have recommended prospective randomized trials, which certainly would strengthen the evidence for these findings.

### Impact of Tai Chi on Blood Pressure

Although the potential impact of tai chi on balance and prevention of falls in older adults is the therapist's primary interest, the client also has hypertension. In the initial database search for articles about tai chi the therapist notices a number related to cardiovascular system effects in general, in addition to a few specifically related to its impact on hypertension. The therapist also selects two reports of RCTs related to these interests[45,46] and one intervention study that specifically investigated the effect of tai chi on balance and hypertension,[34] which is summarized in the following section. For previously sedentary older adults with borderline hypertension (not yet on medication), participation in light intensity tai chi was as effective as aerobic exercise in reduction of blood pressure.[45] After a 12-week intervention, tai chi participants experienced an average reduction of 7.0 mm Hg systolic and 3.2 mm Hg diastolic pressure. Tsai et al[46] reported even greater reductions of BP with use of moderate exercise intensity, with a decrease in systolic blood pressure of 15.6 mm Hg and diastolic pressure of 8.8 mm Hg. Thornton, Sykes, and Tang[34] reported similar results for middle-aged women (35 to 55 years) who were sedentary but normotensive. Taken as a group, these findings provide support for the beneficial effects of tai chi on blood pressure.[25,34,45,46]

The therapist may not always have time to do such an extensive search. Instead she may use a targeted PICO approach.

---

### PICO BOX

For community-dwelling older adults does the use of tai chi improve balance?

P: Community-dwelling older adults
I: Tai chi
O: Balance

The therapist combines the search terms and finds only one relevant article.[32] She then broadens the term *community-dwelling older adults* to *aged* and finds 52 articles. She reads through the 52 articles (which overlaps mostly with her original set except for at least one additional article[49] and eliminates people with pathology and frail elderly to arrive at her final set.

---

P = **Population** (patient/client, problem, person condition or group attribute)
I = **Intervention** (the CAM therapy or approach)
C = **Comparison** (standard care or comparison intervention)
O = **Outcomes** (the measured variables of interest)

---

## CLINICAL DECISION MAKING

### Generate a Clinical Hypothesis

The therapist uses the data gathered and presented in the client case description to develop a clinical hypothesis and a plan of care. Her clinical hypothesis is that the combined effects of age-associated changes in the neuromuscular system (such as strength loss), plus a recent decline in physical activity, may place Rose at increased risk for falls. The therapist decides to add tai chi to the plan of care developed for Rose. She expects that this client will demonstrate improved balance and increased confidence in movement after participation in tai chi.

### Examine

Based on the examination data provided in the client case description, the therapist has identified specific risk factors for falls. She decides to use the following outcome measures to monitor the impact of participation in tai chi for this individual: fear of falling, multidirectional reach test (including forward reach, lateral reach, and backward lean), TUG vs. TUG Manual, and the Berg. All are reliable measures of balance performance, and several have normative values for comparison. In addition, these measures are able to predict fall risk for community-dwelling older adults. Finally, these assessment approaches are practical to administer and require equipment readily available in most clinics.

### Intervene

The review of the evidence supports the use of tai chi for Rose's plan of care as a mechanism to improve her balance and reduce her risk for falls. A wide variation exists in the frequency and duration of tai chi programs presented in the literature, although the majority ranged from 8 to 16 weeks.[22,23] In the FICSIT trials, a modest intervention of one to two times per week for 15 weeks reduced falls in older adults.[27,36] On the other hand, Tsang and Hui-Chan[32] found that as little as 4 weeks of intensive tai chi practice (six times per week) resulted in improved balance in older adults.

After reviewing the available resources and discussing options with her, Rose decides to attend an "introduction to tai chi" program offered by physical therapists who are presenting group exercise sessions at the community center. She chooses this option because she lives in a small community, and limited local resources exist. This option will allow her to see if she enjoys tai chi through the introductory class offered. If so, she can decide to explore options for further participation in tai chi.

A local physical therapist with an interest in tai chi is offering health promotion classes at the community center. One offering is an introduction to tai chi class, based on community needs and interest in the topic. The presentations include a background of the history of tai chi, its potential benefits for seniors, and guidelines to assist seniors in finding the appropriate class, instructor, or resource to suit their needs and abilities. The presentations feature small classes of 8 to 12 participants, which meet twice a week for an hour for 8 weeks. This format allows seniors to try tai chi in a supervised setting and modify the activities based on their needs and abilities. Exercise classes include an overview of the principles and philosophy of tai chi, warm-up exercises, and demonstration and practice of basic moves, in addition to individual tai chi forms. Examples of class activities are included in Figures 9-2 and 9-3. Each session includes review and practice of previously learned moves and gradual introduction of new ones with approximately one new form added each week. At the conclusion of the introduction to tai chi class, the

therapist educated the clients on issues related to adapting tai chi for older adults. The therapist also provided participants with a resource list including various websites to explore at the community library to try to locate an instructor if they wished to continue their practice (see Appendix 1).

## Adapting Tai Chi for Older Adults

Traditional forms of tai chi require whole body coordination and sometimes use intricate upper or lower body movements, or single limb postures. In a number of instances reported in the literature, tai chi has been modified to suit the needs of various target groups. Li et al[6] noted that "from a safety standpoint, not every tai chi posture is physically appropriate for seniors" (p. 210). According to the China National Sports Commission[47] tai chi can be performed in a high, medium, or low stance dependent on the age and ability of the practitioner. The low stance is a semi-squatting position with knees bent almost to 90 degrees. The high stance is recommended for seniors because it places less stress on the joints and muscles of lower extremities.[1]

A second consideration is the complexity of traditional long or short versions (e.g., 24-, 48-, 88-, or 108-form Yang style), which may prove challenging to learn and remember for seniors. Wolf

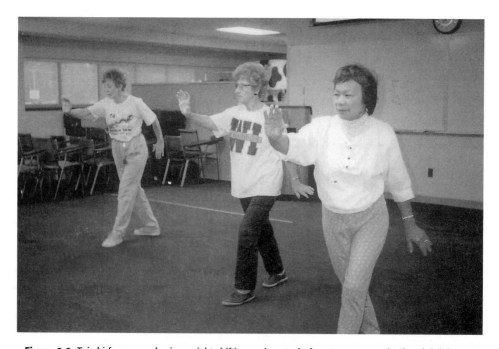

**Figure 9-2** Tai chi forms emphasize weight shifting and control of posture as seen in "brush left knee."

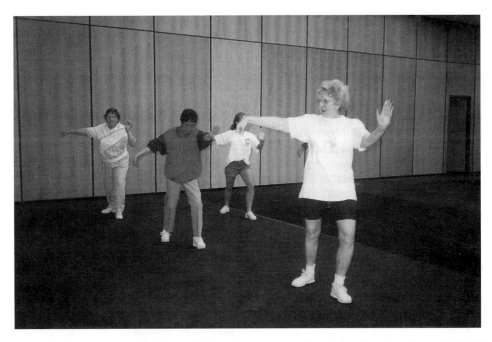

**Figure 9-3** Older adults participating in tai chi exercise group complete the form known as "grasp bird's tail."

et al[25] modified the original 108-form Yang style to a 10-form sequence, which reduced the complexity and was more appropriate for independent community-dwelling older adults. For a more detailed discussion of the program, in addition to diagrams and descriptions of the 10-form version, readers are referred to the literature.[48] However Li et al[1] felt that some of the 10-form movements were still too challenging for seniors (e.g., the heel kicking movement with single limb support). They called for additional modifications and further reduction of the number of movements to accommodate a wider audience, including healthy or frail older adults and individuals with physical impairments or mobility challenges.

This was the basis for development of "A Simpler Eight-Form Easy Tai Chi for Elderly Adults."[1] The 8-form tai chi sequence was designed to be performed while standing but also can be done seated. It was recommended for older adults regardless of activity level and for use as part of a rehabilitation program in research or clinical settings for frail seniors and others with impairments or functional limitations. The authors also presented some preliminary data from ongoing research using the program, with promising results on various measures of functional ability. Additional information about this exercise program can be found on the authors' website, described in the Appendix.

Another example of modifying tai chi to reach a wider audience was presented by Skelton and Dinan,[16] who developed the Falls Management Exercise (FaME) Programme for community-dwelling older adults with a history of falls. They used an adapted tai chi sequence, beginning with chair exercises and progressing to standing practice of the various forms. The initial phase of standing activity also was adapted by using a chair or wall for support, with a gradual progression to unsupported standing activities.

## Choosing an Instructor

Skelton and Dinan[16] also recommended that tai chi instructors be trained and experienced at adapting moves for older people, particularly when working with individuals with a history of falls. A list of guidelines for consumers in choosing an instructor was found on the Yahoo Health website (see Appendix) and is presented below. Although no certifying organization exists for tai chi instructors, some helpful guidelines to consider follow:

Choose an environment that appears clean and safe
Ask how long the facility has been operating
Observe a class before joining or signing up
Does the instructor communicate clearly? Is the

instructor attentive to students' individual abilities?

Is the instructor experienced in all forms of tai chi, from beginner's level to more advanced?

Do you get a good feeling about the class?

Although these guidelines are directed toward the general population of consumers, it is particularly important for older adults to find an instructor who is client-centered and willing to modify activities appropriately to ensure participant safety. These guidelines can be shared with clients interested in participating in tai chi.

## Outcomes

The client is seen for a follow-up visit at the conclusion of the 8-week tai chi classes. Outcome measures are presented in Table 9-2. All of the areas have shown improvement with the exception of blood pressure, which was unchanged. The client reports an increased confidence in her movements and is no longer fearful of falling. A notable improvement occurred in her reach scores, and they now fall within the average values reported in the literature.[4] Her gains are comparable with those reported in a study by Thornton, Sykes, and Tang,[34] who reported a mean increase in forward reach of 7.2 cm (approximately 2.8 inches). In addition, her forward reach score is approaching the 10-inch cutoff reported in the literature.[5] She also made

gains in her Berg score, which translates into a reduced risk of falls. For example, she was able to assume a tandem stance position and successfully complete the alternate stool step tasks for the full score. In addition, she was able to maintain single limb stance for 5 to 10 seconds, thus meeting the criteria for a score of three out of four on this item.

Rose reports that she is able to easily complete the exercises in the home program originally issued during her initial consultation with the physical therapist. She reports exploring websites (see Appendix) to locate a tai chi instructor, but none were located in her town. At this point she has decided to purchase a video for home use to continue practicing tai chi and has begun to explore other opportunities for group exercise in her community.

## Report the Outcomes

The therapist decides that her original clinical hypothesis was correct, namely that age-associated changes in the neuromuscular system combined with a recent decline in physical activity had placed Rose at an increased risk of falls. She incorporated tai chi into her original plan of care that included client education and a home exercise program for lower extremity strengthening. The intended outcomes of improved balance, increased confidence in movement, and decreased risk of falls were achieved for this client. The therapist decides to

## Table 9-2     Outcomes After 8-Week Tai Chi Exercise Program

| TEST/MEASURE | BASELINE SCORE | POST EXERCISE | CHANGE |
|---|---|---|---|
| Forward reach | 7 inches | 9.5 inches | +2.5 inches |
| Lateral reach | 4 inches | 6 inches | +2 inches |
| Backward lean | 3 inches | 4.5 inches | +1.5 inches |
| TUG | 11 sec | 10 sec | −1 sec |
| TUG Manual | 14 sec | 12 sec | −2 sec |
| TUG–TUG Manual | 3 sec | 2 sec | −1 sec |
| Berg balance scale | 52/56 | 55/56 | +3 |
| Fear of falling | Yes | No | Increased Confidence |
| Strength | Hip ext 3+/5 | Hip ext 4/5 | $\frac{1}{2}$ grade increase |
|  | Knee ext 4/5 | Knee ext 4+/5 | $\frac{1}{2}$ grade increase |
| Blood pressure | 126/88 | 126/88 | Unchanged |

Note: items listed in the table are common clinical measures and were described in the patient case and evaluation section.
*TUG*, Timed up and go. *TUG Manual*, timed up and with a manual task added, such as carrying a glass of water.

report the results of this case study to encourage clinicians to consider using complementary therapies such as tai chi, to promote health and wellness in older adults who may be at risk for falls. A possible venue for this type of case report would be the journal *Physiotherapy Theory and Practice*.

## SUMMARY

Tai chi is a moderate-intensity exercise that has support in the literature for improvement of balance and postural control in community-dwelling older adults. In addition, tai chi has been shown to reduce falls in seniors who may be at risk for falls. For this particular individual tai chi appeared to be a desirable option in a plan for wellness that included fall prevention. The decision to add tai chi to this client's plan of care was based on evidence and practicality. Tai chi is a low-cost intervention that enhances self-confidence in movement ability. No specialized equipment is required other than comfortable clothing and shoes. Once learned, tai chi can be performed anywhere. As group exercise tai chi has the potential benefit of increased social interaction for older adults. Given the benefits of tai chi practice for community-dwelling older adults, a number of groups have modified the forms to meet the needs of persons with varied levels of functional ability.

## REFERENCES

1. Lundin-Olsson L, Nyberg L, Gustafson Y: Attention, frailty, and falls: the effect of a manual task on basic mobility, *J Am Geriatr Soc* 46:758-61, 1998.
2. Newton R: Validity of the multi-directional reach test: a practical measure for limits of stability in older adults, *J Gerontol* 56A(4):M248-52, 2001.
3. Duncan P et al: Functional reach: predictive validity in a sample of elderly male veterans, *J Gerontol* 47: M93-8, 1992.
4. Shumway-Cook A et al: Predicting the probability for falls in community-dwelling older adults, *Phys Ther* 77:812-9, 1997.
5. APTA: Guide to physical therapist practice, *Phys Ther* 81(1):1-768, 2001.
6. Li F et al: A simpler eight-form easy tai chi for elderly adults, *J Aging Phys Act* 11:206-18, 2003.
7. Zwick D et al: Evaluation and treatment of balance in the elderly: a review of the efficacy of the Berg balance test and tai chi *Quan, NeuroRehabilitation* 15:49-56, 2000.
8. Chaline E: *Tai chi for body mind and spirit: a step-by-step guide to achieving physical and mental balance*, New York, 1998, Sterling Publishing.
9. Hooton C: *T'ai chi for beginners*, New York, 1996, The Berkley Publishing Group.
10. Carradine D, Nakahara D: *Tai chi workout: the beginner's program for a healthier mind and body*, New York, 1995, Henry Holt and Company.
11. Liao W: *The essence of t'ai chi*, Boston, 1995, Shambhala Publications.
12. Yu T: *Tai chi mind and body*, London, 2003, DK Publishing.
13. Yu T, Johnson J: *Tai chi fundamentals: health care professionals and instructors manual*, Madison, Wis, 1999, Uncharted Country Publishing.
14. McKenna M: The application of tai chi chuan in rehabilitation and preventive care of the geriatric population, *Phys Occup Ther Geriatr* 18(4):23-33, 2001.
15. Bottomley JM: The use of tai chi as a movement modality in orthopaedics, *Orthop Phys Ther Clin North Am* 9:3, 2000.
16. Skelton DA, Dinan SM: Exercise for falls management: rationale for an exercise programme aimed at reducing postural instability, *Physiother Theory Pract* 15:105-20, 1999.
17. Gillespie LD et al: Interventions for preventing falls in elderly people, *Cochrane Database of Systematic Reviews* 3:CD000340, 2001.
18. Gillespie LD et al: Interventions for preventing falls in elderly people, *Cochrane Database of Systematic Reviews* 4:CD000340, 2003.
19. Li JX, Hong Y, Chan KM: Tai chi: physiological characteristics and beneficial effects on health, *Br J Sports Med* 35:148-56, 2001.
20. Sherrington C, Lord SR, Finch CF: Physical activity interventions to prevent falls among older people: update of the evidence, *J Sci Med Sport* 7:43-51, 2004.
21. Verhagen AP et al: The efficacy of tai chi chuan in older adults: a systematic review, *Fam Pract* 21:107-13, 2004.
22. Wang C, Collet JP, Lau J: The effect of tai chi on health outcomes in patients with chronic conditions, *Arch Intern Med* 164:493-501, 2004.
23. Wu G: Evaluation of the effectiveness of tai chi for improving balance and preventing falls in the older population: a review, *J Am Geriatr Soc* 50:746-54, 2002.
24. Gatti JC: Which interventions help to prevent falls in the elderly? *Am Fam Phys* 65(11):2259-60, 2002.
25. Wolf SL et al: Reducing frailty and falls in older persons: an investigation of tai chi and computerized balance training, *J Am Geriatr Soc* 44:489-97, 1996.
26. Li F et al: Tai chi and fall reductions in older adults: a randomized controlled trial, *J Gerontol Med Sci* 60A(2):187-94, 2005.

27. Wolf SL et al: The effect of tai chi quan and computerized balance training on postural stability in older subjects. Atlanta FICSIT group. Frailty and injuries: Cooperative studies on intervention techniques, *Phys Ther* 77(4):371-84, 1997.

28. Taggart HM: Effects of tai chi on balance, functional mobility, and fear of falling among older women, *Appl Nurs Res* 15(4):235-42, 2002.

29. Li F et al: An evaluation of the effects of tai chi on physical function among older persons: a randomized controlled trial, *Ann Behav Med* 23(2):139-46, 2001.

30. Li F et al: Tai chi enhances self-efficacy and exercise behavior in older adults, *J Aging Phys Activ* 9:161-71, 2001.

31. Yan JH: Tai chi practice improves senior citizens' balance and arm movement, *J Aging Phys Activ* 6:271-84, 1998.

32. Tsang WWN, Hui-Chan CWY: Effect of 4- and 8-wk intensive tai chi training on balance control in the elderly, *Med Sci Sports Exercise* 36(4):648-57, 2004.

33. Tse SK, Bailey DM: T'ai chi and postural control in the well elderly, *Am J Occup Ther* 46(4):295-300, 1992.

34. Thornton EW, Sykes KS, Tang WK: Health benefits of tai chi exercise: improved balance and blood pressure in middle-aged women, *Health Promotion Int* 19:33-8, 2004.

35. Nowalk MP et al: A randomized trial of exercise programs among older individuals living in two long-term care facilities: the falls FREE program, *J Am Geriatr Soc* 49:859-65, 2001.

36. Wolf SL et al: Intense tai chi training and fall occurrences in older, transitionally frail adults: a randomized, controlled trial, *J Am Geriatr Soc* 51:1693-701, 2003.

37. Wu G et al: Improvement of isokinetic knee extensor strength and reduction of postural sway in the elderly from long-term tai chi exercise, *Arch Phys Med Rehab* 83:1364-69, 2002.

38. Hakim RM et al: Differences in balance related measures among older adults participating in tai chi, structured exercise, or no exercise, *J Geriatr Phys Ther* 27(1):11-5, 2004.

39. Wong AM et al: Coordination exercise and postural stability in elderly people: effect of tai chi chuan, *Arch Phys Med Rehab* 82:608-12, 2001.

40. Tsang WWN, Hui-Chan CWY: Effects of tai chi on joint proprioception and stability limits in elderly subjects, *Med Sci Sports Exer* 35(12):1962-71, 2003.

41. Tsang WWN et al: Tai chi improves standing balance control under reduced or conflicting sensory conditions, *Arch Phys Med Rehab* 85:129-37, 2004.

42. Xu D et al: Effect of tai chi exercise on proprioception of ankle and knee joints in old people, *Br J Sports Med* 38:50-4, 2004.

43. Tsang WWN, Hui-Chan CWY: Effects of exercise on joint sense and balance in elderly men: tai chi versus golf, *Med Sci Sports Exercise* 36(4):658-67, 2004.

44. Xu D, Li, J, Hong Y: Effect of regular tai chi and jogging exercise on neuromuscular reaction in older people, *Age Ageing* 34:439-44, 2005.

45. Young DR et al: The effects of aerobic exercise and t'ai chi on blood pressure in older people: results of a randomized trial, *J Am Geriatr Soc* 47:277-84, 1999.

46. Tsai J et al: The beneficial effects of tai chi on blood pressure and lipid profile and anxiety status in a randomized controlled trial, *J Altern Compl Med* 9(5):747-54, 2003.

47. Commission CNS: *Simplified taijiquan,* Beijing, China, 1983, People's Sports.

48. Wolf SL, Coogler CE, Xu T: Exploring the basis for tai chi chuan as a therapeutic exercise approach, *Arch Phys Med Rehab* 78:886-92, 1997.

49. Wolfson L et al: Training balance and strength in the elderly to improve function, *J Am Geriatr Soc* 41(3):341-43, 1993.

# APPENDIX 1
## Additional Resources

The following section provides a variety of additional resources for physical therapists interested in incorporating tai chi into the plan of care for their clients. Selected videotapes are presented as resources to help familiarize the clinician with elements of tai chi. In addition, some of the videos may be useful as a home program for clients. Many of these resources are also available in DVD format. Several examples of websites also are discussed as resources to provide general information and assist with locating an instructor or locating items for purchase by therapists and their clients (Box 9-1).

## VIDEOS

A number of videotapes are commercially available with various forms of tai chi for home use. Some are not appropriate for use by older adults, particularly if they previously have been sedentary. Renting a video or DVD before purchase is a good recommendation. The following section highlights a few videos currently available, but this is not an exhaustive list. In addition, the comments that follow the description of the resources are based on the opinion of the author and in no way represent a product endorsement; rather, they are points of consideration for health care professionals who are seeking resources they may recommend to their clients or for their own personal use.

---

### Box 9-1 | Resources for Health Professionals

**VIDEOS**

*Tai Chi for Health,* 1987, Y & R Productions, Inc.
*Tai Chi: The Gift of Balance,* 1996, Tai Chi Health and Science Research Center
*Tai Chi Fundamentals: Health Care Professionals and Instructors*
*Tai Chi Fundamentals: Simplified Exercises for Beginners*
*Tai Chi for Older Adults,* 1998, East Action Video, Wellspring Media

---

## Tai Chi for Health

This video presents basic principles and guidelines, an introduction to arm movements and tai chi stepping, warm-up exercises, and demonstration of tai chi forms. It includes demonstrations of each new move from front, side, and back views, followed by periodic reviews of a small set of previous moves in sequence. The video concludes with a demonstration of the entire set of 17 moves in sequence. The narrator recommends that beginners learn only one or two moves per week and practice them daily. This is good advice because trying to learn too many moves at a time gets confusing. The narrator also cautions beginners not to bend their knees too much, and most forms are demonstrated using a "high stance."

This video is user friendly for beginners and older adults. The program begins with double-limb support and weight shifting and progresses to single-limb support as a transition of weight shifting. It is modified easily for use by older adults. For example, during tai chi stepping, older adults can take smaller steps forward and back. In addition, the single-limb support demonstrated as a transition of weight shifting in the video can be modified by touching down the toe or heel midway through the step for support. Finally, providing a view from behind the instructor makes learning new moves less confusing.

*Running time:* 50 minutes. 1987. Y & R Productions, Inc.; ISBN 55873-203-9

## Tai Chi: The Gift of Balance

This video features Tai Chi Master Tingsen Xu, PhD, who selected 9 forms specifically for seniors from the 108-form Yang style tai chi. It opens with scenes of Dr. Xu performing tai chi against the backdrop of a waterfall, a meadow, and the Great Wall of China, during introductory comments about the history and philosophy of tai chi. The exercise program begins with warm-up exercises, followed by demonstration of each of the 9 forms individually, and concludes with a demonstration of all of the movements in sequence.

This simplified form of tai chi was developed specifically with seniors in mind and has been tested in research studies. Each form is demonstrated slowly and clearly and repeated several times to the right and left.

*Running time:* 60 minutes. 1996. To order or for further information contact:

Tai Chi Health and Science Research Center
P.O. Box 98426
Atlanta, GA 30359
Note: this resource is not available from websites like many of the others.

## Tai Chi Fundamentals: Health Care Professionals and Instructors

*Tai Chi Fundamentals* was developed by Tricia Yu, MA, and Jill Johnson, MS, PT, GCS. This video can be purchased individually or as part of a "Professional Set" consisting of the 100-minute video with an accompanying 126-page manual. Yu is the Director of the Tai Chi Center in Madison, Wisconsin, with 28 years' experience teaching Yang style tai chi. Johnson is a physical therapist and a tai chi practitioner who uses elements of the program for her geriatric clients. In addition these authors developed a video/DVD for daily home use to enhance client and student learning called *Tai Chi Fundamentals: Simplified Exercises for Beginners* (87 minutes). The Tai Chi Fundamentals Form was developed by adapting movements of traditional Yang style tai chi to bring the benefits of tai chi to individuals with a wide range of abilities. It is intended for use by health professionals with their clients, including older adults and individuals with various "limiting conditions." A third resource is *Tai Chi Fundamentals: Mastering Tai Chi Basics*, which is also available in video and DVD formats.

Information available on the website, promotional materials, and a short demo tape were reviewed, but the full-length videotapes were not reviewed by this author. A wide variety of books, videos, and DVDs are available for purchase through the website *http://www.taichihealth.com* (see additional information listed under description of websites).

## Tai Chi for Older Adults

Dr. Paul Lam, an Australian family physician and tai chi practitioner, modified traditional Yang style tai chi for adults over age 50. The video includes an introduction to tai chi, warm-up exercises, five standard movements, four additional movements, and sitting qigong (breathing exercises). The video includes scenes of older adults performing tai chi in a park, in addition to testimonials from participants. Warm-up exercises are demonstrated with older adults standing next to a sturdy chair for support as needed. The following sequence is used to instruct each of the new movements: first, Dr. Lam demonstrates a move; second, he instructs a client; third, Dr. Lam and the client perform the movement together while the viewer watches from behind; and fourth, the client or class demonstrates the move.

The video included frequent reminders to ensure safety, and participants are advised to consult their physicians with any questions about specific activities in the video. The narrator reminds participants to bend knees slightly and adopt a comfortable stance. Each of the movements is broken down into parts, each part is demonstrated and repeated, and finally the entire sequence is demonstrated and repeated. The evenly paced approach and view from behind provided by the instructor help make tai chi easier to learn, practice, and remember.

*Running time:* 110 minutes. 1998, East Action Video at Wellspring Media; ISBN 1-885538-91-X. Videos available at *http://www.taichiproductions.com*

## T'ai Chi for Health: Yang Short Form with Terry Dunn

The video includes a demonstration of the 37-posture Yang style short form. It begins with a philosophical introduction to tai chi and warm-up exercises, followed by an introduction to basic tai chi postures, and step-by-step instruction with an inset view from a different angle to facilitate learning.

The video opens with a demonstration of tai chi set against beautiful scenery near the water's edge on a rocky coastline, accompanied by soothing background music. Although artistically impressive, some of the postures demonstrated may be inappropriate for older adults. For example, deep squats, lunges, and "low stance" postures are depicted, and instructions often include assuming a stance that is twice shoulder width. Clinicians would need to make significant modifications of the stances and postures for use by older adults, or they could recommend this video instead for younger more active adults.

*Running time:* 120 minutes. Healing Arts Home Video; ISBN 0-945671-05-9

## WEBSITES

### Tai Chi Health
### http://www.taichihealth.com

This site is a useful resource for background information about tai chi and includes resources for the public and for health professionals, such as professional training workshops, books, videos, DVDs, and audiotapes. A variety of products, including the *Tai Chi Fundamentals* videotapes and DVDs, are available for online purchase.

### American Tai Chi Association–Tai Chi & Health Information
### http://www.americantaichi.net

The Tai Chi and Consumer Health Information Center website is sponsored by the American Tai Chi Association (ATCA), which is a nonprofit organization for tai chi professionals in the United States. The purpose of the website is to provide a source of reliable and credible information about tai chi and its health benefits. The website provides a link to help consumers locate a tai chi coach in their area.

### Tai Chi Network http://www.taichinetwork.org

This site provides a geographical listing of teachers and centers with name, address, phone number, and the center's major interest (e.g., Yang style of tai chi). The site describes itself as an online community of teachers and students seeking instructors. Teachers and students can become members and receive notices of interest, such as a new listing of instructors in their area.

### Healthy Aging Center–Health World
### http://healthyaging.ori.org

The authors'[1] website provides a video clip of the "8-Form Easy Tai Chi" performed in standing and sitting, a list of the names of the 8 forms, and an instructor's training manual. The seated version uses the same series of forms but focuses on upper extremity movements, trunk rotation, and seated weight shifting. This routine was derived from the contemporary 24-form simplified Yang-style tai chi (China National Sports Commission, 1983[47]). It is designed specifically for the elderly or for individuals with mobility challenges or physical impairments. The instructor's training manual, designed for use in research projects, provides detailed movement description of 8-form easy tai chi, in addition to guidelines for a typical training session and progression through the program.

# CHAPTER 10

## Overview of Biologically Based Therapies in Rehabilitation

*Susan Gerik, John Maypole*

---

Biologically based therapies are among the most popular forms of complementary and alternative medicine (CAM). The use of biologically based therapies is widespread in the United States and is increasing.[1]

## CONSUMER USE OF BIOLOGICALLY BASED THERAPIES

Results from a recent survey by Kelly and colleagues[1] that tracked weekly herb and dietary supplement use in 8476 American adults from 1998 to

2002 demonstrated that overall use of these biologically based therapies increased from 14.2% to 18.8%. Further, the results showed that herb and dietary supplement use in the older population doubled.[1] In North America, a 2002 National Health Interview Survey (NHIS)[2] interviewed more than 31,000 adult Americans and found high levels of CAM use when persons are healthy and sick.

Overall, the NHIS survey found that 36% of adults are using some form of CAM. When megavitamin therapy and prayer specifically for health reasons are included in the definition of CAM, that number rises to 62%.[2] About one fifth of the adults surveyed by the NHIS used some form of natural product within the preceding 12 months. From the survey, CAM in general most often was used to treat and/or prevent musculoskeletal conditions or other conditions that involve chronic or recurring pain, issues particularly salient to care providers with clients needing rehabilitative services.[2] Those more likely to use CAM therapies, including biological therapies, were women, those who had completed a higher level of education, adults who had been hospitalized recently, and former smokers.[2]

The use of CAM by parents or caregivers is the single best predictor of CAM use in children, and herbal use by children is on the rise, with 28% to 40% of children exposed to herbals for conditions such as asthma, anxiety, insomnia, and attention-deficit hyperactivity disorder (ADHD).[3] In children with complex or chronic illnesses, such as cancer or autism, the rate of biological therapy use parallels that of adults with similar conditions, approaching 100%.

Trends in CAM use vary among different socioeconomic sectors and minorities in the United States. The NHIS data (Figure 10-1) provide some broad information on CAM use in general.

Research continues in the effort to characterize national trends in CAM use by minorities. To date, generalizations about CAM use are limited by geographical differences in demographics and influ-

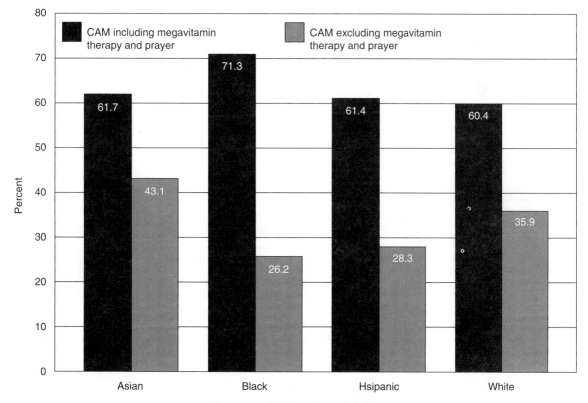

**Figure 10-1** CAM use by race/ethnicity.
Source: from: http://nccam.nih.gov/news/camsurvey fs1.htm#natural

ences between and among minority and ethnic communities. However, differences have been identified in limited or smaller scale studies. For example, in a survey of outpatient clinics in Houston, Texas, approximately half of Hispanics and half of Asians used herbs compared with 41% of Caucasians and 22% of African Americans.[4] Also, clients were more likely to use herbs if they had an immigrant family history or if other family members used herbs. More Caucasians (67%) disclosed their herbal use to their health care providers than African Americans (45%), Hispanics, (31%), or Asians (31%).[4] As of 2002, the top 10 botanical or natural products used by American adults in the NHIS survey are identified in Figure 10-2.

Internationally, the use of botanical medicines is generally higher than in the United States. For example, 70% of "Western-trained" doctors in Japan prescribe kampo drugs daily.[6] In Britain, recent investigations have shown that herbal medicine has been used by about 31% of the adult population.[7] About 80% of the world's population relies primarily on traditional medicines, including biologically based therapies, for their health care needs.[8]

## KEY TERMS AND DEFINITIONS

According to the National Center for Complementary and Alternative Medicine (NCCAM) at the National Institutes of Health (NIH), biologically based therapies "include, but are not limited to, botanicals, animal-derived extracts, vitamins, minerals, fatty acids, amino acids, proteins, prebiotics and probiotics, whole diets, and functional foods."[9] Clarification of these terms is key to understanding

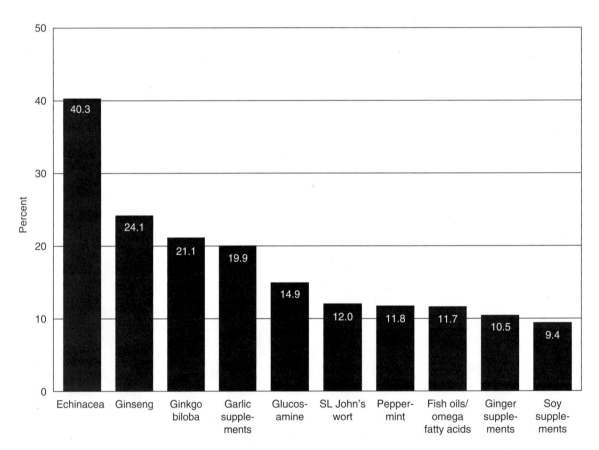

*The percentage for each product represents its rate of use among U.S. adults who use natural products.

**Figure 10-2** Top 10 natural products.
from: http://nccam.nih.gov/news/camsurvey fs1.htm#natural

their uses, composition, safety, oversight, and regulation.

## Botanical Products

Even for a particular class of product, a variety of terms may be used. Botanical drug products also may be known as herbal products or nutriceuticals. Botanical drug products are intended for use in the diagnosis, cure, mitigation, treatment, or prevention of disease in humans. A botanical drug product consists of vegetable materials, which may include plant materials, algae, macroscopic fungi, or combinations of these. These products may be available in a variety of forms, including a solution (e.g., tea), powder, tablet, capsule, elixir, topical, or injection. By distinction, fermentation products (e.g., alcohol) and highly purified or chemically modified botanical substances are not considered botanical drug products.[10]

## Dietary Supplements

The Dietary Supplement Health and Education Act of 1994 (DSHEA) defines a dietary supplement as a product (other than tobacco) taken *in addition to* a normal diet. More on this key legislation is mentioned below. Further, dietary supplements must contain one or more dietary ingredients (including vitamins; minerals; herbs or other botanicals; amino acids; and other substances such as enzymes, organ tissues, glandular materials, and metabolites). The U.S. Food and Drug Administration (FDA) oversees supplement use and regulation. The FDA characterizes and regulates botanicals and dietary supplements according to their use, not according to their composition. If the intended use is to "promote health," the agent is viewed as a dietary supplement. By contrast if the intended application of a product is to treat or prevent a disease, the agent is considered to be a drug. To meet labeling requirements, a dietary supplement must be intended to be taken by mouth as a pill, capsule, tablet, or liquid.[11]

## Herbs

An herb is the above-ground part of a nonwoody plant that does not persist through the winter. It also is known commonly as a crude drug, or as a flavoring used in cooking.[12] Other terms are used synonymously for herbs or herbal products, including *botanicals, nutriceuticals,* and *phytopharmaceuticals.*

## Functional Foods

Functional foods are defined broadly as foods that provide more than simple nutrition. They supply additional physiological benefit to the consumer, through properties that promote health and/or disease prevention. Many, if not most, vegetables can be considered functional foods because they deliver benefits beyond basic nutrition. Tomatoes, for example, provide lycopene, a phytochemical with powerful antioxidant properties.

## Probiotics

Probiotics are bacteria-containing foods, such as milk and milk solids, yogurt, and kefir, which may favorably alter the floral composition of the gut through competition of one type of culture with another.

## Prebiotics

Prebiotics are biologically based therapies used to alter the bacterial composition of the intestines, not by adding bacteria, but by changing the type of substrate provided to the existing mixture.[13]

## Special Diets

Special diets, such as those advocated by Atkins, Ornish, Weil, and others, purport to prevent or mitigate the symptoms of illness and/or to promote wellness. Orthomolecular therapies include the use of specific types of ingredients, such as minerals, or high-dose vitamins to prevent or treat illness, or to enhance wellness.[14]

## REGULATION AND SAFETY OF HERBS AND DIETARY SUPPLEMENTS

The DSHEA of 1994 has proven to be a landmark piece of legislation for the ongoing manufacture, safety, and use of biologically based therapies. Per this legislation, herbs and dietary supplements are regulated as foods rather than drugs. This means, unlike pharmaceuticals, herbs and dietary supplements are not required to meet the strict standards of safety, effectiveness, and quality established by the FDA. Knowing the distinction between the regulation of biologically based therapies and the regulation of pharmaceutical products has consequences for the consumer and clinician.

## Safety

Unlike a pharmaceutical product DSHEA does not require that research establish an herb or dietary supplement's safety for consumers before its release in the market.

## Effectiveness

Manufacturers do not have to prove that an herb or dietary supplement is effective. Rather, the manufacturer can say that the product addresses a nutrient deficiency, supports health, or reduces the risk of developing a health problem, if that is true. If the manufacturer does make a claim, it must be followed by the statement, "This statement has not been evaluated by the Food and Drug Administration. This product is not intended to diagnose, treat, cure, or prevent any disease."[15]

## Quality

A manufacturer does not have to prove an herb or dietary supplement's purity or caliber. The FDA is not required to analyze the content of herbal or dietary supplement products. Manufacturers who want to demonstrate a commitment to the quality of their products can voluntarily follow the FDA's stricter—but optional—Good Manufacturing Practices or GMPs for drugs.[15] The designation "GMP" on a supplement's label ensures product quality, although it does not indicate safety or efficacy.

The Federal Trade Commission (FTC) also oversees advertising of herbs and dietary supplements. It requires that all information about supplements be truthful and without misleading information. However, limited enforcement resources and manpower, and the explosion of information outlets on the Internet and in the media blunt the impact of these efforts. Given the multitude of avenues through which vendors can disseminate claims and advertising, the enforcement resources of the FDA are underequipped for the task. Removal of problematic or unsafe biologically based therapies, as in the case of the dietary supplement ephedra, does occur. However, the number of products removed has been relatively limited. Given limited government oversight of

biologically based therapies in the United States, consumers may have limited information regarding the risks or effectiveness of a variety of products. It is a caveat emptor scenario for clinicians and consumers.

## Adverse Events and Reactions

The MedWatch system of the FDA allows health care professionals and consumers to report serious adverse events, potential and actual product use errors, and product quality problems associated with FDA-regulated drugs, biologicals (including human cells, tissues, and cellular and tissue-based products), medical devices (including in vitro diagnostics), special nutritional products, and cosmetics. Reporting instructions and forms can be accessed at http://www.fda.gov/medwatch/how.htm

The MedWatch system has been used in limited fashion for adverse event reporting for herb/dietary supplement use since 2004.[16] Websites for the Office of Dietary Supplements at the NIH[17] contain searchable information on warnings and safety postings from the FDA and false advertising claims from the FTC. Other surveillance systems include information on biologically based therapies such as the American Association of Poison Control Centers (AAPCC) incident database known as the Toxic Exposure Surveillance System (TESS).[18]

The reporting of adverse events, toxicity, or contamination in botanical or biological products is an issue of public health and safety. To address this on a national scale, the TESS database monitors, identifies, and responds to emerging contaminations or poisonings. This effort is a partnering of multiple agencies, including the Centers for Disease Control and Prevention, and the AAPCC, with 62 regional and local poison control centers (PCCs).

As described on the CDC website, the TESS database is a flexible and adaptable system that can be used by government and health agencies to do the following:

- Identify emerging problems that may be associated with newly introduced household products (including botanical or biological products), pharmaceuticals, or pesticides
- Identify early indicators for chemical exposures occurring at multiple sites throughout the United States
- Identify illnesses resulting from intentional or unintentional chemical exposures at a single site or across multiple locations

- Monitor the frequency of reports involving potentially abused substances

As such, the TESS database serves as a portal for the reporting of suspected cases for concern by consumers or clinicians. TESS is not intended to function as a searchable database for an individual in practice, however. Individuals in the United States can contact the PCC in their area by calling 800-222-1222, where they will be referred directly to their local or regional center.

## SOURCES OF INFORMATION

### Research

In laboratory settings, plant extracts have been shown to have a variety of physiological effects and act like pharmacological agents. These effects include antiinflammation vasodilation and antimicrobial, anticonvulsant, sedative, and antipyretic effects. However, because of limited research on the biological therapies, the mechanism of action of many herbs, and dietary supplements, biological therapies remains unknown or incompletely understood.

A number of issues have influenced the dissemination of information regarding the effectiveness and safety of biologically based therapies. The efficacies of herbal medicines that have been tested in clinical trials are of varying methodological quality. Fortunately or unfortunately, the gold standard of allopathic medicine for measuring the effectiveness of a therapy is the randomized controlled trial (RCT), yet RCTs on biologically based therapies are relatively limited in number. Despite an increased interest in biologically based therapies, research funding in this area is limited when compared with the budgets of the pharmaceutical sector. Even if many more RCTs on biologically based therapies were conducted, generalizing the data may be difficult because investigations may use several different botanical features and preparations to determine efficacy.[19]

As Ernst and others noted, analysis of the evidence for recent overviews of rigorous trials of herbal medicines has had mixed results: of 23 systematic reviews of herbal therapies, 11 came to a positive conclusion, nine yielded promising but not convincing results, and three were negative.[20] Despite these inconsistencies, sensible recommendations can be made based on appraisal of the existing literature and rational risk-benefit analysis.

## Commission E Monographs

In 1978 the German Ministry of Health established Commission E, a panel of experts charged with evaluation of the safety and efficacy of the herbs available in pharmacies for general use. The Commission reviewed more than 300 herbal drugs. This collection is known as the Commission E Monographs. The monographs are intended to provide guidelines for the general public, health practitioners, and companies applying for registration of herbal drugs. In general, they do not contain standards for assaying the quality and purity of herbal drugs, and they differ from North American and British publications in that some of their outcome measures do not use RCTs. For some clinicians and investigators, this may limit their use as a resource. Following the Commission E Monograph in Germany, the European Scientific Cooperative on Phytotherapy (ESCOP) evolved in Europe over the 1990s and reviews the therapeutic uses of herbal medicinal products. In all, 60 ESCOP monographs were published.[21]

## National Center for Complementary and Alternative Medicine

In North America, the largest source of funding remains the NCCAM at the National Institutes of Health. NCCAM has declared that its future research portfolio will have an increased emphasis on studies of the mechanisms underlying CAM approaches, including biologically based therapies.[22] For the busy clinician, the NCCAM website gives an overview of the government funded research in CAM (Box 10-1) and general

| Box 10-1 | Areas of Special Interest for NCCAM Research |
|---|---|

Anxiety and depression*
Cardiovascular diseases *
Ethnomedicine
HIV/AIDS and immune modulation/enhancement*
Inflammatory bowel disease and irritable bowel syndrome*
Insomnia
Liver
Obesity/metabolic syndrome*
Respiratory diseases*

*A number of these conditions are seen in clients seeking physical therapy or rehabilitative services.

information regarding and summaries of different forms of complementary therapies. For the health care provider or consumer, this Internet resource can be a helpful starting point to access general yet accurate and timely information about vitamins, minerals, herbs, and dietary supplements.

## ConsumerLab.com

Health care providers concerned with the quality and safety of commercially prepared biologically based products may want to investigate ConsumerLab.com (CL), a private certification organization that evaluates products related to health, wellness, and nutrition, including herbal products, vitamins, minerals, functional foods, and dietary supplements. Companies can have their products tested through CL's Product Reviews and Voluntary Certification Program. Products that "pass" the products review and certification program are eligible to carry the CL seal of approval. Health care providers and consumers who see the CL seal of approval on the label or packaging of an herbal product, vitamins, minerals, or dietary supplements are ensured that the product has undergone unbiased testing and has met standards of safety and quality. However, consumers should note that the manufacturer incurs the expense of the voluntary submission and testing. So, if a product does not have a CL seal of approval, a consumer does not know if a manufacturer has chosen not to submit the product for testing, or if the product has failed to meet the standards for the CL seal. To obtain the test results of product reviews, including pass/fail lists and a list of products that have achieved the CL seal of approval, a consumer or health care provider must purchase a subscription through ConsumerLab.com.

## Natural Standard

Natural Standard, which can be accessed, online at http://www.naturalstandard.com/, is an international, multidisciplinary collaboration of clinicians and researchers founded to provide high-quality, evidenced-based information about complementary and alternative therapies. Natural Standard has developed several databases including Herbs & Supplements, Interactions, Brand Names, Condition Center, Complementary Practices, and Dictionary. For each therapy or botanical product included in the databases, an impartial research team has systematically gathered scientific data and expert opinions. Then, using a validated rating scale, the quality of the evidence is evaluated. Monographs written by the research team are then peer-reviewed before inclusion in the databases. The databases are organized so that a subscriber can read a comprehensive evidenced-based systematic review that provides details of efficacy, adverse effects, interactions, dosing, and more, or a simple "flashcard." The flashcard has been adapted from a comprehensive review and provides a quick look-up and easy reading that can be used as a client handout. Another feature of Natural Standard's databases is the "Condition Center-Comparative Efficacy Chart." For these charts, medical conditions are cross-referenced across the evidence-based monographs and the interventions are arranged hierarchically by level of evidence for efficacy. Although Natural Standard appears to a valuable resource for user-friendly and highly credible information on complementary and alternative therapies, individual subscriptions to the databases are currently not available. According to the website, all database access and content licensing agreements need to be made between an organization, institution, or corporation.

## USE OF BIOLOGICALLY BASED THERAPIES IN REHABILITATION MEDICINE

Herbs are used in many different contexts, and clients who seek treatment from rehabilitation teams may inquire about biologically based therapies or already may be using them. It is helpful for health care providers to be acquainted with the more common herbs and supplements and know how to access reliable information so that they may serve as informed intermediaries for their clients. For the rehabilitation professionals, the greatest amount of evidence in biologically based therapies is found in research on herbs and dietary supplements. For the purposes of this chapter, this review is focused on the evidence of the use of herbs and dietary supplements.

Approaching the literature search for botanicals used in rehabilitation medicine may yield very different results depending on the choice of search terms and the database selected. Table 10-1 demonstrates a representative literature search for the body of information presented below. CAM on PubMed provides the most fruitful source of information specific to the botanical approach to treating these conditions.

| Table 10-1 | **Literature Search Results** | | |
|---|---|---|---|
| | CAM ON PUBMED (MARCH 8, 2006) | CINAHL (1982-MARCH 2006) | COCHRANE DATABASES (MARCH 8, 2006) |
| Botanical | 1099 | 167 | 90 |
| Dietary supplements | 10,064 | 251 | 1923 |
| Herbs | 2565 | 888 | 258 |

In this section, 20 common conditions for which clients seek rehabilitative therapy are addressed. The common herbs and supplements used for those conditions are listed. These botanicals have been classified based on the availability and quality of scientific evidence for their use in these conditions. The evidence for most of the botanicals listed has been evaluated in HealthNotes and classified into one of the three following categories:

1. Reliable and relatively consistent scientific data showing substantial health benefit
2. Contradictory, insufficient, or preliminary studies suggesting a health benefit or minimal health benefit
3. Supported by traditional use but minimal or no scientific evidence (for herbs); little scientific evidence of minimal health benefit (for supplements)

Herbs and supplements in the first category (reliable, consistent evidence) and the second category (contradictory or preliminary) are emphasized and placed in Table 10-2. Botanicals in the last category are deemphasized. Table 10-2 summarizes the herbs and supplements mentioned for the selected conditions. Doses and preparations used in clinical trials are listed. Special precautions or concerns are listed under Notes.

## Acute Sports Injuries and Muscle Soreness

Sprains and strains are frequent occurrences for athletes. Some preparations can be helpful in addition to the traditional RICE (rest, ice, compression, and elevation) approach.

Trypsin and chymotrypsin have been shown to be efficacious in healing minor injuries. They are proteolytic enzymes that have some antiinflammatory effect. Some clients report less pain and swelling with use of these enzymes.[23,24]

Other supplements, such as bromelain and vitamins A and C, have shown some benefit.[25-27] L-carnitine, in particular, seemed to reduce muscle soreness after exercise for some athletes.[28] Horse chestnut is an herb used topically for sprains. It acts as an antiinflammatory and reduces swelling.[29] Arnica, considered by many to be a homeopathic remedy, also is proposed to be beneficial for managing joint and muscle soreness after exercise or injury. A case study in which arnica is included in a client's plan of care is described in Chapter 6.

## Age-Related Cognitive Decline

A number of nutritional supplements have been purported as helpful for deterioration of memory and concentration in the elderly. Acetyl-L-carnitine, phosphatidylserine, and vinpocetine have shown some promise. Acetyl-L-carnitine delays the onset of age-related cognitive decline and seems to improve cognitive function in the elderly.[31,32]

Phosphatidylserine from bovine brain phospholipids has been shown to improve memory and mood in two trials.[33] Vinpocetine, found in Vinca minor, a ground cover more commonly known as periwinkle, was found to improve symptoms of dementia in clients with a variety of brain diseases.[34,35]

The herb ginkgo biloba also has been found to be safe and effective in a number of double-blind trials. One study failed to show specific improvement, but subjects did not decline either, which suggests possible treatment effect.[36] The decision-making process used to include ginkgo biloba in management of a client with Alzheimer's disease is described in Chapter 11.

High homocysteine levels have been demonstrated to be associated with cognitive decline and cerebral atrophy. Folic acid has been used to attempt to lower homocysteine levels, so a theoretical role also exists for its use in age-related cognitive decline.[37]

## Amputations

Cayenne topically applied has provided some relief for clients who experience phantom limb pain.[38]

**Table 10-2    Supplements and Herbs Commonly Used in Rehabilitation Medicine**

| CONDITION | SUPPLEMENT/HERB | DOSE | NOTES |
|---|---|---|---|
| Acute sports injuries | Trypsin and chymotrypsin | 4-8 tablets per day | |
| | Horse chestnut | Topically 2% gel | Applied every 2 hr until swelling subsides |
| Age-related cognitive decline | Acetyl-L-carnitine | 1500 mg per day | Effect lasted 30 days after discontinued |
| | Phosphatidylserine | 300 mg per day | |
| | Vinpocetine | 60-80 mg per day | |
| | Ginkgo biloba | | |
| Amputation | Cayenne | Topically 0.025% to 0.075% cream | Four times daily |
| Arthritis | Glucosamine sulfate | 1500 mg per day | |
| | Chondroitin sulfate | 1200 mg per day | |
| | SAMe | 1200 mg per day | |
| | Cat's claw | 100 mg per day | |
| | Cayenne | Topically 0.025% to 0.075% cream | Four times daily |
| | Ginger | 255 mg twice per day × 6 wks | |
| Burns | Vitamin C | 2000-3000 mg per day | |
| | Vitamin D | | |
| | Aloe | Topically | |
| Bursitis | None | | No strong scientific evidence |
| Cancer | Beta glucans | 1-2 mg 1-2 times per week × 1 yr | Reduces risk |
| | Fish oil | 1 gm per week | Reduces risk |
| | Melatonin | 20 mg per day | |
| | Vitamin B6 | Not stated | |
| Chronic fatigue | L-carnitine | 1 gm three times per day | |
| | NADH | 10 mg per day | |
| | Vitamin B12 | 2500-5000 mcg every 2-3 days | |
| COPD | N-acetyl cysteine | 200 mg three times per day | |
| | Essential fatty acids | 760 mg gamma-linolenic acid, 1200 mg alpha-linolenic acid, 700 mg eicosapentaenoic acid, 340 mg of docosahexaenoic acid | Not certain which components are most responsible for improvement in exercise capacity |
| Fibromyalgia | 5-HTP | 100 mg three times per day | Under medical supervision |
| | SAMe | 800 mg per day × 6 wks | |
| HIV/AIDS | Arginine + HMB + glutamate | 8 gm arg, 7 gm glut, 1.5 gm HMB | |
| | Selenium | 400 mcg per day × 8 days | In deficiency |
| | DHEA | 200-500 mg per day × 8 wks | |
| Low back pain | Trypsin and chymotrypsin | 4-8 tablets per day | |
| | Colchicine | 0.6-1.2 mg per day | Under medical supervision |
| Macular degeneration | Lutein | 10 mg per day | |
| | Zinc | 45 mg per day | |
| Multiple sclerosis | Vitamin D | 400 IU per day | |
| Myocardial infarction | Coenzyme Q10 | 60 mg twice per day | |
| | L-carnitine | 4-6 gm per day | |
| | Vitamin C | 100-200 mg per day | |
| | Folic acid | | |
| Neuropathic pain | | | |
| Parkinson's disease | Coenzyme Q10 | 1200 mg per day × 16 months | |
| | Methionine | 5 gm per day | |
| | NADH | 5 mg twice per day | Mixed results |
| | Vitamin B2 | 30 mg three times per day | |
| | Vitamin E and C | 3200 IU vitamin E with 3 gm vitamin C | In combination |

| Table 10-2 | Supplements and Herbs Commonly Used in Rehabilitation Medicine—cont'd | | |
|---|---|---|---|
| CONDITION | SUPPLEMENT/HERB | DOSE | NOTES |
| Stroke | Vinpocetine | IV injection | Within 72 hr of stroke |
| Tendonitis | DMSO | Topically 10% gel | Under medical supervision |
| Wounds | Vitamin E | 400 IU | |
| | Vitamin C | 1-3 gm per day | |
| | Essential fatty acids | | |
| | Zinc | 135-150 mg per day | |
| | Aloe | Topically | Mixed results |
| | Gotu kola | Topically 1%-2% extract | |
| Athletic performance | Creatine monohydrate | 15-20 gm per day | |
| | Vitamin E and C | Vitamin C 400 mg per day with vitamin E 800-1200 IU per day | |
| | Rhodiola | 200 mg 1 hr before exercise | Only occasional use |

*Doses listed were used in clinical trials and do NOT necessarily represent recommended doses for routine use.

## Arthritis

Osteoarthritis represents joint disease from aging and injury. Treatment is aimed at symptom control. Some excellent evidence supports the use of a number of nutritional supplements and herbs for osteoarthritis.

Glucosamine sulfate and chondroitin sulfate are used widely by many clients to treat arthritic pain, swelling, and joint function. Many trials have supported the effectiveness of glucosamine and chondroitin in addressing these symptoms[39-46] and are reviewed in the case of women with osteoarthtitis in Chapter 12.

S-adenosyl methionine (SAMe) acts as an antiinflammatory. Although the mechanism is not known, SAMe seemed to reduce the severity of symptoms in clinical trials.[47-51]

Herbs such as boswellia (an antiinflammatory) in combination with aswagandha, turmeric, and zinc have shown some promise for the treatment of pain and stiffness caused by osteoarthritis.[52] Cat's claw has been shown to be significantly more effective than placebo in relief of osteoarthritis pain.[53] Topical cayenne creams reduce pain and tenderness of joints caused by osteoarthritis.[54-56] Ginger also has been used for arthritis. Trials have shown efficacy of ginger extracts in clients with osteoarthritis of the hip or knee.[57]

## Burns

Burns may result from extreme heat, chemicals, or electricity. Vitamin C in combination with vitamin E has been used because of the antioxidant properties. They may help protect against sunburns resulting from ultraviolet rays.[57] Vitamin E alone used topically on minor burns is a popular remedy, but its use is not supported by scientific evidence.

Clients with extensive burns may suffer vitamin D deficiency when a large surface area of the skin is damaged.[58] Such clients may benefit from supplemental vitamin D. Because vitamin D is a fat-soluble vitamin, it may accumulate in the body, so supervision by an experienced health care provider is recommended during its use.

Chymotrypsin has been used to reduce tissue destruction in some settings.[59] Honey seems to improve formation of granulation tissue when applied to dressings. The effect is comparable to silver sulfadiazine and polyurethane dressings.[60] Oral ornithine ketoglutarate may be helpful in improvement of wound healing in burn clients.[61] Zinc supplementation has been found to improve the outcomes of burn clients when administered in combination with other trace minerals. Recipients seemed to have fewer pulmonary infections and a shorter ICU stay.[62]

Aloe is a popular herbal remedy for surface burns. Scientific evidence proving its efficacy is preliminary, and a small number of clients may experience contact dermatitis from its use.

Probiotics also have been used in burn clients to reduce the risk of bacterial translocation. In a small animal study, probiotics reduced bacterial translocation and decreased intestinal mucosal atrophy after thermal burn injury.[63]

## Bursitis

Bursitis is associated with pain and tenderness in addition to limited range of motion. Little evidence supports nutriceuticals for bursitis. A preliminary study suggested that intramuscular injections of vitamin B12 may relieve symptoms of shoulder bursitis, but more studies are needed.[64]

## Cancer

Many different nutritional supplements and herbal remedies have been used for reducing the risk of developing cancer, enhancing quality of life with cancer, or attempting to cure or arrest the progression of cancer. The literature is replete with evidence that supports a healthy diet as a major contributor to cancer risk reduction. A few nutritional supplements and herbs are mentioned here to give a sample of some of the biologically based therapies used.

Beta-glucans such as lentinan appear to increase survival in people with advanced cancer.[65] Fish oil 1 gram per week decreases the general risk of cancer.[66] Folic acid supplementation appears to reduce the risk of colon cancer.[67] Garlic supplements reduce the risk of prostate cancer in preliminary studies.[68] Taking pyridoxine orally appears to reduce the risk of lung cancer.[69]

## Chronic Fatigue Syndrome

Chronic fatigue syndrome (CFS) is characterized by extreme fatigue often accompanied by muscle or joint pain, short-term memory loss, sleep disturbances, and lymphadenopathy. The symptoms typically last for more than 6 months and can be disabling.

Magnesium seemed to improve the symptoms of CFS when administered via intramuscular injection, particularly in clients with low red blood cell magnesium.[70]

Several nutritional supplements have been used to try to avert the symptoms. L-carnitine participates in the energy production within cells. One preliminary trial showed an improvement in symptoms in clients with CFS.[71] Nicotinamide adenine dinucleotide (NADH) also helps with energy production. One trial showed an improvement in quality of life for clients who receive NADH. More research is needed.[72]

Vitamin B12 deficiency may contribute to fatigue, but several trials have shown that even clients who are not vitamin B12 deficient respond to supplementation with increased energy. The research in this area is preliminary but shows some promise. Intramuscular injections of B12 are required for adequate effect because gastrointestinal absorption is limited.[73]

Other supplements such as DHEA, fish oil, and magnesium have been used but have minimal or no supporting scientific evidence. Similarly, herbs such as Asian ginseng, eleuthero, and licorice have been used but have not proven to be efficacious in clinical trials. Asian ginseng and eleuthero theoretically work on the basis of their immunomodulating activity and reportedly help support the hypothalamic-pituitary-adrenal axis.

## Chronic Obstructive Pulmonary Disease

Chronic obstructive pulmonary disease (COPD) is represented by chronic bronchitis and emphysema leading to poor ventilation and oxygenation. COPD leads to substantial decrease in function and is frequently fatal.

Eating foods high in beta-carotene content seems to be associated with lower prevalence of bronchitis and dyspnea in male smokers with COPD[74]; however, beta-carotene supplementation has been associated with an increased risk of lung and prostate cancer in persons with a history of smoking and asbestos exposure. Intravenous magnesium has been potentially helpful for treating COPD exacerbations.[75]

N-acetylcysteine has been used for clients with bronchitis. It acts as a mucolytic and has some antioxidant activity.[76] In clients with moderate COPD, taking N-acetyl cysteine orally may reduce frequency of exacerbations by 40%.[77] L-carnitine has proved helpful in clients with chronic lung disease who wish to exercise.[78]

Increasing intake of essential fatty acids has been linked to reduced risk for the development of COPD.[79] Some evidence from one trial suggested that fatty acid supplements given to clients who already were diagnosed with COPD improved exercise tolerance.[80]

One double-blind trial showed that an extract of ivy leaf was as effective as a prescription mucolytic in clients with chronic bronchitis.[81]

## Fibromyalgia

Fibromyalgia causes pain and has no known cause or cure. Clients with fibromyalgia who have low serotonin levels may benefit from supplementation with 5-HTP. Trials have shown improvement of symptoms in such clients. Clients who take 5-HTP orally seem to experience improvement in pain, morning stiffness, and sleeplessness.[82,83] Topical capsicum cream reduces pain at tender points when applied four times per day for 4 weeks.[84] Gamma-hydroxybutyrate also seems to help alleviate fibromyalgia-associated pain, fatigue, and sleep disturbance.[85]

S-adenosylmethionine (SAMe) given intravenously provided some pain relief and improved mood and stiffness for clients suffering from fibromyalgia when tested for 6 weeks. In two other studies, SAMe taken orally seemed to improve symptoms.[86]

## HIV/AIDS-Related Muscle Atrophy

Beta-glycans were used successfully to improve immune function in preliminary trials.[87] Coenzyme Q10 also seems to improve immune function.[88] Glutamine has been used to enhance the intestinal absorption of nutrients and improve weight gain in individuals with HIV/AIDS.[89,90] Marijuana also seems to improve weight gain by increasing appetite in clients with AIDS.[91]

Broad-spectrum nutritional supplements also may be helpful because many clients with HIV infection and/or AIDS have multiple nutritional deficiencies.[92] Selenium deficiency seems to be associated with high mortality in AIDS clients, so selenium supplementation may be warranted.[93] Supplementation with dehydroepiandrosterone sulfate may improve fatigue and depression in HIV-positive clients.

Arginine in combination with the amino acid derivative hydroxymethylbutyrate and glutamine has been used for preservation of lean body mass. In a double-blind trial, AIDS clients who had lost 5% of their body weight in the 3 months preceding the study were given a placebo or 1.5 gm hydroxymethylbutyrate, 7 gm L-glutamine, and 7 gm of L-arginine for 8 weeks. Those taking the supplement mixture gained an average of 3 pounds, 85% of which was lean body weight.[94] In an initial trial, an 8-week course of DHEA supplementation reported improvement in low mood and low energy.[95] Several other vitamins have been used to allay various symptoms and conditions associated with HIV infection and AIDS and to slow disease progression.

Several herbs also have been used in clients with HIV infection. They are used principally to directly kill HIV (e.g., boxwood and licorice), to modulate the immune system (e.g., Asian ginseng, echinacea, mistletoe, and turmeric), and to fight infection (e.g., garlic and tea tree oil).

## Low Back Pain

Low back pain (LBP) is a common, chronic condition for many Americans. Causes of LBP include disc herniation, compression fractures, poor posture, scoliosis, muscle spasms, and other musculoskeletal disorders.

Enzymes such as chymotrypsin and trypsin in combination have been used in a number of trials for clients with chronic LBP conditions with some benefit.[96]

Devil's claw has been found to be helpful to reduce nonspecific LBP as well as prescription medications do.[97] One trial suggested that large amounts of willow bark may relieve clients' LBP.[98]

Other nutritional supplements such as D,L-phenylalanine and vitamins B1, B6, and B12 in combination have less definitive evidence for effectiveness.

Colchicine may be helpful for LBP associated with a herniated disc. A review of several double-blind trials showed that colchicine was associated with relief of pain, muscle spasm, and weakness.[99] Colchicine may have potentially severe side effects so should be taken only under the supervision of a health care provider skilled in herbal medicine.

## Macular Degeneration

Nutritional supplements such as lutein and zinc have contradictory evidence regarding their potential health benefit; however, they are likely safe.[100,101] Ginkgo biloba may help early-stage macular degeneration according to a small preliminary study.[102]

Beta-carotene orally when combined with vitamin C, vitamin E, and zinc seemed to provide a 27% risk reduction for visual loss resulting from macular degeneration and may contribute to arresting progression to advanced macular degeneration.[103,104] Similarly, lutein seems to be related to a lower risk of macular degeneration, particularly when it is consumed through dietary intake.[105] Taking 10-mg lutein per day for 12 months may improve some symptoms of macular degeneration in preliminary trials.[106]

## Multiple Sclerosis

Multiple sclerosis (MS) is a progressive neurological disorder in which clients develop paresthesias, muscle weakness, visual disturbances, loss of coordination, and disturbance of mood. Unfortunately, little scientific evidence supports the health benefits of nutritional supplements and herbs in the treatment of multiple sclerosis.

A cannabis-based product called Sativex was given as a mouth spray to clients with neuropathic pain associated with MS. The spray significantly reduced the pain, spasticity, muscle spasms, and sleep disturbances in these clients.[107] Marijuana taken orally or smoked seems to be effective in reduction of tremor and spasticity.[108]

Aconiti had a pain-relieving effect in one animal study.[109] Other products that have been used but lack strong scientific data include calcium, fish oil, vitamin E, magnesium, and ginkgo biloba.

In one study, vitamin D supplementation appeared to be associated with a 40% decreased risk of MS in women. The effect seemed to depend on cumulative dose, requiring at least 400 IU per day for protective effect.[110]

## Myocardial Infarction

Disease of the coronary arteries, which feed the heart muscle, frequently contributes to myocardial ischemia or infarction. Several nutritional supplements have been found to help with arresting or slowing the development of coronary artery disease.

Coenzyme Q10 is important in energy metabolism. Its use is associated with lower lipoprotein levels, which reduce cardiac risk. Use of coenzyme Q10 in clients who recently had survived a myocardial infarction seemed to reduce the number of recurrent infarctions and reduced the cardiac death rate.[111]

L-carnitine is an amino acid that helps in fatty acid transport. Trials suggest that taking L-carnitine regularly is associated with a higher chance of surviving a myocardial infarction.[112]

Vitamin C also seems to have some protective mechanism for blood vessels.[113] Scientific evidence attempting to prove cardioprotection is inconsistent, however.[114]

Fish oil is an important source of the essential omega-3 fatty acids EPA and DHA. Fish oil has been linked to reversal of atherosclerosis and reduction in number of fatal heart attacks.[115] Dietary recommendations for omega-3 fatty acids can be found on the American Heart Association website at *http://www.americanheart.org*.

Magnesium has shown mixed results in clinical trials for heart attack victims. Similarly, the relationship of selenium and cardioprotection is not certain. No herbs have shown particular promise in the treatment or prevention of myocardial infarction.

## Neuropathic Pain

Neuropathic pain can be tremendously difficult to alleviate. Little scientific evidence with human subjects is available for the effects of biologically based therapies on neuropathic pain other than traditional pharmaceuticals. A promising trial used a processed Aconiti tuber to produce analgesia in rats with neuropathic pain after partial nerve injury.[107]

Several studies suggest that marijuana and other cannabinoids have therapeutic potential for relief of pain among other symptoms. More research is needed, however.[116]

Intravenous magnesium has had some benefit in relieving neuropathic pain associated with cancer. A 500 mg to 1 gm dose seemed to relieve pain up to 4 hours in one trial.[117]

## Parkinson's Disease

Parkinson's disease (PD) affects primarily older adults. A number of supplements have shown some promise in the treatment of PD. Black tea, green tea, coffee, and caffeine have been linked to a decreased risk for PD.[118,119]

Coenzyme Q10 supplementation slowed the progression of the disease.[120] Vitamin E also is associated with a reduced risk of PD.[121] Vitamins C and E appear to reduce or delay the need for medication intervention.[122] Vitamin E intake must be high to achieve adequate levels in the brain.[123]

Methionine has been associated with some symptom improvement in preliminary trials.[124] Nicotinamide adenine dinucleotide (NADH) raises the level of dopamine in the brain, which suggests a theoretic use for it in the treatment of PD.[125] Vitamin B2 (riboflavin) supplementation was given to clients who were deficient in B2 and had PD. After 3 months of treatment, all subjects had some improvement in their movement, which was sustained at 6 months.[126] A small study showed improvement in motor control after supplementation with D-phenylalanine.[127]

## Stroke

Stroke is the third leading cause of death in the United States. Most strokes do not result in death but rather disability such as reversible or permanent paralysis. Nutritional supplements proposed for stroke prevention are aimed at the underlying risk factors for stroke, such as hypertension, diabetes, hypercholesterolemia, and atherosclerosis.

Increasing dietary calcium may decrease risk of stroke in women.[128] Fish oil also seems to reduce stroke risk by 27%.[129] Magnesium may reduce the risk for stroke in men.[130]

Taking glycine may have some neuroprotective effect for stroke clients when given within 6 hours of onset of symptoms.[131]

Vinpocetine given parenterally improved some biochemical measures of brain function in some trials involving stroke victims.[132] More research is needed, however.

Some clients at high risk for stroke are given anticoagulants such as aspirin. Herbs and supplements with anticoagulant activity include garlic, fish oil, ginkgo biloba, and vitamin E. These should be used with caution in clients receiving prescription anticoagulants such as warfarin because of the risk of bleeding.

## Tendonitis

Tendonitis is often a result of overuse, which may result in inflammation of the connective tissue. Dimethyl sulfoxide (DMSO) has been used as a topical antiinflammatory. One trial showed a significant reduction in pain and inflammation in clients with elbow and shoulder tendonitis when 10% DMSO was applied.[133]

Proteolytic enzymes such as bromelain theoretically should help based on their antiinflammatory action.[134]

## Wounds

Many nutritional supplements have been used successfully for treatment of clients with decubitus ulcers because nutritional deficiencies impair wound healing.

Antioxidants frequently are depleted in healing wounds. Oral supplementation of flavonoids, folic acid, vitamin C, vitamin E, and oral and topical zinc has been shown to promote and accelerate wound healing in some settings.[135-140]

Trypsin applied topically may be helpful to cleanse necrotic tissue in wounds and enhance healing.[141]

Herbs such as aloe vera, gotu kola, and comfrey[30] are used topically to accelerate wound healing. Research on gotu kola has been primarily through in vitro and animal studies. Although aloe vera has been used traditionally for wound healing, scientific evidence is mixed.[142]

Topical essential fatty acids have been used successfully to prevent pressure ulcers in malnourished individuals. Gotu kola and hyaluronic acid have been used, but further research is needed.[143,144]

## Enhancing Athletic Performance

Many clients seek the advice of health care providers for health optimization rather than treatment of conditions. Individuals trying to achieve peak performance frequently turn to nutritional supplements and herbs.

Creatine monohydrate is used widely to enhance high-intensity performance and to build muscle. It is used in energy production for muscle cells. Creatine may increase gain of lean body mass. Many well-designed studies have shown that creatine supplementation improves performance in short-duration, high-intensity exercise.[145] Of note, chronic high doses of creatine may be injurious to the kidney. Whey protein also can be helpful for building lean body mass.

Vitamins C and E are used to reduce pain and promote recovery after athletic injuries.[146]

Other supplements used include citrate, DHEA, glutamine, and beta-hydroxy beta-methylbutyrate (HMB). Pyruvate has been used to enhance exercise performance. Many other supplements are used but lack scientific evidence for enhancement of athletic performance. Some of the more common products are arginine/ornithine, chromium, coenzyme Q10, L-carnitine, pyruvate, and zinc. Herbs that have been found to be effective in some settings include Asian ginseng, eleuthero, and rhodiola rosea.

## SUMMARY

A great deal of data are available that support the use of botanical products in a number of conditions treated by physical therapists. Those therapies for which reliable, consistent data support their safety and efficacy may be recommended. Therapies that have insufficient or contradictory data should prompt conversation and consideration. Therapies that lack data may still offer some benefit but should be approached with caution. Health care professionals are expected to act as informed intermediaries for clients so that they have access to reliable information regarding their health care. Being familiar with biologically based therapies that have the potential to address clients' diagnoses, symptoms, and goals is important for all health care providers. Knowledge of the potential adverse effects of herbs and other biologically based therapies, including drug interactions, is also of the utmost importance.

Using appropriate key terms for searching the scientific literature and complete and unbiased resources available through texts and online resources, therapists can assist their clients with decisions regarding biologically based therapies.

## REFERENCES

1. Kelly JP et al: Recent trends in use of herbal and other natural products, *Arch Intern Med* 165:281-6, 2005.
2. National Center for Complementary and Alternative Medicine: The Use of Complementary and Alternative Medicine in the United States. Available at: *http://nccam.nih.gov/news/camsurvey_fs1.htm #natural*. Accessed January 17, 2007.
3. Hrastinger A et al: Is there clinical evidence supporting the use of botanical dietary supplements in children? *J Pediatr* 146:311-7, 2005.
4. Kuo ST et al: Factors associated with herbal use among urban multiethnic primary care patients: a cross-sectional survey. *BMC Compl Altern Med* 4:18, 2004. Available at: http://www.biomedcentral.com. Accessed January 17, 2007.
5. National Center for Complementary and Alternative Medicine: The use of complementary and alternative medicine in the United States. Available at: *http://nccam.nih.gov/news/camsurvey_fs1.htm# natural*. Accessed December 5, 2005.
6. Watanabe S et al: Unique place of Kampo (Japanese traditional medicine) in complementary and alternative medicine: a survey of doctors belonging to the regional medical association in Japan, *Tohoku J Exp Med* 194:55-63, 2001.
7. Thomas KS, Nicoll JP, Coleman P: Use and expenditure on complementary medicine in England: a population based survey, *Complement Ther Med* 9:2-11, 2001.
8. Tesch BJ: Herbs commonly used by women: an evidence-based review, *Am J Obstet Gynecol* 188(suppl 5):S44-55, 2003.

9. National Center for Complementary and Alternative Medicine: Backgrounder: biologically based practices: an overview. Available at: *http://nccam.nih.gov/health/backgrounds/biobasedprac.htm*. Accessed January 17, 2007.
10. Botanical Review Team, Center for Drug Evaluation and Research, U.S. Food and Drug Administration: What is a botanical drug? Available at: *http://www.fda.gov/cder/Offices/ODE_V_BRT/botanicalDrug.htm*. Accessed January 17, 2007.
11. National Center for Complementary and Alternative Medicine: Considerations for NCCAM Clinical Trial Grant Applications. Available at: *http://nccam.nih.gov/research/policies/clinical-considerations.htm#skipnav*. Accessed January 17, 2007.
12. *Webster's medical desk dictionary*, Springfield, Massachusetts, 1986, Merriam Webster.
13. Jones P: Clinical nutrition: 7. Functional foods—more than just nutrition, *J Can Med Assoc* 166:1555-63, 2002.
14. The University of Texas MD Anderson Cancer Center: About Complementary/Integrative Medicine. Available at: *http://www.mdanderson.org/departments/CIMER/dIndex.cfm?pn=7B632E4A-56B2-11D5-812100508B603A14*. Accessed January 17, 2007.
15. U.S. Food and Drug Administration, Center for Food Safety and Applied Nutrition: Current Good Manufacturing Practices (CGMP's). Available at: *http://www.cfsan.fda.gov/~dms/dscgmps3.html*. Accessed January 17, 2007.
16. Kroll D: ASHP statement on the use of dietary supplements, *Am J Health Syst Pharm* 61:1707-11, 2004.
17. Office of Dietary Supplements: Health Information. Available at: *http://dietary-supplements.info.nih.gov/health_information/health_information.aspx*. Accessed January 17, 2007.
18. Centers for Disease Control: Toxic Exposure Surveillance System. Available at: *http://www.cdc.gov/mmwr/preview/mmwrhtml/su5301a74.htm*. Accessed January 17, 2007.
19. Ernst E et al: *The desktop guide to complementary and alternative medicine*, Edinburgh, 2001, Mosby.
20. Ernst E: Herbal medicines put into context, *Br Med J* 327:881-2, 2003.
21. What is ESCOP? The European Scientific Cooperative on Phytotherapy (ESCOP). Available at: *http://www.escop.com*. Accessed December 12, 2005.
22. National Center for Complementary and Alternative Medicine: Research funding priorities. Available at: *http://nccam.nih.gov/research/priorities/index.htm#5*. Accessed December 15, 2005.
23. Trickett P: Proteolytic enzymes in treatment of athletic injuries, *Appl Ther* 6:647-52, 1964.

24. Deitrick RE: Oral proteolytic enzymes in the treatment of athletic injuries: a double-blind study, *Pennsylvania Med J*, October 1975, pp 35-7.

25. Cirelli MG: Five years experience with bromelains in therapy of edema and inflammation in postoperative tissue reaction, skin infections and trauma, *Clin Med* 74(6):55-9, 1967.

26. Tiidus PM, Houston ME: Vitamin E status and response to exercise training, *Sports Med* 20:12-23, 1995.

27. Ringsdorf WM Jr, Cheraskin E: Vitamin C and human wound healing, *Oral Surg Oral Med Oral Pathol* 53:231-6, 1982.

28. Giamberardino MA et al: Effects of prolonged L-carnitine administration on delayed muscle pain and CK release after eccentric effort, *Int J Sports Med* 17:320-4, 1996.

29. Guillaume M, Padioleau F: Veinotonic effect, vascular protection, anti-inflammatory and free radical scavenging properties of horse chestnut extract, *Arzneimittelforschung* 44:25-35, 1994.

30. Weiss R: *Herbal medicine*, Gothenburg, Sweden: Ab Arcanum and Beaconsfield, UK, 1988, Beaconsfield Publishers, p 342.

31. Cipolli C, Chiari G: Effects of L-acetylcarnitine on mental deterioration in the aged: initial results, *Clin Ter* 132(suppl 6):479-510, 1990 [in Italian].

32. Salvioli G, Neri M: L-acetylcarnitine treatment of mental decline in the elderly, *Drugs Exp Clin Res* 20(4):169-76, 1994.

33. Maggioni M et al: Effects of phosphatidylserine therapy in geriatric patients with depressive disorders, *Acta Psychiatr Scand* 81:265-70, 1990.

34. Hindmarch I, Fuchs HH, Erzigkeit H: Efficacy and tolerance of vinpocetine in ambulant patients suffering from mild to moderate organic psychosyndromes, *Int Clin Psychopharmacol* 6:31-43, 1991.

35. Balestreri R, Fontana L, Astengo F: A double-blind placebo controlled evaluation of the safety and efficacy of vinpocetine in the treatment of patients with chronic vascular senile cerebral dysfunction, *J Am Geriatr Soc* 35:425-30, 1987.

36. Schneider LS et al: A randomized, double-blind, placebo-controlled trial of two doses of Ginkgo biloba extract in dementia of the Alzheimer's type, *Curr Alzheimer Res* 2:541-51, 2005.

37. Troen A, Rosenberg I: Homocysteine and cognitive function, *Semin Vasc Med* 5:209-14, 2005.

38. Cannon DT, Wu Y: Topical capsaicin as an adjuvant analgesic for the treatment of traumatic amputee neurogenic residual limb pain, *Arch Phys Med Rehabil* 79:591-3, 1998.

39. Qiu GX et al: Efficacy and safety of glucosamine sulfate versus ibuprofen in patients with knee osteoarthritis, *Arzneimittelforschung* 48:469-74, 1998.

40. Drovanti A, Bignamini AA, Rovati AL: Therapeutic activity of oral glucosamine sulfate in osteoarthritis: a placebo-controlled double-blind investigation, *Clin Ther* 3:260-72, 1980.

41. Vaz AL: Double-blind clinical evaluation of the relative efficacy of ibuprofen and glucosamine sulphate in the management of osteoarthritis of the knee in outpatients, *Curr Med Res Opin* 8:145-9, 1982.

42. Pujalte JM, Llavore EP, Ylescupidez FR: Double-blind clinical evaluation of oral glucosamine sulphate in the basic treatment of osteoarthrosis, *Curr Med Res Opin* 7:110-4, 1980.

43. Verbruggen G, Goemaere S, Veys EM: Chondroitin sulfate: S/DMOAD (structure/disease modifying anti-osteoarthritis drug) in the treatment of finger joint OA, *Osteoarthritis Cartilage* 6(Suppl A):37-8, 1998.

44. Bucsi L, Poór G: Efficacy and tolerability of oral chondroitin sulfate as a symptomatic slow-acting drug for osteoarthritis (SYSADOA) in the treatment of knee osteoarthritis, *Osteoarthritis Cartilage* 6(Suppl A):31-6, 1998.

45. Pipitone V et al: A multicenter, triple-blind study to evaluate galactosaminoglucuronoglycan sulfate versus placebo in patients with femorotibial gonarthritis, *Curr Ther Res* 52:608-38, 1992.

46. Morreale P et al: Comparison of the antiinflammatory efficacy of chondroitin sulfate and diclofenac sodium in patients with knee osteoarthritis, *J Rheumatol* 23:1385-91, 1996.

47. Domljan Z et al: A double-blind trial of ademetionine vs naproxen in activated gonarthrosis, *Int J Clin Pharmacol Ther Toxicol* 27:329-33, 1989.

48. Müller-Fassbender H: Double-blind clinical trial of S-adenosylmethionine versus ibuprofen in the treatment of osteoarthritis, *Am J Med* 83(suppl 5A):81-3, 1987.

49. Vetter G: Double-blind comparative clinical trial with S-adenosylmethionine and indomethacin in the treatment of osteoarthritis, *Am J Med* 83(suppl 5A):78-80, 1987.

50. Maccagno A: Double-blind controlled clinical trial of oral S-adenosylmethionine versus piroxicam in knee osteoarthritis, *Am J Med* 83(suppl 5A):72-7, 1987.

51. Montrone F et al: Double-blind study of S-adenosyl-methionine versus placebo in hip and knee arthrosis, *Clin Rheumatol* 4:484-5, 1985.

52. Kulkarni RR et al: Treatment of osteoarthritis with a herbomineral formulation: a double-blind, placebo-controlled, cross-over study, *J Ethnopharmacol* 33:91-395, 1991.

53. Piscoya J et al: Efficacy and safety of freeze-dried cat's claw in osteoarthritis of the knee: mechanisms

of action of the species *Uncaria guianensis*, *Inflamm Res* 50:442-8, 2001.

54. Altman RD et al: Capsaicin cream 0.025% as monotherapy for osteoarthritis: a double-blind study, *Semin Arth Rheum* 23(suppl 3):25-33, 1994.

55. Deal CL et al: Treatment of arthritis with topical capsaicin: a double-blind trial, *Clin Ther* 13:383-95, 1991.

56. Schnitzer T, Morton C, Coker S: Topical capsaicin therapy for osteoarthritis pain: achieving a maintenance regimen, *Semin Arth Rheum* 23(suppl 3):34-40, 1994.

57. Eberlein-Konig B, Placzek M, Przybilla B: Protective effect against sunburn of combined systemic ascorbic acid (vitamin C) and d-alpha-tocopherol (vitamin E), *J Am Acad Dermatol* 38:45-8, 1998.

58. Klein GL et al: Synthesis of vitamin D in skin after burns, *Lancet* 363:291-2, 2004.

59. Latha B et al: Serum enzymatic changes modulated using trypsin: chymotrypsin preparation during burn wounds in humans, *Burns* 23:560-4, 1997.

60. Subrahmanyam M: A prospective randomized, clinical and histological study of superficial burn wound healing with honey and silver sulfadiazine, *Burns* 24:157-61, 1998.

61. De Bandt JP et al: A randomized controlled trial of the influence of the mode of enteral ornithine alpha-ketoglutarate administration in burn patients, *J Nutr* 128(3):563-9, 1998.

62. Berger MM et al: Trace element supplementation modulates pulmonary infection rates after major burns: a double-blind, placebo-controlled trial, *Am J Clin Nutr* 68:365-71, 1998.

63. Gun F et al: Effect of probiotic supplementation on bacterial translocation in thermal injury, *Surg Today* 35:760-4, 2005.

64. Klemes IS: Vitamin B12 in acute subdeltoid bursitis, *Ind Med Surg* 26:290-2, 1957.

65. Matsuoka H et al: Lentinan potentiates immunity and prolongs the survival time of some patients, *Anticancer Res* 17:2751-5, 1997.

66. Tavani A et al: n-3 polyunsaturated fatty acid intake and cancer risk in Italy and Switzerland, *Int J Cancer* 105:113-6, 2003.

67. Baron JA et al: Folate intake, alcohol consumption, cigarette smoking, and risk of colorectal adenomas, *J Natl Cancer Inst* 90:57-62, 1998.

68. Key TJ et al: A case-control study of diet and prostate cancer, *Br J Cancer* 76:678-87, 1997.

69. Hartman TJ et al: Association of the B-vitamins pyridoxal 5′-phosphate (B6), B12, and folate with lung cancer risk in older men, *Am J Epidemiol* 153:688-94, 2001.

70. Cox IM, Campbell MJ, Dowson D: Red blood cell magnesium and chronic fatigue syndrome, *Lancet* 337:757-60, 1991.

71. Plioplys AV, Plioplys S: Amantadine and L-carnitine treatment of chronic fatigue syndrome, *Neuropsychobio* 35:16-23, 1997.

72. Forsyth LM et al: Therapeutic effects of oral NADH on the symptoms of patients with chronic fatigue syndrome, *Ann Allergy Asthma Immunol* 82:185-91, 1991.

73. Lapp CW, Cheney PR: The rationale for using high-dose cobalamin (vitamin B12), *CFIDS Chronicle Physicians' Forum* Fall:19-20, 1993.

74. Rautalahti M et al: The effect of alpha-tocopherol and beta-carotene supplementation on COPD symptoms, *Am J Respir Crit Care Med* 156:1447-52, 1997.

75. Skorodin MS et al: Magnesium sulfate in exacerbations of chronic obstructive pulmonary disease, *Arch Intern Med* 155:496-500, 1995.

76. Van Schayck CP et al: Are anti-oxidant and anti-inflammatory treatments effective in different subgroups of COPD? A hypothesis, *Respir Med* 92:1259-64, 1998.

77. Pela R et al: N-acetylcysteine reduces the exacerbation rate in patients with moderate to severe COPD, *Respiration* 66:495-500, 1999.

78. Dal Negro R et al: Effects of L-carnitine on physical performance in chronic respiratory insufficiency, *Int J Clin Pharmacol Ther Toxicol* 26:269-72, 1988.

79. Shahar E et al: Dietary n-3 polyunsaturated fatty acids and smoking-related chronic obstructive pulmonary disease, *N Engl J Med* 331:228-33, 1994.

80. Broekhuizen R et al: Polyunsaturated fatty acids improve exercise capacity in chronic obstructive pulmonary disease, *Thorax* 60:376-82, 2005.

81. Meyer-Wegner J: Ivy versus ambroxol in chronic bronchitis. *Zeits Allegemeinmed* 69:61-6, 1993 [in German].

82. Puttini PS, Caruso I: Primary fibromyalgia syndrome and 5-hydroxy-L-tryptophan: a 90-day open study, *J Int Med Res* 20:182-9, 1992.

83. Caruso I et al: Double-blind study of 5-hydroxytryptophan versus placebo in the treatment of primary fibromyalgia syndrome, *J Int Med Res* 18:201-9, 1990.

84. McCarty DJ et al: Treatment of pain due to fibromyalgia with topical capsaicin: a pilot study, *Semin Arthr Rheum* 23:41-7, 1994.

85. Scharf MB et al: Effect of gamma-hydroxybutyrate on pain, fatigue, and the alpha sleep anomaly in patients with fibromyalgia. Preliminary report, *J Rheumatol* 25:1986-90, 1998.

86. Tavoni A et al: Evaluation of S-adenosylmethionine in primary fibromyalgia. A double-blind crossover study, *Am J Med* 83:107-10, 1987.

87. Gordon M et al: A placebo-controlled trial of the immune modulator, lentinan, in HIV-positive patients: a phase I/II trial, *J Med* 29:305-30, 1998.

88. Folkers K et al: Coenzyme Q10 increases T4/T8 ratios of lymphocytes in ordinary subjects and relevance to patients having the AIDS related complex, *Biochem Biophys Res Commun* 176:786-91, 1991.

89. Noyer CM et al: A double-blind placebo-controlled pilot study of glutamine therapy for abnormal intestinal permeability in patients with AIDS, *Am J Gastroenterol* 93:972-5, 1998.

90. Shabert JK et al: Glutamine-antioxidant supplementation increases body cell mass in AIDS patients with weight loss: a randomized, double-blind controlled trial, *Nutrition* 15:860-4, 1999.

91. Goldschmidt RH, Dong BJ: Treatment of AIDS and HIV-related conditions: 2000, *J Am Board Fam Pract* 13:274-98, 2000.

92. Mustafa T et al: Association between exercise and HIV disease progression in a cohort of homosexual men, *Ann Epidemiol* 9:127-31, 1999.

93. Chariot P, Perchet H, Monnet I: Dilated cardiomyopathy in HIV-infected patients [letter; comment], *N Engl J Med* 340:732 (discussion 733-745), 1999.

94. Clark RH et al: Nutritional treatment for acquired immunodeficiency virus-associated wasting using beta-hydroxy beta-methylbutyrate, glutamine, and arginine: a randomized, double-blind, placebo-controlled study, *JPEN J Parenter Enteral Nutr* 24:133-9, 2000.

95. Rabkin JG et al: DHEA treatment for HIV+ patients: effects on mood, androgenic and anabolic parameters, *Psychoneuroendocrinology* 25:53-68, 2000.

96. Hingorani K: Oral enzyme therapy in severe back pain, *Br J Clin Pract* 22:209-10, 1968.

97. Chrubasik S et al: Comparison of outcome measures during treatment with the proprietary Harpagophytum extract doloteffin in patients with pain in the lower back, knee or hip, *Phytomedicine* 9:181-94, 2002.

98. Chrubasik S et al: Treatment of low back pain exacerbations with willow bark extract: a randomized double-blind study, *Am J Med* 109:9-14, 2000.

99. Rask MR: Colchicine use in five hundred patients with disk disease, *J Neurol Orth Surg* 1(5):1-19, 1980.

100. Richer S et al: Double-masked, placebo-controlled, randomized trial of lutein and antioxidant supplementation in the intervention of atrophic age-related macular degeneration: the veterans LAST study (Lutein Antioxidant Supplementation Trial), *Optometry* 75:216-30, 2004.

101. Newsome DA et al: Oral zinc in macular degeneration, *Arch Ophthalmol* 106:192-8, 1988.

102. Lebuisson DA, Leroy L, Reigal G: Treatment of senile macular degeneration with *ginkgo biloba* extract: a preliminary double-blind study versus placebo. In Fünfgeld FW, editor: *Rokan (ginkgo biloba): recent results in pharmacology and clinic*, Berlin, 1988, Springer-Verlag, pp 231-6.

103. Age-Related Eye Disease Study Research Group: A randomized, placebo-controlled, clinical trial of high-dose supplementation with vitamins C and E, beta carotene, and zinc for age-related macular degeneration and vision loss. AREDS report no. 8, *Arch Ophthalmol* 119:1417-36, 2001.

104. Age-Related Eye Disease Study Research Group: Potential public health impact of age-related eye disease study results: AREDS report no. 11, *Arch Ophthalmol* 121:1621-4, 2003.

105. Pratt S: Dietary prevention of age-related macular degeneration, *J Am Optom Assoc* 70:39-47, 1999.

106. Richer S et al: Double-masked, placebo-controlled, randomized trial of lutein and antioxidant supplementation in the intervention of atrophic age-related macular degeneration: the veterans LAST study (Lutein Antioxidant Supplement Trial), *Optometry* 75:216-30, 2004.

107. Perras C: Saltivex for the management of multiple sclerosis symptoms, *Issues Emerg Health Technol* 72:1-4, 2005.

108. Zajicek J et al: Cannabinoids for treatment of spasticity and other symptoms related to multiple sclerosis (CAMS study): multicentre randomised placebo-controlled trial, *Lancet* 362:1517-26, 2003.

109. Xu H et al: Pain-relieving effects of processed Aconiti tuber in CCI-neuropathic rats, *J Ethnopharmacol* Sept 22: epub, 2005.

110. Munger KL et al: Vitamin D intake and incidence of multiple sclerosis, *Neurology* 62:60-5, 2004.

111. Singh RB et al: Effect of coenzyme Q10 on risk of atherosclerosis in patients with recent myocardial infarction, *Mol Cell Biochem* 246:75-82, 2003.

112. Singh RB et al: A randomized, double-blind, placebo-controlled trial of L-carnitine in suspected acute myocardial infarction, *Postgrad Med J* 72:45-50, 1996.

113. Davini P et al: Controlled study on L-carnitine therapeutic efficacy in post-infarction, *Drugs Exp Clin Res* 18:355-65, 1992.

114. Klipstein-Grobusch K et al: Dietary antioxidants and risk of myocardial infarction in the elderly: the Rotterdam study, *Am J Clin Nutr* 69:261-6, 1999.

115. Von Schacky C et al: The effect of dietary omega-3 fatty acids on coronary atherosclerosis. A randomized double-blind, placebo-controlled trial, *Ann Intern Med* 130:554-62, 1999.

116. Corey S: Recent developments in the therapeutic potential of cannabinoids, *P R Health Sci J* 24(1):19-26, 2005.

117. Crosby V, Wilcock A, Corcoran R: The safety and efficacy of a single dose (500 mg or 1 g) of intrave-

nous magnesium sulfate in neuropathic pain poorly responsive to strong opioid analgesics in patients with cancer, *J Pain Symptom Manage* 19:35-9, 2000.

118. Ross GW et al: Association of coffee and caffeine intake with the risk of Parkinson's disease, *JAMA* 283:2674-9, 2000.

119. Ascherio A et al: Prospective study of caffeine intake and risk of Parkinson's disease in men and women, *Proc 125th Ann Mtg Am Neurological Assoc*, Boston, Mass, 2000, Oct 15, 2000, pp 18-42.

120. Shults CW et al: Effects of coenzyme Q10 in early Parkinson disease: evidence of slowing of the functional decline, *Arch Neurol* 59:1541-50, 2002.

121. de Rijk MC et al: Dietary antioxidants and Parkinson disease: the Rotterdam study, *Arch Neurol* 54:762-5, 1997.

122. Fahn S: A pilot trial of high-dose alpha-tocopherol and ascorbate in early Parkinson's disease, *Ann Neurol* 32:S128-32, 1992.

123. Vatassery GT, Fahn S, Kuskowski MA: Alpha tocopherol in CSF of subjects taking high-dose vitamin E in the DATATOP study. Parkinson Study Group, *Neurology* 50:1900-2, 1998.

124. Smythies JR, Halsey JH: Treatment of Parkinson's disease with l-methionine, *South Med J* 77:1577, 1984.

125. Cotzias GC et al: Nicotinamide ineffective in parkinsonism, *N Engl J Med* 287:147, 1972.

126. Coimbra CG, Junqueira VB: High doses of riboflavin and the elimination of dietary red meat promote the recovery of some motor functions in Parkinson's disease patients, *Braz J Med Biol Res* 36:1409-17, 2003.

127. Heller B, Fischer E, Martin R: Therapeutic action of D-phenylalanine in Parkinson's disease, *Arzneimittelforschung* 26:577-79, 1976.

128. Iso H et al: Prospective study of calcium, potassium, and magnesium intake and risk of stroke in women, *Stroke* 30:1772-9, 1999.

129. Iso H et al: Intake of fish and omega-3 fatty acids and risk of stroke in women, *JAMA* 285:304-12, 2001.

130. Suter PM: The effects of potassium, magnesium, calcium, and fiber on risk of stroke, *Nutr Rev* 57:84-8, 1999.

131. Gusev EI et al: Neuroprotective effects of glycine for therapy of acute ischaemic stroke, *Cerebrovasc Dis* 10:49-60, 2000.

132. Szakall S et al: Cerebral effects of a single dose of intravenous vinpocetine in chronic stroke patients: a PET study, *J Neuroimaging* 8:197-204, 1998.

133. Kneer W et al: Dimethylsulfoxide gel in treatment of acute tendopathies. A multicenter, placebo-controlled, randomized study, *Fortschritte Med* 112:142-6, 1994.

134. Cirelli MG: Treatment of inflammation and edema with bromelain, *Delaware Med J* 34:159-67, 1962.

135. Palmieri B, Gozzi G, Palmieri G: Vitamin E added silicone gel sheets for treatment of hypertrophic scars and keloids, *Int J Dermatol* 34:506-9, 1995.

136. Vaxman F et al: Can the wound healing process be improved by vitamin supplementation? Experimental study on humans, *Eur Surg Res* 28:306-14, 1996.

137. Mazzotta MY: Nutrition and wound healing, *J Am Podiatr Med Assoc* 84:456-62, 1994.

138. Blonstein J: Control of swelling in boxing injuries, *Practitioner* 203:206, 1960.

139. Pories WJ et al: Acceleration of healing with zinc sulfate, *Ann Surg* 165:432-6, 1967.

140. Hunt TK: Vitamin A and wound healing, *J Am Acad Dermatol* 15:817-21, 1986.

141. Latha B et al: The efficacy of trypsin: chymotrypsin preparation in the reduction of oxidative damage during burn injury, *Burns* 24:532-8, 1998.

142. Schmidt JM, Greenspoon JS: Aloe vera dermal wound gel is associated with a delay in wound healing, *Obstet Gynecol* 78:115-7, 1991.

143. Brinkhaus B et al: Chemical, pharmacological and clinical profile of the east Asian medical plant Centella asiatica, *Phytomedicine* 7:427-48, 2000.

144. King SR, Hickerson WL, Proctor KG: Beneficial actions of exogenous hyaluronic acid on wound healing, *Surgery* 109:76-84, 1991.

145. Mesa JL et al: Oral creatine supplementation and skeletal muscle metabolism in physical exercise, *Sports Med* 32:903-44, 2002.

146. Jakeman P, Maxwell S: Effect of antioxidant vitamin supplementation on muscle function after eccentric exercise, *Eur J Appl Physiol* 67:426-30, 1993.

## ADDITIONAL RESOURCES

Atkins RC: Dr. Atkins' New Diet Revolution, New York *2002 M. Evans and Company, Inc.*

American Heart Association

Botanical Review Team, FDA Office of Drug Evaluation

CAM use in the US, 2002. pdf file. From CDC Advance Data in Health Statistics, May 2004

ConsumerLab.com

DSHEA text

FDA Consumer Hotline

HealthNotes

MedWatch

Ornish D. Eat More, Weigh Less: Dr. Dean Ornish's Life Choice Program for Losing Weight Safely While Eating Abundantly New York, 2001 *Dean* HarperCollins Publishers Inc.

Weil A. Eating Well for Optimum Health New York 2000 Alfred A Knopf

NCCAM

NCCAM herbal supplement safety information

Use of Dietary Supplements in the United States, 1988-94: Data From the National Health Examination Survey, the National Health and Nutrition Examination Surveys, and the Hispanic Health and Nutrition Examination Survey (PHS) 99-1694.

Office of Dietary supplements, NIH

Natural Standard

Natural Medicine Comprehensive Database

# CHAPTER 11

## Ginkgo Biloba

*Ellen D. Mandel*

---

### CASE

Robert is a 66-year-old retired accountant who is currently receiving outpatient physical therapy for a muscle strain in his low back. He recently was diagnosed with early Alzheimer's disease (AD) and is considering taking ginkgo biloba extract (GBE) to help improve his cognition. The therapist had had clients who have used GBE for enhancement of circulation and memory but is uncertain of GBE's safety and efficacy given Robert's past and current medical condition. Knowing that Robert's family physician assistant (PA) is knowledgeable about botanicals and has prescribed herbal and dietary supplements for other clients, the therapist suggests that Robert and his wife make an appointment with her to discuss the use of GBE. The therapist also seeks permission to contact the PA to discuss the effect GBE may have on Robert's outcomes in physical therapy. The following examination and clinical decision-making process is offered by Robert's PA.

### ■ Initial Examination

**Client and Family Report:** The client has difficulty with recall, including events within 1 week of their occurrence. He often pauses for long periods to find a particular word and forgets the names of common household items. He has difficulty managing his checkbook and has been getting lost while driving in his usual neighborhood.

**Client Goals:** To improve memory, problem solving, and mental clarity

**Employment:** Retired accountant

**General Health:** Positive for mild benign prostatic hypertrophy (BPH) associated with a reduction in urinary stream with some dribbling. Complains of difficulty sleeping and has been receiving physical therapy for a muscle strain in his low back. Denies all other medical conditions including hypertension (HTN), diabetes mellitus (DM), and coronary artery disease (CAD) and has never experienced seizures, palpitations, symptoms of neuropathy, intermittent claudication, tremors, or changes in gait.

**Medications:** Diphenhydramine HCl (Benadryl) three times per week to assist with sleep

**Laboratory Studies:** Normal head CT scan and laboratory tests; negative for neurosyphilis

**Cardiopulmonary:** *Vitals:* BP=140/78; HR=80, normal rhythm, without murmur; RR=14, lungs clear to auscultation

**Neuromuscular:** ROM: Within normal limits throughout; Force generation: 5/5 throughout; DTRs: 2+ with downward plantar reflex, no frontal release signs; sensation and cranial nerve exams: normal

**Function:** Normal gait pattern; c/o discomfort and tenderness at right paraspinals in

when standing or walking for more than 30 minutes
**Cognition/Mental Status:** Mini Mental State Examination (MMSE) = 22/30; requires assistance to manage finances and to remember to change from pajamas to daytime clothing in the morning; denies hallucinations and alterations of mood

### Evaluation

The physical examination, imaging, and lab studies did not reveal any overt pathology to explain Robert's impaired cognitive status and difficulty with instrumental activities of daily living (IADL), which supports the diagnosis of early AD.
**Plan of Care:** Robert and his family were provided with information about AD and were referred to

a support group that can provide them with a network of support services and practical suggestions for living with AD. Because Robert also is showing signs of impaired IADL, his wife and son were offered some suggested behavioral changes for management of these and other issues that may arise. Robert was advised to discontinue his periodic use of Benadryl and to work to establish a sleep hygiene approach with his wife.

### Incorporating CAM into the Plan of Care

The PA was familiar with some of the studies conducted on GBE and believes that GBE may address Robert's desire to try an herbal supplement for his cognitive status. To verify the safety and efficacy of GBE, the PA invesigates the literature.

## INVESTIGATING THE LITERATURE

To become familiar with the application of GBE in persons similar to Robert and to verify the recommended dose and potential outcomes, the PA uses two strategies to investigate the scientific literature. The first is a detailed approach in which preliminary background reading is performed on the management of AD and GBE. This is followed by search of the databases and evaluation of the literature with use of reviews and primary sources for use of GBE with AD. The second is the use of the PICO format for a focused search to answer the clinical questions generated by the case.

AD is a complex, progressive neurological disorder with no known cure. Reliable and current information regarding assessment, diagnosis, progression, and treatment is critical to clinicians to be able to offer clients and their families the most current, comprehensive, and compassionate care available. Because of the complexity of management of persons with AD a review of the literature should include overview information on dementia, assessment, diagnosis, and interventions.

### Preliminary Reading: Overview of Dementia

Dementia is defined as a clinical syndrome involving a sustained loss of intellectual functions and memory that results in dysfunction in daily living.[1] Dementia falls into two broad categories: reversible and nonreversible. AD is a type of nonreversible dementia, yet it is especially important to rule out reversible dementia early to attain the best possible outcomes. Reversible dementia accounts for less than 20% of all causes of dementia. One particular disorder, depressive pseudodementia, is an example of a readily treatable reversible dementia. This alteration in cognitive function is more closely related to the underlying depression than to a true neurological impairment. It is a challenge to diagnose because one third of clients with dementia also have co-existing depression. Other examples of potentially reversible dementia include neoplasms; autoimmune disorders such as multiple sclerosis and disseminated lupus erythematosus; toxins such as those incurred with alcoholism; infections; trauma such as subdural hematoma; nutritional disorders such as vitamin B12 deficiency; and specific drugs or polypharmacy. Many categories of drugs may contribute to or cause dementia, including anticholinergics, digoxin, steroids, and drugs used in the treatment of Parkinson's disease, anxiety, ulcers, and cardiovascular disease.

Nonreversible dementias fall into four broad categories: degenerative diseases of the central nervous system, vascular disorders, trauma, and infections. AD, a neurodegenerative disease, accounts for about two thirds of dementia in the geriatric population.[1] It was first described by Alois Alzheimer, who reported on a 56-year-old female who presented with a rapidly progressive memory loss of 5 years' duration and delusions about being killed. At the time of her institutionalization she had great difficulty reading, writing, naming, and acquiring new information with the backdrop of a totally normal neurological exam. Upon autopsy her brain showed atrophy, and Bielschowsky silver staining revealed neuronal changes now called "neurofibrillary tangles," and "miliary foci" now known as *senile* or *neuritic plaque*. Alzheimer noted the presenile nature of the dementia, and his name lives on with his early diagnosis.[2]

AD is considered to be the most common dementia, with nearly 10% of the population older than age 65 being affected.[2] It is suggested that 7.1% of all deaths in 1995 were attributable to AD, which places it on par with cerebrovascular disease as the third leading cause of death. The prevalence of AD doubles every 5 years beyond age 65 and affects approximately 4.5 million Americans. By 2050, it is estimated that some 13.5 million Americans will have AD. Financial estimates put the annual national direct and indirect costs of caring for persons with AD at $100 billion.[3] Thus interventions that improve quality of life and minimize expense can play a significant role in the treatment of this disease.

Research has shown an increased risk of AD with first-degree relatives, and recently several genes have been directly linked. Chromosomes 1, 14, and 21 all carry a potentially linked gene.[2] Chromosome 19 codes for the gene for ApoE, a plasma protein better known for triglyceride and cholesterol transport. Those individuals who carry the ApoE E4 allele have an estimated risk of developing AD of 45% to 60%. This is a fruitful area of research, and future efforts will undoubtedly uncover other genetic links.[2]

### Assessment of Alzheimer's Disease

Physicians list five required areas in the initial assessment of AD[4]:

1. Instrumental activities of daily living (IADL)
2. Cognition, most commonly assessed using the Mini Mental State Examination (MMSE)
3. Co-morbid medical conditions
4. Disorders of mood and emotion
5. Caregiver status

Assessment of IADL determines the client's ability to perform the complex tasks necessary for independent function, such as the ability to use the telephone, travel alone, shop, cook, take medication, and manage money. Clients are scaled as fully independent, need assistance, or dependent in all areas.[4] As an example, Robert exhibits deficiencies in IADL because he requires assistance managing finances and remembering to change from his pajamas to daytime clothing in the morning. IADL assessment also revealed dependence in traveling secondary to his known history of getting lost while driving in familiar places.

The Mini Mental State Exam (MMSE[5]) scales an individual's neurocognitive function in areas such as orientation, immediate and delayed recall, attention, naming, following a command, reading, and writing. The results are 24 to 30 (maximum score is 30) as normal, 20 to 23 as mild, 10 to 19 as moderate, and 1 to 9 as severe. A score of 23 or less places an individual at likely risk of a neurocognitive deficit and is suggestive of AD, although additional testing and evaluation to discriminate the type of dementia are recommended.[4,5] Robert's score on the MMSE was 22 out of a maximum score of 30 as a result of lost points in the areas of orientation, immediate recall, naming, and attention.

The client in this case has minimal co-morbid medical conditions except for mild insomnia, which may be related to the AD, benign prostatic hypertrophy, and a lumbar muscle strain. Some concern exists regarding the use of Benadryl, an antihistamine, also classified as an anticholinergic, because it may worsen the symptoms of dementia. Geldmacher and Whitehouse[6] report that many commonly used drugs such as analgesics, anticholinergics, antihypertensives, psychotropics, and sedative-hypnotics can interfere with cognition, and so discontinuing this medication was indicated for Robert. Robert's risk of vascular dementia from stroke is very low because he has no history of hypertension or coronary artery disease and denies any mood alterations. These findings help to minimize the diagnosis of pseudodementia, in which clients are aware of a slowing of cognition but are often unaware of their own depressive symptoms.[6]

Robert is fortunate to have a healthy wife, secure financial status, and supportive family and friends. These areas of support will be called upon in many ways over the next few years. Specific scales exist to measure caregiver burden. AD ultimately has a more profound effect on the caregiver than the client. The client withdraws to another place in the past, while the caregiver often is rooted in the reality of the present. These scales measure the severity of caregiver stress associated with the common AD neuropsychiatric problems in addition to others such as sleep-wake cycle shifting. They may assist with caring for the caregiver as needed.[4] Hallucinations, often of the visual variety, occur in up to 25% of clients with AD, and delusions affect about 50%. Symptoms of depression and anxiety occur in up to 40% of cases and may be the presenting signs of the disease. These psychological disturbances can wreak havoc on the caregiver and cause burnout.[6]

### *Laboratory Studies*

Kawas[7] stresses the importance of the laboratory workup to ensure the absence of a reversible dementia in the newly diagnosed client. In addition to a careful history and physical and neurological exam, the client should have some type of brain imaging such as a non–contrast-enhanced computed tomographic (CT) scan or magnetic resonance imaging (MRI). Measurement of electrolytes and hepatic, thyroid, and renal functions in addition to vitamin B12 and folate levels is recommended. Testing for HIV and neurosyphilis (tertiary, irreversible form) is suggested based upon risk assessment. A lumbar puncture should be performed in clients with a history or signs of cancer or infection. Some physicians[8] recommend a urinalysis and complete blood count. Abnormalities found through imaging and/or laboratory screening require further testing and assessment relative to the risk of reversible dementia. Indiscriminate testing has a low yield and large economic burden. In this case, Robert's CT and laboratory tests were normal and a neurosyphilis test was negative.

### *Diagnosis*

The definitive reference for classifying mental illness, including dementia, is the *Diagnostic and Statistical Manual of Mental Disorders*.[9] Based upon Robert's history, physical and cognitive testing, and laboratory/imaging assessments, the diagnosis of

dementia of the Alzheimer's type appears to be appropriate. He fits more closely to the mild stage in terms of his AD symptoms and is a candidate for behavioral and pharmacological intervention.[8]

### *Overview of Interventions*

AD is a far-reaching disorder without a cure. Many clients survive up to 10 years, often with a slow and steady decline in cognition and function. These changes must be addressed initially and on an ongoing basis. Providing such care is emotionally, financially, and physically stressful.

### Behavioral Therapeutics

Major areas of concern include making changes and providing a framework for the caregiver to have control over such potentially dangerous events as wandering and hazardous driving of a vehicle. Assessment of this function has not been well clarified, especially in early dementia.[1] Clients who wander should be registered in the Alzheimer's Association Safe Return Program and may require locked doors and gates.[10] Other areas that benefit from a behavioral or combined behavioral and pharmacological approach include incontinence, day-night reversal, and general agitation.

Family therapy is recommended to deal with feelings of anger, guilt, and such unavoidable issues as durable power of attorney, handling of assets, and the possible need for the hiring of a health aid or being institutionalized for care. End-of-life decisions should be discussed as early as possible in the diagnosis of AD, while the client can still participate. It is difficult for the family to realize the imperative and reality of end-of-life care until their family member no longer recognizes them. Family members should be encouraged to seek respite periodically and may benefit from AD support groups.[1]

### Standard Medication Options

Cummings et al[10] report that the cholinesterase inhibitors have been shown to provide a modest improvement in symptoms, temporary stabilization of cognition, or reduction in the rate of cognitive decline in some clients with mild to moderate AD. These agents work by raising acetylcholine levels in the brain by inhibiting the acetylcholinesterase enzyme, which normally degrades acetylcholine. Studies show that as many as one third of clients exhibit a seven-point improvement on neuropsychological tests. This is equated to a 5% to 15% benefit over placebo. The translation of these results to the family requires discussion to avoid any misinterpretation or false hopes of remission in the classic sense because these agents do not halt the progression of the disease.

Currently four drugs are in this class: donepezil (Aricept), rivastigmine (Exelon), galantamine (Razodyne, previously marketed as Reminyl), and tacrine (Cognex). No true head-to-head studies have been performed to compare these agents. Selection depends upon side effect profiles and administration regimens. Principles of geriatric psychopharmacology suggest starting at low dosages and slow titration with careful monitoring for side effects and outcome.[10]

Donepezil (Aricept), a daily dosed medication, has demonstrated clinically meaningful improvements in cognitive and global function with an efficacy of up to 4.9 years. Rivastigmine (Exelon), dosed twice daily, has been shown to be effective in temporarily slowing cognitive decline, improving function, and reducing behavioral and psychopathology in mild to moderate AD. However, the side effect profile may make the more efficacious higher doses difficult to implement. Galantamine (Razodyne) also is dosed twice daily and has similar effects and the same concern of side effects with higher doses. Tacrine (Cognex) although still available, is no longer marketed by the manufacturer, and is considered a second line agent because of its potential for elevation in liver enzymes in 40% of treated clients. Tacrine (Cognex) is also dosed four times per day and frequent liver enzyme assessment is required. The cholinesterase class of medication should be discontinued if adherence is poor, if untoward side effects occur, or if deterioration of function remains at the pretreatment rate after a 6-month to 12-month trial. In these cases, clients may benefit from a trial with another drug in this class.[10] Further, nonsteroidal antiinflammatory drugs (NSAIDS) should be used with caution due to the potential for increased stomach ulcer risk when combined with the acetylcholinesterase class of medications. Namenda (memantine HCl) is a new class of medication used in the treatment of the symptoms of moderate to severe Alzheimer's disease. Unlike the other agents, this medication targets another chemical associated with memory and learning called glutamate. Due to its different mode of action, it may be added to the acetylcholinesterase class of medications. Dosing, with or without food, must be carefully titrated, and it is contraindicated in severe kidney disease. Namenda has not been tested in those with seizure disorder. Its side effects include confusion, constipation, coughing, dizziness, hallucinations, headache, high blood pressure, pain, sleepiness, and vomiting.

## Preliminary Reading: Overview of Ginkgo Biloba

Ginkgo biloba (GB), also known as duck foot tree (based upon the leaf shape), maidenhair tree, and silver apricot, has been popular in Europe and more recently the United States for its suspected neuroprotective properties. GB comes from the ginkgo tree, the world's most ancient tree, thought to originate 200 million years ago. A standard preparation of GB is 24% ginkgo flavonol glycosides and 6% terpene lactones, which is referred to as ginkgo biloba extract (GBE) or EGb761. (See Figures 11-1 and 11-2.)

Information about how to obtain and use GBE can be found in a wide range of sources including the Internet, published textbooks, articles, and advertisements by companies that produce and distribute herbal therapies, in addition to practitioners of herbal therapies. Information found on the Internet can be obtained through reliable sources such as the National Institute of Health and peer-reviewed newsletters in addition to less-than-reliable advertisers masquerading as legitimate research bodies. Caution is recommended with use of popular Internet search engines because their criteria for rank-ordering their search list are based upon the number of times the website has been

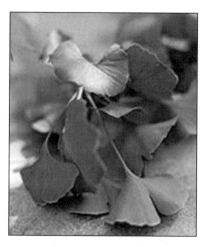

**Figure 11-1** Ginkgo biloba leaves. (From Life Extension Foundation.)

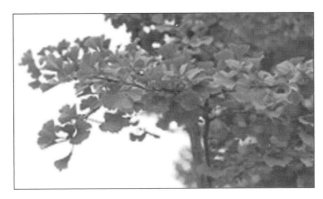

**Figure 11-2** Ginkgo biloba tree. (From Alive Publishing Group, Inc.)

accessed during a prescribed period of time. This means that an interesting, graphically well-designed, and easy-to-navigate website may be listed at the top of the search results regardless of the accuracy of the information it provides. Search engines routinely sell advertising space to provide search services to the consumer for no cost. They do not endorse their advertisers; they merely offer them a service.

An underused resource for information on herbs and other botanicals is the network of home economists and extension services known as the Cooperative State Research, Education, and Extension Service (CSREES). This agency, created by Congress in 1994, is within the U.S. Department of Agriculture and can be accessed online at http://www.csrees.usda.gov.

Another source of information about GBE and many other herbal therapies can be found in The Complete German Commission E Series Monographs: Therapeutic Guide to Herbal Medicines (see Chapter 10).[11] The Commission E Monographs have a long history that began in Germany, with the Imperial Decree of 1901, which permitted the trade of many botanical drugs outside pharmacies. These monographs may be purchased in full or as a condensed version and are available on CD-ROM. Two monographs exist for GBE. One is a negative or unapproved monograph of various ginkgo preparations that did not conform to standardized preparations. These preparations included crude ginkgo leaf and extracts made with ethanol or methanol. The positive or approved monograph included standardized ginkgo extracts made with acetone and water, which clinical studies determined to have positive benefits.[12]

The condensed Commission E Series,[12] a compendium of herbal medicine, approves the internal use of GBE for the symptomatic treatment of disturbed performance in organic brain syndrome in such cases as dementia, including primary dementia and other types such as vascular and mixed forms. It is recommended in the treatment of memory deficits and disturbances in concentration. The Commission E notes GBE's benefits in other areas related to improved blood flow in the brain and retina, microcirculation, antagonism of platelet-activating factor, and inactivation of toxic oxygen radicals.[12]

## Searching the Databases and Evaluating the Literature

The PA reviews current information about the diagnosis of AD and common interventions for AD to be sure that her plan of care is appropriate for Robert. She also reads about the general safety and proposed uses of GBE and proceeds in a search of the scientific literature to find more specific evidence that may support or refute the use of GBE in persons with AD. The results of the literature search are summarized in Table 11-1.

### Reviews

From the Evidence-Based Medicine (EBM) databases a couple of relevant reviews were identified. Ernst and Pittler[13] reviewed nine studies in which GBE preparations were tested for symptomatic treatment of AD and multi-infarct dementia. All the studies used double-blind, randomized, placebo-controlled designs with dosages of GBE equal to 120 mg or 140 mg. The studies ranged in

**Table 11-1    Literature Search Results**

| | GINKGO BILOBA | COGNITION | GINKGO AND COGNITION | ALZHEIMER'S DISEASE | ALZHEIMER'S DISEASE AND GINGKO BILOBA |
|---|---|---|---|---|---|
| MEDLINE (1966-April 2005) | 711 | 52,186 | 56 | 42,332 | 68 |
| CINAHL (1982-April 2005) | 293 | 6959 | 42 | 5181 | 43 |
| PsycINFO (1806-April 2005) | 155 | 25,635 | 13 | 16,315 | 27 |
| CAM on PubMed (April 2005) | 827 | 70,105 | 76 | 32,675 | 89 |
| All EBM Reviews (April 2005) | 315 | 4384 | 41 | 1851 | 17 |

duration from 4 to 52 weeks. The results from eight of nine studies demonstrated an improvement in dementia symptoms in the GBE groups compared with the placebo group. Of the four studies that reported adverse events, three reported no adverse effect for the GBE groups compared with the placebo groups, whereas one study reported the occurrence of a suspected acute stroke.

Birks and Grimley-Evans'[14] systematic and critical literature review was conducted to assess the efficacy and safety of GBE for the treatment of clients with dementia or cognitive decline. They critically assessed 33 randomized, double-blind studies, which ranged in duration from 3 to 52 weeks with dosages ranging from 80 to 600 mg/day for inclusion criteria and number of subjects, methods, outcome measures, and statistical analysis. The authors reported that subgroup analysis on a specific category such as AD was difficult to conduct because precise diagnoses were not always available. In addition, small sample sizes and unsatisfactory methods plagued some of the earlier studies included in the review. The meta-analysis, however, provided some promising evidence of improvement in cognition and function associated with GBE use as compared with placebo, with no significant adverse events.

Literature reviews that included randomized, controlled, double-blind studies with subjects who specifically had a diagnosis of AD also were obtained through MEDLINE and PsycInfo.[15,16] Analysis revealed that 3 to 6 months of therapy with 120 to 240 mg of GBE per day had a small but significant positive effect on cognitive function in subjects' AD. Improvement in daily functioning and ADL was less clear because of differences in the functional outcome used by the studies.

Although published literature reviews[13-16] suggest that GBE may be helpful to improve cognitive function in persons with AD and other forms of demen-

tia, obtaining and reading primary sources may inform decisions to be made about Robert's use of GBE.

### Primary Sources

Two experimental studies[17,18] included in the review by Oken, Storzback, and Kaye[15] were conducted with more than 200 subjects, including men with AD. In one study[17] the experimental group received 120 mg of GBE per day. The experimental group in the other study received 240 mg/day.[18] Both groups demonstrated modest differences in stabilization and improvement of cognitive function when compared with a placebo. Le Bars et al[17] also reported improvement in daily living and social behaviors in persons who received GBE. Adverse events were not statistically different from placebo in either study.[17,18] A considerably smaller clinical trial conducted by Maurer et al[19] also demonstrated that persons with mild to moderate AD had significant improvement of attention and memory after 3 months of daily GBE.

In contrast, a large, multicenter clinical trial conducted by van Dongen et al[20] found that subjects with AD, vascular dementia, or age-associated memory impairment (AAMI) who received 160 mg or 240 mg of GBE per day for 24 weeks did not demonstrate statistically significant improvement on psychometric tests when compared with placebo. The authors have suggested that recruitment of subjects from 39 nursing homes may have caused an overrepresentation of the very old (mean age = 84 years) and a high level of co-morbidities, which may help to explain why their outcomes regarding GBE and cognitive functioning were inconsistent with previous findings. Table 11-2 provides a summary of the investigations into the use of GBE with dementia.

Although a literature search for experimental studies regarding the use of GBE in persons with

Derby Hospitals NHS Foundation
Trust
Library and Knowledge Service

AD renders many relevant citations, a closer look at the primary sources reveals that several researchers have published more than one report per clinical trial by retrospective analysis of the data obtained from their original GBE trial. Intent-to-treat, subject classification based on the condition severity, and duration of treatment have been addressed and analyzed, yet no remarkable differences in outcomes have been observed.[18,20-24] All the studies presented in Table 11-2 include adverse effect information and conclude that the use of GBE had few, if any, negative side effects. Nevertheless, concern for adverse events and drug interactions is present whether an agent is derived from a plant or chemically purified in a laboratory. Maidment[16] reported that although GBE is generally well tolerated as studies demonstrate, a small number of case reports exist of hemorrhage or prolonged bleeding, with an association of GBE potentiating the anti-coagulant effect of aspirin and warfarin. Physicians frequently suggest that it be avoided in clients with clotting disorders, those taking anticoagulation medications, or those awaiting surgery.

The available scientific literature on the use of GBE in persons with AD and other forms of dementias includes randomized, double-blind, placebo-controlled studies; review articles; and a meta-analysis. The reported outcomes of these studies suggest that persons with dementia who took GBE demonstrated improvement in cognitive functioning when compared with persons who received a placebo. According to one review,[15] the effect size was comparable with the cognitive improvement observed in clients with AD who received donepezil.[25] Limitations in study comparison have included inconsistent classification of subjects according to their dementia or level of cognitive functioning and the mixed use of non-standardized and standardized primary outcome measures. Dosage of GBE was also variable, although most researchers used ginkgo extract Egb761 that contained 22% to 27% flavone glycoside and 5% to 7% terpene lactones[16] and was administered at either 240 mg[18] or 120 mg[17] per day with similar outcomes. Schulz[26] reports that treatments with the acetylcholinesterase inhibitors cost five times the amount of GBE and are associated with 10 times more common adverse drug reactions, which furthers the likelihood that the public will use nonprescription agents to promote cognitive functioning. Although issues such as proper

dosing and GBE's potential for anticoagulant effects need to be investigated, clients such as Robert may benefit from including GBE in their plan of care.

A more focused search of the literature using the PICO strategy reveals three relevant clinical trials.[14,17,22] However, two articles[20,21] considered during the PA's clinical decision-making process were not obtained through the PICO approach of searching the literature. The therapist may not always have time to do such an extensive search. Instead she may use a targeted PICO approach.

## PICO BOX

For clients with Alzheimer's disease, does ginkgo biloba improve cognitive function and activities of daily living?

P: People with Alzheimer's disease
I: Ginkgo biloba
C: No comparison
O: Cognitive function
O: Activities of daily living

A MEDLINE search combining all the terms was performed on October 23, 2006 and yielded three references,[14,17,22] all of which are relevant for this case. This targeted search did not, however, identify the studies by Van Dongen et al,[20,21] which informed the clinician's clinical decision-making process.

P = **Population** (patient/client, problem, person condition or group attribute)
I = **Intervention** (the CAM therapy or approach)
C = **Comparison** (standard care or comparison intervention)
O = **Outcomes** (the measured variables of interest)

## CLINICAL DECISION MAKING

The reported studies included men of Robert's age group and demonstrated the possibility of either modest or no improvement without any degradation of cognition. Potential adverse events exist yet seem small in light of Robert's general good health, absence of chronic disease, or daily medication usage. He has no known coagulopathy and uses no platelet-related medications. The family's dislike of conventional medications and the results of the available research on GBE,[15] which demonstrate potentially similar outcomes as those observed with donepezil (Aricept),[25] lead the PA to suggest that

**Table 11-2  Ginkgo Biloba and Alzheimer's Disease Research**

| SOURCE | SUBJECTS | DESIGN | INTERVENTIONS | OUTCOME MEASURES | RESULTS/CONCLUSIONS |
|---|---|---|---|---|---|
| Van Dongen et al[20] | n=214 AD, VD, or AAMI | Multicenter RCT | 5 groups: • 240 mg EGb: 24 weeks • 160 mg EGb: 24 weeks • Placebo: 24 weeks • 240 mg EGb: 12 weeks • Placebo: 12 weeks • 16 mg EGb: 12 weeks • Placebo: 12 weeks | CGI SKT NAI-NAA | No statistically significant benefit of EGb over placebo, regardless of dose, in persons with AD, VD, AAMI |
| Kanowski et al[18] | n=216 Mild to moderate AD or MID | Multicenter RCT | 2 groups: • 240 mg EGb: 24 weeks • Placebo: 24 weeks | CGI SKT NAB | Statistically significant benefits of EGb over placebo in psychopathology (GCI) and attention and memory (SKT) in persons with mild to moderate AD or MID. Performance on NAB not significantly different. |
| LeBars et al[17] | n=202 Mild to severe AD or MID | Multicenter RCT | 2 groups: 120 mg EGb: 52 weeks Placebo: 52 weeks | CGI ADAS GERRI | Statistically significant benefits of EGb over placebo in cognitive functioning (ADAS-cog) and caregiver ratings of cognitive, social, and emotional behaviors (GERRI) in persons with mild to moderate AD or MID. |
| Maurer et al[19] | n=20 Mild to moderate AD | RCT | 2 groups: 240 mg EGb: 12 weeks Placebo: 12 weeks | SKT ADAS CGI ZVT | Statistically significant benefits of EGb over placebo in attention and memory (SKT) in persons with mild to moderate AD. No statistically significant improvement in psychometric tests (ZVT and ADAS), but not significant |

AD, Alzheimer's disease; VD: Vascular dementia; AAMI: Age-associated memory impairment
MID: Multi-infarct dementia
EGb: Gingko biloba
CGI: Clinical Global Impression of Change
SKT: Syndrom-Kurz Test
NAB: Nernberger Alters Beobachtungsskala
ADAS: Alzheimer's Disease Assessment Scale
ADAS-Cog: Alzheimer's Disease Assessment Scale-Cognitive Subscale
NAI-NAA: Nurnberger Alters Inventar-Instrumental Activities of Daily Living
GERRI: Geriatric Evaluation by Relative's Rating Instrument
ZVT: Zahlen-Verbingdungs Test

GBE may be helpful in addressing Robert's cognitive decline.

## Generate a Clinical Hypothesis

The PA hypothesizes that the rate of cognitive decline will slow, and Robert will maintain a more stable lifestyle, which will give his family time to reconcile the diagnosis and include Robert in key decisions about his quality of life and potential end of life. The PA is uncertain if the use of GBE will affect Robert's sleep, BPH, or muscle strain but hypothesizes that if Robert's decline in cognitive status slows or improves, his ability to follow through with instructions from his family and physical therapist will remain intact.

## Intervene and Evaluate

The PA explained the state of literature to Robert and his family and described the potential risks, benefits, and cost of GBE. Since medication options are rather slim, and GBE offers some potential benefits with minimal risk, Robert and his family agreed to initiate GBE and carefully monitor Robert's condition. The PA recommended to start therapy conservatively with the lower dose used in the available studies of GBE 120 mg/day. The PA then assisted with the selection of the GBE product to be sure that it met the established standards for the active ingredient and for purity. Increasing the dose of GBE to 240 mg/day would be an option if either no response or a small improvement occurs. Robert's tolerance and potential side effect profile must be considered because the limited number of studies did not demonstrate a remarkable dose effect response. This decision would require careful consideration. The use of standardized tools such as the MMEE,[5] Alzheimer's Disease Assessment Scale (ADAS),[27] and Geriatric Evaluation by Relative's Rating Instrument (GERRI)[28] to assess changes in Robert's cognition and functional status will be helpful to provide some objective data for determining the effects of GBE. Discontinuation of the GBE would be encouraged if no improvement occurs in 6 months or if cognition worsens at any time.

Robert should receive quarterly follow-up with his primary care provider with attention to routine medical care, accepted laboratory measurement, and prevention of chronic medical conditions.

## Report the Outcomes

Regardless of the client's outcome, the PA may want to present her experience to peers in the medical community by writing a case report to describe the intervention and the cognitive, psychological, and medical outcomes that Robert experienced. Collaboration with Robert's physical therapist for information regarding his outcomes in physical therapy also may contribute to objective measures of physical impairments and functional limitations. In addition, the PA could reflect on the caregiver's potential stress reduction, knowing that the family offered an intervention that may have extended the quality of life for this family member. These positive memories may offer some solace when the ravages of AD are at their most severe.

## SUMMARY

Eisenberg and colleagues[29] reported on perceptions of adults who use complementary therapies and conventional therapies. Overall prevalence of use of complementary therapies increased significantly between 1990 and 1997 in the United States with estimated expenditures totaling $21 billion. In this chapter Robert and his family wanted to participate in the management of his condition by using GBE to address some of his symptoms of AD. The PA, in keeping with the principles of evidence-based practice, sought to support the use GBE and searched the scientific literature to learn about the potential risks and benefits for the client. The available literature is limited and the outcomes are mixed, yet the practitioner established a plan of care that respects the client's desires by including a trial of GBE. By maintaining an open, supportive relationship with the client, the PA would be able to monitor the client's status and make adjustments to treatment when medically necessary. Clinicians must pay attention to available medical research, be aware of potentially adverse consequences of using prescription medications and nonprescription medications or herbs, and encourage clients to discuss their personal treatment ideas and plans.

## REFERENCES

1. Kane RL, Ouslander JG, Abrass IB: Delirium and dementia. In *Essentials of clinical geriatrics,* ed 5, Columbus, Ohio, 2004, McGraw-Hill.
2. Cummings JL, Mendez MF: Alzheimer's disease and other disorders of dementia. In Goldman L, Auisello

D, editors: *Cecil textbook of medicine,* ed 22, Philadelphia, 2004, WB Saunders, pp 2253-5.

3. UAB Health System, Physician On-Line Resource Center: Predictors of Longevity in Alzheimer's Disease. Available at: *http://www.health.uab.edu/4docs/show.asp?durki=66673.* Accessed June 7, 2004.

4. Cummings JL et al: Guidelines for managing Alzheimer's disease: Part I Assessment, *Am Fam Physician* 65:2263-72, 2002.

5. Folstein MF, Folstein SE, McHugh PR: Mini-mental state: a practical method for grading the cognitive state of patients for the clinician, *J Psychiatr Res* 12:189-98, 1975.

6. Geldmacher DS, Whitehouse PJ: Evaluation of dementia, *N Engl J Med* 335:330-6, 1996.

7. Kawas CH: Early Alzheimer's disease, *N Engl J Med* 329:1056-63, 2003.

8. Buckles VD, Coats M, Morris JC: Dementia. Best Practices of Medicine, November 1, 2000. Available at: *http://merck.praxis.md/index.asp?page=bpm_brief&article_id=bpm01NE09.* Accessed June 3, 2004.

9. American Psychiatric Association: *Diagnostic and statistical manual of mental disorders,* ed 4, Washington, DC, 1994, The Association.

10. Cummings JL et al: Guidelines for managing Alzheimers disease: Part II Treatment, *Am Fam Physician* 65:2525-34, 2002.

11. Blumenthal M et al, editors: *The complete German Commission E series monographs: therapeutic guide to herbal medicines,* Austin, TX, 1998, American Botanical Council.

12. Blumenthal M, Goldberg A, Brinckmann J: Gingko bilobal leaf extract. In Blumenthal M, Goldberg A, Brinckmann J, editors: *Herbal medicine: expanded Commission E monographs,* Newton, Mass, 2000, Integrative Medicine Communications, pp 160-9.

13. Ernst E, Pittler MH: Ginkgo biloba for dementia: a systematic review of double-blind, placebo-blind, placebo-controlled trials, *Clin Drug Invest* 17:301-8, 1999.

14. Birks J, Grimley Evans J: Ginkgo biloba for cognitive impairment and dementia, *The Cochrane Database of Systematic Reviews,* 2005, The Cochrane Library.

15. Oken BS, Storzbach DM, Kaye JA: The efficacy of ginkgo biloba on cognitive function in Alzheimer disease, *Arch Neurol* 55:1409-15, 1998.

16. Maidment I: The use of Ginkgo biloba in the treatment of dementia, *Psychiatr Bull* 25:353-6, 2001.

17. Le Bars PL et al: A placebo-controlled, double-blind, randomized trial of an extract of Ginkgo biloba for dementia. North American EGb study group, *JAMA* 278:1327-32, 1997.

18. Kanowski S et al: Proof of efficacy of the ginkgo biloba special extract Egb 761 in outpatients suffering from mild to moderate primary degenerative dementia of the Alzheimer type of multiinfarct dementia, *Pharmacopsychiatry* 29(2)47-56, 1996.

19. Maurer K, Ihl R, Dierks T, Forlich L: Clinical efficacy of ginkgo biloba special extract EGb761 in dementia of the Alzheimer type, *J Psychiatr Res* 31:645-55, 1997.

20. van Dongen M et al: Gingko for elderly people with dementia and age-associated memory impairment: a randomized clinical trial, *J Clin Epidemiol* 56:367-76, 2003.

21. van Dongen M et al: The efficacy of gingko for elderly people with dementia and age-associated memory impairment: new results of a randomized clinical trial, *JAGS* 48(10):1183-94, 2000.

22. Kanowski S, Hoerr R: Gingko biloba extract EGb 761 in dementia: intent-to-treat analyses of a 24-week, multi-center, double-blind, placebo-controlled, randomized trial, *Pharmacopsychiatry* 36(6):297-303, 2003.

23. LeBars PL et al: Influence of the severity of cognitive impairment on the effect of the ginkgo biloba extract EGb761 in Alzheimer's disease, *Neuropsychobiology* 45:19-26, 2002.

24. LeBars PL: Response patterns of EGb761 in Alzheimer's disease: influence of neuropsychological profiles, *Pharmacopsychiatry* (Suppl 1):S50-S55, 2003.

25. Rogers SL et al: A 24-week double-blind placebo-controlled trial of donepezil in patients with Alzheimer's disease, *Neurology* 50:136-45, 1998.

26. Schulz V: Ginkgo extract or cholinesterase inhibitors in patients with dementia: what clinical trials and guidelines fail to consider, *Phytomedicine* 10(suppl): 74S-79S, 2003.

27. Rosen WG, Mohs RC, Davis KL: A new rating scale for Alzheimer's disease, *Am J Psychiatry* 141:1356-64, 1984.

28. Schwartz GE: Development and validation of the geriatric evaluation by relative's rating instrument (GERRI), *Psychol Rep* 53:479-88, 1983.

29. Eisenberg DM et al: Perceptions about complementary therapies relative to conventional therapies among adults who use both: results from a national survey, *Ann Intern Med* 135:344-51, 2001.

## ADDITIONAL RESOURCES

### Alzheimer's Disease

Administration on Aging

National Association of Area Agencies on Aging

Alzheimer's Association

Family Caregiver Alliance

Alzheimer's Disease Education and Referral Center

**Ginkgo Biloba**
American Botanical Council
American Herbal Pharmacopeia
Cooperative State Research, Education, and Extension
    Service (CSREES)

National Library of Medicine's Medline search system
NIH National Center for Complementary and
    Alternative Medicine

# CHAPTER 12

## Glucosamine Chondroitin

*Diane Rigassio Radler*

CASE

John is a 71-year-old man in good health. He was educated as a mechanical engineer and worked in industry until retirement 6 years ago. He is married and lives with his wife in an adult community. The couple has three adult children, two who live within 50 miles of them. John tries to remain fairly active and enjoys fishing from his boat and walking to the community center. Lately, walking and boarding his boat have become challenging because of his osteoarthritis pain.

### Initial Examination

John is in excellent health for his age. He currently has mildly elevated prostate specific antigen (PSA), which is monitored every 6 months, and hypertension, which is controlled with captopril and hydrochlorothiazide. He has a history of diverticulitis, which has required hospitalization three times in the past 8 years. He was taking rofecoxib for his osteoarthritis pain and was switched to naproxen when rofecoxib was removed from market use. He is concerned about adverse events of gastrointestinal (GI) bleeding and seeks an alternative.

**Client Report:** John's bilateral knee osteoarthritis limits his daily activities and is increasingly limiting his favorite recreation activities of boating, fishing, and walking to the recreation center in the community. He states that when he is sitting and watching television or socializing with friends, his knees really do not bother him. However, when he bears weight, the pain in his knees increases to a moderate level. Extensive walking (more than one-half mile) or climbing stairs causes significant pain.

**Client Goals:** To reduce the pain in his knees so that he can continue to enjoy fishing from his boat and walking to the recreation center

**Employment:** John is a retired engineer. His wife is also retired.

**General Health:** Good

**Medications:** Captopril, hydrochlorothiazide, naproxen

**Anthropometrics:** Height: 6 feet, 0 inches; weight: 192 lbs; body mass index: 26; no recent weight change

**Laboratory:** Normal except for PSA 6 mg/ml

**Radiographs:** Narrowing of joint space and osteophyte formation

**Integumentary:** Mild swelling bilaterally

**Cardiopulmonary:** BP 143/80, HR 72

**Neuromusculoskeletal ROM:** Limited into extension by 5/5 degrees bilaterally, pain upon palpation and crepitus. Decreased quadriceps and hip extensor strength 4/5 bilaterally

**Function:** Limited by pain rating of 2/10 at rest, increasing to 6/10 with elevations and ambulation

### ■ Incorporating CAM into the Plan of Care

John is not satisfied with the relief he has received using naproxen and is wary of the possible adverse event of GI bleeding. He would like to be able to do his daily activities without limitation and with reduced pain. According to John's BMI, he may be classified into the "overweight" category (BMI of 26 to 29). For John to be at the desirable BMI of 25, he would need to weigh 184 pounds, which would require a weight loss of 8 pounds. Although weight loss is advocated in people with arthritis who are overweight, John is at his usual weight with significant pain that may not be considerably affected by a 4% weight loss. Adding the dietary supplement containing glucosamine and chondroitin will be explored.

Information about herbals and supplements is prevalent in the popular press. Clients often ask their physical therapist for information about use of such supplements. Physical therapists in collaboration and consultation with other health care providers such as physicians and dietitians can serve as a resource for client education. In this chapter a physical therapist and a dietitian interact to educate a man with osteoarthritis (OA) of the knee, whose medication for pain secondary to arthritis, Vioxx, was withdrawn from the market. He wants to learn more about how the dietary supplement containing glucosamine and chondroitin may be used to alleviate his arthritis pain. He is interested in combining the dietary supplement with the appropriate exercise to improve his mobility.

## INVESTIGATING THE LITERATURE

### Preliminary Reading

Once the therapist is comfortable with understanding the patient's diagnosis and the current management of OA, he does some preliminary reading on glucosamine and chondroitin to obtain some background information before investigating the literature. The background information will help the therapist develop a strategy for the literature review.

Glucosamine and chondroitin are over-the-counter products and are considered dietary supplements. A logical place to begin is an online database with an unbiased perspective on dietary supplements. Two helpful resources are the Natural Medicines Comprehensive Database, an evidence-based resource particular to dietary supplements used by clinicians of conventional and complementary medicine, and the PDR*health* site by Thomson Healthcare (see Additional Resources) that includes a database of nutritional supplements. Because glucosamine and chondroitin are used by people with OA, another resource for background information is the Arthritis Foundation (see Additional Resources). These resources may be accessed for overview information summarizing original research. A more comprehensive literature review may follow the preliminary reading.

Glucosamine, as the name implies, is an amino glucose. It is a component of cartilage proteoglycans and essential for the synthesis of glycoproteins, glycolipids, and glycosaminoglycans in the human body.[1] Supplements of glucosamine are derived from exoskeletons of marine life or are manufactured synthetically. Glucosamine sulfate is the form most widely available and used in clinical trials.

Glucosamine is thought to stimulate the metabolism of chondrocytes of articular cartilage and the synovial cells of synovial tissue and is purported to rebuild damaged cartilage and promote antiinflammatory and analgesic activity.[1,2] By these actions, glucosamine may help provide relief of symptoms and slow the progression of OA.

Chondroitin, as chondroitin sulfate, is classified as a glucosaminoglycan, which is composed of glucuronic acid and galactosamine.[1] Supplements of chondroitin are derived from shark or bovine cartilage.[3] Chondroitin plays a role in the formation of joint matrix structures in mammals and may protect cartilage degradation in OA.[1,3]

Glucosamine and chondroitin are naturally occurring substances and fall under the category of dietary supplements. Hence, preliminary reading also should include background knowledge on the regulation of dietary supplements in the United States. The popularity of dietary supplements in the last decade has been the result of several factors, including the plethora of supplements available on the market in stores and through Internet sales.

The abundance of supplement manufacturers and the relative ease of getting a product to market are the result of the passage of the Dietary Supplement Health and Education Act of 1994 (DSHEA, pronounced "De-shay"). DSHEA was an amendment to the Food, Drug, and Cosmetic Act, which made dietary supplements and dietary supplement ingredients exempt from the regulations that apply to food and drugs.[4] The DSHEA stipulated that the dietary supplement must include a disclaimer statement on the product label that the product has not been evaluated by the Food and Drug Administration (FDA); however, it conveys no judgment from an authoritative source that the product is effective or safe. At times the allowable "structure-function" claims on dietary supplements are confusing to consumers in that no regulation exists regarding the claims to health and wellness.

In practice, if a person wishes to use dietary supplements, the best choice is to buy from a reputable manufacturer and look for voluntary analyses by independent agencies. If a product undergoes and passes quality standards by an independent agency, the product can bear the seal of approval. A sample of four popular agencies and their corresponding seals are depicted in Table 12-1.

## Searching the Databases

After becoming familiar with the dietary supplements, the therapist reviews the available data for efficacy and safety of glucosamine and chondroitin. His search strategy begins with the health-related literature using MEDLINE, CINAHL, PsycINFO, and CAM on PubMed. As a busy clinician he chooses to evaluate efficacy and safety, targeting evidence-based reviews and meta-analyses. He searches evidence-based reviews on the Cochrane Central Register of Controlled trials, Cochrane Database of Systematic Reviews, Database of Abstracts of Reviews of Effects, and InfoPOEMs-InfoRetriever.

The initial search strategy for finding research on the use of glucosamine and chondroitin for OA is conducted on MEDLINE. A general search is done initially using the term *osteoarthritis* and including all the subcategories. Likewise, the terms *glucosamine* and then *chondroitin* are searched. Because this evaluation is to include the use of *glucosamine* and *chondroitin*, the terms are combined. Finally the terms *glucosamine and chondroitin* were combined with *osteoarthritis*. This search strategy is

| Table 12-1 | Sample of Independent Agencies Assessing the Quality of Dietary Supplements | |
| --- | --- | --- |
| AGENCY | URL | QUALITY SEAL |
| ConsumerLab | http://www.consumerlab.com | Be Sure It's CL Approved |
| NSF International | http://www.nsf.org | Contents Tested & Certified www.nsf.org |
| Shuster Labs | http://www.shusterlabs.com | Technically Advanced Quality Assurance (TAQA) program |
| US Pharmacopia | http://www.usp.org | |

repeated in CINAHL, PsycINFO, CAM on PubMed, and all evidence-based reviews. Search results then may be further refined to return articles only with human participants and in the English language. As desired the search also can be limited to review articles, those available with full text online, or most recent publication dates. For purposes of this search, articles are limited to evidence-based reviews. See results of the search in Table 12-2.

Depending on the time available for research, clinicians may be satisfied with the levels of evidence and clinical practice guidelines researched and summarized by an evidence-based review tool such as those provided by InfoPOEMs-InfoRetriever. Clinicians using electronic handheld devices should be aware that evidence-based databases such as InfoRetriever are available for personal digital assistants (PDAs). Downloads may be available on a free trial basis followed by subscription for continuous current updates.

## Evaluating the Literature

Given that the intent of this search is to find the strongest evidence for using or not using glucosamine and chondroitin for the management of OA, an evidence-based approach is the most logical. The literature search was limited to full text and clinical trial or meta-analysis. Three pertinent reviews were retrieved: two on glucosamine and chondroitin and one on just glucosamine for OA.

In 2000 McAlindon et al published a meta-analysis and systematic quality assessment of clinical research of glucosamine and chondroitin for symptoms of OA of the knee or hip.[5] For a clinical trial to meet their review, the intervention must have been blinded, include a placebo group, and have a duration of at least 4 weeks. Fifteen clinical trials

met the stipulations for inclusion from which the reviewers concluded that glucosamine and chondroitin had a moderate to large treatment effect on symptoms of OA. However, the reviewers warned that the actual efficacy may be more modest because of the variability in methodology of some studies, that is, the outcome could be pain or function, and the measurement tool could be the visual analog scale, Western Ontario McMaster University Osteoarthritis Index (WOMAC), (described later in the chapter)[6] or Lequesne Index. (a radiographic measure to evaluate the joint space).[7] In addition, the effect size was smaller if measured at 4 weeks of treatment, which suggests that the greatest therapeutic benefit may be realized after 1 month of supplementation with glucosamine and chondroitin. Nevertheless, the authors conclude that some benefit without reported adverse events may exist.

Richy et al[8] in 2003 published a meta-analysis to assess the effect of glucosamine and chondroitin in OA of the knee. The researchers conducted individual meta-analyses on the effects of the dietary supplements on pain and physical functioning as measured by the WOMAC Index,[6] joint space narrowing measured with the Lequesne Index,[7] and visual analog scales for pain, mobility, safety, and response to treatment. The selection criteria stipulated that the clinical trials must have been designed as randomized and blinded, with a placebo group; the assessment was specific to the knee or hip; and the treatment period was 4 weeks or more. The initial set of clinical trials was 36; 15 met the inclusion criteria. The authors concluded that orally administered glucosamine was effective after several weeks of treatment for all outcomes; chondroitin was effective according to the visual analog scale for pain and mobility, and the Lequesne Index. They further concluded that both supplements were as

| Table 12-2 Literature Search Results | | | | | |
|---|---|---|---|---|---|
| | GLUCOSAMINE | CHONDROITIN | OSTEOARTHRITIS | GLUCOSAMINE AND CHONDROITIN | GLUCOSAMINE, CHONDROITIN, AND OSTEOARTHRITIS |
| MEDLINE (1966-June 2005) | 13,004 | 11,032 | 27,179 | 850 | 125 |
| CINAHL (1982-June 2005) | 260 | 153 | 2646 | 122 | 84 |
| PsycINFO (1872-June 2005) | 14 | 13 | 372 | 2 | 2 |
| CAM on PubMed (June 2005) | 534 | 284 | 920 | 4 | 0 |
| All EBM reviews (June 2005) | 138 | 163 | 2422 | 20 | 19 |

safe as the placebo because no significant differences in adverse events were reported. Even though glucosamine and chondroitin often are combined in one dietary supplement, additional research is warranted to determine if the combination is superior to the individual components.

Most recently, Towheed et al published a systematic review of the effectiveness and toxicity of glucosamine in OA.[2] The researchers included studies of orally administered glucosamine for the treatment of OA at any joint except the temporomandibular joint and included studies that were randomized trials, including a placebo group. The outcomes assessed were symptomatic relief and structural integrity of the joint. The authors reported that in 20 trials, glucosamine was superior to placebo in alleviation of pain and improvement of function when assessed with the Lequesne Index,[11] and safety was excellent as measured by adverse events. Additionally, two clinical trials using a specific brand of glucosamine sulfate, Rotta brand (Rotta Pharm, Monza, Italy), demonstrated that glucosamine slowed progression of knee OA as observed by radiographs.

The therapist has already performed a specific search. This can be further refined with a targeted PICO approach. With the PICO approach the therapist uses terms that are relevant to the clinical question.

### Literature Relevant to Clinical Considerations

Although the incidence of adverse events is reported in the research to be not significantly different than placebo, the clinician should still monitor a client who decides to take glucosamine and chondroitin supplements for adverse events that may occur. Reported adverse events include gastrointestinal disturbances such as nausea, diarrhea, and constipation.

Adverse events are believed to be related to the organic nature of glucosamine and chondroitin. Glucosamine is derived from the exoskeleton of shellfish. People with shellfish allergies have been warned about reactions; however, none have been reported in the literature. Theoretically, glucosamine may have adverse events related to metabolism such as elevated cholesterol, blood pressure, or glucose; however, no cases have been reported in the literature. The theoretical concern with the use of glucosamine is with regard to its possible effect on glucose metabolism, specifically by decreasing glucose-induced insulin secretion or by impairing

---

**PICO BOX**

For persons with OA of the knee, does the ingestion of chondroitin sulfate and or glucosamine decrease pain and improve mobility?

P: Persons with OA
I: Chondroitin sulfate and/or glucosamine
O: Pain
O: Mobility

A search conducted in October of 2006 using MEDLINE (from 1996 forward) yields five articles for glucosamine and four for chondroitin. Of these articles only one (the same one in both searches) is an evidence-based review and was identified by the therapist in a previous section of the search. The original search performed by the therapist was done more than a year before (June 2005) the PICO that is described here. However, the therapist has continued to monitor the literature and has identified a large multicenter, randomized trial sponsored by the NCCAM to try to answer the questions of efficacy of chondroitin sulfate and glucosamine administered separately and in combination to decrease pain in people with OA of the knee.[9] In this paper the therapist did not find definitive support for the use of either glucosamine or chondroitin in reducing pain for persons with OA. Several commentaries on the paper[10-12] question the validity of the findings.

The use of the PICO approach to search for information on this particular case illustrates the relevance of continually updating searches and evaluating the findings in the literature.

P = **Population** (patient/client, problem, person condition or group attribute)
I = **Intervention** (the CAM therapy or approach)
C = **Comparison** (standard care or comparison intervention)
O = **Outcomes** (the measured variables of interest)

---

glucose uptake and metabolism in muscle.[1] Scroggie, Albright, and Harris[13] evaluated the effect of glucosamine and chondroitin supplements on glycosylated hemoglobin in people with type 2 diabetes mellitus. In an outpatient setting, elderly men and women with type 2 diabetes were randomized to receive 1500 mg glucosamine hydrochloride and 1200 mg chondroitin sulfate or placebo for 90 days. Glycosylated hemoglobin levels were not significantly different between the two groups, either before or after treatment. The authors conclude that the use of glucosamine and chondroitin does not appear to alter glucose metabolism in people with type 2 diabetes. Chondroitin is derived from bovine cartilage, and it is speculated that chondroitin supplements could be manufactured from animals contaminated with bovine spongiform encephalopathy. At this time no cases have been reported, and the risk of transmission seems to be low. In addition, chondroitin and glucosamine are chemically similar to heparin and may have an additive anticoagulant action when combined with warfarin. No hematological variations have been reported; however, monitoring of patients on warfarin who add over-the-counter supplements or prescribed medications is always advocated.[14]

## CLINICAL DECISION MAKING

### Generate a Clinical Hypothesis

After reviewing the literature and consulting with a dietitian, the clinician is better prepared to have an open discussion about the use of dietary supplements with John to involve him in the decision-making process. The clinician wants to be sure to inform John of the benefits that seem to outweigh the risks from what is known about the supplements in human use and as it applies to his condition. Glucosamine and chondroitin appear to be beneficial for pain and function in OA of the knee and also appear to have minimal risk based on safety reports. However the most recent reports on glucosamine and chondroitin efficacy are not favorable. John decides that he does want to try glucosamine and chondroitin in place of his NSAID even though the most recent studies are not favorable.

Based on the review of the literature and the clinician's previous knowledge of OA management he hypothesizes that the client will have increased strength and improved mobility as a result program of exercise. The addition of dietary supplements may reduce the pain. Based on the literature the expected outcome will occur no sooner than 4 weeks.[15]

### Evaluate

Based on the review of the literature the therapist adds the WOMAC index to his examination and evaluation of the client. The WOMAC index is a multidimensional measure of pain, stiffness, and physical functional disability that has been shown to be valid and reliable for individuals with OA.[16-20] The pain dimension has five items that include pain at rest or with activity. The function dimension asks about the degree of difficulty in 17 activities. The items are rated on a numerical rating scale (in cm)

ranging from 0 ("no symptoms/no limitation") to 10 ("maximal symptoms/maximal limitation"). It is considered a measure of physical function in addition to health-related quality of life.[21,22]

### Intervene

A joint approach is used for the intervention of this patient. Because no curative treatments exist for OA, the physical therapist and dietitian team uses a combined exercise and dietary supplement approach to manage the knee pain and improve functional mobility.[23,24] Based on his reading the therapist decides to use a combination of aerobic walking and a home exercise program of quadriceps strengthening. Both have been reported to be equally effective at reduction of pain and disability from OA.[25] He explains to the client that exercise adherence[26] and weight loss[27] have been shown to correlate with improvements for individuals with OA and urges him to be vigilant with his program.

The most common dose for glucosamine is 1500 mg and is best divided into three doses. For chondroitin, the recommended dose is 400 mg taken three times per day for a total of 1200 mg per day. The out-of-pocket cost for the suggested dose is approximately a dollar per day. John agrees to begin a regimen of 500 mg glucosamine with 400 mg chondroitin three times per day. The dietitian teaches John about buying the supplements from a reputable company and to look for a supplement that has been evaluated by an independent agency, such as those listed in Table 12-1.

### Report the Outcomes

The physical therapist and dietitian believe that the management rather than the specific outcomes of this client's case may be of interest to other physical therapists and dietitians. Although the management of patients with OA is familiar to most therapists, the consideration of an alternative to an NSAID for pain relief may not be. In addition, the combined approach of exercise and the use of glucosamine chondroitin, and importantly, the length of time it takes for the therapist and client to see some change would be of interest to other therapists. Finally, other therapists may be interested in the resources for evaluation of the quality of dietary supplements. For all these reasons the therapist chooses to submit a case report to the geriatric section of the APTA for the combined sections meeting. Although this is primarily a musculoskeletal condition, the client of advanced age is likely to be seen by a therapist with a practice in geriatrics in addition to one in orthopedics.

## SUMMARY

In this chapter clinical decision making is applied to a case of an older man with OA of his knees who is interested in using glucosamine and chondroitin for relief of pain and for improvement in function. After searching the databases for research regarding the use of the dietary supplements in OA, the physical therapist, dietitian, and client decide on a trial of glucosamine 1500 mg per day and chondroitin 1200 mg per day for at least 4 weeks. The client is instructed to buy the supplements from a reputable vendor and to seek out supplements that have met the quality standards of independent agencies. The client is monitored for improvement in function and pain symptoms using a visual analog scale and the WOMAC index and also is monitored for adverse events. Findings of the case are submitted as an abstract for a combined sections meeting.

## REFERENCES

1. Jellin JM et al: *Pharmacist's letter/prescriber's letter natural medicines comprehensive database*, Stockton, Calif, 2005, Therapetic Research Faculty.
2. Towheed TE et al: Glucosamine therapy for treating osteoarthritis, *Cochrane Database Syst Rev* The Cochrane Library Volume 2:CD002946, 2005.
3. Das A Jr, Hammad TA: Efficacy of a combination of FCHG49 glucosamine hydrochloride, TRH122 low molecular weight sodium chondroitin sulfate and manganese ascorbate in the management of knee osteoarthritis, *Osteoarthritis Cartilage* 343-50, 2000.
4. Dietary Supplement Health and Education Act of 1994. Available at: *http://vm.cfsan.fda.gov/~dms/dietsupp.html.* Accessed June 30, 2005.
5. McAlindon TE et al: Glucosamine and chondroitin for treatment of osteoarthritis: a systematic quality assessment and meta-analysis, *JAMA* 1469-75, 2000.
6. The Western Ontario and McMaster Universities Osteoarthritis Index (WOMAC): a review of its utility and measurement properties, *Arthritis Rheum* 45:453-61, 2001.
7. Lequesne MG et al: Indexes of severity for osteoarthritis of the hip and knee. Validation–value in comparison with other assessment tests, *Scand J Rheumatol* (suppl)65:85-9, 1987.
8. Richy F et al: Structural and symptomatic efficacy of glucosamine and chondroitin in knee osteoarthritis: a comprehensive meta-analysis, *Arch Intern Med* 1514-22, 2003.
9. Clegg DO et al: Glucosamine, chondroitin sulfate, and the two in combination for painful knee osteoarthritis, *N Engl J Med* 354:795-808, 2006.
10. Ernst E: Glucosamine and chondroitin sulfate for knee osteoarthritis. (Comment. Letter) *New Engl J Med* 2006;354:2184-2185; author reply 2184-5, 2006, May 18.
11. Vassiliou VS: Glucosamine and chondroitin sulfate for knee osteoarthritis. (Comment. Letter) *New Engl J Med* 2006;354:2184-2185; author reply 2184-5, 2006, May 18.
12. Pelletier JP: Glucosamine and chondroitin sulfate for knee osteoarthritis. (Comment. Letter) *New Engl J Med* 354:2184-5; author reply 2184-5, 2006, May 18.
13. Scroggie DA, Albright A, Harris MD: The effect of glucosamine-chondroitin supplementation on glycosylated hemoglobin levels in patients with type 2 diabetes mellitus: a placebo-controlled, double-blinded, randomized clinical trial, *Arch Intern Med* 1587-90, 2003.
14. Scott GN: Interaction of warfarin with glucosamine-chondroitin, *Am J Health-Syst Pharm* 61:1186, 2004.
15. Iudica AC: Can a program of manual physical therapy and supervised exercise improve the symptoms of osteoarthritis of the knee? *J Fam Pract* 49:466-7, 2000.
16. Bellamy N, Buchanan WW: A preliminary evaluation of the dimensionality and clinical importance of pain and disability in osteoarthritis of the hip and knee, *Clin Rheumatol* 5:231-41, 1986.
17. Bellamy N et al: Validation study of WOMAC: A health status instrument for measuring clinically important patient relevant outcomes to antirheumatic drug therapy in patients with osteoarthritis of the hip or knee, *J Rheumatol* 15:1833-40, 1988.
18. Bellamy N: Pain assessment in osteoarthritis: experience with the WOMAC osteoarthritis index, *Semin Arthritis Rheum* 18(suppl 2):14-7, 1989.
19. Bellamy N et al: Signal measurement strategies: are they feasible and do they offer any advantage in outcome measurement in osteoarthritis? *Arthritis Rheum* 33:739-45, 1990.
20. Bellamy N et al: Double blind randomized controlled trial of sodium meclofenamate (Meclomen) and diclofenac sodium (Voltaren): post validation reapplication of the WOMAC osteoarthritis index, *J Rheumatol* 19:153-9, 1992.
21. Angst F et al: Responsiveness of the WOMAC osteoarthritis index as compared with the SF-36 in patients with osteoarthritis of the legs undergoing a comprehensive rehabilitation intervention, *Ann Rheum Dis* 60:834-40, 2001.

22. Salaffi F, Carotti M, Grassi W: Health-related quality of life in patients with hip or knee osteoarthritis: comparison of generic and disease-specific instruments, *Clin Rheumatol* 24:29-37, 2005.

23. American Academy of Orthopaedic Surgeons: *AAOS Clinical practice guideline on osteoarthritis of the knee,* Rosemont, Ill, 2003, American Academy of Orthopaedic Surgeons, 2003.

24. Bennell K, Hinman R: Exercise as a treatment for osteoarthritis, *Curr Opin Rheumatol* 17(5):634-40, 2005.

25. Roddy E, Zhang W, Doherty M: Aerobic walking or strengthening exercise for osteoarthritis of the knee? A systematic review, *Ann Rheum Dis* 64:544-8, 2005.

26. van Gool CH et al: Effects of exercise adherence on physical function among overweight older adults with knee osteoarthritis, *Arthritis Rheum* 53:24-32, 2005.

27. Messier SP et al: Weight loss reduces knee-joint loads in overweight and obese older adults with knee osteoarthritis, *Arthritis Rheum* 52:2026-32, 2005.

## ADDITIONAL RESOURCES

Arthritis Foundation
InfoPOEMs-InfoRetriever
Natural Medicines Comprehensive Database
PDRhealth site

# CHAPTER 13

## Energy Therapy

*Ellen Zambo Anderson*

---

The purpose of this chapter is to provide the reader with an overview of energy medicine/therapy, one of the major domains of complementary and alternative medicine (CAM), as identified by the National Center for Complementary and Alternative Medicine (NCCAM).[1] Different types of energies and energy therapies are defined, and the available scientific literature is described. Assumptions for subtle energy or biofield-based energy approaches are reviewed, and several interventions are described in general terms. Therapies and interventions likely to be used by clients receiving physical therapy services, such as therapeutic touch (TT), qigong, and reiki, are described in greater detail through case studies found in Chapters Chapters 14, 15, and 17, respectively. A brief description of bioelectromagnetic energy modalities, their application in health and medicine, and a description of the relevant literature also are provided. The application of static magnets in

rehabilitation and details about this intervention are described in a case study in Chapter 16.

## DEFINITIONS

Energy medicine or energy therapy is based on the assumption that all living things possess energy, emit energy, and are affected by external energies within and outside the electromagnetic spectrum. Electromagnetic or "bioelectromagnetic"[1] forms of energy are considered by the NCCAM to be *veritable* energies because they can be measured.[2] Electromagnetic energies include vibration, light, magnetism, and rays from other parts of the electromagnetic spectrum. They have been used in instruments such as the electrocardiogram (ECG) and the electro-encephalogram (EEG) to measure or describe the functioning of the heart and the brain, respectively. Radiation therapy, laser surgery, and cardiac pacemakers are interventions that have used external sources of veritable energy to treat disease and abnormal conditions.

External energies, which fall outside of the electromagnetic spectrum, sometimes are called *subtle energies* and are thought to be a basic life force or vital energy that flows within and through all living things. Adequate and unrestricted subtle energy, known as *chi or qi, prana, manna, ki,* or *ether* in different cultures, is thought to be necessary for optimal health and function. The NCCAM considers subtle energy or "biofields"[1] to be putative. Putative energy fields are those that have, up to now, defied reliable measurement.[2]

A challenge to the field of energy medicine as a major domain of CAM is the debate among experts regarding the terminology used to classify and describe energy-based therapies, conflicted opinions about reliable and valid measures of different forms of energy, and a limited body of scientific literature dominated by investigations into the effects of bioelectromagnetic forces on the body and bioelectromagnetic modalities with comparatively few studies on subtle energy therapies. Table 13-1 demonstrates a search of the scientific literature with key words that attempt to identify different types and applications of energy medicine.

## Key Words

The terms *energy medicine* and *energy therapy* render a similar number of results, with the most citations found in CINAHL. A few observations can be made with a quick scan of the titles and abstracts. It appears that the larger number of CINAHL citations found with key words *energy therapy* instead of *energy medicine* were due to the inclusion of articles about diet and nutritional therapies and their role in improvement of energy and performance and would not be considered an energy therapy according to the NCCAM. In all databases,

descriptive articles and editorials dominated the results. In CINAHL, limiting the search of energy therapy with the word *research* reduced the number of citations from 176 to 77. Of these articles, 73 were about diet therapy or physical therapy and their role in energy expenditure, energy conservation, and metabolic energy requirements, which makes them irrelevant in an investigation of energy therapy. Of the four relevant articles, all were reports on the use of bioelectromagnetic forms of energy. Three were related to the application of acoustic energy for wound management[3-5] and one article was about the use of pulsed radiofrequencies in the treatment of temporomandibular joint pain and dysfunction.[6] No articles about biofield therapies were identified.

As expected, a more targeted search of *electromagnetic medicine* and *electromagnetic therapy* rendered several citations in which bioelectromagnetic energies were investigated. Of the 40 articles in MEDLINE, only 10 were either a case report or a clinical trial. When the 50 CINAHL citations were limited to *research*, only 12 articles met the limitation. Of the 102 articles found through the CAM on PubMed database, seven articles met the limitation of "clinical trial."

From the search of just the key words in Table 13-1, it appears that although several descriptive reports and discussions about energy medicine or energy therapy can be found in the scientific literature, only a few scientific studies have been conducted. The majority of those studies appear to be on the use of bioelectric modalities for the management of wounds. Searching key words alone suggests almost a complete void of research on subtle energy or biofield therapies. If, however, the key words in Table 13-1 are mapped to subject headings, and those terms are searched, many relevant citations are identified. An example is provided in Table 13-2.

| Table 13-1 | Results of Literature Search Using Key Words | | | |
|---|---|---|---|---|
| | MEDLINE (1966-SEPTEMBER 2005) | CINAHL (1982-SEPTEMBER 2005) | PSYCINFO (1806-SEPTEMBER 2005) | CAM ON PUBMED (SEPTEMBER 2005) |
| Energy medicine | 28 | 121 | 10 | 30 |
| Energy therapy | 27 | 176 | 14 | 3 |
| Subtle energy | 12 | 13 | 20 | 10 |
| Biofield medicine | 0 | 0 | 0 | 6 |
| Biofield therapy | 1 | 1 | 0 | 17 |
| Electromagnetic medicine | 1 | 8 | 0 | 102 |
| Electromagnetic therapy | 40 | 50 | 1 | 31 |

| Table 13-2 | Results of Literature Search Using Key Words Mapped to Subject Headings | | |
|---|---|---|---|
| DATABASE | KEY WORD | RELEVANT SUBJECT HEADING | CITATIONS |
| CINAHL | Energy medicine | Bioenergy therapies | 137 |
| | | Energy field | 222 |
| | | Electromagnetics | 111 |
| | Energy therapy | Reiki | 131 |
| | | Alternative therapies | 8247 |
| | | Energy field | 222 |
| | | Electric stimulation | 2216 |
| | Electromagnetic medicine | Electromagnetic fields | 413 |
| | | Energy field | 222 |
| | Electromagnetic therapy | Magnet therapy | 258 |
| | | Electromagnetics | 111 |
| | | Electric stimulation | 2216 |
| | | Electromagnetic fields | 415 |
| | | Electrotherapy | 210 |
| | | Alternative therapies | 8247 |

## Subject Headings

Citations obtained with use of the subject headings were scanned for title and purpose. Once again, a search of the subject headings rendered predominantly descriptive articles, although more research and case study reports were identified when subject headings were used as compared with the key words in Table 13-1. For example, when the term *bioenergy therapies* was searched, descriptive articles dominated the results, yet several research and case study reports were identified. Of these articles, the majority reported on outcomes, that is, the effects or changes observed when an energy therapy was the independent variable.[7-12] Other researchers investigated the potential mechanism for changes observed with energy therapy[13] and the attributes of energy medicine practitioners.[14-16]

When the subject heading *energy field* was limited to *research*, 35 articles were identified. When limited further with use of the term *case study*, 16 articles were found. Although not all the articles were reports of research or case studies or were relevant to the domain of energy medicine, several articles were reviewed for purpose and findings. Six were found to be outcome studies,[17-22] whereas one article included information about outcomes and potential mechanisms.[23] Articles written about the attributes of energy medicine practitioners included those identified with the subject heading *bioenergy therapies*[14-16] plus one additional study by Nelson and Schwartz.[24] New with this search was the identification of a few articles written about the development and application of tools for measuring energy fields.[25-28]

As expected, a search of bioelectromagnetic energies with use of a subject heading such as *electromagnetic fields* rendered many more research articles than did searches of putative energies. As seen in Table 13-2, 415 articles were found when the term *electromagnetic fields* was searched in the CINAHL database. Of those articles, 127 were peer-reviewed research articles. Thirty-nine, or slightly more than 30%, were studies in which researchers investigated the potential interference of electromagnetic fields on the function of medical equipment such as pacemakers and internal cardiac defibrillators. Epidemiological studies made up 20%, in which researchers investigated the relationship between exposure to electromagnetic fields and cancer, sleep disorders, and other conditions. In the area of therapeutic or medical interventions, however, less than 25 articles were identified. Six of the articles were reports on potential mechanisms of action for a range of energy therapies. Eighteen articles included reports of experiments in which the researchers measured the outcomes of treatment that use electrical stimulation for the treatment of a variety of conditions, including tendonitis, pain, and open wounds.

## Summary of the Literature Search

Finding relevant research articles about energy medicine or energy therapy requires familiarity with many terms related to this broad area of CAM, including an understanding that different types of energies currently are being used and investigated in health and medicine. Searching the key words and subject headings in Tables 13-1 and 13-2 reveals literature dominated by descriptive articles, although outcomes research and several mechanism studies have been identified. NCCAM has acknowledged that up to now its research portfolio has been somewhat limited to studies of biologically based practices and whole medical systems.[29] In its 2005-2009 Strategic Plan, however, the NCCAM has identified the need to "recruit multidisciplinary teams to investigate energy medicine" and has called for researchers in energy medicine to (1) apply in studies of energy medicine the same standards used in designing experiments in physics, chemistry, and other scientific disciplines, (2) accelerate progress in understanding the source of biological effect of putative energy fields, and (3) enhance understanding of what transpires in the course of energy healer-client interactions.[29] Currently, however, additional articles relevant to energy therapies can be found when the specific approach or modality is searched in the scientific literature. A review of biofield and bioelectromagnetic therapies follows.

## BIOFIELD THERAPIES

Practitioners and proponents of biofield therapies accept the assumptions and tenets of native American medicine and ancient Eastern medical systems such as Ayuveda, the Japanese Kampo system, and traditional Chinese medicine (TCM), which, for thousands of years, have proposed the existence of a vital life force or energy. This life force, known as *qi* or *chi* in Chinese, *prana* in Sanskrit, and *ki* in Japanese, provides the basis for dynamic and interactive energy systems of life. A healthy state is achieved when vital energy flows harmoniously throughout the mind and body. Disease, illness, or impairment is thought to occur when energy is low or when the flow of energy is restricted or unbalanced. Complete explanations of these assumptions can be found in Chapter 4, Whole Medical Systems. A few biofield therapies such as Healing Touch (HT) and polarity therapy will be described here, whereas other therapies including TT, qigong, and reiki will be detailed through client cases in subsequent chapters (Chapters 14, 15, and 17).

## Qigong

Eastern medicine systems propose similar yet different mechanisms by which qi or prana travels throughout a living organism. TCM suggests that qi travels through the body via a complex network of channels and meridians. The 12 major meridians are aligned with specific organ-energy systems so that energy flows along these meridians and channels and vitalizes tissues and organs. Qigong, a biofield approach, assumes that vital energy can be manipulated through internal and external mechanisms and that the practice of qigong promotes the filling of channels with vital energy.[30] A full explanation of the principles, proposed benefits, and practice of qigong can be found in Chapter 15. A review of the available scientific literature related to qigong is applied to a client who has a history of cardiac disease, pain, and anxiety.

## Therapeutic Touch

In Ayurveda, a whole medical system described in Chapter 4, the subtle energy system that exists in all persons is a network of nadis and chakras, through which prana circulates. Nadis are the energy channels interwoven with the physical nervous system.[31] Connected to the channels are seven psychoenergetic centers known as *chakras*. Chakras are viewed as specialized energy centers from which energy is absorbed and distributed,[31] with each chakra linked to a different region of the body. Therapeutic touch is a contemporary energetic healing practice developed in the 1970s that is based on the ancient concepts of prana and chakras and the assumption that dysfunction reflects imbalance or interruption of life energy.[32] A more detailed explanation of TT and the scientific investigations into the use of TT for pain management can be found in Chapter 14.

## Healing Touch

Similar to TT, Healing touch began in the nursing profession as a contemporary energetic healing practice. Developed in the early 1980s by Janet Mentgen, HT is a holistic therapy that proposes to work through the human energy biofields to clear blockages and restore the balance of energy within the body.[33,34] According to Wilkinson et al,[33] HT actually includes techniques from TT and other healing therapies. The clinical practice of HT begins with a systematic assessment of a client's symptoms and a process in which practitioners become "centered" or "fully present."[33] Next, practitioners assess the client's energy field by moving their hands a few inches above the entire length of the client's body. Energy imbalance and blockages are identified and treated by practitioners who use techniques to transfer and manipulate a client's energy fields based on the client's need for self-healing.[35]

In 1996 Healing Touch International, Inc., (HTI) was formed as an educational and professional membership organization that seeks to promote HT as a holistic healing intervention and offers instruction and certification in HT.[34] Training in HT involves multilevel education taught by a certified HT instructor. Over the five levels of training, HT students are provided with increasingly more complex didactic and experiential learning experiences. This training can culminate with certification as an HT practitioner after the student has demonstrated competency in the practice of HT.[35] HTI is made up of more than 2000 members,[34] with more than 200 certified instructors and nearly 2000 certified HT practitioners. Worldwide, estimates suggest that more than 67,000 individuals, mostly health care professionals, have taken HT classes.

Wardell and Weymouth reviewed and analyzed publications about HT that are found in peer-reviewed journals, a research survey compiled by HTI, HT newsletters, theses, dissertations, textbooks, and electronic databases. They provided a table and narrative summary of the publications in a 2004 article.[36] Their findings were categorized by condition or study area, which included pain, cancer, endocrine-immune-HIV, cardiovascular, elderly, mental health, and "other," which suggests that HT has been fairly well investigated. Of note, however, is that of 27 references presented as outcome studies of HT, only five have been published in peer-reviewed journals. The others have been published either in the *Healing Touch Newsletter* or are unpublished papers or manuscripts. In addition, the authors of the review article state, "Full studies were usually not available to the authors, and incomplete reporting and lack of consistency was often found in the summary documents."[36] So, despite the findings of a few researchers that suggest HT may be helpful in reduction of pain, stress, and fatigue and improvement of the quality of life,[33,35,37] much more rigorous research is necessary before any conclusions or recommendations can be made regarding the safety and efficacy of HT.

## Reiki

Reiki is an energy-based approach to healing that originated in ancient Tibetan Buddhist teachings. Reiki was "rediscovered" in the 1800s and, consistent with other therapies based on Asian medical systems, assumes that physical and emotional impairments are linked to abnormalities of a person's energy or biofields. A more complete description of Reiki, including its history, its application in health and healing, and a review of its scientific literature, is presented in Chapter 17, along with a discussion of integrating Reiki into a plan of care for a person with a history of breast cancer.

## Polarity Therapy

In addition to the assumptions of vital life force, biofield fields, energy flow, and balance, Eastern medical approaches propose the concepts of universal elements and polarity. According to *The Yellow Emperor's Classic of Internal Medicine*,[38] an ancient Chinese text considered to be the world's earliest medical textbook, every form, object, and event in the universe consists of a relationship between yin and yang. Yin, known as the negative pole of an electromagnetic field, is associated with feminine, passive, dark, and inner qualities. The positive pole, known as yang, is associated with masculine, active, light, and outer qualities. The five elemental energies—metal, water, wood, fire, and earth—reflect the activities of yin and yang and account for the influences that the cyclical changes in nature can have on life. Degrees of elemental "fullness" and "emptiness" and their relationship with each other contribute to the relative balance of yin and yang.[30] A more detailed explanation of yin and yang can be found in Chapter 4.

Polarity therapy, an energy therapy developed by Dr. Randolf Stone in the mid 1900s, is based on the assumption of a dynamic relationship between positive and negative charges within every system and at every level of life. The intention of polarity therapy is to balance the rhythmic flow of energy between the poles of positive and negative charge within the body. Balancing the flow of energy is done primarily through different forms of manual touch, pressure, and oscillating movements. The practitioner also may offer recommendations to eat certain foods and perform specific exercises so that a balanced flow of energy can be maintained.[39]

Despite an extensive body of writings left behind by Dr. Stone, a paucity of experimental studies exists in the area of polarity therapy. Beneford et al[40] did investigate the fluctuation of electromagnetic fields during polarity therapy and reported a reduction in gamma radiation at four different treatment sites, but an explanation and implications for the reduction have not been well described.

## BIOELECTROMAGNETIC ENERGIES

Whereas biofield therapies are rooted in the ancient principles of universal energy and vital life force, *bioelectromagnetic* therapies use electrical currents, mechanical vibrations, sound, visible light, and the manipulation of electromagnetic fields to facilitate health and healing. Some bioelectromagnetic therapies have been well investigated and are considered part of standard care for a variety of conditions. Other therapies, such as sound, music, phototherapy, and laser therapy, require additional study. Several studies of static magnet therapy have been conducted and will be discussed in Chapter 16.

### Electrical Stimulation

In the book *The Body Electric*[41] Robert Becker details his study of salamander regeneration and how this work led to the realization that bioelectrical currents exist throughout the body and nervous system. Since then, various forms of electrical stimulation such as capacitively coupled electrical stimulation (CCEST) have been used for tissue healing including cases of nonunion fractures,[42,43] chronic wounds,[44-46] and spinal fusions.[47-49] Transcutaneous electrical nerve stimulation (TENS), another form of electrical stimulation, which is delivered to motor or nerve points through topical electrodes, has been used to manage pain in a variety of client conditions.[50-52] Unlike TENS, which is noninvasive, percutaneous electrical nerve stimulation (PENS) is applied through the insertion of acupuncture-like needles into a client's soft tissue. Researchers have found PENS to be helpful in reduction of pain in persons with chronic low back pain,[53,54] sciatica,[55] and headache.[56]

In addition to the interventions for tissue healing and pain management, many other uses of bioelectromagnetic fields are considered part of standard care. Examples include radiation therapy for various forms of cancer,[57] ultraviolet light for psoriasis,[58] and laser surgery to improve vision.[59] Diagnosing disease and pathology also has been advanced by the use of energy fields in magnetic resonance imaging (MRI)[60] and electrocardiograms (ECG).[61]

### Sound and Music

Sound therapy, in which auditory and vibratory inputs are used to influence a person's physiological and/or psychological state, includes sound healing, vibroacoustic sound therapy, music, and music therapy. Practitioners of sound healing may use chimes, chanting, or drumming to create particular sound frequencies at specific intervals in an effort to promote health and healing of the mind and body.[62] Vibroacoustic sound therapy is a sound technology that uses audible sound vibrations to decrease stress, promote relaxation, and improve health.[63] Sound frequencies within the range of human hearing are directed to the body through a system of transducers imbedded in soft furniture. Proponents of this approach suggest that the primary outcome of vibroacoustic therapy is initiation of a relaxation response as described by Harvard professor Herbert Benson in *The Relaxation Response*,[64] although few clinical trials on the effects of vibroacoustic therapy have been published.[65,66]

In contrast, to sound therapy, a fair amount of research has been conducted to investigate the possible effects of music and music therapy. Several researchers have found that listening to certain types of music can lower blood pressure and heart rate,[67-69] reduce pain,[67,70-73] decrease anxiety,[71-75] and improve sleep.[76] Although there have been some studies in which music therapy has not been helpful in improving quality of life (QOL) scores,[77] improving memory,[78] or reducing depression,[77] the literature generally supports music as a useful therapeutic intervention for different client populations. Investigators have agreed that advancing music and music therapy research requires studies with more subjects, consistent outcome measures, and more rigorous designs.[79,80]

### Light

Phototherapy is the use of light for the purpose of facilitation of a therapeutic effect. A review of 11 animal studies suggests that phototherapy may be helpful in promotion of recovery from posttraumatic and postoperative peripheral nerve injuries,[81] whereas low-level laser therapy (LLLT) has been reported to promote healing and repair of connective tissue such as muscles, tendons, and ligaments.[82-85]

Systematic reviews of LLLT in persons with osteoarthritis (OA),[88] rheumatoid arthritis (RA),[89] and chronic joint disorders[90] report mixed results from a large sample of studies. Favorable results regarding pain control have been reported for subjects with RA[89] and chronic joint pain,[90] although the systematic review of LLLT for OA reports conflicting results.[88] In two small double-blinded clinical trials, subjects with temporomandibular disorders[86] and rotator cuff tendonitis[87] did not benefit more than the control group on pain and functional measures. Researchers recommend that optimal treatment procedures, including wavelength, duration, dosage, and site application, be investigated in randomized clinical trials to determine the effectiveness of LLLT.[88-90]

Outcomes from studies on the application of phototherapy for cutaneous wound healing also have been mixed.[91,92] A review of research related to the use of Irlen tinted lenses, colored overlays, and optometric phototherapy (syntonics) suggests that these therapies cannot be proved or disproved and that a valid theoretical hypothesis is required for further investigations.[93] Bright light therapy has produced positive effects in the treatment of depression in older adults[94] and seasonal affective disorder,[95] although standard procedures for application of this modality need to be established. Typically, bright light therapy requires clients to sit in front of a light box that emits very high fluorescent light (typically 10,000 lux) from 15 minutes to 3 hours, one or two times per day, depending on the equipment used and the client's condition. The use of ultraviolet light for treatment of psoriasis and other dermatological conditions is well supported in the scientific literature[96,97] and for many health care providers is considered a part of standard care.

## Magnets

The use of magnetism, in particular the use of static magnets, has been fairly well accepted by the general population as an energy modality for pain management. The medical community, however, has been slow to recommend magnet therapy as a viable alternative for standard pain management interventions in part because of questions about a magnet's polarity and power and its magnetic field penetration and flux density.[98] A detailed explanation of static magnet therapy and the scientific literature relevant to the application of magnets for musculoskeletal pain can be found in Chapter 16.

## SUMMARY

Energy therapies are approaches or interventions that use different forms of energy to promote health and healing. Therapeutic and diagnostic uses of light and electrical energy are fairly well established in modern Western medicine. Approaches that assume the existence of a universal life force and involve a healing intention to promote biofield interaction and energy balance are consistent with ancient Eastern medical systems and Native American medicine, yet are not considered to be part of standard care in the West. Some physicians, known to many as practitioners of integrative medicine, have suggested that if Western medicine wants to consider a more holistic approach to client care, principles of energy systems and their application to medicine and wellness will need to be fully explored.[99-102] To date, evidence to support these approaches varies widely. More specific therapy chapters in this section take the reader through a decision-making process in which scientific literature for TT, qigong, Reiki, and magnet therapy is identified as it relates to specific client conditions and goals.

## REFERENCES

1. National Center for Complementary and Alternative Medicine: What is CAM? Available at: *http://nccam.nih.gov/health/whatiscam/*. Accessed June 30, 2005.
2. National Center for Complementary and Alternative Medicine. Backgrounder. Energy Medicine: An Overview. Available at: *http://nccam.nih.gov/health/backgrounds/energmed.htm*. Accessed June 30, 2005.
3. Klucinec B et al: Effectiveness of wound care products in the transmission of acoustic energy, *Phys Ther* 80:469-776, 2000.
4. Klucinec B, Denegar C, Mahmood R: The transducer pressure variable: its influence on acoustic energy transmission, *Sport Rehabil* 6:47-53, 1997.
5. Klucinec B: The effectiveness of the Aquaflex gel pad in the transmission of acoustic energy, *Athl Train* 3:313-7, 1996.
6. Al-Badawi EA et al: Efficacy of pulsed radio frequency energy therapy in temporomandibular joint pain and dysfunction, *Cranio: The Journal of Craniomandibular Practice* 22:10-20, 2004.

7. Shin Y, Lee MS: Qi therapy (external qigong) for chronic fatigue syndrome: case studies, *Am J Chin Med* 33:139-41, 2005.

8. Shannon AR: Jin Shin Jyutsu outcomes in a patient with multiple myeloma, *Altern Ther Health Med* 8:126-8, 2002.

9. Koopman BG, Blasband RA: Case reports: two case reports of distant healing: new paradigms at work? *Altern Ther Health Med* 8:116-9, 2002.

10. Omura Y: Special sunrise and sunset solar energy stored papers and their clinical applications for intractable pain, circulatory disturbances and cancer: comparison of beneficial effects between special solar energy stored paper and Qigong energy stored paper, *Acupunct Electrother Res* 29:1-42, 2004.

11. Creath K, Schwartz GE: Measuring the effects of music, noise, and healing energy using a seed germination bioassay, *J Altern Complement Med* 10:113-22, 2004.

12. Lee MS et al: Effects of Qi-therapy on blood pressure, pain and psychological symptoms in the elderly: a randomized controlled pilot trial, *Complement Ther Med* 11:159-64, 2003.

13. Lee MS et al: Effects of in vitro and in vivo Qi-therapy on neutrophil superoxide generation in healthy male subjects, *Am J Chin Med* 3:623-8, 2003.

14. Warber SL et al: Biofield energy healing from the inside, *J Altern Complement Med* 10:1107-13, 2004.

15. Yount G et al: Biofield perception: a series of pilot studies with cultured human cells, *J Altern Complement Med* 10:463-7, 2004.

16. Schwartz GE et al: Biofield detection: role of bioenergy awareness training and individual differences in absorption, *J Altern Complement Med* 10:167-9, 2004.

17. Mansour AA et al: The experience of Reiki: five middle-aged women in the Midwest, *Altern Complement Ther* 4:211-7, 1998.

18. Gilbert B, Gilbert L: Qigong technologies: effective energy therapies for emotional trauma and associated physical pain, part I: Emotional Freedom Technique (EFT), *Acupunct Today* 4:28, 2003.

19. Leviton R: The ideal clinic: energy medicine for healing psoriasis, *Altern Med* 23:40-4, 46-7, 1998.

20. Mills A: Therapeutic touch-case study: the application, documentation and outcome, *Complement Ther Med* 4:127-32, 1996.

21. Olson K, Hanson J: Using Reiki to manage pain: a preliminary report, *Cancer Prev Control* 1:103-13, 1997.

22. Vaughan S: The gentle touch, *J Clin Nurs* 4:359-68, 1995.

23. Shah S et al: A study of the effect of energy healing on in vitro tumor cell proliferation, *J Altern Complement Med* 4:359-65, 1999.

24. Nelson LA, Schwartz GE: Human biofield and intention detection: individual differences, *J Altern Complement Med* 11:93-101, 2005.

25. Borg H: Alternative method of gifted identification using the AMI: an apparatus for measuring internal meridians and their corresponding organs, *J Altern Complement Med* 9:861-7, 2003.

26. Crawford CC et al: Alterations in random event measures associated with a healing practice, *J Altern Complement Med* 9:345-53, 2003.

27. Sancier KM: Electrodermal measurements for monitoring the effects of a qigong workshop, *J Altern Complement Med* 9:235-41, 2003.

28. Koizumi H, Reeves AL: A pilot study of electroencephalographic changes associated with ki, *J Altern Complement Med* 5:349-52, 1999.

29. National Center for Complementary and Alternative Medicine: National Institutes of Health. Expanding Horizons of Health Care Strategic Plan 2005-2009, Washington, DC, 2004, Government Printing Office, pub no 04-5568.

30. Reid D: *The complete book of Chinese health and healing,* Boston, 1994, Shambhala.

31. Gerber R: *Vibrational medicine for the 21st century,* New York, 2000, HarperCollins.

32. Krieger D: *Therapeutic touch inner workbook: ventures in transpersonal healing,* Santa Fe, NM, 1997, Bear and Company.

33. Wilkinson DS et al: The clinical effectiveness of healing touch, *J Altern Complement Ther* 8:33-47, 2002.

34. Healing Touch International: History. Available at: *http:www1.healingtouchinternational.org.* Accessed December 19, 2006.

35. Cook Loveland CA, Guerrerio JF, Slater VE: Healing touch and quality of life in women receiving radiation treatment for cancer: a randomized controlled trial, *Altern Ther Health Med* 10(3):34-41, 2004.

36. Wardell DW, Weymouth KF: Review of studies of healing touch, *J Nurs Scholar* 36:147-54, 2004.

37. Post-White J et al: Therapeutic massage and healing touch improve symptoms in cancer, *Integr Cancer Ther* 2:322-44, 2003.

38. Veith I: The *Yellow Emperor's Classic of Internal Medicine,* (Veith, Trans.). Los Angeles, 1970, University of California Press.

39. Kitts B: Polarity therapy. In Tappan FM, editor: *Healing massage techniques: holistic, classic, and emerging methods,* Norwalk, Conn, 1988, Appleton & Lange, pp 197-218.

40. Benford MS et al: Gamma radiation fluctuations during alternative healing therapy, *Altern Ther Health Med* 5(4):51-66, 1999.

41. Becker RO, Selden G: *The body electric,* New York, 1985, William Morris.

42. Zamora-Nevis F et al: Electrical stimulation of bone malunion with the presence of a gap, *Acta Orthop Belg* 61:169-76, 1995.

43. Abeed RI, Naseer M, Abel EW: Capacitively coupled electrical stimulation treatment: results from patients with failed long bone fracture unions, *J Orthop Trauma* 12:510-3, 1998.

44. Kloth LE, McCulloch JM: Promotion of wound healing with electrical stimulation, *Adv Wound Care* 95:42-5, 1996.

45. Baker LL et al: Effects of electrical stimulation on wound healing in patients with diabetic ulcers, *Diabetes Care* 20:405-12, 1997.

46. Gardiner SE, Frantz RA, Schmidt F: Effect of electrical stimulation on chronic wound healing: a meta-analysis, *Wound Repair Rejuvenation* 7:495-503, 1999.

47. Kane WJ: Direct current electrical bone growth stimulation for spinal fusion, *Spine* 13:363-65, 1988.

48. Mooney V: A randomized double blind prospective study of the efficacy of pulsed electromagnetic fields for interbody lumbar fusions, *Spine* 15:708-12, 1990.

49. Goodwin CB et al: A double-blind study of capacitively coupled electrical stimulation as an adjunct to lumbar spinal fusions, *Spine* 14:1349-56, 1999.

50. Yurtkuran M, Kocagil T: TENS, electroacupuncture and ice massage: comparison of treatment for osteoarthritis of the knee, *Am J Acupunct* 27:133-40, 1999.

51. Fagade OO, Obilade TO: Therapeutic effect of TENS on post-IMF trismus and pain, *Afr J Med Med Sci* 32:391-94, 2003.

52. Cheing GL, Luk ML: Transcutaneous electrical nerve stimulation for neuropathic pain, *J Hand Surg [Br]* 30:50-5, 2005.

53. Ghoname EA et al: Percutaneous electrical nerve stimulation for low back pain: a randomized crossover study, *JAMA* 281:818-23, 1999.

54. Weiner DK et al: Efficacy of percutaneous electrical nerve stimulation for the treatment of chronic low back pain in older adults, *J Am Geriatr Soc* 51:599-608, 2003.

55. Ghoname EA et al: Percutaneous electrical nerve stimulation: an alternative to TENS in the management of sciatica, *Pain* 83:193-9, 1999.

56. Ahmed HE et al: Use of percutaneous electrical nerve stimulation (PENS) in the short-term management of headache, *Headache* 40:311-5, 2000.

57. Tisdale BA: When to consider radiation therapy for your patient, *Am Fam Phys* 59:1177-84, 1999.

58. Pardasani AG, Feldman SR, Clark AR: Treatment of psoriasis: an algorithm-based approach for primary care physicians, *Am Fam Phys* 61:725-33, 2000.

59. Bower KS, Weichel ED, Kim TJ: Overview of refractive surgery, *Am Fam Phys* 64:1183-90, 2001.

60. Matsuoka H et al: Preoperative evaluation by magnetic resonance imaging in patients with bowel obstruction, *Am J Surg* 18:614-7, 2002.

61. Wiviott SD, Braunwald E: Unstable angina and non-ST-segment elevation myocardial infarction: Part I. Initial evaluation and management, and hospital care, *Am Fam Phys* 70:525-32, 2004.

62. Bittman BB et al: Composite effects of group drumming music therapy on modulation of neuroendocrine-immune parameters in normal subjects, *Altern Ther Health Med* 7:38-47, 2001.

63. Boyd-Brewer C, McCaffrey R: Vibroacoustic sound therapy improves pain management and more, *Holist Nurs Pract* 18:111-9, 2004.

64. Benson H, Klipper MZ: *The relaxation response,* New York, 1976, Avon Books.

65. Patrick G: The effects of vibroacoustic music on symptom reduction: inducing the relaxation response through good vibrations, *IEEE Eng Med Biol* 18:97-100, 1999.

66. Standley JM: The effect of vibroatactile and auditory stimuli on perception of comfort, heart rate and peripheral finger temperature, *J Music Ther* 28:120-34, 1991.

67. Baranson S, Zimmerman L, Nieveen J: The effects of music interventions on anxiety in the patient after coronary artery bypass grafting, *Heart Lung* 2:124-33, 1995.

68. White JM: Effects of relaxing music on cardiac autonomic balance and anxiety after acute myocardial infarction, *Am J Crit Care* 8:220-30, 1999.

69. Chafin S et al: Music can facilitate blood pressure recovery from stress, *Br J Health Psychol* 9:393-403, 2004.

70. Schorr A: Music and pattern change in chronic pain, *Adv Nurs Sci* 15(4):27-36, 1993.

71. Voss JA et al: Sedative music reduces anxiety and pain during chair rest after open-heart surgery, *Pain* 112:197-203, 2004.

72. Good M et al: Relaxation and music reduce pain following intestinal surgery, *Res Nurs Health* 28:240-51, 2005.

73. Nilsson U, Unosson M, Rawal N: Stress reduction and analgesia in patients exposed to calming music postoperatively: a randomized controlled trial, *Eur J Anaesthesiol* 22:96-102, 2005.

74. Lopez-Cepero Andrada JM et al: Anxiety during the performance of colonoscopies: modification using music therapy, *Eur J Gastroenterol Hepatol* 16:1381-86, 2004.

75. Lee OK et al: Music and its effect on the physiological responses and anxiety levels of patients receiv-

ing mechanical ventilation: a pilot study, *J Clin Nurs* 14:609-20, 2005.

76. Lai HL, Good M: Music improves sleep quality in older adults, *J Adv Nurs* 49:234-44, 2005.

77. Schmid W, Aldridge D: Active music therapy in the treatment of multiple sclerosis patients: a matched control study, *J Music Ther* 41:225-40, 2004.

78. Hirokawa E: Effects of music listening and relaxation instructions on arousal changes and the working memory task in older adults, *J Music Ther* 41:107-27, 2004.

79. Kneafsey R: The therapeutic use of music in a care of the elderly setting: a literature review, *J Clin Nurs* 6:341-46, 1997.

80. LeScouarnec R et al: Use of biaural beat tapes for treatment of anxiety: a pilot study of tape preference and outcomes, *Altern Ther Health Med* 7:58-63, 2001.

81. Gigo-Benato D, Geuna S, Rochkind S: Phototherapy for enhancing peripheral nerve repair: a review of the literature, *Muscle Nerve* 31:694-701, 2005.

82. Amaral AC, Parizotto NA, Salvini TF: Dose-dependency of low-energy HeNe laser effect in regeneration of skeletal muscle in mice, *Lasers Med Sci* 16:44-51, 2001.

83. Reddy GK, Stehno-Bittel L, Enwemeka CS: Laser photostimulation of collagen production in healing rabbit Achilles tendons, *Lasers Surg Med* 22:281-7, 1998.

84. Stasinopoulos D: The use of polarized polychromatic non-coherent light as therapy for acute tennis elbow/lateral epicondylalgia: a pilot study, *Photomed Laser Surg* 23:66-9, 2005.

85. Fung DT et al: Therapeutic low energy laser improves the mechanical strength of repairing medial collateral ligament, *Lasers Surg Med* 31:91-6, 2002.

86. Conti PC: Low level laser therapy in the treatment of temporomandibular disorders (TMD): a double-blind pilot study, *Cranio: The Journal of Craniomandibular Practice* 15(2):144-9, 1997.

87. Vecchio P et al: A double-blind study of the effectiveness of low level laser treatment of rotator cuff tendinitis, *Br J Rheumatol* 32:740-2, 1993.

88. Brosseau L et al: Low level laser therapy (Classes I, II and II) for treating osteoarthritis, *Cochrane Database Syst Rev* 3, 2004.

89. Brosseau L et al: Low level laser therapy (Classes I, II and II) for treating rheumatoid arthritis, *Cochrane Database Syst Rev* 4, 2005.

90. Bjordal JM et al: A systematic review of low level laser therapy with location-specific doses for pain from chronic joint disorders, *Austr J Physiother* 39:107-16, 2003.

91. Taly AB et al: Efficacy of multiwavelength light therapy in the treatment of pressure ulcers in subjects with disorders of the spinal cord: a randomized double-blind controlled trial, *Arch Phys Med Rehabil* 85:1657-61, 2004.

92. Mendez TM et al: Dose and wavelength of laser light have influence on the repair of cutaneous wounds, *J Clin Laser Med Surg* 22:19-25, 2004.

93. Evans BJ, Drasdo N: Tinted lenses and related therapies for learning disabilities—a review, *Ophthal Physiol Optics* 11:206-17, 1991.

94. Tsai YF et al: The effects of light therapy on depressed elders, *Int J Geriatr Psychiatry* 19:545-8, 2004.

95. Golden RN et al: The efficacy of light therapy in the treatment of mood disorders: a review and meta-analysis of the evidence, *Am J Psychiatry* 162:656-62, 2005.

96. Hamzavi I, Lui H: Using light in dermatology: an update on lasers, ultraviolet phototherapy, and photodynamic therapy, *Dermatol Clin* 23:199-207, 2005.

97. Simon JC, Pfieger D, Schopf E: Recent advances in phototherapy, *Eur J Dermatol* 10:642-5, 2000.

98. Eccles NK: A critical review of randomized controlled trials of static magnets for pain relief, *J Altern Complement Med* 11:495-509, 2005.

99. Gerber R: *Vibrational medicine: new choices for healing ourselves,* rev ed, Santa Fe, NM, 1988, Bear & Co.

100. Dossey L: *Reinventing medicine: beyond mind-body to a new era of healing,* New York, 1999, HarperCollins.

101. Pelletier KR: *The best alternative medicine,* New York, 2000, Simon and Schuster.

102. Weil A: *Health & healing—understanding conventional & alternative medicine,* Boston, Mass, 1983, Houghton Mifflin.

# CHAPTER 14

## Therapeutic Touch

*Ellen Zambo Anderson*

John is a 40-year-old former football player with osteoarthritis of his right knee. He is a pharmaceutical representative. His recreational activities include coaching a youth soccer team and playing basketball on a YMCA men's team. Physical therapy has helped to improve his strength and range of motion. Although his pain has been reduced, it continues to limit him when he coaches his son's soccer team. He asks his physical therapist if adding TT to his physical therapy and exercise program will help to reduce his pain.

### Initial Examination

***Client Report:*** John was referred to physical therapy after his physician discontinued the painkillers he was taking because they started to cause severe stomach distress.

***Client Goal:*** To decrease pain so that he can continue to coach his son's soccer team

***General Health:*** Good

***Medications:*** None

***Musculoskeletal:*** ROM: Trunk, bilateral upper extremities, left lower extremity=WNLs throughout; right knee extension/flexion=5 to 110 degrees; posture: WNLs

***Neuromuscular:*** Force generation: trunk and bilateral upper extremities=5/5 throughout; left lower extremity=5/5 throughout; right hip flexors/extensors, abductors/adductors=5/5;

right hip internal/external rotators, right knee flexors/extensors=4/5; right ankle=4/5 throughout

***Function:*** Pain: Right knee pain, at rest=4/10; standing=5/10; after walking 1/4 mi.=7/10; running=8-9/10

### Evaluation

The therapist determined that the client's limited right knee ROM, pain, and weakness were consistent with a diagnosis of osteoarthritis of the knee. The therapist informed John that he can benefit from physical therapy interventions that address his knee pain and strength impairments at his knees and ankles.

### Plan of Care

John attended four physical therapy sessions, which included ice and high-voltage electrical stimulation to the right knee, along with isokinetic exercises of both lower extremities. He also started a group aquatic exercise program at the local pool two times per week. He reported that the combination of physical therapy and the underwater exercise was helping him gain some lower extremity strength and muscular endurance, but he was frustrated that the pain relief he got from therapy did not last. He was instructed to ice his knee whenever he felt pain, but John reported that this was not always possible.

## Reevaluation

A reexamination after eight sessions of physical therapy over 4 weeks demonstrated an improvement in the client's lower extremity strength and reduction of pain at rest (3/10), after ambulating $1/4$ mi (5/10), and after running 1/8 mi. (7/10), but the pain was still too limiting for coaching his son's soccer team. Transelectrical nervous stimulation (TENS) was then tried as an intervention to help John manage his pain, but he found it to be too cumbersome for the minimal pain relief it provided. John informed the therapist he had heard about TT from a friend and was wondering if it may help his knee pain.

## Incorporating Cam into the Plan of Care

The therapist was aware that TT was a complementary therapy most often used with persons experiencing stress or anxiety but was uncertain of its application in persons with pain. The therapist considered the possibility that John may benefit from receiving TT as an adjunct to his rehabilitation program. She decided to find out more about TT by searching the scientific literature and contacting a TT practitioner whom she had met at a health care provider seminar at the local community center.

The therapist had developed a plan of care that included ice, high-voltage electrical stimulation, isokinetic exercise, and TENS and supported the client's twice weekly aquatic exercise program. Although the client's impairments of strength, pain, and muscular endurance were improving, he was still not able to achieve adequate long-term pain management necessary for coaching his son's soccer team. To evaluate the appropriateness of a recommendation of TT for this client, the therapist needed to become familiar with TT and evaluate the evidence supporting its use in clients whose diagnosis or impairments were similar to John's.

## INVESTIGATING THE LITERATURE

The therapist uses two strategies to investigate the literature. The first is a detailed approach in which preliminary background reading is performed on TT. This is followed by a search of databases and evaluation of the literature using reviews and primary sources for TT and arthritic pain. The second is the use of the PICO format for a focused search to answer the clinical questions generated by the case.

## Preliminary Reading

Several books written about TT[1-4] describe TT as a complementary therapy developed in the 1970s by Delores Krieger, RN, PhD, and Dora Kunz to promote health and healing. Persons with pain, anxiety, and a variety of other conditions are reported to benefit from receiving TT. Four assumptions form the basis for how and why TT is thought to facilitate health and healing. The first assumption as described by Krieger[1] is that the body is an open energy system, in which energy flows within and through the body in a dynamic interface with the environment. The second assumption suggests that individuals are bilaterally symmetrical so that the right and left sides of the body and the front and back mirror each other, which allows for a balanced flow of energy. The third assumption is that impairment in biological functioning, illness, or disease is associated with an imbalance of energy or an irregularity of energy flow through the body. The fourth assumption suggests that the body can achieve a process of self-healing through manipulation of subtle energy fields and restoration of appropriate energy levels and flow.[1]

All the assumptions underpinning TT's approach and process to healing have their roots in the ancient Hindu concepts of prana and chakras.[3,5] Prana, equivalent to chi or qi, is considered to be a universal life energy that circulates through the universe and all living things. Chakras are energy centers positioned at strategic, vital areas of the human energy field that are associated with an endocrine gland and major nerve plexus. Chakras are able to receive, transform, and send prana through a vast network of interconnecting channels, known as nadis. A blockage, interruption, or imbalance of energy flow is thought to exist when disease or pathology exists within a bodily system or systems. Restoring or rebalancing an individual's personal energy field or energy flow is important for the promotion of his or her own inner healing capabilities. Following a stepwise process, a TT practitioner can assess and modulate a client's energy field with the intention of promoting self-healing.

Familiarity with how TT is applied or offered is important in consideration of its use. A practitioner administers TT in a four-step process. The first step, called *centering,* is a process in which practitioners center their consciousness so that a state of integration and quiet can be achieved.

From this state of centeredness, practitioners begin the assessment phase by placing their hands 2 to 3 inches from the client's head and moving their hands down the client's body, making note of the client's energy field and acknowledging how the energy is perceived. A practitioner, for example, may describe a client's energy as blocked or sluggish in a particular area.[4] Or the energy may be perceived as vibratory, tingly, hot, or cold in some areas and not others. These observations may suggest that the practitioner should return to these areas later in the process (Figure 14-1).

Krieger[1] has described the next step in the TT procedure as "unruffling the field." During this activity, TT practitioners sweep away bound up or congested energy, which allows the final step of the process to begin with a client's energy field being open and unrestricted (Figure 14-2). During the final stage of the TT process, practitioners can direct and modulate their own energy and/or the client's energy in a specific manner to improve energy flow and balance. The intention is for the client's energy flow to be balanced and the energy field to be symmetrical so that healing can occur (Figure 14-3).

During a typical TT session, clients remain fully clothed and are seated in a chair. Sessions usually take approximately 20 to 30 minutes to complete, although practitioners report that some clients may require an hour-long session to achieve a relative state of energy balance. Frail clients and children may benefit from just 5 to 8 minutes of TT.[6]

Licensed health care providers and consumers should be aware if specific credentials or training

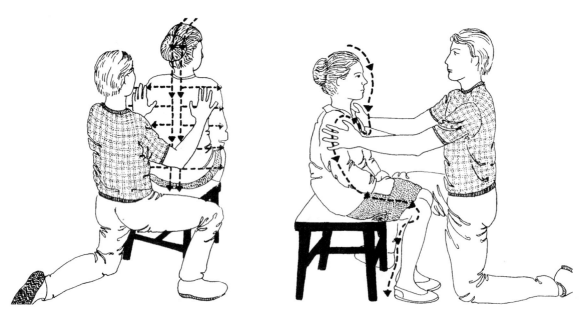

**Figure 14-1** Assessing the energy field.

are required to ensure the appropriate application of a therapeutic approach or modality. Despite the similarities between TT and the "laying-on-of hands" approach to healing, Krieger and Kunz do not believe that people need to be "chosen" by a higher entity to be a healer. They suggest that everyone is capable of developing a keen awareness of health and dysfunction and that anyone can heighten their perception of subtle energy if they desire to do so.[1] Krieger has been successful in integrating the teaching of TT into many nursing school curriculums across the United States and has endorsed the teaching of TT to anyone who is committed to helping others heal. According to Nurse Healers Professional-North America (NHP-NA), an organization that promotes the work and teaching of TT, more than 85,000 people have learned TT worldwide. Basic TT concepts are taught in 12-hour weekend workshops, although practice is required to develop proficiency and skill. NHP-NA recommends those practitioners wanting to practice in a medical or health care environment complete a 1-year mentorship with a qualified TT practitioner or teacher and participate in an intermediate level workshop. Although no standard requirements or certification to be a TT practitioner exist, the Self-Evaluation Tool of Therapeutic Touch Scale (SETTS), developed by Krieger and Patricia Winstead-Fry, PhD, RN, can be used to assist clients in discriminating between experienced and proficient practitioners and those who are less experienced.[2]

Another way to determine a practitioner's level of proficiency is to inquire if the TT practitioner is a qualified to-be instructor. To be recognized by

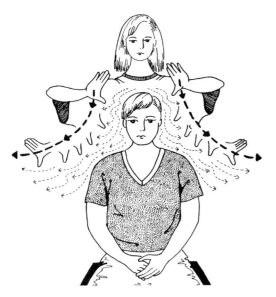

**Figure 14-2** Unruffling the energy field.

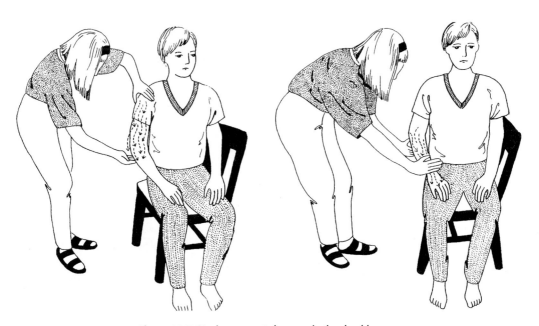

**Figure 14-3** Moving congested energy in the shoulder area.

NHP-NA as a qualified TT instructor, the practitioner needs to have practiced TT regularly for 5 years, had 1 year of mentorship, completed two advanced workshops, and had 1 year of teaching mentorship with a qualified TT instructor.

## Searching Databases

Having read about the assumptions, suggested applications, and training of TT practitioners, the therapist searches the Cochrane Collection of Databases to determine if any critical reviews of TT studies have been published. The key word "therapeutic touch" was searched in the Evidence-Based Medicine (EBM) databases. A review of TT for acute wound healing was found in the Cochrane Database of Systematic Reviews (CDSR), but this application of TT was not relevant for the client. The Database of Abstracts of Reviews of Effectiveness (DARE) renders two analyses of published TT reviews,[7,8] which evaluated reviews by Winstead-Fry and Kijek[9] and Peters,[10] respectively. The critique of one review suggests that the moderate effect of TT reported by the authors is not supported by the evidence. Analysis of the review by Peters, however, indicates that some preliminary evidence may support the use of TT for physiological and psychological outcomes, including reduction of pain and anxiety, but the reviewers suggest that more rigorous research is necessary to establish a solid body of evidence on the effectiveness of TT.

### Primary Sources

The existence of critical reviews on and about TT suggests that this intervention may have a fairly large literature and that investigations into the use of TT for arthritic pain may be available. So a search of four databases, MEDLINE, CINAHL, PsycINFO, and CAM on PubMed, is conducted (Table 14-1). Using the key words *therapeutic touch*, the search renders nearly 500 MEDLINE citations, more than 700 in the CINAHL database and 93 PsycINFO citations. When duplicates are eliminated, a total of 1083 references remained, with the majority found in CINAHL. The finding that most of the citations are indexed in CINAHL is expected because TT most often is practiced by nursing, a discipline whose literature is indexed most widely in CINAHL.

To reduce the large number of articles found with the key words *therapeutic touch*, the search is limited to "review." This allows a more efficient view of the kinds of studies that had been conducted on TT and determine if it had been investigated for pain management (see Table 14-1). A scan of the review articles suggests that outcomes research in TT can be divided into three broad categories: reduction of stress and anxiety, reduction of pain, and wound healing.[9-15] Attempts to investigate possible mechanisms of TT included physiological measures such as blood pressure, EMG activity, and immunoglobulin levels.

Because John was wondering if TT may be helpful in reducing knee pain that was due to osteoarthritis, the literature search is refined by combining the key words *arthritis* and *pain*, respectively, with *therapeutic touch*. This search strategy identifies studies in which TT is applied in subjects with either pain or arthritis. Duplicate studies are removed and titles are scanned visually to determine if the articles are relevant for the client and his goals, When the key words *therapeutic touch* and *pain* are combined, a few articles are found to be about touch therapies different than TT, such as Healing Touch (HT) and Reiki. The other articles include TT, but the subjects had pain related to burns,[16] carpal tunnel syndrome,[17] tension headache,[18] cancer,[19] phantom limb pain,[20] or chronic pain[21] and not specifically arthritic pain. A quick read of these abstracts indicates that for the most part, TT appears to be helpful in reducing subjects'

| Table 14-1 Literature Search Results | | | | | | |
|---|---|---|---|---|---|---|
| | THERAPEUTIC TOUCH | REVIEW | ARTHRITIS | PAIN | TT AND PAIN | TT AND ARTHRITIS |
| MEDLINE (1966-January 2004) | 466 | 90 | 73,125 | 195,151 | 66 | 2 |
| CINAHL (1982-January 2004) | 743 | 48 | 3774 | 28,390 | 82 | 4 |
| PsycINFO (1806-January 2004) | 93 | NA | 2163 | 26,986 | 13 | 3 |
| CAM on PubMed (January 2004) | 469 | 91 | 3461 | 13,721 | 70 | 7 |

reports of pain and in many studies a reduction in anxiety also was observed. In addition, Quinn and Strelkauskas[22] considered the physiological effects TT may have on the practitioner, an avenue of research that warrants further investigation. Fortunately, this search also reveals three studies[23-25] that appeared to be particularly relevant to John's case because the subjects were persons with osteoarthritis. Combining the search terms *therapeutic touch* and *arthritis* render the same articles. Although searching *TT* and *arthritis* may have been more efficient, therapists would benefit from the broader *TT* and *pain* search because this also would address the application of TT for pain with different etiologies. A PICO approach is a similarly efficient yet limited strategy for searching the available literature on TT, osteoarthritis, and pain.

The therapist may not always have time to do such an extensive search. Instead she may use a targeted PICO approach.

---

### PICO BOX

For persons with osteoarthritis of the knee does the use of TT reduce pain?

P: Persons with osteoarthritis (OA) of the knee
I: Therapeutic Touch
C: No comparison
O: Pain

A MEDLINE search conducted in December 2006 using all of the search terms yielded the articles by Eckes Peck[23,24] and Gordon[25] reviewed in the chapter. No other articles relevant to this case were found. This finding suggests that this targeted approach may be useful for therapists familiar with TT who are interested in a specific client population and outcome and that no new studies investigating TT for osteoarthritic pain have been indexed.

---

P = **Population** (patient/client problem, person, condition, or group attribute)
I = **Intervention** (the CAM therapy or approach)
C = **Comparison** (standard care or comparison intervention)
O = **Outcome** (the measured variable of interest)

---

## EVALUATING THE LITERATURE

In the first study conducted to investigate the effect of TT in persons with arthritis, Eckes Peck[23] ran-domly assigned 82 noninstitutionalized older adults (51 to 90 years old) with arthritis to receive either TT or progressive muscle relaxation (PMR) treatments. Subjects served as their own control while receiving routine care for arthritis during a 4-week baseline period. Routine care was not manipulated and continued during the intervention period of the study. Subjects received either six sessions at 1-week intervals of TT from a qualified TT practitioner, validated by the practitioner's SETTS score,[2] or six sessions of PMR treatment with a nurse trained in PMR and assessed by the researcher before the study. Visual analog scales (VAS) were used at baseline and post–sixth treatment to measure pain and distress. Significant differences from baseline to post–sixth session were found within groups. Subjects who received TT reported a decrease in pain ($t=7.60$, $p<0.001$) and distress ($t=7.08$, $p<0.001$). PMR decreased pain ($t=6.58$, $p<0.005$) and distress ($t=6.90$, $p<0.001$). Between-group analysis showed that, although no significant baseline differences exist between the two groups, subjects who received PMR demonstrated a significantly greater reduction in distress ($F[2, 75]=5.6$, $p=0.005$) and approached significance for pain ($F[2, 76]=2.8$, $p=0.06$), compared with subjects who received TT.

The design and procedures used in this study offer benefits and limitations. A strength of the study is that the independent variables (TT and PMR) were applied as full sessions not constrained by time, and multiple sessions were included in the trial. This application or procedure represents a more standard or typical practice of TT as compared with other studies, in which TT has been limited to one or two 10-minute sessions. One of the serious limitations of this study's design is that the researchers did not include a control group and therefore cannot address the concern that treatment results were due to a placebo effect rather than because of either TT or PMR.

This limitation is also evident in another publication by Eckes Peck.[24] This article appears to be a report of some other outcome measures collected and analyzed from the original study of older adults with osteoarthritis described in the previous paragraphs. Improvement in functional mobility such walking and bending, in addition to hand functioning, was observed in subjects who received either TT or PMR, although the subjects in the trial were much older than John and the outcomes did not address the high demands of his goal to coach youth soccer.

In a study that did include a control group and subjects that were closer to John's age, Gordon et al[25] randomly assigned subjects who were 40 to 80 years of age with osteoarthritis of the knee to TT, mock TT, or standard care. The dependent variables were pain and its impact on general well-being and health status measured by standardized, validated instruments, and a qualitative, in-depth interview. Before the study, actual and mock TT treatment sessions were videotaped and reviewed to ensure that objective observers could not tell the difference between the two interventions. The groups received either TT or mock TT once a week for 6 weeks. Baseline measures were recorded for all three groups during weeks one and seven and then again at week 13. The researchers found that the TT group had significantly decreased pain (p=0.002 and p=0.002) and improved general activity (p=0.001 and p=0.0005) as compared with the mock-TT (placebo) and control groups, respectively. Although Gordon's sample size (n=25)[25] was smaller than Eckes Peck's (n=82),[23] Gordon's inclusion of placebo and control groups and the use of standardized, validated outcome instruments help to support the authors' conclusions that, based on their results, TT may offer a means of symptom control for persons with osteoarthritis.

Although several studies have supported the use of TT for reduction of pain in a variety of conditions, little TT research has been conducted in persons with osteoarthritis. Nevertheless, the results of one two-group longitudinal study[23] and one randomized, single-blinded controlled trial[25] suggest that persons with osteoarthritis can experience a significant reduction of pain with the application of TT. Therapist and clients should be aware that further research, with larger sample sizes, is recommended highly and that the long-term effects of TT and mechanism of effect have not been well investigated.

After reviewing the available scientific literature, the therapist believes that some evidence supports TT as an intervention that may be helpful in decreasing John's arthritic knee pain. In addition, no adverse events of TT were reported in any of the articles reviewed. Thus far, standard interventions used for pain reduction, including ice, high-voltage electrical stimulation, and TENS, have not provided the client with adequate pain relief, so adding TT for pain management seems to be a reasonable recommendation.

## CLINICAL DECISION MAKING

### Generate a Clinical Hypothesis and Relevant Outcome Measures

Having decided to recommend TT as an intervention, the therapist generates a clinical hypothesis. In this case, the therapist hypothesizes that TT will aid the client in pain management and thereby allow him to resume coaching soccer. Before the client begins TT, the therapist conducts a reexamination of the client to include two standardized tools: the Multidimensional Pain Inventory (MPI), a valid and reliable measure of clinical pain[26,27] that was used as an outcome measure in Gordon,[25] and the Western Ontario McMaster Osteoarthritis Index (WOMAC), a self-administered health survey designed to measure disability of clients with osteoarthritis of the hip or knee.[28] These objective measures establish a baseline for the client's pain and function before the initiation of TT and allow the therapist to measure and evaluate changes after TT has been integrated into the client's plan of care.

### Intervene and Evaluate

The physical therapist explains the state of the TT literature to John so that he is able to ask questions and participate in the decision about whether to add TT to his plan of care. The therapist then verifies the credentials of the TT practitioner she had met at the community center and receives written permission from John to contact the practitioner for updates on the TT sessions. After four sessions of physical therapy that include ice, electrical stimulation, and progressive lower extremity exercises and four sessions of TT, the client is reexamined and the therapist evaluates the outcome of including TT in the client's plan of care. The client reports that his pain during ambulation is now a 3 out of 10 after walking $\frac{1}{2}$ mile and that he is able to jog $\frac{1}{4}$ mile before the pain increases to a 6 out of 10. A full reexamination is scheduled in 3 weeks, but the client calls and cancels his appointment because he is exercising on his own and is learning to apply TT himself. He reports that his pain has not completely resolved, but he is confident he can be an assistant soccer coach next season.

### Report the Outcomes

The therapist should consider writing a case report to describe (1) how and why a complementary therapy was incorporated into the client's plan of care and (2) whether the client's outcomes support the therapist's clinical hypothesis. Dissemination of the therapist's findings can add to the TT literature and its potential use for reduction of pain in clients with arthritis. In addition, case reports of this nature, in which a complementary therapy has been integrated into a client's plan of care, can encourage a dialog about the use of complementary therapies in the management of pain in a client population frequently encountered by rehabilitation professionals. A possible venue for this type of paper may be *The Journal of Orthopedic and Sports Physical Therapy.*

## SUMMARY

In this chapter, John, a client with osteoarthritis of the knee, inquired about trying TT because even though his knee strength and range of motion were improving with physical therapy and exercise, pain still was limiting his ability to coach his son's soccer team. The client's therapist investigated and evaluated the available literature on TT and determined that TT appeared to be effective in reduction of pain in a variety of subjects, including those with osteoarthritis. The therapist verified the credentials of a local TT practitioner, obtained permission from John to speak to the practitioner about his condition, and initiated a collaborative client care plan. The client discharged himself from therapy when he felt confident that he could manage his knee pain through a home exercise program and self-applied TT.

## REFERENCES

1. Krieger D: *The therapeutic touch: how to use your hands to help or heal,* New York, 1979, Simon and Schuster.
2. Krieger D: *Accepting your power to heal: the personal practice of therapeutic touch,* Santa Fe, NM, 1993, Bear and Company.
3. Krieger D: *Therapeutic touch inner workbook: ventures in transpersonal healing,* Santa Fe, NM, 1997, Bear and Company.
4. Macrae J: *Therapeutic touch: a practical guide,* New York, 1987, Alfred A Knopf.
5. Lansdowne ZF: *The Chakras and esoteric healing,* Delhi, India, 1993, Motilal Banarsidass Publishers.
6. Claire T: Bodywork. *What type of massage to get and how to make the most of it,* New York, 1995, William Morrow and Company. Chapter 12 Therapeutic Touch: Modulating the Human Energy Field
7. Database of Abstracts of Reviews of Effectiveness (DARE) NHS Centre for Reviews and Dissemination: *An integrative review of meta-analysis of therapeutic touch,* York, UK, 2003, University of York.
8. Database of Abstracts of Reviews of Effectiveness (DARE) NHS Centre for Reviews and Dissemination: *The effectiveness of therapeutic touch: a meta-analytic review,* York, UK, 2003, University of York.
9. Winstead-Fry P, Kijek J: An integrative review and meta-analysis of therapeutic touch research, *Altern Ther Health Med* 5:56-67, 1999.
10. Peters RM: The effectiveness of therapeutic touch: a meta-analytic review, *Nurs Sci Q* 12:52-61, 1999.
11. Easter A: The state of research on the effects of therapeutic touch, *J Holistic Nurs* 15:158-75, 1997.
12. Spence JE, Olsen MA: Quantitative research of therapeutic touch: an integrative review of the literature 1985-1995, *Scand J Caring Sci* 11:183-90, 1997.
13. Meehan TC: Therapeutic touch as a nursing intervention, *J Adv Nurs* 28:117-25, 1998.
14. Ramnarine-Singh S: The surgical significance of therapeutic touch, *Assoc Operating Room Nurs* 69:358-69, 1999.
15. Ireland M, Olson O: Massage therapy and therapeutic touch in children: state of the science, *Altern Ther Health Med* 6:54-63, 2000.
16. Turner JG et al: The effect of therapeutic touch on pain and anxiety in burn patients, *J Adv Nurs* 28:10-28, 1998.
17. Blankfield RP et al: Therapeutic touch in the treatment of carpal tunnel syndrome, *J Am Board Fam Pract* 14:335-42, 2001.
18. Keller E, Bzdek VM: Effects of therapeutic touch on tension headache pain, *Nurs Res* 35:102-6, 1986.
19. Samarel N et al: Effects of dialogue and therapeutic touch on preoperative and postoperative experiences of breast cancer surgery: an exploratory study, *Oncol Nurs Forum* 25:1369-76, 1998.
20. Leskowitz ED: Phantom limb pain treated with therapeutic touch: a case report, *Arch Phys Med Rehab* 81:522-4, 2000.
21. Lin Y, Taylor AG: Effects of therapeutic touch in reducing pain and anxiety in an elderly population, *Integrative Med* 1:155-62, 1998.
22. Quinn JF, Strelkauskas AJ: Psychoimmunologic effects of therapeutic touch on practitioners and recently bereaved recipients: a pilot study, *Adv Nurs Sci* 15:13-26, 1993.
23. Eckes Peck SD: The effectiveness of therapeutic touch for decreasing pain in elders with degenerative arthritis, *J Holist Nurs* 15:176-98, 1997.
24. Peck SD: The efficacy of therapeutic touch for improving functional ability in elders with degenerative arthritis, *Nurs Sci Q* 11:123-32, 1998.

25. Gordon A et al: The effects of therapeutic touch on patients with osteoarthritis of the knee, *J Fam Pract* 47:271-6, 1998.

26. Bernstein IH, Jaremko ME, Hinkley BS: On the utility of the West Haven-Yale Multidimensional Pain Inventory, *Spine* 20:956-63, 1995.

27. Riley JL et al: Empirical test of the factor structure of the West Haven-Yale Multidimensional Pain Inventory, *Clin J Pain* 15:24-30, 1999.

28. Bellamy N et al: Validation study of WOMAC: a health status instrument for measuring clinically important patient relevant outcomes to antirheumatic drug therapy in patients with osteoarthritis of the hip or knee, *J Rheumatol* 15:1833-40, 1988.

# CHAPTER 15

## Qigong

*Bill Gallagher, Richard Lund*

Penelope is a 55-year-old female sculptor who had a myocardial infarction followed by a triple coronary artery bypass graft 1 month ago. She has completed phases I and II of a cardiac rehabilitation program. Penelope has developed low back pain (LBP) and has been referred for outpatient physical therapy to address her pain and progress her home exercise/walking program.

### Initial Examination

*Client Report:* The client reports mild panic attacks when needing to go to the hospital or social gatherings and complains of LBP. She is concerned that she may not be able to continue to work on large sculpture pieces because of her cardiac status and back pain.

*Client Goals:* To eliminate back pain, increase activity level, and reduce her situational anxiety

*Medications:* Inderal, Coumadin, Lipitor, Xanax

*Cardiovascular and Pulmonary:* Vitals: HR: 82; BP: 130/80; RR: chronic hyperventilation (26 breaths/minute at rest); walks $2\frac{1}{2}$ mph × 45 minutes without cardiac symptoms. Reports breathing is much more rapid during panic attacks. Demonstrates high thoracic respiration—unable to demonstrate diaphragmatic respiration despite verbal and tactile cues. Blood values: cholesterol 280, triglycerides 206, HDL 22 and LDL 150.

*Musculoskeletal:* Upper extremities: limited shoulder elevation (130 degrees) bilaterally; lower

extremities: positive Thomas test bilaterally, which indicates psoas tightness; posture: excessive thoracic kyphosis and forward head, hyperlordotic lumbar spine; palpation: moderate myofascial dysfunction noted in quadratus lumborum, scalenes, upper trapezius, and pectorals

*Neuromuscular:* Strength: 5/5 throughout except quadriceps, hamstrings, dorsiflexor, and gluteus medius strength 4–/5, abdominals 3+/5, short neck flexors 3–/5; back pain: sitting 1/10, standing 4/10, walking level ground 4/10, walking uphill 3/10, walking downhill 5/10, reaching overhead 5/10.

**Affect:** an affiliated psychologist suggested the Beck Anxiety Inventory to track progress of the client's anxiety symptoms (score=38/63).

### Evaluation

Based on the pain behavior (worse with extension) and palpation, the LBP appears to be generated (primarily) by facet joint arthritis. This is exacerbated by thoracic and scapular immobility, myo-fascial dysfunction, impaired abdominal strength, poor posture, hyperventilation, mental stress, and improper body mechanics.

### Plan of Care

Penelope attended six physical therapy sessions, which included (1) manual therapy to gently mobilize the thoracic spine to increase extension and address limited scapular mobility and myofascial dysfunction; (2) therapeutic exercise to strengthen the quadriceps, hamstrings, dorsiflexors, gluteus medius, abdominals, and short neck flexors; and (3) neuromuscular reeducation to facilitate diaphragmatic respiration, correct posture, and relaxation.

### ■ Reevaluation

After eight sessions over a period of 4 weeks the client demonstrated a reduction of anxiety (Beck Anxiety Inventory=27/63) and reduction of back pain (pain sitting 0/10; standing 2/10; walking level surface 2/10; walking uphill 1/10; walking downhill 3/10; reaching for objects overhead 3/10) in addition to improvements in posture and strength.

Although the client felt that the diaphragmatic breathing facilitation had helped the pain and panic attacks, allowing her to use the Xanax less frequently, she still found herself reverting to shallow, rapid chest breathing when pressured. Her respiration rate at rest is now 19/minute (down from 26). The client's friend recommended she try qigong with a local teacher to further address her pain and anxiety, and so she asked the therapist's opinion regarding the safety and efficacy of this therapy.

### Incorporating Cam into the Plan of Care

The therapist, completely unfamiliar with qigong yet intrigued by the idea of incorporating qigong into the client's plan of care, decides to investigate and evaluate qigong's safety and efficacy before he gives recommendations to his client.

## INVESTIGATING THE LITERATURE

The therapist uses two strategies to investigate the literature. The first is a detailed approach in which he does preliminary background reading of qigong and consults with a qigong instructor. This is followed by a search of the databases and evaluation of the literature using reviews and primary sources for qigong, in addition to meditation and breathing. The second strategy is the use of the PICO format for a focused search to answer the clinical questions generated by the case. In this case two PICOs are generated: one for LBP and the other for anxiety.

### Preliminary Reading

Qigong (pronounced *chee-gung* and also known as chi kung or chi gung) is one of the five pillars of traditional Chinese medicine along with herbology, nutrition, acupuncture, and manual therapy. This tradition is based on the concept of qi. The word *qi* usually is translated as "vital energy" or "breath" and is closely related, if not identical, to the yogic concept of "*prana,*" the Greek "pneuma," the

Hebrew "*ruach,*" the Native American "great spirit," and the Judeo-Christian "breath of life." This concept of vital energy is multifaceted and pervades traditional Chinese culture, including medicine, martial arts (wushu), and environmental design and placement (feng shui). When qi is sufficient and flows harmoniously in the mind-body, respiratory, cardiovascular, orthopedic, metabolic, and emotional health is optimal. Indeed, traditional Chinese medicine, unlike allopathic Western medicine, does not segregate psychological problems from physiological in evaluation and treatment, because both are manifestations of disordered qi flow (see Chapter 4).[1] Correct biomechanical function allows qi to flow properly and that qi flow, in turn, allows ideal body mechanics and posture. Meanwhile, skeptics criticize the concept of qi as a worthless construct consistent with magical thinking.[2] This skepticism is supported by the plethora of ways that the word *qi* is used, which makes it a hard concept for the Western mind to accept.

The first written record of qigong, defined as the science of vital energy accumulation, balance, and circulation, dates back to the Zhou dynasty, which ruled China from 1122 to 934 BC. Written during this era, the classic *Tao Te Ching* refers to breathing techniques that "concentrate Qi and achieve softness." Over centuries of development, emperors, philosophers, scholars, clergy, martial artists, and doctors have contributed to the broad field of knowledge encompassed by the term *qigong*. Yoga practices from India and Tibetan practices were gradually cross-pollinated with qigong indigenous to China.[3]

Qigong, true to its substantially Taoist heritage, resists the scientific and scholarly impulse to reduce it to neatly defined categories. It can be categorized as an energy-based system, as a mind-body approach, or more accurately as belonging to both categories. In the same way, it is impossible to break qigong into mutually exclusive subcategories. However, several ways do exist to group similar practices together to help analyze the field.[4,5]

Qigong can be differentiated by the purpose for which it has been developed. Spiritual qigong, for example, focuses primarily on attainment of enlightenment, yet it can take different forms. Practice in a Buddhist tradition emphasizes the achievement of Buddhahood or cultivation of the ability to see through illusion and relinquish attachment, whereas Taoist qigong tradition emphasizes longevity and harmony between the practitioner and the environment.

Martial qigong assumes that harmonious qi flow is facilitated and in turn allows for movement that minimizes excess muscle tension and effort. Martial qigong practices such as tai chi and bagua seek to develop "internal power," whereas Iron Shirt was developed to make the body impervious to blows. The Iron Palm Technique conditions the hands and other parts of the body to improve striking ability and decrease sensitivity to pain. Medical qigong emphasizes healing and regulates the energy circulation to prevent illness and cure diseases.

Another way to categorize qigong is by the dichotomy of internal versus external. Internal qigong seeks to accumulate and circulate qi in a the practitioner's own body through static meditation, breathing exercises, and movement. External qigong includes healing emission qigong and martial emission qigong. Healing emission qigong is thought to involve the exchange of energy from the practitioner to the client to address energetic deficiency and harmonize qi flow, whereas martial emission qigong is meant to train the practitioner to discharge qi to cause pain or subdue an opponent.

A third way to classify qigong is under the heading Nei Dan or Wai Dan.[4] In Nei Dan (internal elixir), vital energy is gathered in the dantien (abdominal area) via breathing practices, movement, and mental focus and then lead by the mind to other parts of the body, especially the extremities. In Wai Dan, qi is drawn to the extremities and flow is stimulated by mental focus and muscular activity. When the qi flow is sufficient, it is thought to overflow into the rest of the meridian system to invigorate qi flow in general.

A fourth way to categorize qigong is by whether the body is still or moves (static versus dynamic) or what position is assumed (supine, sitting, or standing).

Again, these categories are by no means mutually exclusive. For example, tai chi chuan, a practice primarily focused on building martial prowess, is also considered to improve health. In fact, many practice this martial art only for health purposes and therefore have no idea of its martial application. In the same way, the spiritual qigong path includes a focus on health and longevity to improve the practitioner's chance of achieving enlightenment in the present lifetime. Those who practice any style report tingling sensations, heat, or a flow of warm water through the body, thought to be manifestations of qi flow. It is thought that qi can be led to any part of the body for the purpose of healing. According to qigong theory, many qigong practitioners believe that the will leads the mind, the mind leads the qi, and the qi leads the blood. At the functional level, qi leads strength.

Although many forms of qigong exist, most, if not all, styles seek to cultivate a calm and quiet mind and the ability to release unnecessary muscular tension. They also teach correct posture, with the meaning of "correct" dependent on the style. Qigong also is meant to facilitate balance and stability and emphasizes, at least in initial training, breathing into the lower *dantien*. The dantien or sea of qi is located below (caudal and deep to) the navel and is meant to be the source of all movement. The lower dantien also is known as the *hara* in Japanese and as the *navel chakra* in Ayurvedic mind-body energetics. Broadly defined, qigong can encompass mental imagery, supine/seated/standing meditation, breath work, self-massage, intense shaolin-based practice,[6] and exercises associated with internal martial arts, including tai chi chuan. Qigong styles that emphasize relaxation and equanimity, minimal to moderate exertion, and regulated breathing are thought to address stress-related

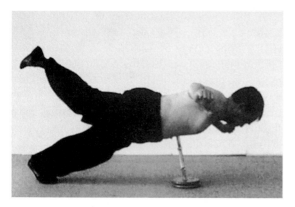

**Figure 15-1** A potentially dangerous qigong technique. (From Liang S, Wu W: *Qigong empowerment: a guide to Medical Taoist Buddhist Wushu and energy cultivation,* East Providence, Rhode Island, 1997, Way of the Dragon.)

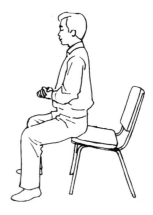

**Correct sitting position**

**Figure 15-2** Sitting meditation. (From Mantak Chia, Iron Shirt Chi Kung I, Huntington, NY, 1983, Healing Tao Books.)

problems, including mild to moderate hypertension. Qigong on the gentle end of the spectrum seems well suited for phase III and IV cardiac rehabilitation because of its apparent low risk of inducing myocardial ischemia or musculoskeletal injury. Because qigong healers may use a variety of practice approaches and employ a wide spectrum of techniques, some of which may be potentially dangerous (Figure 15-1) for Penelope,[5-7] the therapist decides to contact the qigong instructor for a description of a typical qigong session before proceeding with a more specific search of the scientific literature. She obtains written permission from Penelope to discuss her issues with the qigong teacher and arranges a meeting with him.

## Consulting with the Qigong Instructor

The qigong instructor explained and demonstrated how he would work with Penelope using several types of qigong exercise.

### Sitting Meditation

The training would start with sitting meditation on a chair to begin the process of calming the mind and bringing moment-to-moment awareness of the body and breath (Figure 15-2). This instructor would encourage slow, continuous, diaphragmatic breathing through the nose. He would also teach her to be aware of her sitting posture and continuously adjust it according to qigong principles. By promoting physical relaxation and correct alignment, sitting meditation facilitates the circulation of blood and qi. Penelope would be instructed to

focus on the breath and, when the mind wanders (as it is sure to do), gently return the focus to the sensation of respiration and spinal elongation. When the mind is calm and the posture is correct, qi flows more smoothly, evenly, and continuously.

### Self-Massage

This part of the program would consist of self-applied massage to help relax the muscles, move lymph and blood, disperse qi stagnation, and stimulate smooth energy flow (Figure 15-3). Special attention would be given to certain acupuncture points, where qi flow can be manipulated easily, and the major channels through which qi flows.

### Medical Qigong

This part of the qigong program would consist of exercises to help address the more specific qi stagnation and imbalance that Penelope's history suggests is likely in her heart, kidney, and lung organ meridian system. Certain qigong movements, breathing, and mental awareness techniques promote the release, circulation, and balance of qi in these organs (Figure 15-4). The movements also apply gentle pressure and relax the organs and surrounding fascia, which provides a gentle massage that promotes circulation, increases respiratory efficiency, and balances function. All of these stretching and twisting movements would be performed gently and slowly. An example of these types of qigong movements would be forward and backward swing arms, in which she would swing her arms forward (shoulder flexion) while extend-

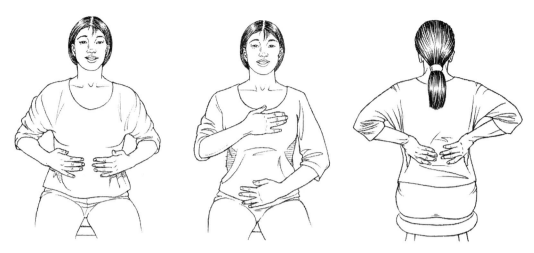

**Figure 15-3** Self-massage. (From Jahnke R: *The healer within,* San Francisco, 1997, Harper.)

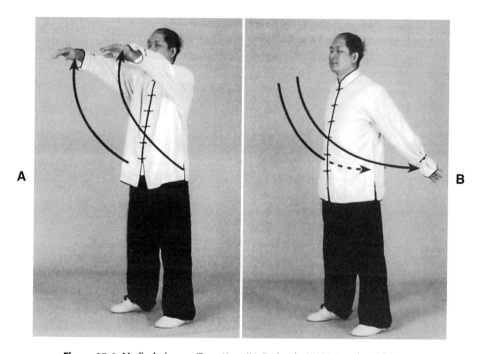

**Figure 15-4** Medical qigong. (From Yang JM: Back pain, YMAA, Jamaica Plain, MA.)

ing her thoracic spine and then swing her arms back (shoulder extension) while flexing her spine. Some of these qigong exercises also use sounds to help relax and nourish the organs. The heart sound ("Hawwwww") is repeated subvocally as a mantra to help the heart be open and balanced.

### Standing Meditation

The purpose of this practice is to gather and enhance circulation of qi while building strength and endurance, especially in the lower half of the body (Figure 15-5). This practice also teaches the practitioner to

"root" herself to the ground to build stability and balance. This is a way to stimulate and regulate the function of the viscera, muscles, ligaments, and bones. Various processes, such as blood circulation, heart rate, breathing, and functioning of the nervous system, are thought to be optimized.

The instructor would first ask Penelope, as she initiates the standing meditation, to calm the mind and adjust her posture according to the principles of qigong. Furthermore, she would be instructed to bend her knees while allowing the pelvis to tilt slightly posteriorly and the tailbone to release

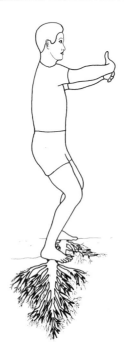

**Figure 15-5** Standing meditation. (From Chia M: *Iron Shirt Chi Kung I*, Huntington, NY, 1986, Healing Tao Books.)

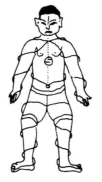
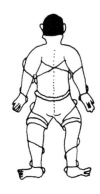

**Figure 15-6** Chan su qigong. (From the Dao Foundation.)

toward a point between her heels. At the same time, he would ask her to focus on spinal elongation. The image of the head floating up as if suspended by a string would be used. He would explain that expanding downward (the coccyx) and upward (the occiput) simultaneously would reduce curvature of the spine and lengthen it to improve circulation. As she relaxes into the posture, she would feel her center of gravity descend. He would instruct Penelope to allow unnecessary muscular and mental tension to "drop down" into the ground with each exhalation and to imagine that she had "roots" growing from her feet, deep into the earth. This image would help promote stability and relaxation while standing.

### Chan Su Qigong

The most vigorous exercise that Penelope would be taught is Chan Ssu Chin, also known as *tai chi qigong* or *silk reeling energy practice* (Figure 15-6). Taking its name from the movements of the silk worm as it makes silk, Chan Su Chin is the circular, spiraling component of tai chi mechanics. The rotation should feel like the extremities are twisting in a wringing motion, like gently squeezing water from a wet towel while the spine is elongated in a neutral position. The teacher states that this would increase Penelope's qi and allow it to flow smoothly while developing strength, flexibility, and improved coordination.

One of the spiraling energy qigong exercises that would be taught to her is called "wave hands like clouds." This movement is performed while standing, with her feet about hip width apart. The arms make circling motions in front of her body, as she turns her waist and shifts her weight at the same time. She would be taught to spiral her hands, arms, and legs in coordination with the turning of the dantien (pelvis). This creates the circular, spiral motion of Chan Su Chin.

The teacher expects the feelings of tranquility experienced during qigong to gradually permeate all areas of Penelope's life. She would be able to cope with challenging circumstances more calmly and develop a profound sense of confidence and contentment.

When asked about his credentials, the qigong instructor stated that he founded his own school, teaching classes and workshops in wellness through tai chi. He has written several training manuals and articles and produced three tai chi videos. He also stated that he began training in tai chi and qigong in 1979 and continues training with a high-level master. He completed a nondegree program in exercise science and is certified in health fitness instruction by the American College of Sports Medicine. He has taught tai chi to sedentary executives at Fortune 500 corporations and to sick people in a nearby hospital. In addition, he provides the therapist with testimonials, letters of recommendation, and a list of clients.

The teacher reports that qigong is being incorporated by licensed therapists into physical therapy to increase coordination, balance, and confidence. He has experience working with clients with chronic, therapy-resistant back pain. He attributes his good results with this population to improved circulation of qi and blood. He also believes qigong could stimulate damaged nerves, which would result in healing and reduction in inflammation and pain. He emphasizes that these exercises provide functional movement through multiple ranges and planes of motion, which results in improvements in strength, flexibility, stability, balance, and coordination. Finally, he assures the physical therapist that he understands necessary precautions for a client like Penelope and that he would not teach any techniques likely to precipitate cardiac issues or irritate the spine.

## Searching the Databases and Evaluating the Literature

### Critical Reviews

After familiarizing himself with the theoretical and practical application of qigong, the therapist searches the Cochrane collection of databases to see if any critical reviews of qigong studies have been published. Because those databases have no information on qigong, and the qigong teacher indicated that he would teach meditation, breathing exercises, and movements derived from the yang tai chi form, he decides to search the database for critical reviews of the terms *tai chi, meditation*, and *breathing exercise*. From the reviews it appears that tai chi may be an effective intervention for fall prevention (see Chapter 9).[9] No Cochrane reviews pertinent to meditation exist. A Cochrane review in which breathing exercises were found to be helpful for asthma provides some support for the benefits of this part of qigong practice.[10] A Cochrane review of mind-body therapies for LBP concludes that the

evidence indicates that these therapies, on average, have a moderately positive effect on pain intensity.[11] A review of mind-body interventions can be found in Chapter 7.

### Primary Sources

To fully assess a potentially large body of literature, a search of four databases, MEDLINE, CINAHL, PsycINFO, and CAM on PubMed, is conducted. The key word *qigong* is searched. Because a large number of articles are identified, the search is limited to reviews (Table 15-1). A scan of the review articles indicates that qigong has been investigated for pulmonary disease, cardiac disease, cancer, pain, and panic disorder. The additional key words *back pain, anxiety, myocardial infarction*, and *coronary artery bypass* are chosen because they are pertinent to Penelope. When the key words *qigong* and *myocardial infarction* OR *coronary artery bypass* are combined, several articles are found to be on "breathing exercise" and "relaxation technique" instruction, so these terms are not searched separately. Skepticism regarding the potency of breathing exercises after coronary artery surgery is supported by one study.[12] Another found complications after open-heart surgery less prevalent in participants who received breath training.[13] One study found in this search reported improved outcomes in participants who had survived myocardial infarction who were taught breathing and relaxation techniques.[14] When the key words *qigong* and *cardiac* are combined, several studies examining the effect of qigong on cardiac psychophysiology are revealed. A review of these abstracts indicates that qigong

| Table 15-1 | Literature Search Results | | | |
|---|---|---|---|---|
| | MEDLINE (1966-JUNE 2004) | CINAHL (1982-JUNE 2004) | PSYCINFO (1872-JUNE 2004) | CAM ON PUBMED (JUNE 2004) |
| Qigong | 82 | 17 | 5303 | 19,851 |
| Review | 0 | 0 | 411 | 1855 |
| Myocardial infarction OR coronary artery bypass surgery AND rehabilitation | 33 | 7 | 1353 | 1681 |
| Back pain | 1638 | 166 | 265 | 1718 |
| Anxiety | 74,648 | 3853 | 67,042 | 5124 |
| Qigong AND myocardial infarction OR coronary artery bypass surgery | 16 | 0 | 0 | 16 |
| Qigong and back pain | 11 | 0 | 0 | 3 |
| Qigong and anxiety | 4 | 0 | 0 | 62 |

appeared to elicit beneficial physiological responses, including reduction in blood pressure and catecholamine levels,[15] improved heart rate variability,[16] reduced heart rate, and respiratory rate.[17]

When the key words *qigong* and *back pain* are searched, no clinical studies evaluating the effectiveness of qigong for LBP are found. One poorly controlled study found improvements, including a reduction of back pain, in a group of participants with fibromyalgia who were taught a combination of qigong, relaxation/meditation, and cognitive-behavioral techniques.[18] When the search is expanded to *pain* and *qigong*, several abstracts indicate that qigong was helpful for pain. Lee,[19] in a retrospective survey on therapeutic efficacy of qigong in Korea, found that 43.1% of the respondents found qigong helpful for pain. Astin et al,[20] in a randomized controlled trial, found no statistical difference in pain between participants with fibromyalgia who attended a mind-body training program that included qigong and subjects in an education support group that served as the control. Potts et al,[21] in an uncontrolled trial, found that group treatment that included education, relaxation, breathing training, graded exposure to activity and exercise, and challenging automatic thoughts about heart disease was helpful for chest pain with normal coronary arteries. Wu et al[22] evaluated the effect of internal qigong instruction and external qigong emission from a "qigong Master" in a block-random placebo-controlled clinical trial. Of the experiment's participants, 91% reported pain reduction, whereas only 36% of control participants reported pain relief.

When the key words *qigong* and *anxiety* are searched, most of the studies focus on breathing exercise in general. At least one study found better anxiety reduction in participants taught breathing exercises.[23] One study found changes in stress hormones.[24] Many studies indicate a connection between chronic hyperventilation and anxiety and panic syndromes.[25-35] This connection between two client complaints (anxiety and chronic hyperventilation) prompts the therapist to explore possible connections between *back pain* and *anxiety*. Again, this search reveals multiple studies that suggest a link between Penelope's back pain and anxiety.[36-39]

Because the teacher plans to teach Penelope seated, standing, and moving meditation, the key word *meditation* is combined with *pain* and then combined with *cardiac*. Again, this search generates evidence that various forms of meditation are helpful for pain and heart disease.[40] Because the qigong training would include imagery, a search for *guided imagery* and *pain* or *cardiac* is conducted. Studies that suggest that guided imagery can be helpful for people with coronary artery disease, pain, and anxiety are found.[41-43] Likewise, a search on the key words *coronary heart disease* and *anxiety* generates several articles that indicate that anxiety can have a negative impact on cardiac health.[44-46]

Using the PICO strategy, the therapist performs targeted searches using the client's different impairments (low back pain and anxiety). This strategy allows the therapist to compare the search results and easily identify studies that include subjects similar to Penelope's and have investigated outcomes consistent with Penelope's goals.

---

### PICO BOX

For persons with low back pain does the use of qigong reduce pain and anxiety and improve breathing?

P: Persons with LBP
I: Qigong
C: No comparison
O: Pain
O: Anxiety
O: Breathing

For persons with anxiety does the use of qigong reduce pain and anxiety and improve breathing?

P: Persons with anxiety
I: Qigong
C: No comparison
O: Pain
O: Anxiety
O: Breathing

In July 2006 a MEDLINE search combining the terms *qigong, back pain* or *pain*, and *anxiety* rendered three articles.[22,62,63] Two of the three references were not identified in the therapists' original search[62,63] because these were published 1 year after he executed it. The addition of these two references is not particularly relevant to the case. They do, however, indicate that the literature has been updated. Adding the term *breathing* did not change the search results.

---

P = **Population** (patient/client, problem, person, condition, or group attribute)
I = **Intervention** (the CAM therapy or approach)
C = **Comparison** (standard care or comparison intervention)
O = **Outcomes** (the measured variables of interest)

## CLINICAL DECISION MAKING

Several good-quality studies indicate that qigong and each of its components, taught by the local teacher, are safe and effective for participants with cardiac issues. Qigong also appears to have the potential to address Penelope's complaint regarding anxiety. Part of qigong practice is to release unnecessary tension in muscles. It is believed that muscles offer an excellent way to assess mental stress because anxiety amplifies muscle tension. Mental tension is increased by proprioceptive input found in conditions of high musculoskeletal tension, contributing to anxiety, so learning to release excess muscle tension through qigong would have a calming effect on the mind and decrease psychophysiological arousal. Furthermore, the ability to notice that a stress response has occurred and to reverse it will allow Penelope to return to a relatively relaxed state more quickly, thereby reducing the possibility of mental stress to exacerbate her heart disease or back pain. Qigong also is expected to have a more direct effect on Penelope's anxiety. By focusing the mind on the body and breath while scanning for inappropriate muscle tension, troubling thoughts will arise less frequently and be easier to let go of as they arise. This practice of maintaining focus on the body and motion and letting go of distracting thoughts is in agreement with the definition of a relaxation technique developed by the U.S. National Institutes of Health[47] and relaxation technique authorities.[20,48,49] Therefore the therapist hypothesizes that the calming effect attributed to qigong will address directly Penelope's panic attacks and may improve cardiac function[47,50,51] and reduce LBP.[52-54] The postures and respiratory and movement patterns taught by the local teacher are in complete agreement with the therapist's understanding of correct body mechanics to minimize Penelope's facet-generated LBP.

### Generating a Clinical Hypothesis

The therapist concludes that the available qigong training is likely to work synergistically with a standard physical therapy program to maximize function and minimize pain. He hypothesizes that by reducing anxiety through breath work and mental imagery, the qigong will improve cardiac function and reduce low back muscle tension and thereby decrease the LBP. By eliciting a relaxation response, the suboccipital and paraspinal muscles will carry less tension and decrease any tendency for these muscles to spasm and reduce the compressive forces on the spine. A relaxation response also may improve motor control to optimize posture, alignment, breathing patterns, and muscle activity to minimize mechanical stress on the spine. Diaphragmatic respiration also will allow transversus abdominus, the deepest abdominal muscle, to be in a more powerful length-tension relationship. The therapist reasons that lumbar stability[46,55] and diaphragmatic respiration require coordination between the diaphragm, pelvic floor, and transversus abdominus. Improved diaphragmatic excursion may enhance movement of quadratus lumborum and psoas through fascial connections and decrease the tendency of these muscles to shorten.[54] Tightness of quadratus lumborum and psoas is part of Penelope's pattern of LBP and postural dysfunction.

The LBP also will be helped by the practice of standing meditation because it reinforces ideal posture for relief of zygoapophysial arthritis.[56] By learning to flex the knees and "drop the tailbone," hyperlordosis and kyphosis will be reduced. Also, this flattened lumbar spine stretches the lumbodorsal fascia. Because this fascia acts on a longer lever arm relative to the center of rotation (in the discs) than the erector spinae, this posture reduces the compressive force on the spine.[57] The tai chi qigong will help Penelope build leg strength and help her learn to maintain her lumbar spine in a neutral range, especially in the horizontal plane, because a key component of tai chi qigong is to drive all movement in the transverse plane via pelvic axial rotation and translation in the transverse plane. The hip rotators, including the posterior fibers of gluteus medius, drive pelvis rotation on the femurs and the thoracic rotation in the same direction and at the same time. By controlling segmental spinal rotation, Penelope will keep her low back in a neutral position in the transverse plane, which will minimize the contact stress in the zygoapophysial joints.[58] In addition, tai chi qigong's characteristic wide and deep stances afford a large base of support. This stable base of support is consistent with correct lifting, pushing, and pulling, and these stances also tend to strengthen the lower extremities, which facilitates lumbar stabilization. Likewise, because maintenance of postural control correlates with good outcome in subjects with LBP[58] the balance improvements expected with tai chi qigong training and practice also may reduce Penelope's LBP.

Finally, because Penelope appears to be enthusiastic about the initiation of qigong training, the therapist considers it likely that the training would elicit a beneficial and clinically significant placebo response. This potential beneficial psychophysiological response could further improve her cardiovascular function and reduce back pain[59,60] and panic attacks.[61] Penelope's positive expectation regarding this intervention is also likely to facilitate adherence to the qigong program. This venerable practice hopefully will engage Penelope on the physical, mental, social, and spiritual/philosophical levels. Research and therapist intuition indicate a pattern of disharmony (Figure 15-7) that includes interconnections among the breathing pattern disorder, the panic disorder, the coronary artery disease, and the LBP.

## Relevant Outcome Measures

During Penelope's initial evaluation and reevaluations the therapist recorded her vital signs, observed her breathing pattern and posture, and measured her strength and flexibility. He also recorded the client's report of pain using a VAS and her Beck Anxiety Inventory score. All of these examination procedures can be performed during a subsequent reevaluation following the incorporation of qigong into her plan of care.

## Intervene and Evaluate

The therapist explains the potential benefits of qigong to Penelope and refers her to the qigong instructor he interviewed. Penelope gives permission for the therapist and instructor to speak with each other so that they can coordinate exercises and activities and assist Penelope in achieving her goals.

## Reporting the Outcomes

Regardless of the outcome, the therapist should consider writing a case report to describe (1) how and why qigong was integrated into the plan of care and (2) whether the outcome observed supports his clinical hypothesis. Dissemination of the therapist's findings can add to the qigong literature and help others evaluate its use for cardiac rehabilitation, back pain, and anxiety. In the same way, case reports such as this can encourage an open dialogue regarding the integration of unorthodox therapies into the management of cardiac disease, back pain, and excessive anxiety in the population frequently treated by rehabilitation professionals. Possible venues for this type of paper would be *Spine*, *The American Heart Journal*, or *Alternative Therapies in Health and Medicine*.

## SUMMARY

In this chapter the clinical decision-making process is applied to help a therapist determine whether qigong is a reasonable practice to recommend for a client with a history of myocardial infarction, triple coronary artery bypass surgery, back pain, and anxiety. After evaluating the available literature on qigong and meeting with a qigong instructor to learn about the specific qigong approach that would be offered to the client, the therapist is optimistic that the client will benefit from including qigong in a rehabilitation plan of care.

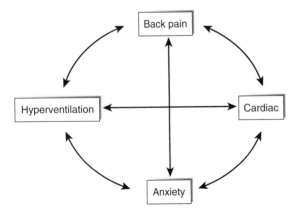

**Figure 15-7** Interconnections among disorders. (From Integrative Rehab: Tai Chi & Qigong Course Manual, Bill Gallagher, East West Rehabilitation Institute, New York, 2004.)

## REFERENCES

1. Kaptchuk T: *The web that has no weaver*, Illinois, 1983, Congdon & Weed.
2. Huston P: China, chi, and chicanery: examining traditional Chinese medicine and chi theory, *Skeptical Inquirer*, September/October 1995.
3. History of QiKung. Available at: *http://www.acupuncture.com/QiKung/History.htm*. Accessed July 14, 2004.
4. Yang YM: *The root of qigong*, Jamaica Plain, Mass, 1997, YMAA Publication Center.
5. Liang SY, Wu WC: Qigong empowerment: a guide to medical Taoist Buddhist wushu and energy cultivation, Rhode Island, 1997, Way of the Dragon, pp 263-5.

6. Ng BY: Qigong-induced mental disorders: a review, *Aust N Z J Psychiatry* 33:197-206, 1999.

7. Chia M: *Awaken healing energy through the Tao,* Santa Fe, 1983, Aurora.

8. Jou TH: *The Tao of Tai-Chi Chuan: way to rejuvenation,* Warwick, NY, 1980, Tai Chi Foundation.

9. Gillespie LD et al: Interventions for preventing falls in elderly people (Cochrane Review) From The Cochrane Library, Issue 2, 2004.

10. Holloway E, Ram FSF: Breathing exercises for asthma (Cochrane Review). In: The Cochrane Library, Issue 2, 2004.

11. van Tulder M et al: Behavioural treatment for chronic low back pain: a systematic review within the framework of the Cochrane Back Review Group, *Spine* 25:2688-99, 2000.

12. Jenkins SC et al: Physiotherapy after coronary artery surgery: are breathing exercises necessary? *Thorax* 44:634-9, 1989.

13. Vraciu JK, Vraciu RA: Effectiveness of breathing exercises in preventing pulmonary complications following open heart surgery, *Phys Ther* 57:1367-71, 1977.

14. van Dixhoorn J: Favorable effects of breathing and relaxation instructions in heart rehabilitation: a randomized 5-year follow-up study, *Ned Tijdschr Geneeskd* 15:530-4, 1997.

15. Lee MS et al: Qigong reduced blood pressure and catecholamine levels of clients with essential hypertension, *Int J Neurosci* 113:1691-701, 2003.

16. Lee MS et al: Effects of Qi-training on heart rate variability, *Am J Chin Med* 30:463-70, 2002.

17. Lee MS et al: Effect of Qi-training on blood pressure, heart rate and respiration rate, *Clin Physiol* 20:173-6, 2000.

18. Creamer P et al: Sustained improvement produced by nonpharmacologic intervention in fibromyalgia: results of a pilot study, *Arthritis Care Res* 13:198-204, 2000.

19. Lee MS: Retrospective survey on therapeutic efficacy of qigong in Korea, *Am J Chin Med* 31:809-15, 2003.

20. Astin JA et al: The efficacy of mindfulness meditation plus qigong movement therapy in the treatment of fibromyalgia: a randomized controlled trial, *J Rheumatol* 30:2257-62, 2003.

21. Potts SG et al: Group psychological treatment for chest pain with normal coronary arteries, *Quarterly Journal of Medicine* 92:81-6, 1999.

22. Wu WH et al: Effects of qigong on late-stage complex regional pain syndrome, *Altern Ther Health Med* 5:45-54, 1999.

23. Hibbert GA, Chan M: Respiratory control: its contribution to the treatment of panic attacks. A controlled study, *Br J Psychiatry* 154:232-6, 1989.

24. Ryu H et al: Acute effect of qigong training on stress hormonal levels in man, *Am J Chin Med* 24:193-8, 1996.

25. Han JN et al: Medically unexplained dyspnea: psychophysiological characteristics and role of breathing therapy, *Chin Med J (Engl)* 117:6-13, 2004.

27. Willeput R et al: Hyperventilation syndrome: evaluation of voluntary hypoventilation programs in two rehabilitation centers, *Rev Mal Respir* 18:417-25, 2001.

28. Han J, Zhu Y, Li S: Occurrence of hyperventilation syndrome in Chinese patients, *Zhonghua Jie He He Hu Xi Za Zhi* 21:98-101, 1998.

29. Ley R: The modification of breathing behavior: Pavlovian and operant control in emotion and cognition, *Behav Modif* 23:441-79, 1999.

30. Han JN et al: Influence of breathing therapy on complaints, anxiety and breathing pattern in patients with hyperventilation syndrome and anxiety disorders, *J Psychosom Res* 41:481-93, 1996.

31. Tweeddale PM, Rowbottom I, McHardy GJ: Breathing retraining: effect on anxiety and depression scores in behavioural breathlessness, *J Psychosom Res* 38:11-21, 1994.

32. Fensterheim H, Wiegand B: Group treatment of the hyperventilation syndrome, *Int J Group Psychother* 41:399-403, 1991.

33. Cowley DS, Roy-Byrne PP: Hyperventilation and panic disorder, *Am J Med* 83:929-37, 1987.

34. Hibbert GA, Chan M: Respiratory control: its contribution to the treatment of panic attacks. A controlled study, *Br J Psychiatry* 154:232-6, 1989.

35. Rapee RM: A case of panic disorder treated with breathing retraining, *J Behav Ther Exp Psychiatry* 16:63-5, 1985.

36. Pfingsten M, Schops P: Low back pain: from symptom to chronic disease, *Z Orthop Ihre Grenzgeb* 142:146-52, 2004.

37. Vowles KE et al: Pain-related anxiety in the prediction of chronic low-back pain distress, *J Behav Med* 27:77-89, 2004.

38. Slesinger D, Archer RP, Duane W: MMPI-2 characteristics in a chronic pain population, *Assessment* 9:406-14, 2002.

39. Grachev ID, Fredrickson BE, Apkarian AV: Brain chemistry reflects dual states of pain and anxiety in chronic low back pain, *J Neural Transm* 109:1309-34, 2002.

40. Zamarra JW et al: Usefulness of the transcendental meditation program in the treatment of patients with coronary artery disease, *Am J Cardiol* 77:867-70, 1996.

41. Halpin LS et al: Guided imagery in cardiac surgery, *Outcomes Manag* July-September 132-7, 2002.

42. Mannix LK et al: Effect of guided imagery on quality of life for patients with chronic tension-type headache, *Headache* 39:326-34, 1999.

43. Tusek DL: Guided imagery: a powerful tool to decrease length of stay, pain, anxiety, and narcotic consumption, *J Invasive Cardiol* 11:265-67, 1999.

44. Buselli EF, Stuart EM: Influence of psychosocial factors and biopsychosocial interventions on outcomes after myocardial infarction, *J Cardiovasc Nurs* 13:60-72, 1999.

45. Ulmer D: Stress management for the cardiovascular patient: a look at current treatment and trends, *Prog Cardiovasc Nurs* 1:21-9, 1996.

46. Grace SL et al: Cardiac rehabilitation I: review of psychosocial factors, *Gen Hosp Psychiatry* 24:121-26, 2002.

47. Integration of Behavioral and Relaxation Approaches into the Treatment of Chronic Pain and Insomnia. NIH Technology Statement Online 1995 Oct 16-18, 1-34.

48. Benson H: *The relaxation response,* New York, 1975, William Morrow and Company.

49. von Kanel R et al: Effects of depressive symptoms and anxiety on hemostatic responses to acute mental stress and recovery in the elderly, *Psychiatry Res* 126:253-64, 2004.

50. Sapolsky R: *Why zebras don't get ulcers: an updated guide to stress-related diseases, and coping,* New York, 2001, WH Freeman.

51. Ornish D et al: Intensive lifestyle changes for reversal of coronary heart disease, *JAMA* 280:2001-7, 1998.

52. Sarno JE: *Healing back pain,* New York, 1991, Warner.

53. Kabat-Zinn J, Lipworth L, Burney R: The clinical use of mindfulness-meditation for the self- regulation of chronic pain, *J Behav Med* 8:163-90, 1985.

54. Chaitow L, Bradley D, Christopher G: *Multidisciplinary approaches to breathing pattern disorders,* Edinburgh, 2002, Churchill Livingstone.

55. Jin P: Changes in heart rate, noradrenaline, cortisol and mood during Tai Chi, *J Psychosom Res* 33:197-206, 1989.

56. Gallagher B: Tai chi chuan and qigong: physical and mental practice for functional mobility. *Top Geriatr Rehab* 19:172-82, 2003.

57. Adams M et al: *The biomechanics of back pain,* Edinburgh, 2002, Churchill Livingstone.

58. Lout S et al: One-footed and externally disturbed two-footed postural control in patients with chronic low back pain and healthy control subjects. A controlled study with follow-up, *Spine* 23:2081-9, 1998.

59. Benedetti F, Arduino C, Amanzio M: Somatotopic activation of opioid systems by target-directed expectations of analgesia, *J Neurosci* 19:3639-48, 1999.

60. Solomon S: A review of mechanisms of response to pain therapy: why voodoo works, *Headache* 42:656-62, 2002.

61. Piercy MA et al: Placebo response in anxiety disorders, *Ann Pharmacother* 30:1013-9, 1996.

62. Cheung BM et al: Randomized controlled trial of qigong in the treatment of mild essential hypertension, *J Hum Hypertens* 19(9):697-704, 2005.

63. Lee MS, Jang HS: Two case reports of the acute effects of Qitherapy (external qigong) on symptoms of cancer: short report, *Complement Ther Clin Pract* 11(3):211-3, 2005.

## ADDITIONAL RESOURCES

The National Qigong Association
The Qigong Association of America
The Qigong Institute
Qi: Journal of Traditional Eastern Health and Fitness

# CHAPTER 16

## Magnets

*Ellen Zambo Anderson, Cathy Caro-Scarpitto*

---

### CASE

Susan is a 21-year-old female student and singer who presents with a gradual onset (approximately 1 year) of pain in both sides of her jaw, clicking when opening her mouth very wide, and "cracking" in her neck. More recently, Susan is experiencing numbness in the left TMJ region when singing. She was referred to a physical therapist by her dentist. Upon examination by a physical therapist, it is determined that Susan has musculoskeletal impairments consistent with temporomandibular joint (TMJ) syndrome. After two sessions of standard physical therapy the therapist decides to add static magnets to Susan's plan of care.

#### ■ Initial Examination

***Medical History:*** Right wrist fracture 3 years ago; extraction of four wisdom teeth 1 week ago

***Client Report:*** The client's primary complaint is pain in the TMJ region bilaterally, clicking at end range opening of opening her mouth, and "cracking" in the neck. She denies episodes of jaw locking. Susan reports that her dentist made an intraoral splint to address her complaints and then referred her to physical therapy.

***Client Goals:*** Eliminate pain and increase mouth opening

***Employment:*** Receptionist involving computer entry; student

***Recreational Activities:*** Church choir

***General Health:*** Good

***Medications:*** None

***Musculoskeletal:*** Posture and alignment: forward head alignment, rounded shoulders with increased lumbar lordosis. Left shoulder, eye, and cheek bone higher on the right. With teeth closed, mandible was slightly deviated to the left. ROM: Cervical AROM limited in lateral flexion right 0 to 30 degrees, lateral flexion left 0 to 35 degrees, rotation right 0 to 65 degrees, rotation left 0 to 40 degrees. Mandibular depression was limited to 25 mm of opening with a slight deviation to the left. Lateral mandibular deviation was asymmetrical: 7 mm right, 13 mm left; protrusion was WNL with a slight deviation to the left. A mild click was noted in the left TMJ at the end of opening. AROM in both UE's was WNL. TMJ loading was negative for reproduction of symptoms.

***Palpation:*** Trigger nodules and pain were noted at suboccipitals, cervical paraspinals L>R, left masseter, left internal pterygoid, and mylohyoid bilaterally. Tenderness was noted upon external palpation of the TMJ bilaterally with teeth together and apart.

***Neuromuscular:*** Force generation: Bilateral upper extremities=4+/5 throughout; cervical musculature=4+/5, with the exception of the right sternocleidomastoid=3/5. (See Function for pain status.)

***Function:*** Jaw pain has interfered with singing and eating.

Pain: Jaw pain, at rest=2-3/ 10; when singing and eating=4-5/10

## ▰ Evaluation

The therapist determines that the client presents with a classic TMJ syndrome L>R and a mild class II occlusion, including altered mandibular dynamics, trigger nodules in the TMJ and cervical musculature, decreased cervical ROM and weakness, and poor posture and body mechanics.

## ▰ Plan of Care

Susan attends physical therapy two times per week, which includes moist heat and transelectrical nervous stimulation (TENS) to the cervical paraspinal musculature and upper trapezius bilaterally and moist heat to the TMJ, followed by ultrasound to the left TMJ and masseter for 5 minutes at 1.0 w/cm² continuous. Massage and myofascial release techniques were performed to the masseter, upper trapezius, cervical paraspinals, levator scapulae, and internal pterygoids. The client is instructed in proper posture and body mechanics in addition to a home exercise program, including postural, ROM, and specific TMJ exercises. A cervical pillow is recommended.

### Incorporating cam into the Plan of Care

During Susan's third visit, the therapist decides to add static magnets to her plan of care, knowing that he has successfully incorporated the use of static magnets for pain control and healing into several other clients' plans of care. A small magnet with a strength of 1700G was placed over the left TMJ during the application of moist heat for 20 minutes. Susan also is given the magnet to take home so that she can apply it with tape several times a day, especially when she is experiencing pain.

The therapist develops a plan of care, which includes moist heat, TENS, ultrasound, massage, myofascial release, and client education. She then decides to add magnets after two sessions based on her clinical expertise and her experience in using static magnets with clients had impairments similar to Susan. The therapist is familiar with some of the scientific magnet studies and decides to search the literature to determine if any researchers have investigated the use of magnets specifically for TMJ dysfunction and pain.

The therapist did not terminate other interventions that may have been helpful in reduction of the client's pain, such as TENS, myofascial release, and ultrasound, and therefore cannot state conclusively that the use of magnets eliminated the client's pain. However, it appears that over the course of therapy the addition of static magnets facilitated a remarkable reduction of pain.

After a total of five sessions, the client subjectively reports a "100%" improvement in her condition. She has no complaints of the pain (0/10) that she had been experiencing for a year and is now able to eat and sing without discomfort (pain=0/10). The client presents an improved posture as compared with the initial examination and she appears to be concentrating on correcting her forward head alignment tendency. With the teeth closed, mandibular alignment is only very slightly deviated to the left and mandibular depression is increased to 40 mm of opening. Lateral mandibular deviation is only slightly asymmetrical, with more deviation to the right. Cervical muscular strength was 5/5 and cervical active range of motion was within normal limits throughout.

## INVESTIGATING THE LITERATURE

The therapist uses two strategies to investigate the literature. The first is a detailed approach in which preliminary reading is performed on magnets. This may be especially important for therapists unfamiliar with the proposed therapeutic benefits of magnets and the theories or principles that underlie their use in medicine and rehabilitation. Background reading is then followed by a search of the databases for critical reviews and primary research reports on magnets and pain. A second strategy is to use the PICO format for a focused search to answer the clinical question generated by the case.

## Preliminary Reading

Books about the healing and therapeutic effects of magnets can be found in libraries, in bookstores, and on various consumer websites.[1-5] Magnetic therapy includes a variety of approaches, which can be divided into electromagnetic or pulsed fields (PEMF) and static magnetic fields (SMF). PEMF requires an electronic circuit or power source to alter electromagnetic fields and has been demonstrated to facilitate a variety of biological effects.[2] SMFs are produced by strong static magnets of varying size, polarity, and strength, which do not require an electrical current. In Susan's case the therapist added static magnets to her plan of care, so the preliminary readings and literature reviews will focus on this type of magnet therapy.

### History

The history of magnet therapy dates back thousands of years, although the use of static magnets for health and healing is classified as a complementary approach of energy medicine by the National Center for Complementary and Alternative Medicine (NCCAM). *The Yellow Emperor's Book of Internal Medicine,*[6] recorded around 2000 BC and considered to be the world's earliest medical textbook, describes the application of lodestone, the Earth's only natural magnet, to the body's energy channels or meridians to treat imbalances. Vedas, the religious scriptures of the Hindus, is another ancient text that includes descriptions of using instruments such as a siktavati or ashmana for healing. Both devices are thought to have been made of lodestone.[3,4] Ancient Greeks and Egyptians also have provided evidence through their writings and drawings of their belief in the healing properties of magnets and their use of magnets in treating a variety of disorders.[2]

In the sixteenth century, a Swiss physician by the name of Paracelsus proposed an interconnectedness between the mind and body through a life force that he called "archaeus." According to Paracelsus, this life force or energy was influenced by

the forces found in magnets. Magnets could therefore be used to treat illness and promote self-healing. Paracelsus used magnets to treat a wide range of ailments, including inflammation, bleeding, diarrhea, and epilepsy. He also had developed ways of preparing lodestones for different client applications and conditions.[3,4]

During the next century, William Gilbert, physician to Queen Elizabeth I, perpetuated the use of magnets to promote health and treat illness. He described in his book, *De Magnete,* the differences between static electricity, magnetism, and electricity.[7] Gilbert suggested that the Earth is a giant magnet, and within his text explained the directions of the Earth's magnetic lines of force and the compass variations they create.[7]

By the middle of the eighteenth century, carbon-steel magnets were readily available in Europe, and the public's interest in the healing properties of magnets grew. Maximilian Hell, a Hungarian-born Jesuit priest and astronomer, shaped magnets to resemble structures of the body that needed treatment and offered magnetism to clients with good results. Hell's ideas and work significantly influenced Franz Anton Mesmer, a colorful physician and scientist who was trained in medicine, mathematics, and law. Like Paracelsus, Mesmer believed in a universal life force and coined the term "animal magnetism" to describe this force in living creatures. Energy concentrated in magnets was defined as mineral magnetism. Mesmer suggested that bodily fluids possessed polarity and that misalignment of these negatively and positively charged poles could result in illness.[8] Mesmer used external magnetic (mineral) forces in addition to animal magnetism emitted from his hands to cure clients from a variety of ailments, including deafness and seizures. Mesmer also believed he could "magnetize" water, wood, almost anything, with his own animal magnetism and that mineral magnets enhanced conduction of universal energy from his hands to the client.[4] Although Mesmer was popular with the general public and treated many clients, the medical community was critical of his work and findings. They successfully portrayed animal and mineral magnetism as nothing more than a sham. Medical authorities advised the public that magnetic healing was due simply to the power of suggestion and was not the result of an observable or measurable biological process.

As Mesmer's popularity in Europe faded, interest in magnet therapy grew in the United States. In 1795 Elisha Perkins, a physician from Connecticut,

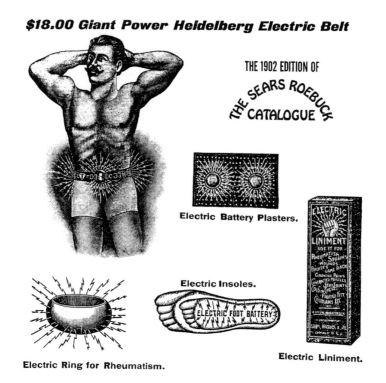

**Figure 16-1** Electrical healing devices listed in the 1902 Catalogue of The Sears Roebuck Company, Chicago, Illinois.

got a patent for his "magnetic tractor," a magnetic device that could remove the cause of an illness by drawing out noxious energy.[4] Perkins was able to convince three medical facilities in the United States and surgeons of the Royal Frederick Hospital in Copenhagen that the magnetic tractor had healing properties and eventually reported 5000 cured cases. The Connecticut Medical Society, however, determined the tractors to be nothing more than a sham.[9] Proponents of magnet therapy and makers of magnetic products including hats, belts, and insoles continued into the early twentieth century with little support from the established medical community (Figure 16-1). After the successes of antibiotic therapy and advances of surgical procedures, magnet therapy moved even further into the shadows of quackery. Now, in the twenty-first century, magnet therapy has once again gained some interest, mainly for chronic conditions and disorders that have not been addressed adequately by standard medical interventions.

### Current Use

The United States Food and Drug Administration (FDA) requires that manufacturers of medical devices receive marketing clearance from the FDA before the devices may be put on the market for purchase or use. To date, the FDA has not cleared static magnets for any medical use, which makes it illegal for magnet manufacturers to advertise that magnets can be used for medical purposes. Nonetheless, magnets are sold and marketed widely in drug stores, in health food stores, and through on-line vendors and direct mail. Costs can range from a few dollars to thousands, depending on the strength of the magnet and the type of product.

Lack of FDA approval has not prevented physicians and other health care professionals from writing books on the use and health benefits of magnets. Although most contemporary authors warn readers that acute or undiagnosed illness or pain requires an examination by a physician and that magnet therapy will not "cure" disease and illness, they have suggested that static magnets be used in combination with other modalities to promote health and healing. In particular, most authors suggest that static magnets are an effective modality for treating a range of pain conditions arising from arthritis, tension, carpal tunnel syndrome, sciatica, post-polio syndrome, fibromyalgia, traumatic injuries, and unknown etiologies.[1-5] Anecdotal reports and endorsements for the use of static magnets for other conditions such as depression[1,3,5] and hypertension[3,5] also can be found in texts about magnetic therapy. Precautions for the use of magnets therapy include the following:

- Pregnancy
- Bleeding or increased risk of bleeding
- Epilepsy
- Implanted devices (pacemaker, insulin pump, metal plate, screws)
- Infection
- Tumor

Although some authors have attempted to report on the scientific literature that supports the application of static magnets in a variety of conditions, details such as research design and study limitations have not been well described.[3,5] In addition, many of the papers and conference reports purported to support the application and positive outcomes of static magnets have not been published in peer-reviewed journals. Research studies that have been published in scientific journals are reviewed in the section on searching the databases later in this chapter.

### Strength

Static magnet strength is determined by the density of magnetic flux lines, or the number of magnetic flux lines per centimeter, and is measured in units called gauss (G) (1 Tesla = 10,000 gauss). Internal gauss indicates the internal strength of the magnet. This measurement or rating may be very different from surface gauss, which indicates the magnetic strength on the external surface of the magnet. Often magnet manufactures report only the internal gauss rating, which is dramatically less than the surface rating. Kahn[3] reported that a product she evaluated had a 12,000 G manufacturer rating and a 1000 to 1500 G surface rating, depending on the area of the surface that was tested. A typical refrigerator magnet measures less than 10 G, whereas therapeutic magnets range from 200 to 3000 G.[3,4] Birla and Hemlin[1] have categorized magnetic field strength as follows:

- Weak = <10 G
- Medium = 10 to 500 G
- Strong = 500 to 2000 G
- Very strong = >2000 G

Magnet therapists consider the depth of the tissue to be treated and the surface area of the magnet when deciding on what gauss of strength to use.

### Other Factors

In addition to the magnet's strength and size, practitioners of magnetic therapy make decisions about the length of exposure, the amount of the body's surface that is exposed to the magnetic field, and whether the magnet is unipolar or bipolar. Some authors suggest that benefits can be realized from a very strong magnet used for a very brief period of time.[1] Others suggest that magnets can be worn all the time and removed when pain relief occurs.[4] For some persons, intermittent use of static magnets is better for pain management than is continuous long-term use over days and months. For others, the opposite is true.

Probably the greatest controversy in magnet therapy concerns the issue of polarity. Magnet products are reportedly available in unipolar and bipolar forms. Bipolar products are designed so that both north and south poles face the body. Unipolar magnet products, sometimes referred to as *unidirectional magnets*, are those in which only one pole, north or south, faces the body. The opposite pole faces away from the body. Some authors of magnet therapy and scientists suggest that a complete unipolar field cannot really exist because every magnet has a north and south pole,[4] and a certain amount of "opposite-pole bleed through" always will occur.[3] Much has been written about which pole should be used to treat different conditions. Some suggest that the north or negative pole is desired if the goal is to reduce pain and swelling and promote relaxation. The south or positive pole is thought to promote swelling and tissue acidity and stimulate wakefulness.[3,5] Because no sound research supports the notion that one pole is more effective than the other, many therapists who use magnets do not differentiate between north and south poles. One author suggests, "If you are using a unipolar magnet and your pain increases, try the other side."[3]

### The National Center for Complementary and Alternative Medicine

Another source of background information on magnets is the National Center for Complementary and Alternative Medicine (NCCAM). A search of the NCCAM website for information about magnets led to a research report entitled, "Questions and Answers About Using Magnets to Treat Pain."[10] This report, written by the NCCAM staff and reviewed by scientific experts from the NCCAM and outside the NCCAM, is available on the website free of charge. The report includes a definition of magnets, a brief history of using magnets for pain management, examples of products using magnets, things consumers should know when considering magnets to treat pain, and beliefs about how magnets may work to produce an analgesic effect. Theories that static magnets may change cell function or increase blood flow have only begun to be tested. The research report also includes brief findings from reviews of scientific studies that were published from August 1999 to August 2003 and randomized clinical trials published from January 1997 to March 2004. A list of magnet studies supported by the NCCAM, which at the time had not yet been published, also is found in the report.

## Searching the Databases

Although the research report by the NCCAM provides some information about the scientific literature available on magnets, the therapist searched scientific databases to access the most recent studies and reviews and to determine if any studies had included subjects with TMJ dysfunction and pain.

### Critical Reviews

The use of magnets in health care has a long history and is proposed by many contemporary physicians and health care providers to be helpful in management of many painful conditions. To determine if any critical reviews of static magnet studies have been published by the Cochrane Collaboration, the therapist searches the Cochrane Database of Systematic Reviews (CDSR) using the key words *magnets* and *pain*. Of the eight reported critical reviews, only one is potentially relevant to the case.[11] Upon a closer inspection of the review the therapist determines that only one article about static magnets[12] is included in a review of interventions for mechanical neck disorders.

Still expecting that review articles on the application of magnets for pain management may be found, the therapist searches two subscription databases, MEDLINE and CINAHL, and a free database, CAM on PubMed, using the key words *magnets* and *pain* and then limits the search to *review articles* (see Table 16-1). He also searches PsycINFO, a subscription database found in the OVID collection of databases, using the key words *magnets* and *pain*, although PsycINFO could not be limited to review articles. Of the reviews that are identified, one was previously noted in the CDSR database[11] and three focus on a variety of interventions, not just magnets, for the management of back pain[13,14] and diabetic neuropathic pain.[15]

The therapist obtains and reads five review articles that show promise for providing relevant information.[16-20] Four of the five articles are reviews of studies that investigated the use of static magnets.[16-19] One article[20] is a descriptive report of magnetic therapy rather than a review of scientific literature. Of the reviews, Eccles'[16] provides the most contemporary information and a specific description of how the primary sources were obtained and analyzed. Eccles' review included 21 randomized controlled trials in which the experimental groups were compared with a placebo or sham group. Each study was assessed for quality using the system suggested by Jadad (see Chapter 2).[21] Of the 21 studies, 13 reported significant pain relief resulting from static magnets. When just the studies considered to be of better quality[18] were assessed, 11 reported positive results, and seven reported insignificant results. These findings appear to offer preliminary support for considering static magnets as a possible intervention for pain management. The three other review articles,[17-19] which were published a few years before Eccles, suggested that inconclusive evidence exists regarding the application of static magnets in medicine and rehabilitation.

Of note is the fact that none of the reviews included studies of subjects with TMJ pain, although all of them contained studies with subjects who had other types of musculoskeletal pain. The results from studies that included subjects with painful orthopedic conditions suggest that static magnets with strength ranging from 850 G to 2000 G may be helpful in pain reduction when compared with sham magnets. To determine the specific treatment protocols and verify the results reported by the reviewers, therapists need to access the complete report for each study, by searching a specific article's title or author found in the reviews' reference list.

### Primary Sources

In addition to searching for primary sources from a critical review's reference list, research articles can be found by searching the scientific databases with key words relevant to Susan's case. Identifying and reading the primary sources would allow for a better understanding of how static magnets were used in each study and also would allow the therapist to appraise the study for design, use of outcome

## Table 16-1    LITERATURE SEARCH RESULTS

|  | MEDLINE (1966-NOVEMBER 2005) | CINAHL (1982-NOVEMBER 2005) | PSYCINFO (1806-NOVEMBER 2005) | CAM ON PUBMED (NOVEMBER 2005) |
|---|---|---|---|---|
| Magnets | 837 | 113 | 76 | 90 |
| Pain | 247,498 | 44,320 | 30,273 | 15,484 |
| Magnets and pain | 40 | 41 | 10 | 32 |
| Review (magnets and pain) | 7 | 2 | Not valid | 7 |
| TMJ pain | 3652 | 444 | 91 | 240 |
| Magnets and TMJ pain | 1 | 0 | 0 | 0 |
| Facial pain | 3978 | 468 | 184 | 332 |
| Magnets and facial pain | 1 | 0 | 0 | 0 |

## PICO BOX

For clients with TMJ pain, does the use of static magnets decrease pain?

P: People with TMJ pain
I: Static magnets
C: Comparison (none)
O: Pain

A search performed in MEDLINE on October 12, 2006, combining all of the terms yielded one reference (22), which had previously been determined as not relevant for this case. Combining *pain* and *magnets* did not render any new or different references from the original search.

P = **Population** (patient/client problem, person condition, or group attribute)
I = **Intervention** (the CAM therapy or approach)
C = **Comparison** (standard care or comparison intervention)
O = **Outcome** (the measured variables of interest)

## Table 16-2    Research Studies on Musculoskeletal Pain Conditions

| AUTHOR (DATE) | CONDITION |
|---|---|
| Harlow et al (2004) | Osteoarthritic hip or knee pain |
| Wolsko et al (2004) | Osteoarthritic knee pain |
| Winemiller et al (2003) | Plantar fasciitis |
| Hinman et al (2002) | Arthritic knee pain |
| Segal et al (2001) | Rheumatoid arthritis |
| Holcomb et al (2000) | Osteoarthritic low back or knee pain |
| Collacott et al (2000) | Arthritic low back pain |
| Kanai et al (1998) | Low back pain |
| Caselli et al (1997) | Plantar fasciitis |
| Hong et al (1982) | Chronic neck and shoulder pain |

measures, analysis, and conclusions. The results of searching the databases using key words are presented in Table 16-1. A more focused search can be performed by narrowing the term *pain* to *temporomandibular joint pain* or *facial pain,* but this strategy reveals only one study[22] that is not relevant to Susan's case. Similarly, the PICO strategy of searching the literature identifies the same citation,[22] which does not provide useful information for the therapist.

## Evaluating the Literature

Research studies found to include subjects with musculoskeletal pain conditions are listed in Table 16-2. All the studies were consistent in that the researchers used a randomized, controlled, double-blind design, with two adding a crossover component. There was, however, variability across the studies regarding the control or placebo group. Some researchers applied identical yet non-magnetic devices, to subjects in the control group. Others used weak magnetic devices in the control group so that blinding could be maintained with subjects who "tested" their device for magnetic properties. All the studies included either or both the Western Ontario and McMaster University arthritic index (WOMAC) and a visual analogue scale (VAS) as primary outcome measures. Both tools are widely accepted as reliable and valid tools for measuring pain and function. These studies did vary, however, in the strength of the magnets that were tested (850 to 2000 G) and when the outcome measures were assessed (1 hour to 12 weeks).

Of 10 studies in Table 16-2, 50% demonstrated a significant analgesic effect with the application of static magnets,[23-27] whereas five studies reported no such effects.[12,28-31] Of the five research studies that reported no significant pain reduction from the use of static magnets, two included subjects with plantar heel pain who received magnetic insoles that were 192 G and worn at least 4 hours daily, four times per week, for 8 weeks[28] or insoles of unknown strength, which were worn during waking hours for 4 weeks.[29] Control subjects in both studies wore nonmagnetic insoles for the same duration. VAS pain scores minimally improved at 4 weeks and 8 weeks[28] for the control and experimental groups. No significant difference existed between the groups, which suggests that magnetic insoles were no better than sham insoles at reducing pain. Caselli et al[29] offered undisclosed randomization, blinding procedures and actual magnet strength as possible reasons for the insignificant results. Winemiller et al[28] suggested that the use of magnets with low strength (192 G) was problematic in their study.

Other researchers who reported insignificant results include Hong et al,[12] who randomly assigned subjects with and without chronic neck and shoulder pain to wear 1300 G or nonmagnetic necklaces continually for 3 weeks. Although 52% of the magnet group reported an analgesic effect, 44% of the placebo group did too, which made the difference between the groups insignificant and suggestive of a large placebo effect.

Two studies that investigated the analgesic effects of static magnets for persons with pain resulting from arthritic conditions were conducted by Collacott et al[30] and Segal et al.[31] In a randomized, double-blind crossover trial, subjects with chronic back pain alternately received nonmagnetic sham devices and magnets of 300 G for 1 week with a 1-week washout period between treatment weeks.[30] Each week, the subjects wore the magnet or the sham for 6 hours each day, 3 days per week. Weekly assessments of pain did not demonstrate a statistically significant effect of the magnets. In the other study,[31] subjects with rheumatoid arthritis and knee pain were assigned randomly to either a treatment group in which subjects wore magnets with a total surface strength of 1900 G or a control group with magnets that measured 720 G. The Rheumatologist and Subject's Global Assessment of Disease Activity (R-GADA, S-GADA), the Modified Health Assessment Questionnaire (MHAQ), and several other measurement tools were performed at baseline, 1 hour, 1 day, and 1 week. Analysis of the data performed by the authors demonstrated a significant reduction of pain in both groups ($p = 0.0001$), but a comparison between the groups was not significant ($p = 0.23$). The authors have suggested that the strength of the "control" magnets may have been sufficient to create analgesic effects in persons with RA and that a nonmagnetic placebo group would have improved the study's design.[31]

Of the five studies that provide support for the analgesic benefits of static magnets four included subjects with arthritis. Wolsko et al[23] used the WOMAC subscale for pain as the primary outcome measure and sought to determine the accuracy of the subjects' belief as to whether they received a magnetic or nonmagnetic device. Subjects in the experimental group (n = 13) were exposed to magnets of 850 G strength and were compared with subjects who were given magnetic devices of the same power but designed to emit the power away from the subject. The comparison revealed a significant reduction in pain in the treatment group ($p = 0.03$) at 4 hours, but no significant difference at 1 or 6 weeks. Although substantial efforts were made to maintain and verify a double-blind, placebo-controlled status throughout the experimental period, the small number of subjects (n = 26) limited the statistical power of the study.

Holcomb, Parker, and Harrison[24] conducted a randomized, double-blind, crossover study to compare the effect of a 2000 G magnetic device to a nonmagnetic placebo with subjects who had chronic back and knee pain with confirmed degenerative disc or joint disease. Subjects were provided with either magnetic or nonmagnetic devices. Outcome measures were assessed at baseline, 1 hour, 3 hours, and 24 hours. After a 7-day washout period, the magnetic and nonmagnetic devices were reversed and pain was reassessed. Use of the magnets was associated with a significant reduction of pain ($p = 0.03$) when compared with the placebo group.

Hinman, Ford, and Heyl[25] included subjects with chronic knee pain resulting from osteoarthritis and used four magnets with a total of approximately 1600 G surface power. Subjects in the control group received nonmagnetic devices. WOMAC scores and times from a 15-meter walk test were recorded at baseline and after 2 weeks. A multivariate analysis of covariance determined a significant treatment effect (p=0.002), in which subjects who wore magnets demonstrated greater reduction in pain (p=0.002) and an improvement in gait speed (p=0.042) than controls. Concerns related to the design of the study include the possibility that subjects in the control group tested their device for magnetic properties and discovered they were in the placebo group and thereby invalidated their status as being blinded to the independent variable.

Harlow et al[26] conducted a randomized, placebo-controlled trial with three parallel groups. Subjects were between the ages of 45 and 80 years with a diagnosis of osteoarthritis of the hip or knee and wore a magnetic bracelet for 12 weeks that was either standard strength (1700 to 2000 G), weak strength (210 to 300 G), or nonmagnetic. Although analysis of variance between the three groups on the WOMAC index showed a difference that was nonsignificant (F=2.90, df=2, 190; p=0.057), analysis of covariance with the baseline WOMAC score entered as a covariate was significant (F=3.24, df=2, 189; p=0.041). Comparison of groups using the Dunnett's test showed a significant mean difference in change in WOMAC A scores between the standard and the nonmagnetic groups (mean difference 1.3; 95% CI 0.09-2.60; p=0.03), but not between the standard and weak groups (mean difference 0.81; −0.44 to 2.07; p =0.26). The researchers addressed issues related to blinding and belief by questioning subjects as to whether they thought they had active or inactive magnetic bracelets. Approximately one third of the subjects in the standard and nonmagnetic groups were correct in their beliefs about their bracelet, and although this did not affect the pattern of the results, the researchers suggest that the validity of the self-reporting of blinding status could be questioned, and therefore a placebo effect could not be ruled out.

Kanai et al[27] conducted a randomized, double-blind study that included subjects with low back pain with mixed etiologies. Magnets of 1800 G were used in the experimental group, and very weak magnets of 100 G were applied in the control group. Pain was assessed at baseline and weekly for 3 weeks. Pain was reduced significantly in the experimental group as compared with the control group after 1 week.

In general, the experimental designs used to test the analgesic effects of static magnets in musculoskeletal disorders were consistently randomized and blinded controlled trials. However, the strength of the magnets was widely varied, with the treatment magnet ranging from 192 G to 2000 G and the control or sham magnet ranging from 0 G to 300 G. Frequency and duration of magnet use, although consistent within each trial, also varied widely, ranging from 6 to 24 hours per day and usage from 1 day to 3 months. Nevertheless, it appears that some evidence supports the use of static magnets for pain reduction in musculoskeletal conditions, and no adverse side effects were reported by any of the researchers. The marked differences in the strength of the therapeutic magnets studied and variations of frequency and duration challenge the clinician to determine an intervention strategy using static magnets that would most likely provide analgesic effects.

## Additional Literature on Static Magnets and Pain

Although a literature search of magnets and pain renders 41and 40 citations in the CINAHL and MEDLINE databases, respectively (see Table 16-1), only studies that included subjects with musculoskeletal disorders were presented in this chapter because they were considered to be the most relevant to Susan's case (see Table 16-2). Many of the other citations were descriptive articles about magnet therapy or the use of magnets in diagnostic equipment and procedures. A few articles were reports on the application of static magnets in healthy subjects[32] or in subjects with conditions unrelated to Susan's case. The results of these studies have been mixed. For example, when compared with a placebo or control group, researchers have found no significant differences in pain relief in subjects with fibromyalgia[33] or a reduction of hot flashes in women with breast cancer.[34] However, four double-blind pilot studies have provided some evidence to support the application of static magnets for the reduction of pain in subjects with post-polio syndrome,[35] painful diabetic neuropathy,[36] dysmenorrhea,[37] and chronic pelvic pain.[38]

## CLINICAL DECISION MAKING

### Generate a Clinical Hypothesis and Relevant Outcome Measures

A review of the literature supports the therapist's use of static magnets for his clients with musculoskeletal pain. Although no studies have included persons with TMJ pain, the therapist hypothesizes that static magnet use will aid Susan in the management of her pain. Although most of the studies reviewed included the WOMAC index and the VAS as measurement tools for pain, Susan does not have arthritis in the hips or knees, so the WOMAC index is not an appropriate outcome measure to use in her case. The therapist does, however, include a VAS as part of the examination for every client with pain and is able to compare Susan's pain during the initial examination with her pain after five sessions of physical therapy that includes magnets. To determine the long-term effects of magnets, he decides to assess the client's pain 1 week after use of the magnets.

### Intervene and Evaluate

To verify the best way to incorporate static magnets into Susan's plan of care, the therapist reviews the studies that demonstrated an analgesic effect with static magnet use. Fortunately, his application of a 1700G magnet directly over Susan's left TMJ is consistent with the average magnet strength used in the studies. Although a majority of the subjects in the research wore magnets for 24 hours per day, the therapist is aware that the magnet can be only partially hidden by the client's hair and suggests that the magnet be worn as much as possible for the next week.

### Report the Outcomes

The therapist may want to consider writing a case report to describe why magnet therapy was considered for inclusion in a client's plan of care and if the client's outcomes supported the therapist's clinical hypothesis. A description of the therapist's decision-making process regarding magnet strength and application informed by the scientific literature also would be helpful to clinicians who want to use an intervention in a safe and efficacious manner. Dissemination of the therapist's findings can add to the literature on static magnets and encourage a discussion about the use of complementary therapies in the management of TMJ pain and dysfunction. Possible journals for this type of report include *The Journal of Orthopedic and Sports Physical Therapy, Dental Abstracts,* and *The Journal of Orofacial Pain.*

## SUMMARY

In this chapter, Susan presented with chronic jaw pain and was diagnosed with bilateral TMJ syndrome, with the left joint more involved than the right. Mandibular dynamics were observed to be impaired, and trigger nodules were noted in the TMJ and cervical musculature. Susan also experienced decreased cervical range of motion and weakness. After two sessions of physical therapy, which included ultrasound, massage, myofascial release, exercise, and client education, the therapist decided to add a static magnet to Susan's plan of care. After 1 week of wearing the magnet as much as possible and continuing with a home exercise program, Susan reported that her pain had been eliminated. A physical examination also revealed improvement in Susan's strength, range of motion, and mandibular dynamics. Although the therapist was unable to find literature that specifically supported the use of static magnets for persons with TMJ syndrome, several studies that supported the use of magnets for pain relief in persons with musculoskeletal disorders were identified. Evidence-based practice requires health care providers to incorporate their clinical expertise, the client's values and goals, and the results of the best *available* scientific literature into the client's plan of care. In this case, the therapist applied these principles and used literature that supports the analgesic benefits of static magnets in persons with orthopedic conditions to verify his decisions regarding the use, optimal magnet strength, and application protocol for his client.

### REFERENCES

1. Birla GS, Hemlin C: *Magnet therapy: the gentle and effective way to balance body systems,* Rochester, Vt, 1999, Healing Arts Press.

2. Gerber R: *Vibrational medicine for the 21st century*, New York, 2000, Harper Collins.

3. Kahn S: *Healing magnets*, New York, 2000, Three Rivers Press.

4. Lawrence R, Rosch PJ, Plowden J: *Magnet therapy: the pain cure alternative*, Rocklin, Calif, 1998, Prima Health.

5. Null G: *Healing with magnets*, New York, 1998, Carroll & Graf Publishers.

6. Veith I: *The yellow emperor's classic of internal medicine*, Los Angeles, 1970, University of California Press (I. Veith, trans.).

7. Gilbert W: *De magnete*, Mineola, NY, 1958, Dover Publications (P. Fleury Mottelay, trans.).

8. Block G, Meserism A: *Translation of the original scientific and medical writings of F.A. Mesmer, MD*, Los Altos, Calif, 1980, William Kaufman.

9. Elisha Perkins. Wikipedia The Free Encyclopedia. Available at: *http://en.wikipedia.org/w/index. php?title=Elisha_Perkins&oldid=17005121*. Accessed January 4, 2006.

10. National Center for Complementary and Alternative Medicine: Questions and Answers About Using Magnets to Treat Pain. Available at: *http://nccam.nih. gov/health/magnet/magnet.htm* May 2004. Accessed January 4, 2006.

11. Kroeling P, Gross A, Houghton PE: Electrotherapy for neck disorders, *Cochrane Database Syst Rev* 2: CD004251, 2005.

12. Hong CZ et al: Magnetic necklace: its therapeutic effectiveness on neck and shoulder pain, *Arch Phys Med Rehabil* 63:462-6, 1982.

13. Maher CG: Effective physical treatment for chronic low back pain, *Orthop Clin North Am* 35:57-64, 2004.

14. Borenstein DG: Epidemiology, etiology, diagnostic evaluation, and treatment of low back pain, *Curr Opin Rheumatol* 13:128-34, 2001.

15. Barbano R et al: Pharmacotherapy of painful diabetic neuropathy, *Curr Pain Headache Rep* 7:169-77, 2003.

16. Eccles NK: A critical review of randomized controlled trials of static magnets for pain relief, *J Altern Complement Med* 11:495-509, 2005.

17. Ratterman R et al: Evidence-based practice. Magnet therapy: what's the attraction? *J Am Acad Nurs Practitioners* 14:347-53, 2002.

18. Hinman MR: The therapeutic use of magnets: a review of recent research, *Phys Ther Rev* 7:33-43, 2002.

19. McLean M, Engstrom S, Holcomb R: Static magnetic fields for the treatment of pain, *Epilepsy Behav* 2(3, part 2):274-80, 2001.

20. Trock DH: Electromagnetic fields and magnets. Investigational treatment for musculoskeletal disorders, *Rheum Dis Clin North Am* 26:51-62, 2000.

21. Jadad AR et al: Assessing the quality of reports of randomized clinical trials: is blinding necessary? *Control Clin Trials* 17:1-12, 1996.

22. Bernhold M, Bondemark L: A magnetic appliance for treatment of snoring patients with and without obstructive sleep apnea, *Am J Orthod Dentofacial Orthop* 113:144-55, 1998.

23. Wolsko PM et al: Double blind placebo controlled trial of static magnets for the treatment of osteoarthritis of the knee: results of a pilot study, *Altern Ther Health Med* 10:36-43, 2004.

24. Holcomb R, Parker RA, Harrison MS: Bipolar magnets for the treatment of chronic low back pain: a pilot study, *JAMA* 283:1322-25, 2000.

25. Hinman MR, Ford J, Heyl H: Effects of static magnets on chronic knee pain and physical function: a double-blind study, *Altern Ther Health Med* 8:50-5, 2002.

26. Harlow T et al: Randomised controlled trial of magnetic bracelets for relieving pain in osteoarthritis of the hip and knee, *Br Med J* 329:1450-4, 2004.

27. Kanai S et al: Therapeutic effectiveness of static magnetic fields for low back pain monitored with thermogaphy and deep body thermometry, *J Jpn Soc Pain Clin* 5:5-10, 1998.

28. Winemiller MH et al: Effect of magnetic vs. sham-magnetic insoles on plantar heel pain: A randomized controlled trial, *JAMA* 290:1474-8, 2003.

29. Caselli MA et al: Evaluation of magnetic foil and PPT Insoles in the treatment of heel pain. *J Am Podiatr Med Assoc* 87:11-6, 1997.

30. Collacott EZ et al: Bipolar permanent magnets for the treatment of chronic low back pain, *JAMA* 283:1322-5, 2000.

31. Segal NA et al: Two configurations of static magnetic fields for treating rheumatoid arthritis of the knee: a double-blind clinical trial, *Arch Phys Med Rehabil* 82:1453-60, 2001.

32. Cahloupka EC, Kang J, Mastrangelo MA: The effect of flexible magnets on hand muscle strength: a randomized double-blind study, *J Strength Cond Res* 16:33-7, 2002.

33. Alfano AP et al: Static magnetic fields for treatment of fibromyalgia: A randomized controlled trial, *J Altern Complement Med* 7:53-64, 2001.

34. Carpenter JS et al: A pilot study of magnetic therapy for hot flashes after breast cancer, *Cancer Nurs* 25:104-9, 2002.

35. Vallbona C, Hazlewood CF, Jurida G: Response of pain to static magnetic fields in postpolio patients: a double-blind pilot study, *Arch Phys Med Rehabil* 78:1200-3, 1997.

36. Weintraub MI: Alternative medicine. Magnetic bio-stimulation in painful diabetic peripheral neuropathy: A novel intervention—a randomized, double-placebo crossover study, *Am J Pain Manag* 9:8-17, 1999.

37. Eccles NK: A randomized, double-blinded, placebo-controlled pilot study to investigate the effectiveness of static magnet to relieve dysmenorrhea, *J Altern Complement Med* 11:681-7, 2005.

38. Brown CS et al: Efficacy of static magnetic field therapy in chronic pelvic pain: a double-blind pilot study, *Am J Obstet Gynecol* 15:82-7, 2002.

# CHAPTER 17

# Reiki

*Ellen Zambo Anderson, Cindy Wolk-Weiss*

## CASE

Betty is a 63-year-old retired physical therapist who was diagnosed with breast cancer in February 2001. After a right mastectomy and a course of chemotherapy, the oncologist declared her "cured" in June of 2002. The following month Betty underwent breast reconstruction surgery. Subsequent to the surgery Betty began to experience breast pain not relieved with pain medications. Her surgeon was unable to identify any abnormality or pathology that could explain her pain. After reading some scientific literature about CAM and cancer and Reiki, Betty sought Reiki as an approach to help facilitate healing and decrease her pain.

### Initial Examination

*Past Medical History:* Breast cancer, mastectomy, chemotherapy, and reconstructive surgery
*Client Goals:* To reduce pain and improve sense of well-being
*Employment:* Retired physical therapist
*General Health:* Good
*Medication:* None
*Tests and Measures:* In this case, the practitioner is not a licensed health care provider and therefore did not complete a screen or examination of the client's cardiovascular, pulmonary, musculoskeletal, or neuromuscular systems.
*Pain:* The client reported breast pain to be 4/10 at rest and as high as 7/10 during active periods throughout the day.

### Evaluation

Knowing that Betty has no reported contraindications to Reiki, that Reiki has no negative side effects, and that Betty's medical status was being monitored adequately and addressed by her physicians, the practitioner agreed to see Betty for Reiki.

### Plan of Care

Having treated many clients with cancer who benefited physically, psychologically, and spiritually from Reiki, the practitioner saw Betty for two Reiki sessions. The practitioner also recommended that the client become trained in performing self-treatments so that she could apply Reiki to herself between professional sessions. Betty complied with this suggestion and was taught to perform self-Reiki by the Reiki practitioner.

### Reevaluation

The client reported that Reiki was helpful for reducing her pain to 2/10 at rest and 5/10 during activity. Nevertheless, Betty decided that reducing the size of the reconstructive surgical implant might make her even more comfortable. She put Reiki on hold and made an appointment to see her surgeon.

## Incorporating CAM into the Plan of Care

Betty underwent more surgery to have the size of the surgical implant reduced. She returned to the Reiki practitioner 4 weeks later and reported that her pain was once again 3/10 at rest and 7/10 during activity. Because the client had a history of pain relief with Reiki, the practitioner proceeded with providing the client with Reiki.

This chapter is a departure from the other therapy chapters in this book in several ways. First, the physical therapist is the client, not the clinician. Second, the client, not the clinician, searches and evaluates the literature before the decision is made to seek out a Reiki practitioner. Lastly, besides surgery, Reiki is provided as a single intervention by a Reiki practitioner and is not incorporated into a standard plan of care. This chapter provides an example of a knowledgeable healthcare consumer who is interested in receiving CAM and investigates the intervention for safety and efficacy. Details of legal, ethical, and cultural issues related to clients who seek therapies and healthcare considered to be CAM can be found in Chapter 3.

## INVESTIGATING THE LITERATURE

Betty and her physicians had been unable to determine a specific cause for her pain. She had tried pharmacological and physical therapy interventions with little success. After someone in Betty's support group had reported that Reiki helped her to "feel so much better," Betty decided to investigate Reiki and find out if this intervention might help her feel better, too. While reading some background information about cancer and CAM, Betty found survey results, which suggests that individuals with chronic conditions tend to seek the services of complementary practitioners for concerns not adequately addressed by standard health care and because they perceive CAM practitioners to have values and beliefs about health and life congruent with their own.[1-3] Persons with cancer were found to use CAM for a variety of reasons, including wanting to boost their immune system, relieve symptoms, improve their quality of life, feel more hopeful, and achieve greater control in their lives.[4] More specifically, women with breast cancer sought CAM to improve their immunity, quality of life, and sense of control; prevent recurrence of cancer; and enhance their conventional medical care.[5,6] Kelner and Wellman[4] determined that people who specifically seek Reiki treatments do so in an effort to deal with emotional issues, address feelings of low energy, and promote health and well-being. Betty identified with the subjects in these studies and continued to search the literature for studies specifically on Reiki. First, she took a detailed approach in which preliminary reading was performed, followed by a search of databases and evaluation of the reviews and primary sources. Then she performed a more focused search of the literature by using the PICO approach.

### Preliminary Reading

The word *Reiki* comprises the two Japanese characters, *rei*, meaning universal spirit, and *ki*, meaning vital life force or energy.[7] A hands-on healing therapy, Reiki is a therapeutic approach in which the practitioner facilitates the delivery of universal energy to an individual to enhance vitality and promote the body's innate ability to heal. The intention of the Reiki practitioner is to act as a conduit for the delivery of universal energy and thereby replenish and restore energy flow and balance.

Acceptance that a universal life force or energy exists is fundamental to understanding Reiki as a healing modality. This subtle energy, known as *ki* in Japanese, *chi* in Chinese, and *prana* in Sanskrit, is the essence that underlies vitality and intelligence of the universe and everything in it.[8] As a pervasive and infinite energy, ki is organized into energy systems and fields that are penetrable and interactive with each other within individuals and between individuals and the environment, which allows universal energy to be received and exchanged.[7,8] Inadequate life force or an imbalance of energy fields or flow is thought to be associated with conditions of disease and emotional distress, which suggests that energetic patterns should be addressed to create an environment for health and well-being.[8]

The system of Usui Reiki Ryoho grew out of the original teachings of Mikao Usui, a Japanese scholar who was born in 1865. Usui studied Japanese Shinto and old Japanese Tendai Buddhist texts, especially those containing forms of Taoism.[9] Many versions of Reiki's history exist, much of which has been revisited and discussed in a texts by Petter[10] and King.[11] Most persons interested in the origins of Reiki agree, however, that Usui studied, fasted, and meditated to seek an understanding of life. At some point during this quest, probably near or on Mt. Kurama, a sacred, spiritual place near Tokyo, Usui dramatically received a powerful form of energy now known as Reiki.[7] He realized that this energy gave him a remarkable ability to heal and that he could easily transfer the ability to access and use this energy to anyone.

Usui's personal experiences and observations about the healing effects of Reiki helped him to realize that healing the spirit was as important as healing the body. Persons who learned responsibility and gratitude through the energy exchange of Reiki were better prepared to achieve and maintain health than persons who were unable to give back for what they received.[7] So, Usui set out to create a system that would assist a person's spiritual progression, healing the mind first.[9] Five principles of Reiki emerged from Usui's studies, practice, and observations (Figure 17-1).[7]

Usui trained many students and elevated between 15 and 20 to the level of master before his death in 1926. Among them, Dr. Chujiro Hayashi, a naval officer and talented healer, established a healing center in Tokyo. Hayashi had kept detailed records of the teachings and treatments he received and adapted Usui's teachings to include the three degrees and the attunement process.[10,12] Over time, Dr. Hayashi continued to modify his style of training and began to focus

**The Ethical Principles of Reiki**

Just for today, do not worry

Just for today, do not anger

Honor your parents, teachers, and elders

Earn your living honestly

Show gratitude for every living thing

**Figure 17-1** The ethical principles of Reiki.

more on the physical healing nature of Reiki rather than emphasize the original spiritual aspects of Usui's system. As Dr. Hayashi taught Usui's original system and his own modified approach, other master students of Usui such as Toshihiro Eguchi did the same. Following the lineage of Reiki masters and their students is beyond the scope of this chapter, but this information can be found in books written about Reiki[10,11] or on the Reiki Threshold website.[12]

Reiki was brought to the West in 1937 by Mrs. Hwayo Takata, a Japanese emigrant. Takata grew up on the island of Kauai, Hawaii, but returned to Japan to inform her parents of her sister's death and to seek treatment for a tumor, gallstones, and appendicitis. Rather than agree to surgery for her condition Takata went to Dr. Hayashi's Reiki clinic to receive daily Reiki treatment. In 4 months she was healed completely and convinced Hayashi to teach her Reiki. He did and followed her to Hawaii the next year, where he initiated her as a Reiki master. Before her death in 1980, Takata initiated 22 Reiki masters, who in turn have initiated Reiki masters throughout North and South America, Europe, New Zealand, and Australia.[13]

A complete Reiki treatment usually takes between 60 and 90 minutes. During this time, clients or receivers lie or sit in any position that is supported and comfortable. Practitioners then position their hands on or over several areas of the client's body, usually beginning at the head and ending at the feet. The intention of the practitioners is for Reiki energy to be pulled through their hands in direct proportion to the needs of the receiver at each area. The practitioner feels the rise and fall of the energy as it surges through their hands and is mindful when the energy is no longer flowing heavily so that the hands can move to the next position. During a typical Reiki session 10 to 20 different hand positions may be applied (Figures 17-2, 17-3, and 17-4). Some practitioners closely follow a prescribed course of hand positions, whereas advanced practitioners, who are able to intuitively determine areas of the client's body that require Reiki energy, may alter the order or the positions based on the client's needs.[14] Although hand placement over the chakra centers was not in the original teaching of Reiki, many newer Reiki masters have added these positions to their practice. Reiki practitioners recommend persons with chronic conditions receive three to four Reiki treatments in a row so that their body can be energized to its fullest capacity. After the initial series of sessions, fre-

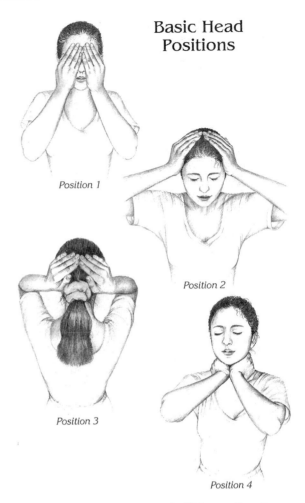

**Basic Head Positions**

*Position 1*

*Position 2*

*Position 3*

*Position 4*

**Figure 17-2** Basic head positions of reiki therapy. (From Petter FA: *Reiki fire,* Twin Lakes, Wisc., 1997, Lotus Light Publications.)

quency of treatment depends on the need of the individual.[14]

Reiki practitioners believe that although everyone has the potential to access Reiki energy, most people are unable to connect with Reiki energy because of a history of trauma, which may have been mental, physical, emotional, or spiritual in nature. This trauma or stress illness has caused energy channels to be blocked. A Reiki master who has been empowered to grant initiations can open these channels and thereby allow Reiki energy to be accessed and received.[7,8] Reiki is taught in three levels or "degrees." Each level includes a series of attunements or initiations intended to open and enhance the channels of Reiki energy within the practitioner.[7,13,14] The first degree of Reiki training usually is taught in four 3-hour sessions. The history and philosophy of Reiki are reviewed, and the stu-

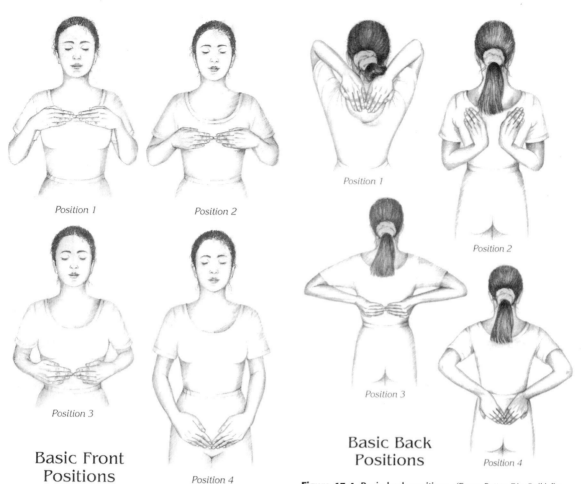

**Figure 17-3** Basic front positions. (From Petter FA: *Reiki fire,* Twin Lakes, Wisc., 1997, Lotus Light Publications.)

**Figure 17-4** Basic back positions. (From Petter FA: *Reiki fire,* Twin Lakes, Wisc., 1997, Lotus Light Publications.)

dents receive four attunements intended to open the higher energy centers including the heart and mind. Once these attunements have been completed, Reiki practitioners believe the student is attuned to Reiki energy for life.[7] Level I training also includes the teaching of the hand positions for working on oneself and others.

Students who complete the first level of Reiki and have a committed practice for several months to a year are eligible to study second-degree Reiki, or Reiki II. Training at the second level enhances the practitioner's ability to perform hands-on treatment through additional attunements. With this training practitioners are better able to assist clients in releasing their habituations and addictions. Level II also includes identification and application of three power symbols that can be used for sending absentee energy and healing intentions.[7]

Third-degree attunement is used to initiate a Reiki master. A final, master symbol, is activated, which increases the power of the practitioner's treatment and is used by the practitioner to help teach Reiki to others.[7,13,14] Reiki treatments do not have to be performed by a Reiki master or by a practitioner who has completed the third-level attunements to be effective. Persons who are interested in teaching Reiki to others, however, should seek well-qualified instructors and consider working with a Reiki master.

Three main organizations seek to promote Reiki as a healing modality and ensure that the principles and teachings of Reiki are taught to others. The Reiki Alliance, which calls its approach to Reiki the *Usui System of Natural Healing,* is headed by Takata's granddaughter and includes several of the original Reiki masters trained by Takata. It is the largest organization of Reiki practitioners. The

American Reiki Masters Association (ARMA) was established by Arthur Robinson, a student of Iris Ishikuro, one of Takata's masters. On her death in 1984, Robinson promised he would work to make Reiki widely available through affordable education and training. The Center for Reiki Training is headed by William Lee Rand and offers Reiki classes and resources for practitioners and clients around the world.[14]

## Searching the Databases

Although good background information about the assumptions, principles, and typical application of Reiki can be found through readily available books and Reiki association websites, the scientific literature was searched to obtain more specific information regarding the application of Reiki for persons with cancer. A review of this literature allowed Betty to learn about the outcome measures that have been used to quantify the benefits of Reiki and if any risks have been identified.

### Critical Reviews

All the evidence-based medicine databases of the Cochrane Library are searched using the key word *Reiki*. Sixteen citations are identified, none of which are a systematic review of Reiki. Several studies included in the Cochrane Central Register of Controlled Trials are about Reiki or distance healing. These articles are scanned for their potential relevance to Betty's goals. The citations for two of the articles are recorded for future reference and reading.[15,16] One of the articles is available online.[17]

### Primary Sources

Additional databases are searched to find case studies, experimental studies, and quasiexperimental studies that include Reiki as the primary inter-vention for persons with pain and/or cancer. Results of the search can be found in Table 17-1. Most of the articles identified by searching the databases are written to provide background information on different approaches of energy medicine, which frequently include Reiki. Several articles, however, are reports of studies conducted by researchers who investigated the possible mechanism[16-18] or outcomes of Reiki.[19-23]

## Evaluating the Literature

Although not all the articles are relevant to Betty's condition or desired outcomes, the volume of literature is small, so all the available articles are reviewed. Shiflett et al[21] conducted a randomized controlled trial (RCT) in which changes in mood were measured, an outcome potentially linked to Betty's goal of enhancing her well-being. The subjects however, were persons diagnosed with a subacute ischemic stroke and not cancer. In this study, subjects received Reiki from either a Reiki master, a first-degree Reiki practitioner, or a sham practitioner. The fourth group included historic controls identified from hospital records. Using the Functional Independence Measure (FIM) and the Center for Epidemiologic Studies-Depression (CES-D) as outcome measures, the authors concluded that Reiki did not appear to be helpful in functional recovery or improvement in mood in persons post stroke.

Another RCT, conducted by Olson, Hanson, and Michaud,[19] included subjects with cancer and pain conditions consistent with Betty's case, although the subjects were considered to be end-stage in the progression of the cancer. The researchers included outcome measures such as pain, quality of life, physiological parameters, and analgesic use more closely aligned with Betty's reasons for seeking Reiki treatments as compared with the outcome

| Table 17-1 | Literature Search Results | | | | |
|---|---|---|---|---|---|
| | ALL EBM DATABASES SECOND QUARTER 2005 | MEDLINE 1966-JUNE 2005 | CINAHL 1982-JUNE 2005 | PSYCINFO 1872-JUNE 2005 | CAM ON PUBMED JUNE 2005 |
| Reiki | 16 | 52 | 137 | 16 | 387* |
| Reiki and cancer | 3 | 4 | 10 | 2 | 10 |
| Reiki and pain | 5 | 11 | 14 | 3 | 16 |

*When limited to "clinical trials" the number of citations was reduced to 44.

tools used for persons post stroke. One group received standard opioid management and rest, the other group received standard opioid management and Reiki. Using the Edmonton Staging System for Cancer Pain and a visual analog scale (VAS), subjects who received Reiki treatments had a significant reduction of pain when compared with subjects who did not receive Reiki, although no differences in analgesic use were observed. These findings were consistent with the results of a pilot study conducted by Olson and Hanson.[20] In addition, subjects who received Reiki had improved scores on the psychological subset of the Quality of Life Measure.

Researchers have investigated the use of Reiki for a person with HIV/AIDs,[22] the combination of Reiki and LeShan for postoperative dental pain,[23] and the combination of Reiki and Transcedental Meditation (TM) for persons with seizure disorders.[18] Although the outcomes from the three studies suggest that Reiki may be helpful in improvement of mood and decrease of pain and seizure activity, these studies have limited validity for supporting Reiki in cases similar to Betty's. Of particular concern is the fact that in two of the studies, Reiki was applied in conjunction with another CAM modality,[18,23] which makes it impossible to determine what effects, if any, were due to the application of Reiki.

Wardell and Engebretson[16] and Mackay, Hansen, and McFarlane[17] studied healthy subjects to investigate the possible mechanism by which Reiki may have an effect. In addition to measuring anxiety, Wardell[16] measured blood pressure, cortisol and secretory IgA levels, and skin temperature and muscle tension, measured through surface electrodes. The results included a decrease in anxiety, systolic blood pressure, and muscle tension, all suggestive of relaxation. A significant increase in the secretory IgA levels indicated a possible increase in immune function. The finding that cortisol levels, which can provide a biochemical measure of stress, were increased for some subjects and decreased for others was not explained by the authors.

Mackay et al[17] did not measure IgA or cortisol, but did measure heart rate (HR), blood pressure (BP), cardiac vagal tone (CVT), cardiac sensitivity to baroreflex (CSB), and respiration rate (RR). In this RCT, in which 45 healthy subjects were divided into three groups, the experimental group received one 30-minute Reiki session, the placebo group received sham Reiki for 30 minutes, and the control group "rested" for 30 minutes. The Reiki and placebo groups had significant changes from baseline, including decreases in HR and RR and increases in CSB and CVT, which suggests that just the presence of a practitioner can influence measures of the autonomic nervous system (ANS). Diastolic BP and mean BP also were decreased significantly in the Reiki group. The authors tested for significant differences *between* the placebo and Reiki groups and found that subjects who received Reiki from a trained practitioner demonstrated significant decreases in HR and diastolic BP as compared with the subjects who received Reiki from a sham or untrained practitioner. The authors suggested that this finding may warrant further exploration into the effects of Reiki on the ANS.

Although the literature on Reiki is somewhat limited, a few interesting observations can be made. First, Reiki has been investigated for its potential mechanism of action in addition to its possible outcomes. Second, Reiki has been investigated in healthy subjects and in subjects with chronic and acute conditions. Last, researchers have begun to investigate standardization procedures that may be done to ensure valid sham Reiki treatments, in an effort to improve the control and quality of future Reiki research.[24]

Betty's status and goals, and the findings from several Reiki studies, suggest that Betty may benefit from receiving Reiki from a qualified practitioner. Although the studies did not include subjects with Betty's specific medical history, Olson et al[19] did demonstrate a significant improvement in psychological scores and a decrease in pain in a sample of subjects who had end-stage cancer. Schmehr[22] also described a decrease in pain with enhanced mood in a case study of a person with HIV/AIDs who had Reiki introduced into his plan of care. Other researchers have found Reiki to be associated with a relaxation response and a reduction of anxiety.[16,17]

A more focused approach for searching the literature is the PICO method. In Betty's situation, this approach would have rendered fewer articles for review and she would not have learned about the levels of training for Reiki practitioners. The PICO method may be a helpful strategy, however, for periodically searching the literature to identify new articles about Reiki, which are relevant to a particular condition.

<table>
<tr><td colspan="2">

## PICO BOX

For persons with cancer does the use of Reiki decrease pain?

P: Persons with cancer
I: Reiki
C: No comparison
O: Reduction of pain

A search combining the terms "Reiki, cancer, and pain" was performed in MEDLINE on September 7, 2007. This search yielded 6 articles. Since the comprehensive search was first conducted in June 2005, only one new article[28] was identified.

---

P = **Population** (Patient/client, problem, person, condition, or group attribute)
I = **Intervention** (the CAM therapy or approach)
C = **Comparison** (standard care or comparison intervention)
O = **Outcome** (the measured variables of interest)

</td></tr>
</table>

## CLINICAL DECISION MAKING

### Generate a Clinical Hypothesis and Relevant Outcome Measures

Betty and the Reiki practitioner have assumed and hypothesized, based on Betty's research and the practitioner's clinical experience, that Reiki would assist Betty in managing her pain and enhance her sense of well-being. Information from several Reiki organizations (see Additional Resources), a variety of books about Reiki, and a few scientific studies have provided some support for this hypothesis. To further test this hypothesis and perhaps advance the literature and practice of Reiki, the practitioner should consider determining Betty's baseline pain and quality of life with standardized measurement tools. The practitioner would then be able to render the tools at predetermined intervals to investigate whether the Reiki sessions are helping the client manage her pain and sense of well-being. From the literature, suggested measurement tools may include the Quality of Life Index for Patients with Cancer,[25] The Edmonton Staging System for Cancer Pain,[26] and a visual analog scale. To administer and interpret the information gained from these tools, the Reiki practitioner may need to collaborate with health care professionals who have expertise in use of these tools.

### Intervene and Evaluate

In this case, Betty sought Reiki from a qualified and experienced Reiki practitioner. Based on her clinical experience, the Reiki practitioner thought Betty could achieve her goals of pain management and an improved sense of well-being through Reiki and proceeded with several Reiki sessions. The client reported that her pain was reduced to a 2/10 after each session and that her pain remained at this level for several days. She returned to the Reiki practitioner for three more sessions over the next 3 months when she felt her pain was increasing and her self-treatment was not always helpful for management of her pain. After one more session, the client reported being essentially pain free. She continued with self-treatment and returned to the Reiki practitioner once every 4 to 6 weeks because she reported that Reiki helped with pain management and was at least in part responsible for an improved sense of well-being. Betty has been pain free for a year and continues to use Reiki as a strategy to enhance her sense of well-being.

Betty's history of cancer and surgery warrant close monitoring of her physical and medical status. She knows that although Reiki may be helping her manage her symptoms, no evidence supports Reiki as a treatment for cancer. She is aware that she should inform her physician about her use of Reiki and to report any new or different observations or complaints to her physician as soon as they occur.

### Report the Outcomes

Betty and the Reiki practitioner should consider collaboration with a researcher in CAM to determine what standardized outcome tools should be used to measure the client's status and offer suggestions regarding the use of those tools. This collaboration also will be helpful for writing a case report that includes specifics regarding the application of Reiki for the management of pain and quality of life in persons with breast cancer. Journals such as *Alternative Therapies in Health and Medicine, Complementary Therapies in Medicine,* and *The Journal of Alternative and Complementary Medicine* may be appropriate publications for this type of report.

### SUMMARY

In this chapter, Betty, a retired physical therapist and breast cancer survivor, investigated the scientific literature about Reiki and found research that offered some support of Reiki as an approach for management of pain and improvement of mood. Based on this literature, Betty decided to use Reiki as an intervention to help manage her pain and sense of well-being. The Reiki practitioner she selected was qualified and experienced in working with clients who had histories of pain and cancer. Betty reported that adding Reiki to her surgical plan of care helped to eliminate her pain and promote a sense of well-being. She continues to use self-administered Reiki energy as a strategy to enhance her quality of life. Betty's case would help to advance the Reiki literature if the practitioner established baseline measures of pain and mood, documented all relevant aspects of the client's plan of care, reevaluated the client's status at regular intervals, and submitted the report for dissemination.

## REFERENCES

1. Vincent C, Furnham A: Why do patients turn to complementary medicine? An empirical study, *Br J Clin Psychol* 35:37-48, 1996.
2. Wolsko PM et al: Use of mind-body medical therapies, *J Gen Intern Med* 19:43-50, 2004.
3. Astin JA: Why patients use alternative medicine: results of a national study, *JAMA* 279:1548-53, 1998.
4. Kelner M, Wellman B: Who seeks alternative health care? A profile of the users of five modes of treatment, *J Altern Compl Med* 3:127-40, 1997.
5. Richardson MA et al: Complementary/alternative medicine use in a comprehensive cancer center and the implications for oncology, *J Clin Oncol* 18:2505-14, 2000.
6. Boon H et al: Use of complementary/alternative medicine by breast cancer survivors in Ontario: prevalence and perceptions, *J Clin Oncol* 18:2515-21, 2000.
7. Horan P: *Empowerment through Reiki,* Twin Lakes, Wis, 2002, Lotus Press.
8. Barnett L, Chambers M: *Reiki: energy medicine,* Rochester, Vt, 1996, Healing Arts Press.
9. Personal communication, Rick Rivard, July 2006.
10. Petter FA: *Reiki fire,* ed 2, Twin Lakes, Wis, 1998, Lotus Press.
11. King D: *O-sensei: a view of Mikao Usui,* China, 2006, Dave King.
12. Rivard RR: Reiki threshold. Available at: *http://www. threshold.ca/reiki/index.html.* Last updated July 6, 2006. Accessed July 12, 2006.
13. Rand WL: *Reiki. The healing touch. 1st & 2nd degree manual,* Southfield, Mich, 1991, Vision Publications.
14. Claire T: *Bodywork: what type of massage to get and how to make the most of it,* New York, 1995, William Morrow and Company.
15. Shore AG: Long-term effects of energetic healing on symptoms of psychological depression and self-perceived stress, *Altern Ther Health Med* 10:42-8, 2004.
16. Wardell DW, Engebretson J: Biological correlates of Reiki Touch (sm) healing, *J Adv Nurs* 33:439-45, 2001.
17. Mackay N, Hansen S, McFarlane O: Autonomic nervous system changes during Reiki treatment: a preliminary study, *J Altern Compl Med* 10:1077-81, 2004.
18. Kumar RA, Kurup PA: Changes in the isoprenoid pathway with transcendental meditation and Reiki healing practices in seizure disorder, *Neurol India* 51:211-4, 2003.
19. Olson K, Hanson J, Michaud M: A phase II trial of Reiki for the management of pain in advanced cancer patients, *J Pain Symptom Manage* 26:990-7, 2003.
20. Olson K, Hanson J: Using Reiki to manage pain: a preliminary report, *Cancer Prev Control* 1:108-13, 1997.
21. Shiflett SC et al: Effect of Reiki treatments on functional recovery in patients in poststroke rehabilitation: a pilot study, *J Altern Complement Med* 8:755-63, 2002.
22. Schmehr R: Enhancing the treatment of HIV/AIDS with Reiki training and treatment, *Altern Ther Health Med* 9:120-1, 2003.
23. Wirth DP et al: The effect of complementary healing therapy on postoperative pain after surgical removal of impacted third molar teeth, *Complement Ther Med* 1:133-8, 1993.
24. Mansour AA et al: A study to test the effectiveness of placebo Reiki standardization procedures developed for a planned Reiki efficacy study, *J Altern Complement Med* 5:1531-64, 1999.
25. Padilla GV et al: Quality of life index for patients with cancer, *Res Nurs Health* 6:117-26, 1983.
26. Bruera E et al: The Edmonton staging system for cancer pain: preliminary report, *Pain* 37:203-9, 1989.
27. Samarel N, Tulman L, Fawcett J: Effects of two types of social support and education on adaptation to early-stage breast cancer, *Res Nurs Health* 25:459-70, 2002.
28. Tsang KL, Carson LE, Olson K: Pilot crossover trial of Reiki versus rest for treating cancer-related fatigue. *Integ Cancer Ther* 6:25-35, 2007.

## ADDITIONAL RESOURCES
### Reiki Organizations
The Reiki Alliance
204 N. Chestnut Street
Kellogg, ID 83837
Phone: (208) 783-3535

The American Reiki Masters Association
(ARMA)
P.O. Box 130
Lake City, FL 32056-0130
Phone: (904) 755-9638

The International Center for Reiki Training
21421 Hilltop Street, Unit #28
Southfield, MI 48034
Phone (toll free): (800) 332-8112
(local): (248) 948-8112

# CHAPTER 18

## Manipulative and Body-Based Therapies

*Judith E. Deutsch*

In this chapter manipulative and body-based therapies are defined and briefly described. These therapies first are discussed relative to the priorities of the National Center for Complementary and Alternative Medicine (NCCAM). Then the quantity and quality of evidence to support the therapies are evaluated. Entire books are devoted to this topic; therefore this chapter is intended only as an introduction.[1]

## DEFINITIONS AND USE

Manipulative body-based therapies are one of the five domains of the NCCAM classification.[2] Manipulative and body-based methods (which in this chapter are referred to as *manual body-based therapies, or MBB therapies*) in complementary and alternative medicine (CAM) are based on manipulation and/or movement of one or more parts of the body. The domain is divided into three categories: osteopathy, chiropractic, and massage and

bodywork. An overview of this domain can be found on the NCCAM website.[3]

The manual body-based (MBB) therapies share the assumption that manipulation or mobilization of the musculoskeletal system (bones, joints, muscle, fascia, and lymph tissue) changes the structure (anatomy) and function (physiology) of the body. Changes in turn may alleviate symptoms related to pathology or eliminate the source of the symptoms. MBB therapies often are applied to manage pain conditions, which are reported to be among the top five reasons individuals seek CAM practitioners (when prayer and megavitamins are excluded from the analysis).[4] Specifically, in the United States individuals seek CAM for back (16.8%), neck (6.6%), joint pain (4.9%), and arthritis (4.9%).[4]

People in the United States visit MBB practitioners frequently. Use of these therapies has been reported to range from 3% to 16% of adults in the United States who receive chiropractic treatment to about 2% to 14% who receive massage therapy in a given year.[3] An early study identified that visits to chiropractors and massage therapists accounted for 50% of the visits to CAM practitioners in 1998.[5] More recent reports show that chiropractic care (7.5%) and massage (5%) are among the top 10 complementary therapies used in the United States.[4] As a domain 10.9% of Americans reported using MBB therapies.[4] However, use of MBB therapies such as Pilates or Rolfing may be underestimated because specific bodywork therapies were not included in this study.

## Osteopathy

Osteopathy is a distinct branch of medicine that in part emphasizes diseases arising from the musculo-skeletal system. This system of practice has been described in detail by Gallagher and Humphrey[6] and is synthesized from their book in this chapter. Dr. Andrew Still, the founder of osteopathy, was trained as a bone-setter. He developed a foundation tenet of the practice about the relationship of structure and function.[7] He viewed the musculoskeletal system as central to the individual's ability to take action.[8] Current teaching of osteopathy is broadened beyond the biomechanical-neuromusculoskeletal to include other models that describe human physiological function and dysfunction. These include the behavioral, energy expenditure and exchange, nutritional, and respiratory-circulatory models.[8]

Osteopaths are trained in manual techniques called *osteopathic manual techniques* (OMTs). OMTs are direct (body part taken in the direction of restriction) or indirect (body part taken in the direction of ease of motion). OMTs applied at the level of the tissue, such as soft tissue and lymphatic treatments, are designed to alter the tone of tissue and increase lymphatic drainage and flow. OMTs at the level of the fascia, such as myofascial release, use the nervous and respiratory systems as a guide for application of the manual technique either directly or indirectly. OMTs at the level of the muscle, such as muscle energy techniques, use the active contraction of the muscle, followed by a stretch to release tissue restrictions. OMTs, such as strain and counterstrain, are based on positioning, in which the passive positioning of the body is used to normalize proprioceptive inputs that may be facilitating the somatic dysfunction. Finally osteopathic manipulations, also named *high-velocity, low-amplitude thrusts*, are applied to restore joint alignment, decrease muscle tension, and stabilize

neural and vascular systems.[8] In all these techniques there is clearly an interplay between the nervous and musculoskeletal systems.

The general approach to apply the OMTs is to position the body and use the manual techniques to change the autonomic nervous system tone to produce tissue relaxation and to increase motion and decrease pain. Ultimately this is done to restore homeostasis in the body so that it may heal itself. These concepts are shared by many of the tissue-based approaches discussed later in this chapter and detailed in the specific therapy chapters found in this section of the book.

Osteopathic medicine as it is practiced in the United States today overlaps with allopathic medicine. Doctors of osteopathy practice in most of the same settings as allopathic MDs. The manual therapy elements of osteopathy are the reason it is listed as a CAM.

## Chiropractic

Chiropractic is an alternative medical system. The originator of this approach, Dr. Palmer, founded the profession in 1895.[9] Like other therapies in the MBB category chiropractic has an emphasis on structure and function. Chiropractors, like osteopaths, believe that disease processes can manifest in the neuromusculoskeletal system and cause somatic dysfunction. Chiropractors, however, emphasize the role of the spinal nerves more than osteopaths. The focus of chiropractic practice is to determine where and when spinal manipulative therapy (SMT) is appropriate and how to then apply an adjustment.[9] Adjustments are in the form of spinal manipulations. The chiropractic examination focuses primarily on joint asymmetry and restrictions, and treatment most often consists of thrust joint manipulation. High-velocity, low-thrust manipulations are the application of a high force applied typically directly over the spine.[10]

Chiropractors now believe that most diseases cannot be cured by spinal manipulation. They now focus their treatments to specifically address spinal impairments.[11] A detailed report on chiropractic and it application to low back pain (LBP) can be found on the NCCAM website.[12] Techniques such as mobilization and muscle energy, used by osteopaths and chiropractors, also are used by physical therapists. In addition, there are derivative approaches from osteopathy and chiropractic such as craniosacral therapies (Chapter 22); these are described in more detail in individual therapy chapters.

## Spinal Manipulation

Spinal manipulation is a specific technique in which the articular capsule is stretched passively by delivering a quick thrust maneuver to the joint.[11] Spinal manipulation techniques are practiced by osteopaths, chiropractors, and other health care practitioners such as physical therapists. Some evidence exists that these techniques originated in Thailand around 1000 BC and in ancient Egypt.[11]

Although not identified as a discrete category of MBB therapies by the NCCAM, spinal manipulation is discussed separately. The rationale for this is based on comprehensiveness of searching and defining a technique that crosses many disciplines. Spinal manipulation is a unique MESH term that yields additional references that would not be found if the search included only chiropractic and osteopathic terms. As such, identification of the complete data set of articles makes interpretation of the application of spinal manipulation techniques comprehensive. The definitions of spinal manipulation by osteopaths have been described in previous sections. The definitions of mobilization and manipulation used by physical therapists can be found in the *Guide to Physical Therapist Practice*.[13] Spinal manipulation is a broad definition describing a continuum of skilled passive movements to the joints and surrounding soft tissues, applied at varying speeds and amplitudes, which include small-amplitude, high-velocity therapeutic movement.[13]

## Massage

Massage is defined by the NCCAM as an assortment of techniques involving manipulation of the soft tissues of the body through pressure and movement.[14] Massage is an ancient healing art that is shared by most of the whole medical systems (traditional Chinese medicine [TCM], Ayurveda, Native American medicine) in addition to Western medicine.

The transfer of massage to the West from China is attributed to French missionaries in the early nineteenth century, who brought Chinese medical books dating to 2700 BC. Many of the terms for massage strokes (effleurage, petrissage) are therefore in French. Massage was incorporated into medical gymnastics in Sweden in the early 1800s and exported to other parts of Europe in the mid-1800s and then New York in 1916. In the United States massage was formalized by Mary McMillan,

who at the time was director of physical therapy at Harvard University.[15]

Massage techniques and applications are varied. Explanations for the effects of massage have been categorized as mechanical, reflex, physiological, psychological, and psychoneuroimmunological.[16,17] Techniques were classified by Andrade and Clifford[18] by the level of the work and the mechanism of action. They are the following:

1. Superficial reflex techniques that stimulate the skin and produce reflex effects such as analgesia
2. Superficial fluid techniques at the level of the skin, superficial fascia, subcutaneous fat, and deep fascia that produce mechanical effects
3. Neuromuscular techniques affecting the muscle and tissue
4. Connective tissue techniques, which involve mechanical stimulation of superficial and deep connective tissue
5. Passive movement techniques that produce tissue and joint motion and affect the fluid flow, connective tissue, and muscle tone
6. Percussive techniques that affect a variety of tissues, depending on the vigor of the stroke[18]

The proposed benefits of massage can be grouped into physiological and psychological effects. These have been summarized by deDomenico and include increased blood and lymph flow, removal of metabolites, resolution of edema, increased extensibility of connective tissue, pain relief, increased joint movement, improved muscle activity, stimulation of autonomic function, removal of lung secretion, and general relaxation.[16] Because massage is regularly included in physical therapy training, it is not covered in detail in this book. For additional textbooks dedicated to massage, refer to the reference section at the end of the chapter.[16,18]

## Bodywork Therapies

Bodywork therapies were identified in early NCCAM classification schemes. These therapies overlap in part with massage and therefore may not be considered by the NCCAM as a separate category. Here they are distinguished from each other for purposes of clarity. Bodywork techniques can be described as being tissue based or movement based.[19] Tissue-based approaches have more in common with massage than movement-based approaches. Tissue-based approaches are those in which work is done directly on the soft tissues of the body. In tissue-based approaches structure is changed to improve function. In contrast, movement-based approaches attend to posture and movement as a means of changing function, which will then have an effect on structure. Many of the approaches discussed in the specific therapies section of this book are movement based, such as Feldenkrais (Chapter 20), Alexander (Chapter 21) and Pilates (Chapter 23). Others are predominantly tissue based such as Rolfing (Chapter 19) and cranial sacral therapy (CST) (Chapter 22). However, some of these therapies, such as Rolfing, involve an interplay between tissue and movement work.

## NATIONAL CENTER FOR COMPLEMENTARY AND ALTERNATIVE MEDICINE RESEARCH PRIORITIES

MBB therapies have not been studied as extensively as other CAM therapies. The NCCAM has identified the following goals for MBB therapy in its 2005-2009 strategic plan[20]:

1. Elucidate mechanisms of action operative in manipulative and body-based practices
2. Determine the disorders and states of wellness for which selected manipulative and body-based practices may offer meaningful benefits and specify the optimal circumstances under which the chosen manipulative and body-based practices are performed
3. Study manipulative and body-based practices to determine their potential therapeutic or wellness benefits
4. Determine the extent to which client expectations before treatment and satisfaction after manipulative and body-based practices are related to objectively measured biological endpoints[20]

Consistent with their strategic plan the NCCAM either has funded or currently is funding a variety of trials in the MBB therapy areas. A search of the NCCAM clinical trials database on currently and previously funded studies indicated a preponderance of massage (15) trials and fewer chiropractic (5), spinal manipulation (4), and osteopathic manipulation (3) trials.[21] No trials were performed on bodyworks.

Massage is being evaluated for its effects on a wide range of clients and conditions. These range from low–birth-weight, preterm infants to people with chronic musculoskeletal pain or pain produced by cancer, sickle cell disease, and HIV to individuals who experience cancer-related fatigue.[22]

Chiropractic research has focused on pain from the low back, migraines, or the temporomandibular joint.[23] Osteopathic research has focused on pulmonary disease, ear infection, and muscle tension for children with cerebral palsy.[24]

In 2005 the National Center for Complementary and Alternative Therapies Institute held a conference on the Biology of Manual Therapies. This group recommended new directions for researching the biological basis of manual therapies.[25] Their recommendations related to understanding the neural, immune, and musculoskeletal basis of manual therapies likely will influence future funding of MBB therapy research.

## INVESTIGATING AND EVALUATING THE LITERATURE

A large discrepancy exists regarding the quantity and quality of the literature published about MBB therapies. A search was conducted using MEDLINE and CINAHL to provide an overview of the state of the literature in these areas. It was limited from 1981 to July 2006. The search terms entered were the names of the therapies outlined in the first column of Table 18-1. These included osteopathy, chiropractic, spinal manipulation (searched Oct 23, 2006), massage, Alexander, Feldenkrais, Rolfing, CST, and Pilates. These terms were selected to parallel the chapters covered in this section. Two different databases were chosen to identify differences in the medical and allied health literatures. Time frames were matched to allow for comparison between the databases. In addition the searches were limited to evidence-based reviews and clinical trials in an effort to qualify the state of the literature. Table 18-1 summarizes the findings of the search.

A review of the table identifies massage as having the greatest number of citations and evidence-based reviews in MEDLINE. In contrast the greatest number of references on chiropractic can be found in the CINAHL database. The importance of searching several databases to identify which may have relevant information is highlighted by the discrepancy in the quantity of articles identified for chiropractic.

A similar format is used to comment on the quality and nature of the findings for each of the topics searched. First, the Cochrane Review findings are reported. Second are comments regarding the randomized clinical trials. This is done using an organization that first reports on outcome studies,

| Table 18-1 | Literature Search Results | | | |
|---|---|---|---|---|
| | MEDLINE | EBM REVIEWS | CLINICAL TRIAL | CINAHL |
| Osteopathic | 2388 | 6 | 40 | 733 |
| Chiropractic | 3260 | 11 | 134 | 10,592 |
| Spinal manipulation | 980 | 7 | 156 (18 CCT) | 461 |
| Massage | 4517 | 20 | 425 (28 CCT) | 3062 |
| Alexander | 24 | 1 | 1 | 56 |
| Feldenkrais | 25 | 0 | 2 | 68 |
| Rolfing | 11 | 0 | 1 | 39 |
| Craniosacral | 12 | 0 | 3 | 129 (43 PR) |
| Pilates | 14 | 0 | 0 | 120 |

*EBM,* Evidence-based medicine (in MEDLINE). *CCT,* Search limited to controlled clinical trials. *PR,* Search limited to peer-reviewed journal.
Search was conducted from 1981 through July 2006 for all terms except the spinal manipulation search was continued through Oct 23, 2006.

followed by validity and reliability studies, and concluding with mechanistic studies. The intent of the following sections is to provide an overview of the literatures, not an in-depth analysis.

## Osteopathy

The terms *osteopathic medicine, osteopathic manipulation,* and *osteopathy* are used in the search for articles related to osteopathy. A total of six Cochrane reviews are found. (Ten total were found, but some were older versions of the same topic.) The Cochrane review articles emphasize two areas in which osteopathy was applied: asthma[26] and dysmenorrhea.[27] Overall no evidence suggests that spinal manipulation is effective for the treatment of primary and secondary dysmenorrhea.[27] Furthermore, insufficient evidence supports or refutes the use of manual therapies for clients with asthma.[26] The reviews were concluded with a familiar recommendation for the need to conduct adequate-size RCTs that examine the effects of manual therapies on clinically relevant outcomes.

Fifty-six clinical trials are found, of which 40 are relevant to osteopathic medicine. Clinical trials are carried out in three general areas: *outcome* trials that evaluated the efficacy and effectiveness of OMT for various conditions, *reliability* studies about cranial sacral constructs, and *mechanistic* studies about osteopathy. Each of these is presented separately.

*Outcomes* of OMT were assessed on a wide range of conditions from musculoskeletal, cardiovascular, and pulmonary to psychological. Osteopathy was reported to improve the functional and impair-

ment level outcomes of clients after hip and knee arthroplasty[28] and to decrease the needs for pain medication postsurgically.[29] Improved short-term and long-term outcomes were reported for clients who received OMT for ankle sprains in the emergency room.[30] The breadth of application of OMTs ranged from the management of depression[31] to reduction of otitis media recurrence.[32]

Osteopathy outcomes also were reported in the cardiovascular and pulmonary domain. OMTs have been shown to improve peak expiratory flow rates in children with asthma[33] and to increase in upper and lower thoracic forced respiratory excursion in adults with asthma.[34] Spinal manipulation also has been studied as an intervention for individuals with hypertension.[35] In a group of hospitalized elderly with acute pneumonia, the use of OMT significantly decreased length of stay and use of antibiotic therapy.[36]

For the management of musculoskeletal and neuromuscular pain, many clinical trials were found, in which osteopathy was compared with other interventions. Results were often favorable for OMT, with some exceptions. For example, OMT produced a similar outcome (reduction of leg pain, back pain, and self-reported disability) to chemonucleosis for individuals with symptomatic lumbar disc herniation who were followed for 12 months[37] and in the management of chronic shoulder pain in the elderly who were managed with standard care.[38] In studies in which clinical outcomes were similar to comparison therapies, authors noted that costs for OMT were lower. This was the case in the use of OMT for clients with subacute back pain, in whom OMT and clinical care had the same clinical results, but use of medication was greater by clients in standard care[39] and for clients with spinal pain followed in primary care.[40] In other instances, however, OMT for chronic nonspecific LBP was not better than the sham condition, although it was better than control,[41] and similarly OMT was found to be the same as shortwave diathermy in the management of nonspecific back pain.[42]

The addition of OMT to the standard of care was reported for conditions that were not related to musculoskeletal pain. For example, OMT (myofascial release and strain counterstrain techniques) was applied to clients with pancreatitis, who were discharged earlier than those receiving standard of care alone.[43] Individuals with fibromyalgia who received OMT added to their standard of care reported a decrease in their pain threshold and perceived pain and improved activities of daily living and perceived functional ability more than those who received only standard care.[44] An interesting report of parents' perception of OMT compared with acupuncture in the management of children with cerebral palsy also was available.[45]

Intrarater and interrater reliability of several cranial sacral concepts associated with OMT was studied. In general, the reliability of intrarater and interrater was found to be poor. Specifically, poor reliability was reported for interexaminer and intraexaminer reliability of the "primary respiratory mechanism,"[46] palpation of the cranial sacral rhythm (CSR),[47] and the relationship of the CSR to respiratory rates.[48] The poor reliability reported in these studies relates to some of the more subtle aspects of measurement in OMT associated with CST.

*Mechanistic* studies examined immune and neurochemical explanations for osteopathic efficacy. The involvement of the endocannabinoid system as an explanation for analgesia was explored.[49] In a double-blind, randomized study the authors reported significant increases for cannabimimetic descriptors on the drug reaction scale for the post-OMT group, which also were associated with blood serum changes.[49] Cutaneous blood flow in the corresponding dermatome was monitored after unilateral high-velocity, low-amplitude thrusts to the lumbosacral junction.[50] The authors reported increases in blood perfusion ipsilaterally and contralaterally, which they interpreted as increased sympathetic outflow resulting from the manipulation.[50] The immune response to an influenza vaccine given in conjunction with OMT also was

explored.[51] An interesting study documented EMG changes consistent with reports of pain reduction associated with menstrual cramping.[52]

In summary, the greatest number of studies related to osteopathy, found in MEDLINE, reported on outcomes related to the application of manipulation to the management of musculoskeletal pain. Outcomes also were reported for the management of cardiovascular and pulmonary in addition to other medical conditions. Outcome studies appear promising. The osteopathy literature also includes studies that address measurement of the CSR construct, which shows poor reliability and mechanistic study that begin to provide neural and immune system explanations for the outcome studies.

## Chiropractic

Searching the terms *chiropractic* and *chiropractic manipulation* in MEDLINE (1981 to 2006) yields 11 Cochrane reviews. Six are the same Cochrane reviews found in the osteopathy search. Five additional reviews include chiropractic as one option for exercise for mechanical disorders of the cervical spine,[53] management of nocturnal enuresis for children,[54] nonsurgical treatment for carpal tunnel syndrome (CTS),[55] and client education and physical modalities for mechanical neck disorders.[56,57] The findings were the following:

- The management of cervical spine disorders responded best to strengthening and combined stretching, but results indicated that mobilization and manipulation in combination with exercise were indicated for cervical pain with and without a headache.[53]
- Chiropractic manipulation was better than sham.[54]
- No benefit was demonstrated for chiropractic in CTS.[55]

The chiropractic techniques were not identified discretely in the two reviews on mechanical neck disorders, which makes it difficult to evaluate those studies relative to chiropractic.[56,57]

Chiropractic clinical trials were carried out in three areas: outcomes research, validation and reliability of osteopathic concepts, and measurements and mechanistic studies. Each area is discussed separately.

The majority of outcome studies focused on the use of chiropractic for the management of LBP. Often these studies compared chiropractic with either physical therapy or standard of care. In an early study published in the *British Medical Journal* chiropractic manipulation was found to be superior to "medical care" using Maitland manipulation or mobilization.[58] Similar findings were reported in a subsequent study when mobilization and manipulation were compared with physical therapy (exercise, massage, and modalities) for clients with chronic low back and cervical pain.[59] In a third study chiropractic manipulation and physical therapy (McKenzie approach) were both found to have comparable outcomes better than client education for individuals with LBP.[60] Most recently findings from the UCLA study have attempted to control for many of the variations in care compared in earlier studies. The UCLA group reported that individuals who received medical care compared with chiropractic care had comparable outcomes in terms of pain complaints and disability. A small decrease in disability occurred for those clients who received medical care and physical therapy.[61] The challenge with interpretation of many of these studies is the different operational definitions of the treatments, in particular those of physical therapy.

Outcome studies also were reported in nonmusculoskeletal areas. These included the application of chiropractic techniques to pediatric clients to alleviate asthma,[62] and a feasibility study for children with otitis media.[63] Chiropractic manipulation combined with nutrition education was found to be comparable with nutrition education provided by a dietitian in the management of hypertension.[64]

Validation and reliability studies were reported in the chiropractic literature. Most of these studies were published in the *Journal of Manipulative and Physiological Therapeutics*. Validation studies were performed on clinical tests for joint dysfunction compared with an x-ray gold standard[65] for measurement tools to quantify cervical range of motion[66] in addition to the pressure of palpation.[67] Studies also were performed to validate sham manipulation procedures that could be used in clinical trials.[68] An effort was made to validate chiropractic constructs such as the cavitation sound that occurs during an adjustment.[69] Reliability studies were performed to test instrument consistency of a spinal compliance meter,[70] interrater and intrarater reliability for determining axial rotations and lateral bending,[71] and interrater and intrarater reliability of a multidimensional spinal diagnostic method commonly used by chiropractors to identify if manipulation is indicated for individuals with chronic LBP,[72] in addition to manual techniques.[73]

Reliability ratings were good to excellent for the rotation tests[71] but poor for the spinal diagnostic method[72] and manual techniques.[73]

Mechanistic studies of chiropractic have focused on the elucidation of underlying neural and musculoskeletal physiology. The neuromuscular reflex response associated with the mechanical force of manually assisted SMT was elucidated by measurement of electromyography during thrusting procedures of the spine.[74] The relationship between pain reduction and spinal manipulation was studied, and experimenters found a small but statistically significant increase in serum beta-endorphin levels in the spinal manipulation group compared with the sham and control groups.[75] In a third study the investigators found that when they induced acute inflammatory pain in the forearms, individuals in the spinal manipulation group experienced less pain and secondary hyperalgesia and allodynia compared with the group that did not receive spinal manipulation. In the absence of blood flow changes the investigators interpreted the effects of the manipulation to be central in origin.[76]

In summary, the comparisons between chiropractic and other modalities to manage LBP show that these techniques can reduce pain and disability but may not be superior to other forms of management, such as physical therapy.[77] Reliability of measurement ranged from poor for manual diagnostics and therapeutics to good for some measurement devices. Mechanisms underlying chiropractic techniques may be neuromusculoskeletal. Of interest is a report from the UCLA group on adverse events. A greater number of adverse events were reported for chiropractic manipulation than for mobilization in individuals with cervical spine pain.[78] The suggestion by the investigators was that chiropractors may choose to use mobilization of the cervical spine over manipulation.

## Spinal Manipulation

Six Cochrane reviews (a total of 10 were found but some were updates on previous reviews) were identified. Of these some overlap occurred with the specific therapy searches, such as the effect of spinal mobilization on LBP. Spinal manipulation was not found to be superior in the relief of acute and chronic LBP when compared with general practitioner care, back school, exercise, physical therapy, or analgesics.[77]

Importantly an article not identified in the chiropractic and osteopathic searches was found that dealt with the use of physiotherapy and manipulation for chronic, recurrent headaches.[79] Chronic headaches were categorized into five types: migraine, tension-type, cervicogenic, a mix of migraine and tension-type, and post-traumatic headache. Support for spinal manipulation for the prophylactic treatment of cervicogenic headache (although this was also the case for low-intensity exercise) was reported. In this review spinal manipulation was not as effective as amitriptyline in the prophylactic management of tension-type headaches; however, short-term effects were stronger for spinal manipulation once treatment was discontinued. No support was found for spinal manipulation for episodic tension-type headache.[79]

In an effort to synthesize the findings across all of the spinal manipulation studies, Ernst and Canter performed a systematic review of the systematic reviews.[80] This review included 15 systematic reviews (not all of them from the Cochrane databases) that related to a variety of conditions: back pain (2), neck pain (2), lower back and neck pain (1), headache (3), nonspinal pain, (1) primary and secondary dysmenorrhea (1), infantile cholic (1), asthma (1), allergy (1), cervicogenic disease (1), and any medical condition (1). The authors concluded that the findings in support for spinal manipulation were largely negative, with the exception of LBP. For people with LBP spinal manipulation appears to be better than a sham condition but comparable to conventional treatments. One of the challenges with evaluation of the effects of spinal manipulation on individuals with LBP is the selection of clients for these studies. Clinical prediction rules that will classify clients to identify them as candidates for manipulation have been validated.[81] Appropriate selection of candidates for spinal manipulation studies may resolve the ambiguous findings.

Clinical trials that evaluated spinal mobilizations were many. Of interest was a comparison between treatment administered by a chiropractor and by a physical therapist.[82] The two groups exhibited no differences in outcomes of pain, health status, and cost. At follow-up, however, subgroups emerged that benefited more from either chiropractic (current pain episode of less than 1 week) or physical therapy (current pain episode of greater than 1 month). More people sought additional treatment in the chiropractic (59%) than the physical therapy (41%) group.[83] These data reinforce the need to classify and triage clients appropriately for spinal manipulation and perhaps evaluate differ-

ences in how these techniques are delivered as part of a comprehensive plan of care.

Ernst reported adverse events for spinal mobilization of the cervical spine.[84] The incidence was high in approximately 50% of the clients who received spinal manipulation but the adverse events were reported to be transient. Serious complications, such as vertebrobasilar accidents, disc herniations, and cauda equina syndrome, occurred in the range of one to two per million manipulations.

To summarize, the literature on spinal manipulation overlaps with that of chiropractic and osteopathy but does have discrete articles associated with it. It appears that application of spinal manipulation for LBP has some promise, and care should be taken to apply manipulation to the cervical spine.

## Massage

The term *massage* was used to search MEDLINE on July 10, 2006. The search yielded 20 reviews from the Cochrane database. Four of these were related to asthma[26] and overlapped with the chiropractic and osteopathic searches. The breadth of the reviews on massage was much greater than either osteopathy or chiropractic.

Cochrane reviews either refuted or did not find support of the use of massage in five articles. Massage was not supported in its application to promote growth and development of preterm babies in either the original[85] or follow-up review.[86] Findings on deep transverse friction massage for the management of tendonitis pain were inconclusive because of small sample sizes.[87] Massage along with all other approaches covered in the review also was found to be inconclusive when used in treatment of adults with upper extremity disorders.[88] Applying massage for well-being and quality of life in clients with lung cancer was inconclusive, with small but not long-lasting effects of reflexology.[89]

Support for massage, in some cases qualified, was found in five of the Cochrane reviews. Massage applied to clients with subacute and chronic nonspecific LBP may be beneficial, especially when combined with exercises and education.[90] Massage was implicated as possibly explaining positive effects of topical agents applied to reduce breast engorgement.[91] Ice massage compared with control was reported to have a statistically beneficial effect on ROM function and knee strength for people with osteoarthritis (OA) of the knee.[92] In clients with cancer, massage and aromatherapy massage had short-term benefits on psychological well-being. The effect on anxiety and physical symptoms was supported by limited evidence. Evidence was mixed regarding whether aromatherapy enhanced the effects of massage.[93] One of the most definitive findings on massage was its application to the perineum before birth. It reduced the likelihood of perineal trauma (mainly episiotomies) and the reporting of ongoing perineal pain. The authors also reported that the massage generally was well accepted by women.[94]

The data set for clinical trials about massage was so large (427) that it was further limited to controlled clinical trials (45) for further review and evaluation. Of these only 29 were relevant to this chapter. The studies could be characterized as focusing on outcomes, validation, or mechanism. Many variations on massage existed.

*Outcome* studies focused on the use of massage to decrease pain and improve well-being. The application of massage ranged from the management of postoperative pain using hand massage and reflexology,[95] to the management of encopresis and chronic constipation in children,[96] to the reduction of nocturnal enuresis.[97] Massage was found to be effective in the first two studies but not in the latter. Massage prevented the deterioration in sleep for cancer clients in an oncology unit who were receiving chemotherapy or radiation.[98] Massage applied by the parents decreased the anxiety of parents and children with contact dermatitis. In addition the children improved significantly on all clinical measures, including redness, scaling, lichenification, excoriation, and pruritus.[99] Negative findings for reflexology were reported for postacute abdominal surgery clients.[100]

Massage was applied in isolation but often in combination with other therapies such as breathing and client education. This was the case, for example, in the application of massage and breathing to decrease pain perception during labor[101] or in combination with aromatherapy to decrease agitation in clients with dementia,[102] and in combination with music therapy to increase weight gain and decrease hospital stays for preterm infants.[103] When compared with other therapies massage was not always found to be the most effective intervention. For example, in the management of chronic neck pain, acupuncture was found to be superior to massage.[104]

The only *validation* study found in this subset of studies was on reflexology. Two experienced reflex-ologists compared their diagnoses to the client's known medical conditions. Using receiver operator curves the investigators found that their diagnostic accuracy was poor. Reliability of the findings also was low.[105]

*Mechanistic* studies implicated the neural, musculoskeletal, and immune systems. Links between the benefits of massage and changes in the immune system were found in a group of women with breast cancer who massaged their breasts. An increase in natural killer (NK) cells and lymphocytes in addition to decreases in depressed moods and anxiety was reported.[106] In men with HIV infections who received massages, a correlation between significant decreases in anxiety with increases in NK cells was reported. They also found a decrease in blood cortisol levels.[107] Newborns massaged by their mothers were found to have a better sleep cycle, which was attributed to effects of rhythms on melatonin secretion of the massaged infants.[108] Modulation of the ANS system was implicated in a study with a controlled cutaneous stimulus that simulated massage. The authors reported nonspecific effects such as temperature increases in addition to specific effects such decreased muscle tension (at least for some muscle sites) and increased sympathetic activation.[109]

In summary, massage was studied in a variety of ways and for diverse conditions. It was used in isolation or in combination with other therapies to reduce anxiety and pain and to promote relaxation. The neural, musculoskeletal, and immune systems were shown to be modulated by massage. When compared with other interventions such as acupuncture for pain reduction, it was not as effective.

## Bodywork Therapies

The literature commented on in this section is sparse. Because each of these therapies has a specific chapter in which the literature relative to the case is reviewed, here only a brief comment on the remaining literature is included. The reader is referred to the individual therapy chapters for richer detail on the therapy and the relevant literature.

The terms searched for the bodywork section corresponded to each of the approaches (Alexander technique, Feldenkrais method, Rolfing, CST, and Pilates) covered in the individual therapy chapters (see Table 18-1). In contrast with osteopathy, chiropractic, and massage, the quantity of the body of literature about bodywork was reduced. Notable in many of the therapies there were more references in CINAHL than in MEDLINE. With the exception of the Alexander technique[110] no Cochrane or reviews on bodywork therapies and few clinical trials were found. The literature indexed in PubMed and EMBASE on movement awareness therapies was reviewed and evaluated by Mehling, DiBlasi, and Hecht.[111] They identified limitations in the literature that included lack of blinding, credible placebos, and poor recruitment.[111]

The application of the Alexander technique (AT) to a client with OA of the knee is presented in Chapter 21. Additional literature is commented on here. AT was evaluated in a critical review by Ernst and Canter.[112] They found that AT was effective in the management of people with Parkinson's disease (PD)[113] and LBP.[114] For the individuals with PD a program of AT improved the Self-Assessment Parkinson's Disease Disability Scale scores at people's best and worst times, the group was less depressed and had an improved attitude relative to those individuals who did not receive the AT.[113] Other work that was not included in the Ernst review is of interest because it was designed to test some of the assumptions of the AT. A Cochrane review of use of AT to improve breathing for people with asthma found no evidence to support the claim.[110] In contrast, healthy people who received 20 AT lessons demonstrated improvements across a series of pulmonary function tests, which included peak expiratory flow, mean expiratory and inspiratory pressures, and mean ventilatory volume.[115] Most recently a case report illustrated the connection between decreases in pain and improvements in postural coordination for an individual with chronic LBP.[116] (For more information on AT, see Chapter 21.)

The literature on the Feldenkrais method (FM) applied to a client with multiple sclerosis and balance data is discussed in Chapter 20. The search performed for this overview chapter identified some of the evidence for FM that can be applied to other client populations. For example, the use of FM has been proposed for children with cerebral palsy.[117] Clients with dystonia reported that FM was among the most effective therapies they used.[118] Individuals with nonspecific musculoskeletal disorders reported improved health-related quality of life and self-efficacy of pain in FM and body awareness therapy groups compared with conventional physical therapy.[119] FM was included as a part of a multimodal intervention for people with eating disorders. The goal was to "normalize" a distorted body image. Individuals in the FM group showed greater comfort with the problematic zones of their body and their own health as well as accepting their own body.[120] Cost effectiveness was demonstrated with the addition of FM to the management of clients with LBP.[121]

Studies on healthy people were few. In one a single session of FM was reported to enhance mood. Similar findings were obtained for yoga and swimming but not aerobic dancing or computer use.[122] FM use of sensory imagery was shown to enhance forward reach, which validates the construct that sensory retraining can improve movment.[123] For more information on FM, see Chapter 20.

The literature on Rolfing or the Ida Rolf Method of Structural Iintegration is covered in Chapter 19.

CST and its application to a person with thoracic pain and Meniére's disease are discussed in Chapter 22. The search for this overview chapter yielded a few references in MEDLINE and more than 100 in CINAHL. When these were limited to peer-reviewed articles, the total was 43 (see Table 18-1). Among these articles was a systematic review of CST that evaluated the biological basis, assessment reliability, and clinical effectiveness.[124] The authors concluded that low-grade evidence supports clinical efficacy, and reliability of measurement was poor.[124] Some of the assumptions of CST were supported partially by the review, namely that minute movements occur between cranial bones and that cerebrospinal fluid flows in a pulsing, rhythmic manner. Importantly the authors pointed out that what is missing from the literature is the relationship between cranial bone movement and cerebrospinal fluid flow patterns.[124] CSTs also were included in two more recent reviews of manual therapies.[125,126] For the management of chronic LBP it was determined that CST has unknown efficacy.[126] For the reducing pain from tension-type headache was a single high-quality study that demonstrated positive outcomes for the CV4 CST.[127] For more information on CST assumptions and clinical approach refer to Chapter 22.

Pilates concepts and their application to a client are discussed in Chapter 23. The literature on Pilates in MEDLINE was limited. It consisted of an editorial in *The Lancet*,[128] a couple of general information papers in the *Harvard Women's Newsletter*,[129] two case reports,[130,131] one quasiexperimental study,[132] and a study in which Pilates was part of a regimen to improve athletic performance.[133] Although modest, the literature describes the intervention and lends some support for the assump-

Derby Hospitals NHS Foundation Trust
Library and Knowledge Service

tions of using core muscles to stabilize the trunk and improve motor performance.[133] This, in turn, could alleviate pain.[130] For more information on Pilates see Chapter 23.

## SUMMARY

MBB therapies consist of different approaches and techniques that focus primarily on the structures and systems of the body, including the bones and joints, the soft tissues, and the circulatory and lymphatic systems. The goal of these therapies is to restore structures to their proper alignment and physiological homeostasis to improve function. Each approach varies in intent and application. Some focus more on the skeletal structures, others on the soft tissues, and yet others on posture and movement. The NCCAM has identified these therapies as worthy of study from mechanistic and outcomes perspectives.

The literature on osteopathy, chiropractic, and massage is of greater quantity and quality than that of bodywork therapies. Outcome, mechanistic, and reliability studies were found in all of the literatures, although in differing amounts. The chiropractic literature had an abundance of studies concerned with validation of fundamental concepts and techniques. The massage and osteopathic literatures had more articles on outcomes. A search of these literatures revealed that studies overlapped in the MBB therapies. This was particularly true in the area of manipulation that is practiced by chiropractors, osteopaths, and physical therapists. Information regarding client selection methods and clear definition of techniques rather than approach-specific terms are needed to advance the literature. Collectively the literature points to use of MBB therapies for pain reduction in some chronic musculoskeletal conditions (especially LBP) and movement efficiency and reeducation in some neurological conditions. However, much remains to be elucidated in terms of mechanism. Studies in which MBB therapies are compared with each other and with other complementary therapies are also underway.

## REFERENCES

1. Coughlin P: *Principles and practice of manual therapeutics,* Philadelphia, 2002, Churchill Livingstone.
2. NCCAM Definitions. Available at: *http://nccam. nih.gov/health/whatiscam/#4.* Accessed March 28, 2006.
3. NCCAM: Manipulative and Manual Body Based Practices. Available at: *http://nccam.nih.gov/health/ backgrounds/manipulative.htm.* Accessed April 4, 2006.
4. Barnes PM et al: Complementary and alternative medicine use among adults: United States, 2002, *Adv Data* 343:1-19, 2004.
5. Eisenberg DM et al: Trends on alternative medicine use in the United States, 1990-1997, *JAMA* 280(18):1569-74, 1998.
6. Gallagher RM, Humphrey FJ: *Osteopathic medicine: a reformation in progress,* New York, 2001, Churchill Livingstone.
7. Osborn GG: The beginning: nineteenth century medical sectarianism. In Humphrey FJ, Gallagher RM, editors: *Osteopathic medicine: a reformation in progress,* New York, 2001, Churchill Livingstone, pp 3-29.
8. Jones JM: The present: osteopathic philosophy. In Humphrey FJ, Gallagher RM, editors: *Osteopathic medicine: a reformation in progress,* New York, 2001, Churchill Livingstone, pp 29-56.
9. Redwood D: Chiropractic. In Miccozi MS, editor: *Fundamentals of complementary and integrative medicine,* ed 3, St Louis, 2006, Saunders Elsevier, pp 139-63.
10. Vickers A, Zollman C: ABC of complementary medicine. The manipulative therapies: osteopathy and chiropractic, *Br Med J* 319(7218):1176-9, 1999.
11. Edmond SL: *Mobilization/manipulation, extremity and spinal techniques,* ed 2, St Louis, 2006, Elsevier.
12. NCCAM: Research Report About Chiropractic and Its Use in Treating Low-Back Pain. Available at: *http://nccam.nih.gov/health/chiropractic/#14.* Accessed April 5, 2006.
13. Guide to Physical Therapist Practice, ed 2, *Physical Therapy* 81:9-744, 2001.
14. NCCAM: Definition of Massage on the Manipulative and Body Based Therapies: An Overview Page. Available at: *http://nccam.nih.gov/health/ backgrounds/manipulative.htm.* Accessed April 17, 2006.
15. Holey ECE: *Evidence-based therapeutic massage: a practical guide for therapists,* New York, 2003, Churchill Livingstone.
16. deDomenico GEW: Mechanical, physiological, psychological, therapeutic effects. In *Beards massage,* ed 4, Philadelphia, 1997, WB Saunders, pp 55-71.
17. Tappan FM: The mind body connection. In *Healing massage techniques: holistic, classic and emerging methods,* ed 2, Norwalk, Conn, 1988, Appleton-Lange, pp 35-41.
18. Andrade CK CP: Conceptual frameworks for outcomes based massage. In *Outcome-based massage,* Baltimore, Md, 2001, Lippincott Williams and Wilkins, pp 12-4.

19. Deutsch JE: Introduction to manual and body based approaches, *Holistic Health*, 2002.

20. NCCAM: Expanding Horizons of Health Care: Strategic Plan 2005-2009: U.S. Department of Health and Human Services, National Institutes of Health, 2005.

21. NCCAM: All NCCAM Clinical Trials. Available at: http://nccam.nih.gov/clinicaltrials/alltrials.htm. Accessed March 28, 2006.

22. Medicine NLo. Massage Clinical Trials.gov. Available at: *http://clinicaltrials.gov/search/term=(NCCAM)+%5BSPONSOR%5D+(massage)+%5BTREATMENT%5D?recruiting=false*. Accessed March 28, 2006.

23. Medicine NLo. Chiropractic Clinical Trials.gov. Available at: *http://clinicaltrials.gov/search/term=(NCCAM)+%5BSPONSOR%5D+(chiropractic+therapy)+%5BTREATMENT%5D?recruiting=false*. Accessed March 28, 2006.

24. Medicine NLo. Osteopathy Clinical Trials.gov. Available at: *http://clinicaltrials.gov/search/term=(NCCAM)+%5BSPONSOR%5D+(osteopathic+manipulation)+%5BTREATMENT%5D?recruiting=false*. Accessed March 28, 2006.

25. Khalsa PS et al: The 2005 Conference on the Biology of Manual Therapies, *J Manipulative Physiol Ther* 29(5):341-6, 2006.

26. Hondras MA, Linde K, Jones AP: Manual therapy for asthma [update of Cochrane Database Syst Rev. 2002;(4):CD001002; PMID: 12519548] *Cochrane Database Syst Rev* 2:CD001002, 2005.

27. Proctor ML et al: Spinal manipulation for primary and secondary dysmenorrhoea [update of Cochrane Database Syst Rev. 2001;(4):CD002119; PMID: 11687141] *Cochrane Database Syst Rev* 3:CD002119, 2004.

28. Jarski RW et al: The effectiveness of osteopathic manipulative treatment as complementary therapy following surgery: a prospective, match-controlled outcome study, *Altern Ther Health Med* 6(5):77-81, 2000.

29. Goldstein FJ et al: Preoperative intravenous morphine sulfate with postoperative osteopathic manipulative treatment reduces patient analgesic use after total abdominal hysterectomy, *J Am Osteopath Assoc* 105(6):273-9, 2005.

30. Eisenhart AW, Gaeta TJ, Yens DP: Osteopathic manipulative treatment in the emergency department for patients with acute ankle injuries, *J Am Osteopath Assoc* 103(9):417-21, 2003.

31. Plotkin BJ et al: Adjunctive osteopathic manipulative treatment in women with depression: a pilot study, *J Am Osteopath Assoc* 101(9):517-23, 2001.

32. Mills MV et al: The use of osteopathic manipulative treatment as adjuvant therapy in children with recurrent acute otitis media, *Arch Pediatr Adolesc Med* 157(9):861-6, 2003.

33. Guiney PA et al: Effects of osteopathic manipulative treatment on pediatric patients with asthma: a randomized controlled trial, *J Am Osteopath Assoc* 105(1):7-12, 2005.

34. Bockenhauer SE et al: Quantifiable effects of osteopathic manipulative techniques on patients with chronic asthma, *J Am Osteopath Assoc* 102(7):371-5, 2002.

35. Morgan JP et al: A controlled trial of spinal manipulation in the management of hypertension, *J Am Osteopath Assoc* 85(5):308-13, 1985.

36. Noll DR et al: Benefits of osteopathic manipulative treatment for hospitalized elderly patients with pneumonia, *J Am Osteopath Assoc* 100(12):776-82, 2000.

37. Burton AK, Tillotson KM, Cleary J: Single-blind randomised controlled trial of chemonucleolysis and manipulation in the treatment of symptomatic lumbar disc herniation, *Eur Spine J* 9(3):202-7, 2000.

38. Knebl JA et al: Improving functional ability in the elderly via the Spencer technique, an osteopathic manipulative treatment: a randomized, controlled trial, *J Am Osteopath Assoc* 102(7):387-96, 2002.

39. Andersson GB et al: A comparison of osteopathic spinal manipulation with standard care for patients with low back pain, *New Engl J Med* 341(19):1426-31, 1999.

40. Williams NH et al: Cost-utility analysis of osteopathy in primary care: results from a pragmatic randomized controlled trial, *Fam Pract* 21(6):643-50, 2004.

41. Licciardone JC et al: Osteopathic manipulative treatment for chronic low back pain: a randomized controlled trial, *Spine* 28(13):1355-62, 2003.

42. Gibson T et al: Controlled comparison of shortwave diathermy treatment with osteopathic treatment in non-specific low back pain, *Lancet* 1(8440):1258-61, 1985.

43. Radjieski JM, Lumley MA, Cantieri MS: Effect of osteopathic manipulative treatment on length of stay for pancreatitis: a randomized pilot study, *J Am Osteopath Assoc* 98(5):264-72, 1998. (Erratum, *J Am Osteopath Assoc* 98[7]:408, 1998.)

44. Gamber RG et al: Osteopathic manipulative treatment in conjunction with medication relieves pain associated with fibromyalgia syndrome: results of a randomized clinical pilot project, *J Am Osteopath Assoc* 102(6):321-5, 2002.

45. Duncan B et al: Parental perceptions of the therapeutic effect from osteopathic manipulation or acupuncture in children with spastic cerebral palsy, *Clin Pediatr* 43(4):349-53, 2004.

46. Sommerfeld P, Kaider A, Klein P: Inter- and intraexaminer reliability in palpation of the "primary respiratory mechanism" within the "cranial concept," *Manual Ther* 9(1):22-9, 2004.

47. Moran RW, Gibbons P: Intraexaminer and interexaminer reliability for palpation of the cranial rhythmic impulse at the head and sacrum, *J Manipulative Physiol Ther* 24(3):183-90, 2001.

48. Hanten WP et al: Craniosacral rhythm: reliability and relationships with cardiac and respiratory rates, *J Orthop Sports Phys Ther* 27(3):213-8, 1998.

49. McPartland JM et al: Cannabimimetic effects of osteopathic manipulative treatment, *J Am Osteopath Assoc* 105(6):283-91, 2005.

50. Karason AB, Drysdale IP: Somatovisceral response following osteopathic HVLAT: A pilot study on the effect of unilateral lumbosacral high-velocity low-amplitude thrust technique on the cutaneous blood flow in the lower limb, *J Manipulative Physiol Ther* 26(4):220-5, 2003.

51. Noll DR et al: The effect of osteopathic manipulative treatment on immune response to the influenza vaccine in nursing home residents: a pilot study, *Altern Ther Health Med* 10(4):74-6, 2004.

52. Boesler D et al: Efficacy of high-velocity low-amplitude manipulative technique in subjects with low-back pain during menstrual cramping, *J Am Osteopath Assoc* 93(2):203-8, 1993.

53. Kay TM et al: Exercises for mechanical neck disorders, *Cochrane Database Syst Rev* 3:CD004250, 2005.

54. Glazener CMA, Evans JHC, Cheuk DKL: Complementary and miscellaneous interventions for nocturnal enuresis in children, *Cochrane Database Syst Rev* 2:CD005230, 2005.

55. O'Connor D, Marshall S, Massy-Westropp N: Nonsurgical treatment (other than steroid injection) for carpal tunnel syndrome, *Cochrane Database Syst Rev* 1:CD003219, 2003.

56. Gross AR et al: Physical medicine modalities for mechanical neck disorders, *Cochrane Database Syst Rev* 2:CD000961, 2000.

57. Gross AR et al: Patient education for mechanical neck disorders, *Cochrane Database Syst Rev* 2:CD000962, 2000.

58. Meade TW et al: Low back pain of mechanical origin: randomised comparison of chiropractic and hospital outpatient treatment, *Br Med J* 300(6737):1431-7, 1990.

59. Koes BW et al: A randomized clinical trial of manual therapy and physiotherapy for persistent back and neck complaints: subgroup analysis and relationship between outcome measures, *J Manipulative Physiol Ther* 16(4):211-9, 1993.

60. Cherkin DC et al: A comparison of physical therapy, chiropractic manipulation, and provision of an educational booklet for the treatment of patients with low back pain, *New Engl J Med* 339(15):1021-9, 1998.

61. Hurwitz EL et al: A randomized trial of medical care with and without physical therapy and chiropractic care with and without physical modalities for patients with low back pain: 6-month follow-up outcomes from the UCLA low back pain study, *Spine* 27(20):2193-204, 2002.

62. Bronfort G et al: Chronic pediatric asthma and chiropractic spinal manipulation: a prospective clinical series and randomized clinical pilot study, *J Manipulative Physiol Ther* 24(6):369-77, 2001.

63. Sawyer CE et al: A feasibility study of chiropractic spinal manipulation versus sham spinal manipulation for chronic otitis media with effusion in children, *J Manipulative Physiol Ther* 22(5):292-8, 1999.

64. Goertz CH et al: Treatment of hypertension with alternative therapies (THAT) study: a randomized clinical trial, *J Hypertens* 20(10):2063-8, 2002.

65. Fernandez-de-las-Penas C et al: Validity of the lateral gliding test as tool for the diagnosis of intervertebral joint dysfunction in the lower cervical spine, *J Manipulative Physiol Ther* 28(8):610-6, 2005.

66. Agarwal S, Allison GT, Singer KP: Validation of the spin-T goniometer, a cervical range of motion device, *J Manipulative Physiol Ther* 28(8):604-9, 2005.

67. Marcotte J, Normand MC, Black P: Measurement of the pressure applied during motion palpation and reliability for cervical spine rotation, *J Manipulative Physiol Ther* 28(8):591-6, 2005.

68. Vernon H et al: Validation of a sham manipulative procedure for the cervical spine for use in clinical trials, *J Manipulative Physiol Ther* 28(9):662-6, 2005.

69. Beffa R, Mathews R: Does the adjustment cavitate the targeted joint? An investigation into the location of cavitation sounds, *J Manipulative Physiol Ther* 27(2):e2, 2004.

70. Leach RA, Parker PL, Veal PS: PulStar differential compliance spinal instrument: a randomized interexaminer and intraexaminer reliability study, *J Manipulative Physiol Ther* 26(8):493-501, 2003.

71. Janik T et al: Reliability of lateral bending and axial rotation with validity of a new method to determine axial rotation on anteroposterior cervical radiographs, *J Manipulative Physiol Ther* 24(7):445-8, 2001.

72. French SD, Green S, Forbes A: Reliability of chiropractic methods commonly used to detect manipulable lesions in patients with chronic low-back pain, *J Manipulative Physiol Ther* 23(4):231-8, 2000.

73. Schops P, Pfingsten M, Siebert U: Reliability of manual medical examination techniques of the cervical spine. Study of quality assurance in manual diagnosis, *Zeitschrift fur Orthopadie und Ihre Grenzgebiete* 138(1):2-7, 2000.

74. Colloca CJ, Keller TS: Electromyographic reflex responses to mechanical force, manually assisted

spinal manipulative therapy, *Spine* 26(10):1117-24, 2001.

75. Vernon HT et al: Spinal manipulation and beta-endorphin: a controlled study of the effect of a spinal manipulation on plasma beta-endorphin levels in normal males, *J Manipulative Physiol Ther* 9(2):115-23, 1986.

76. Mohammadian P et al: Areas of capsaicin-induced secondary hyperalgesia and allodynia are reduced by a single chiropractic adjustment: a preliminary study, *J Manipulative Physiol Ther* 27(6):381-7, 2004.

77. Assendelft WJJ et al: Spinal manipulative therapy for low back pain, *Cochrane Database Syst Rev* 1: CD000447, 2004.

78. Hurwitz EL et al: Adverse reactions to chiropractic treatment and their effects on satisfaction and clinical outcomes among patients enrolled in the UCLA Neck Pain Study, *J Manipulative Physiol Ther* 27(1):16-25, 2004.

79. Bronfort G et al: Non-invasive physical treatments for chronic/recurrent headache, *Cochrane Database Syst Rev* 3:CD001878, 2004.

80. Ernst E, Canter PH: A systematic review of systematic reviews of spinal manipulation, *J Royal Soc Med* 99(4):192-6, 2006.

81. Cleland JA et al: The use of a lumbar spine manipulation technique by physical therapists in patients who satisfy a clinical prediction rule: a case series, *J Orthop Sports Phys Ther* 36(4):209-14, 2006.

82. Skargren EI et al: Cost and effectiveness analysis of chiropractic and physiotherapy treatment for low back and neck pain. Six-month follow-up, *Spine* 22(18):2167-77, 1997.

83. Skargren EI, Carlsson PG, Oberg BE: One-year follow-up comparison of the cost and effectiveness of chiropractic and physiotherapy as primary management for back pain. Subgroup analysis, recurrence, and additional health care utilization, *Spine* 23(17):1875-84, 1998.

84. Ernst E: Manipulation of the cervical spine: a systematic review of case reports of serious adverse events, 1995-2001, *Med J Austral* 176(8):376-80, 2002.

85. Vickers A et al: Massage for promoting growth and development of preterm and/or low birth-weight infants, *Cochrane Database Syst Rev* 2:CD000390, 2000.

86. Vickers A et al: Massage for promoting growth and development of preterm and/or low birth-weight infants, *Cochrane Database Syst Rev* 2:CD000390, 2004.

87. Brosseau L et al: Deep transverse friction massage for treating tendinitis, *Cochrane Database Syst Rev* 4:CD003528, 2002.

88. Verhagen AP et al: Ergonomic and physiotherapeutic interventions for treating upper extremity work related disorders in adults, *Cochrane Database Syst Rev* 1:CD003471, 2004.

89. Sola I et al: Non-invasive interventions for improving well-being and quality of life in patients with lung cancer, *Cochrane Database Syst Rev* 4: CD004282, 2004.

90. Furlan AD et al: Massage for low back pain, *Cochrane Database Syst Rev* 2:CD001929, 2002.

91. Snowden HM, Renfrew MJ, Woolridge MW: Treatments for breast engorgement during lactation, *Cochrane Database Syst Rev* 2:CD000046, 2001.

92. Brosseau L et al: Thermotherapy for treatment of osteoarthritis, *Cochrane Database Syst Rev* 4: CD004522, 2003.

93. Fellowes D, Barnes K, Wilkinson S: Aromatherapy and massage for symptom relief in patients with cancer, *Cochrane Database Syst Rev* 2:CD002287, 2004.

94. Beckmann MM, Garrett AJ: Antenatal perineal massage for reducing perineal trauma, *Cochrane Database Syst Rev* 1:CD005123, 2006.

95. Wang H-L, Keck JF: Foot and hand massage as an intervention for postoperative pain, *Pain Manag Nurs* 5(2):59-65, 2004.

96. Bishop E et al: Reflexology in the management of encopresis and chronic constipation, *Paed Nurs* 15(3):20-1, 2003.

97. Sietam KS, Eriksen L: Zone therapy of children with nocturnal enuresis, *Ugeskrift for Laeger* 160(39):5654-6, 1998.

98. Smith MC et al: Outcomes of therapeutic massage for hospitalized cancer patients, *J Nurs Scholar* 34(3):257-62, 2002.

99. Schachner L et al: Atopic dermatitis symptoms decreased in children following massage therapy, *Ped Dermatol* 15(5):390-5, 1998.

100. Kesselring A: Foot reflexology massage: a clinical study, *Forschende Komplementarmedizin* 6(suppl 1):38-40, 1999.

101. Yildirim G, Sahin NH: The effect of breathing and skin stimulation techniques on labour pain perception of Turkish women, *Pain Res Manag* 9(4):183-7, 2004.

102. Snow LA, Hovanec L, Brandt J: A controlled trial of aromatherapy for agitation in nursing home patients with dementia, *J Altern Complement Med* 10(3):431-7, 2004.

103. Whipple J: The effect of parent training in music and multimodal stimulation on parent-neonate interactions in the neonatal intensive care unit, *J Music Ther* 37(4):250-68, 2000.

104. Konig A et al: Randomised trial of acupuncture compared with conventional massage and "sham" laser acupuncture for treatment of chronic neck pain—range of motion analysis, *Zeitschrift fur Orthopadie und Ihre Grenzgebiete* 141(4):395-400, 2003.

105. White AR et al: A blinded investigation into the accuracy of reflexology charts, *Comp Ther Med* 8(3):166-72, 2000.

106. Hernandez-Reif M et al: Natural killer cells and lymphocytes increase in women with breast cancer following massage therapy, *Int J Neurosci* 115(4):495-510, 2005.

107. Ironson G et al: Massage therapy is associated with enhancement of the immune system's cytotoxic capacity, *Int J Neurosci* 84(1-4):205-17, 1996.

108. Ferber SG et al: Massage therapy by mothers enhances the adjustment of circadian rhythms to the nocturnal period in full-term infants, *J Dev Behav Pediatr* 23(6):410-5, 2002.

109. Naliboff BD, Tachiki KH: Autonomic and skeletal muscle responses to nonelectrical cutaneous stimulation, *Percept Mot Skills* 72(2):575-84, 1991.

110. Dennis J: Alexander technique for chronic asthma, *Cochrane Database Syst Rev* 2:CD000995, 2000.

111. Mehling WE, DiBlasi Z, Hecht F: Bias control in trials of bodywork: a review of methodological issues, *J Altern Complement Med* 11(2):333-42, 2005.

112. Ernst E, Canter PH: The Alexander technique: a systematic review of controlled clinical trials, *Forschende Komplementarmedizin und Klassische Naturheilkunde* 10(6):325-9, 2003.

113. Stallibrass C, Sissons P, Chalmers C: Randomized controlled trial of the Alexander technique for idiopathic Parkinson's disease, *Clin Rehabil* 16(7):695-708, 2002.

114. Elkayam O et al: Multidisciplinary approach to chronic back pain: prognostic elements of the outcome, *Clin Exper Rheumatol* 14(3):281-8, 1996.

115. Austin JH, Ausubel P: Enhanced respiratory muscular function in normal adults after lessons in proprioceptive musculoskeletal education without exercises, *Chest* 102(2):486-90, 1992.

116. Cacciatore TW, Horak FB, Henry SM: Improvement in automatic postural coordination following Alexander technique lessons in a person with low back pain, *Phys Ther* 85(6):565-78, 2005.

117. Liptak GS: Complementary and alternative therapies for cerebral palsy, *Ment Retard Dev Disabil Res Rev* 11(2):156-63, 2005.

118. Junker J et al: Utilization and perceived effectiveness of complementary and alternative medicine in patients with dystonia, *Mov Disord* 19(2):158-61, 2004.

119. Malmgren-Olsson E-B, Branholm I-B: A comparison between three physiotherapy approaches with regard to health-related factors in patients with non-specific musculoskeletal disorders, *Disabil Rehabil* 24(6):308-17, 2002.

120. Laumer U et al: Therapeutic effects of the Feldenkrais method "awareness through movement" in patients with eating disorders, *Psychotherapie, Psychosomatik, Medizinische Psychologie* 47(5):170-80, 1997.

121. Lake B: Acute back pain. Treatment by the application of Feldenkrais principles, *Aust Fam Physician* 14(11):1175-8, 1985.

122. Netz Y, Lidor R: Mood alterations in mindful versus aerobic exercise modes, *J Psychol* 137(5):405-19, 2003.

123. Dunn PA, Rogers DK: Feldenkrais sensory imagery and forward reach, *Percept Mot Skills* 91(3 Pt 1):755-7, 2000.

124. Green C et al: A systematic review of craniosacral therapy: biological plausibility, assessment reliability and clinical effectiveness, *Complement Ther Med* 7(4):201-7, 1999.

125. Fernandez-de-Las-Penas C et al: Are manual therapies effective in reducing pain from tension-type headache? A systematic review, *Clin J Pain* 22(3):278-85, 2006.

126. Maher CG: Effective physical treatment for chronic low back pain, *Orthop Clin North Am* 35(1):57-64, 2004.

127. Hanten WP et al: The effectiveness of CV-4 and resting position techniques on subjects with tension-type headaches, *J Manipulative Therapeutics* 7:64-70, 1999.

128. Shand D: Pilates to pit, *Lancet* 363(9418):1340, 2004.

129. Conditioning by Pilates, *Harv Women's Health Watch* 6(5):7, 1999.

130. Blum CL: Chiropractic and pilates therapy for the treatment of adult scoliosis, *J Manip Physiol Ther* 25(4):E3, 2002.

131. Lugo-Larcheveque N et al: Management of lower extremity malalignment during running with neuromuscular retraining of the proximal stabilizers, *Curr Sports Med Rep* 5(3):137-40, 2006.

132. Segal NA, Hein J, Basford JR: The effects of Pilates training on flexibility and body composition: an observational study, *Arch Phys Med Rehabil* 85(12):1977-81, 2004.

133. Hutchinson MR et al: Improving leaping ability in elite rhythmic gymnasts, *Med Sci Sports Exerc* 30(10):1543-7, 1998.

# CHAPTER 19

## The Ida Rolf Method of Structural Integration

*Judith E. Deutsch*

Susan Greene is an 11-year-old girl who was born prematurely and exhibited delayed motor development. She was diagnosed with spastic diplegic cerebral palsy at 10 months. She was referred to physical therapy (PT) with complaints of low back pain (LBP) and difficulty with walking long distances and going up the stairs.

### ■ Initial Examination

**Client Report:** Susan has had LBP for 4 months since she began middle school. She also reports that the distance to ambulate in the school and the number of stairs she has to climb have increased relative to elementary school.

**Client Goals:** Reduce pain, increase ability to efficiently navigate through school environment, including stairs

**Recreational Activities:** Swimming

**General Health:** Good; she is pre-menses

**Medications:** None

**Cardiopulmonary:** Decreased lateral expansion of chest observed at rest and unchanged with deep breathing; circumferential chest measurement 30 inches; reports fatigue at the end of school and sometimes needs to take a nap

**Musculoskeletal Posture:** Pelvic obliquity, excessive lumbar lordosis, adduction, and internal rotation of the lower extremities. Range of motion (ROM): positive Thomas test, hip flexion is 20 to 120 degrees right side and 30 to 120

degrees on the left side. Hip abduction: 0 to 10 degrees (right), 0 to 5 degrees (left); dorsiflexion 0 degrees bilaterally

**Neuromuscular:** Force generation: Left knee and hip extension 3+/5 and right are 4/5; rectus abdominis and obliques are 2/5. Upper extremity strength is within functional limits. Resistance to passive movement of adductors and internal rotators is 1+ on Ashworth Scale.[1,2] Pain Visual Analogue Scale (VAS) is a 4 to 5/10 for her lower back at the end of the day, especially after prolonged walking.

**Function:** Ambulates in school pain free until third period, when symptoms begin. Timed up and go (TUG)[3] used to measure ambulation speed on 10-meter walk test was 10.9 seconds. She required 25 seconds to ascend and descend one flight of nine steps. Independent with activities of daily living (ADL), except donning and doffing shoes requires minimum assistance. On the Gross Motor Function Classification Scheme (GMFCS) she is a Level II.[4]

### ■ Evaluation and Plan of Care

Susan presents with musculoskeletal, cardiopulmonary, and neuromuscular impairments that may be causing her low back symptoms and limited ambulation. Her physical therapy program is designed to reverse some of those impairments and provide task-specific training to improve functional mobility. The plan includes prolonged stretching of erector spinae, quadratus lumborum, and lower extremity tight muscles, lower extremity and abdominal strengthening using endurance training on a bicycle, and incentive spirometry. Ambulation speed and distance at school will be monitored and timed by wearing a pedometer. Stretching and strengthening program to be executed daily with assistance of parent and reevaluation in 2 weeks.

### Reevaluation

After 2 weeks little change has occurred in lower extremity passive and active ROM. Steps in an average day are 7000. Mother feels that the daughter has difficulty complying with stretching. Client reports she likes the strengthening and bike activities, and her symptoms at school are coming on after fourth period.

### Incorporating Cam into the Plan of Care

The therapist hypothesizes that the client's posture and alignment are contributing to her LBP complaints. Because the client is reporting difficulty with stretching the therapist is considering recommending the Ida Rolf Method of SI method to comprehensively address the range and posture deficits. This SI program will complement the existing strength and endurance program.

This chapter describes the case of an 11-year-old child with spastic diplegic cerebral palsy who received the Ida Rolf Method of Structural Integration (SI) to reduce musculoskeletal impairments that were interfering with functional mobility. The therapist who treated the child collaborates with a clinician scientist who studies the use of SI combined with physical therapy for rehabilitation populations. The treating therapist and clinician scientist use resources easily available in the published literature and resources from the organizations that train both SI and Rolfing practitioners to decide if a series of SI sessions should be added to the plan of care.

## INVESTIGATING THE LITERATURE

The therapist uses two strategies to investigate the literature. The first is a detailed approach in which preliminary background reading is performed on the Ida Rolf Method of SI. This is followed by a search of databases and evaluation of the literature using reviews and primary sources for Rolfing (the term SI is not used for searching as it yields many irrelevant sources), cerebral palsy, and pain. The second is the use of the PICO format for a focused search to answer the clinical questions generated by the case.

## Preliminary Reading

The therapist collaborates with a clinician scientist who is familiar with SI because she has performed some research in the area. The preliminary reading provided to the therapist by the scientist consists of writings by Ida Rolf, who is the originator of the approach. Rolf's theoretical framework and concepts supporting the method first were described in an article[5] and then elaborated on in her book, *Rolfing: The Integration of Human Structures.*[6] Additional information about the approach can be gained from a book in which Rolf is interviewed about Rolfing.[7] Other useful sources are brief descriptions of the approach found on the websites of the two main organization that train practitioners, the Guild for Structural Integration and the Rolfing Institute[8,9]; a three-part series on SI published by a Rolfing practitioner in the *Journal of Body Work Movement Therapies*[10-12]; and chapters written in bodywork[13] and complementary therapy books.[14,15]

The Ida Rolf Method of Structural Integration is practiced by individuals trained in two schools of the approach. Members of the Rolfing Institute are called *Rolfers*, and members of the Guild for Structural Integration (SI) are called *SI practitioners*. Both groups practice their manual body-based approach using the principles described by Rolf. This chapter uses the term *SI* when describing Rolfing.

SI is a systematic approach of tissue-based work and elements of movement reeducation designed to improve the alignment and function of the body. Two main organizing principles of the approach are the interaction of the body with gravity and the role of the fascia as a central organ of the body. Rolf believed that the body's alignment was organized with respect to gravity. Through use, disuse, and even abuse optimal alignment is compromised, which leads to pain and movement difficulties. She believed that this process could be reversed by the use of manual techniques to remodel the fascia, which supports all of the tissues in the body.

The 10 sessions of SI are sometimes referred to as a recipe.[7] This statement is accurate, to some extent, because a systematic approach to each examination and intervention is used. The general examination consists of a three-dimensional examination of posture. This is done by observing posture using Rolf's stacked blocks model of the body (Figure 19-1). Alignment of the blocks in three planes is the standard for optimal posture. The pelvis is considered the central block. The second element of the evaluation is observation of tissue appearance. Evidence of pulling and tight-

ness is an indicator of restriction or tonal changes in the tissue. Observation of bony and soft tissue structures also takes place during movement. The SI metaphor used to describe tissue movement is "the sleeve and core." The sleeve corresponds to appendicular structures that are to move freely over the core or axial structures.

Each session has a specific intent; therefore the examination and intervention are adjusted further to focus on a set of soft tissue structures and appropriate movement cues. Specific movements are selected because they relate to the goals of a session. For example, in the first session breathing is observed to begin work on the anterior chest. Identification of deviations in posture and tissue restrictions related to breathing help locate dysfunction and guide practitioners' interventions. The intent of each examination and primary structures addressed for each session are summarized in Table 19-1.

The intervention consists of soft tissue mobilization by application of the amount of pressure required to free restrictions. The goal is to remove any fascial adherences that prevent structures from being in their optimal alignment. For example, during the second session practitioners focus on the alignment of the lower extremities and work primarily on the superficial soft tissue of the feet and leg, such as the retinaculum on the dorsum of the foot; the perimalleolar structures, such as the peroneal tendons; the gastrocnemius muscles; the medial and lateral collateral ligaments; the tibial crest; the Achilles tendon to the calcaneus; and the medial and lateral arch.[15]

The focus of each session, in addition to the depth of the soft tissue work, is varied systematically. Sessions one through six alternate their emphasis on either the upper (odd numbered, 1, 3, and 5) or lower (even numbered, 2, 4, and 6) part of the body. The depth of the work begins superficially in the first session, working on the fascia of the sternocleidomastoid in the neck, and moves to the deepest structures in the fourth session, such as the insertion of the adductors on the pubic ramus. In sessions seven through 10, the work is done on large fascial planes that connect the upper and lower part of the body. The main structures addressed and the depth of the work are summarized in Table 19-1. A more detailed description of the first six sessions can be found in the *Guild News*[16,17] and a description of the entire series can be found in the *Journal of Body Work Movement Therapies*.[10,11,12]

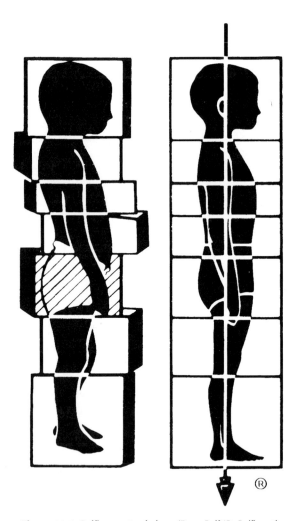

**Figure 19-1** Rolfing postural view. (From Rolf IP: *Rolfing: the integration of human structures,* New York, 1997, Harper & Row, p 33.)

| Table 19-1 | Structural Integration (Rolfing Exercises) | | |
|---|---|---|---|
| SESSION | GOALS | DEPTH | KEY MYOFASCIAL STRUCTURES |
| 1 | Establish a rapport with the client<br>Increase movement with each breath of the thorax and ribs<br>"Horizontalize the pelvis" | Superficial | Rib cage and costal arch |
| 2 | Restore alignment between the calcaneus and the ischial tuberosities<br>Restore balanced movement between the hip, knee, and ankles<br>Direct attention to the relationship of the feet to the ground | Superficial | Periarticular ankle retinaculum, plantar fascia, and lateral arch |
| 3 | Lengthen the lateral line<br>Increase the space between the pelvis and the twelfth rib<br>Release the shoulder and pelvic girdles | Superficial | Quadratus lumborum<br>Twelfth rib |
| 4 | Reduce excessive rotation of the lower limb<br>Align the pelvis in all planes<br>Align the foot with respect to the spine | Deep | Medial retinaculum of the ankle, attachments of the adductors and hamstrings to the pubic ramus |
| 5 | Lengthen the anterior thorax<br>Align the clavicles in all planes<br>Facilitate movement of the arm with proper scapular alignment<br>Facilitate movements of hip flexion | Deep | Psoas, pectoralis minor, rectus abdominis, and diaphragm |
| 6 | Vertically align the lower limb<br>Align the pelvis, sacrum, and spine | Deep | Hip rotators, sacrotuberous ligament<br>Thoracolumbar fascia |
| 7 | Align the head<br>Separate the fascia of the head and arms | Superficial to deep | Sternocleidomastoid, scalenes, masseter, occipital Atlantic ligaments, deep cervical muscles, and cranial fascia |
| 8 and 9 | Focus on either the upper or lower body<br>"Balance and relate the girdles" to the "dorsal lumbar hinge"<br>Relate the limbs to the spine | Varied | Mobility of fascial planes |
| 10 | Integrate a functional whole<br>Maximize movement strategies and efficiency | Varied | Fascial planes across joints |

From Deutsch JE et al: Structural integration applied to patients with chronic pain, *Phys Ther Clin North Am* 9(3):411-27, 2000.

In addition to alignment with respect to gravity and the fascial organization of the body, the role of the parasympathetic nervous system appears to be important in SI. One of the manual techniques used in each session is a pelvic lift. It is performed with the client supine and the knees flexed. One hand is placed on the sacrum, with the fingertips resting on the lumbosacral junction. The second hand is placed on the subject's epigastrum to stabilize the trunk. A cranial traction force is applied, using the hand on the lumbosacral junction to rotate the pelvis posteriorly.[18] Evidence suggests that use of this pelvic lift increases parasympathetic tone and therefore is associated with a relaxation response.[18,19]

Biomechanical alignment with respect to gravity and manipulation of the autonomic nervous system are two of the mechanistic explanations of SI. A third explanation proposed by Oschman is energetic.[20] He described the tissue as having semiconductor properties that could be altered by the soft tissue work. Oschman describes Rolf's work as benefiting from the plasticity of connective tissue.

Sessions typically are performed in 1-week intervals. This is done to allow the body to reorganize itself with respect to gravity. After the 10-session process is completed, individuals may be reevaluated if their symptoms persist. This is more likely to be the case if the person returns to habitual movement patterns and postures that created the original myofascial imbalance. Additional lessons are offered with a greater emphasis on movement reeducation or as tune-up sessions.[21]

## Searching the Databases and Evaluating the Literature

The therapist searches MEDLINE, CINAHL, and PsycInfo. She chooses the first two because they are the databases she is accustomed to searching for research related to rehabilitation, pediatrics, and allied health. Rolf taught her approach to many psychologists, so the therapist also checks PsycInfo. She uses the following search terms: *cerebral palsy, spastic diplegia, pain, flexibility, musculoskeletal, Rolfing,* and *structural integration.* The term *structural integration* yields many extraneous citations, so she does not use it further. She searches the terms separately and then combines them.

The results of her search are summarized in Table 19-2. Very few articles on SI are found; four appear to have some relationship to Susan's case. Three of the articles address pain management with SI, and a fourth relates directly to individuals with cerebral palsy.

Because few articles are found on the approach, the therapist decides to read all of them. Two articles that were published in the 1970s appear to validate basic concepts in SI. Silverman and colleagues[22] used electrophysiological and biochemical measures to quantify the effects of Rolfing on 15 healthy individuals. Significant changes were found in comparison of pre-SI and post-SI measures, which suggests an effect for Rolfing. The authors speculated that a connection exists between the muscular system and the sensory system. In a follow-up study by Hunt and Massey[23] electromyography (EMG) was used to characterize move-

ment efficiency before and after SI. The authors operationally defined movement efficiency using a variety of EMG variables, such as a decrease in duration and an increase in amplitude of contraction in addition to decreases in neuromuscular excitation for areas that were not treated with SI. The authors interpreted these findings as representative of neuromuscular efficiency.

The parasympathetic nervous system is discussed in three articles. Two are quasi-experimental studies that validated the parasympathetic involvement of the pelvic lift manipulation. These two quasi-experimental studies were performed on a group of healthy adults and then compared with another group of elderly adults.[18,19] A third article by some of the same authors is a case study on a person with amyotrophic lateral sclerosis (ALS). The authors speculate that some of the positive outcomes (improved quality of life) of SI use can be attributed to increases in parasympathetic tone, which produced relaxation.[24]

The use of SI for individuals who were experiencing pain is addressed in three articles.[25-27] One is a review article, in which the author concludes that in no clinical trials were pain and function addressed with use of SI.[25] Cottingham and Maitland describe a case report of an individual with LBP in which SI and movement reeducation were used for the management of pain. In this case the authors concluded that it was the movement education component that was essential for recovery of pain-free movement.[26] The article by Deutsch et al was a retrospective chart review of 20 clients who participated in an inpatient rehabilitation program augmented with a 10-session SI series. In that group of clients who had chronic pain had significant decreases in pain reports and improvements of posture and functional mobility.[27]

Only two articles reported in the literature are on Rolfing and children,[28] and of these only in one do the children have cerebral palsy.[29] This quasi-experimental study was performed on a group of 10 individuals with cerebral palsy. They each received a 10-session series of SI. Extensive testing of gait kinematics, kinetics, and cardiopulmonary physiology was performed before and after the training. Severity of the children varied, as did their functional mobility skills. The children with the better outcomes most closely resembled Susan because they were higher functioning and ambulatory. Their outcomes included improved ROM, which was maintained after the SI was discontinued, and improved functional mobility.

| Table 19-2 | Literature Search Results | | |
|---|---|---|---|
| KEY TERMS | MEDLINE | CINAHL | PSYCHINFO |
| Rolfing | 12 | 38 | 18 |
| Rolfing and cerebral palsy | 1 | 0 | 0 |
| Rolfing and pain | 4 | 5 | |
| Rolfing and musculoskeletal system | 3 | 2 | |
| Rolfing and flexibility | 0 | 0 | 0 |

The literature on SI consists primarily of quasi-experimental and descriptive studies. Several are mechanistic validation studies addressing the concepts of neuromuscular efficiency[22,23] and parasympathetic tone.[18,19] The remaining articles describe clinical outcomes for individuals with LBP,[26] chronic pain,[27] ALS,[24] and cerebral palsy.[29] Two published abstracts that did not appear in the search present descriptive results of SI applied to individuals with fibromyalgia[30] and cases of individuals with multiple sclerosis and traumatic brain injury.[31] The two articles related to pain and the one article on individuals with cerebral palsy are rated only as a level III using the criteria of Sackett et al.[32] They are, however, directly applicable to the present case.

The search process and evaluation described may have involved more time than the therapist had if she were working alone. Alternatively she could have implemented a PICO question to drive her search terms. The PICO question is described in the PICO box below.

---

### PICO BOX

Is there any evidence to support the use of Rolfing to reduce low back pain in children with cerebral palsy?

This question was dissected into the PICO categories and generated the search terms listed below.

Population: Children with cerebral palsy
Intervention: Structural integration or Rolfing
Outcome: Low back pain

This search yielded only one reference for the case. This reference is perhaps the most relevant for the case[29], but the other references on pain[26,27] that do not address children with CP would also be useful in the case.

P = **Population** (patient/client, problem, person, condition, or group attribute)
I = **Intervention** (the CAM therapy or approach)
C = **Comparison** (standard care or comparison intervention)
O = **Outcome** (the measured variables of interest)

---

## CLINICAL DECISION MAKING

The therapist decides that she will recommend the use of SI for Susan. The rationale for the decision is based on a combination of client preferences, clinical judgment, and the evaluation of the evidence. The client is reporting difficulty complying with the stretching.

## Generate a Clinical Hypothesis

The therapist hypothesizes that the ROM and alignment issues are central to the elimination of the back pain. She determines that the long-standing muscle length changes from the cerebral palsy will require a systematic approach to reverse. The single article on cerebral palsy presented positive outcomes for children whose symptoms are similar to Susan's. Therefore the therapist hypothesizes that the restoration of ROM and postural alignment provided by the SI, coupled with the abdominal strengthening, will lead to decreased LBP. This, in combination with the fitness program (biking and walking endurance), will also improve Susan's functional mobility.

## Evaluate

To determine if the clinical hypothesis is accurate, the therapist adds several measurements to her previous examination. There is a 1-month wait to see the SI therapist, so she consults with the clinician scientist to get some advice on how to proceed. First, she takes photographs of the client's posture using a standardized procedure and a posture grid in the background. She already has collected information on pain complaints using a VAS scale, ROM using a goniometer, muscle strength using manual muscle testing, circumferential chest measurements, and timed walk and elevations, which she repeats. Third, she adds a quantitative measure of gait endurance by using a 6-minute walk test. She asks a colleague to collect the examination data. The reason for this is to remove any bias that may occur in her measurements as a result of knowing the client's condition and impending intervention. She also decides to take several measurements before the start of the SI series. This will allow her to see how stable the outcome measures are before she initiates the SI intervention. This approach is similar to that of single-subject designs. These types of research designs are more controlled than case reports, are amenable to practice, and have been recommended for use in pediatrics.[33] She is able to implement this approach because of the 1-month wait for the SI intervention to begin.

## Intervene

The SI intervention is completed by an SI practitioner who is also a physical therapist. The process the SI therapist follows is outlined in Table 19-1. Some modifications of the process are necessary because Susan cannot always assume and maintain all of the positions as described in the approach. For example, lesson four, which addresses the inner line, requires that Susan be positioned with additional bolsters and support to assist with decreasing the increased resistance to passive stretch in her adductors. The therapist also applies slower strokes compared with her typical rate of work in treatment of the adductors to avoid triggering a reflexive response that may interfere with elongation of the tight muscles. In addition she makes a conscious decision to emphasize the movement reeducation cues for this client. She does this because of the information in the case report by Cottingham that identifies movement education as an important component for rehabilitation of the person with LBP.[26] The other reason for focusing on movement reeducation is that the client is very active, and some of her pain complaints are related to movement. The movement cues relate to alignment of the lower extremities relative to each other and the lower extremities over the trunk in addition to fluidity of movement.

To identify the SI practitioner, the treating physical therapist used a database posted on the SI website.[34,35] She then follows up with a phone call because she wants the practitioner to have experience with individuals with neurological conditions. She also wants a physical therapist who is trained as an SI practitioner because she feels that the combination of the SI and PT skills is necessary when working with a pediatric client who has a neurologic diagnosis and is presenting with a musculoskeletal condition.

Coordination between the SI therapist and the physical therapist is essential. The SI sessions are scheduled 1 week apart, and the PT sessions are once every 2 weeks to check and update the home exercise program (HEP) and recommend any changes. Because of this coordination, the primary treating therapist identifies that Susan has developed some unexpected balance problems as a result of the changes in her alignment. Therefore the primary treating therapist adds balance examination and interventions to Susan's program.

## Report the Outcomes

After the 10-week SI series Susan is pain free throughout her school day. She no longer requires her naps in the afternoon and has begun an after-school swimming program. Changes in her posture, ROM, 10-meter walk speed, and pedometer readings are summarized in Table 19-3. Follow-up of the child at 6 months revealed some loss of LE ROM and reports of occasional back pain. An additional SI session was performed to integrate the upper and lower trunk and the HEP program was revised to provide some core stabilization exercises. Follow-up at 3-month intervals was recommended. The treating therapist decides that the many interesting aspects to this case would be worth reporting to a larger audience.

## Table 19-3    Examination Findings Across the Episode of Care

| | INITIAL EVALUATION | | AFTER STRETCHING | | AFTER SI | | 6-MONTH FOLLOW-UP | |
|---|---|---|---|---|---|---|---|---|
| Hip flexor range | R 20-120 | L 20-120 | R 20-120 | L 20-120 | R 0-120 | L 0-120 | R 5-120 | L 5-120 |
| Ankle dorsiflexion | R 0 | L 0 | R 0 | L 0 | R 10 | L 10 | R 7 | L 8 |
| Pain (VAS) | 4-5 (after third period) | | 4 (after fourth period) | | 0 Throughout the day | | 1 At the end of school | |
| Abdominal strength | RA 2 Obliques 2 | | RA 2 Obliques 2 | | RA 3 Obliques 3 | | RA 3 Obliques 3 | |
| LE strength | L knee and hip extension 3+ | | Not tested | | L hip and knee extension 4 | | L hip and knee extension 4 | |
| TUG | 10.29 sec | | NT | | 8 | | 8 | |
| Walking | NT | | 5000 steps | | 8000 steps | | 8000 steps | |
| Elevations | 25 sec | | NT | | 15 sec | | 15 sec | |

*SI*, structural integration; *R*, right; *L*, left; *VAS*, visual analogue scale; *RA*, rectus abdominis; *LE*, lower extremity; *sec*, seconds; *TUG*, timed up and go.

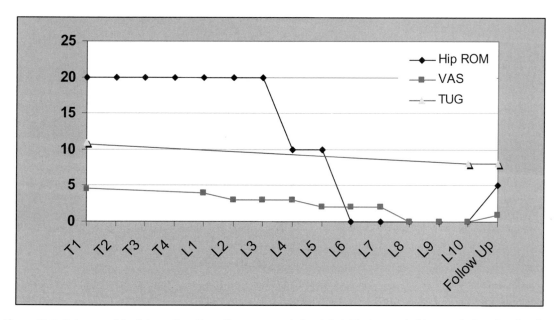

**Figure 19-2 Outcomes of the intervention.** Figure illustrates a gradual and desirable decrease in hip range flexion of motion (lines with diamonds) and pain reports (lines with squares) that begin with SI session 4. A slight increase in pain and loss of ROM are seen at follow up. Walking time decreases (lines with triangles) are maintained. Gains in the timed up and go after SI are maintained at follow up.

Because the intervention had many positive outcomes, but specifically changes occurred at the impairment level, that the therapist speculates are connected to the improvement at the functional level. She tries to illustrate with Figure 19-2 how changes in ROM and pain may be related to the improvements in walking speed and distance. She consults with the clinician scientist about how to proceed. They decide that the SI therapist, clinician scientist, and treating therapist will collaborate to write a paper. The goal will be to submit it to the *Journal of Pediatric Physical Therapy*. They contact the editor to inquire if such a paper would be of interest to the journal. The journal encourages the submission as a single-subject report.

In addition to documenting the details of the intervention they describe the different aspects of clinical decision making: evaluation of the evidence and description of the interaction between the treating therapist, clinician scientist, and SI therapist. The value of follow-up visits for a person who is developing and has a chronic condition is also stressed. The paper is submitted for review to the *Journal of Pediatric Physical Therapy*, in addition to an abstract to the pediatric section for the combined sections meeting of the APTA. Before presenting at the conference they share the information with their colleagues in the clinic and the university.

## SUMMARY

This chapter describes the case of a child with spastic diplegia who reported LBP and difficulty with functional mobility in her middle school setting. After evaluating the evidence, the treating therapist collaborating with a clinician scientist refers the client to an SI practitioner who is also a physical therapist. The three therapists, who function in different capacities, coordinate the examination and intervention of the client. The process of selecting and evaluating the SI intervention is summarized for their clinical colleagues and presented at a professional meeting and submitted as a paper. Follow-up of the client at 6 months reveals some losses of ROM and posture, so a regular follow-up and home exercise program are prescribed.

## REFERENCES

1. Platz T et al: Clinical scales for the assessment of spasticity, associated phenomena, and function: a systematic review of the literature, *Disabil Rehabil* 27(1-2):7-18, 2005.
2. Pandyan AD et al: A review of the properties and limitations of the Ashworth and modified Ashworth Scales as measures of spasticity, *Clin Rehabil* 13(5): 373-83, 1999.

3. Williams EN et al: Investigation of the timed "up & go" test in children, *Dev Med Child Neurol* 47(8):518-24, 2005.

4. Palisano R et al: Gross motor function classification for cerebral palsy, *Dev Med Child Neurol* 39:214-23, 1997.

5. Rolf IP: Structural integration: a contribution to the understanding of stress, *Confin Psychiatr* 16:69-79, 1973.

6. Rolf IP: *Rolfing: the integration of human structures*, New York, 1977, Harper & Row.

7. Feitas R: *Ida Rolf talks,* New York, 1978, Harper and Row.

8. About Structural Integration. Available at: *http://www.rolfguild.org/aboutsi.html.* Accessed March 1, 2006.

9. About Rolfing. Available at: *http://www.rolf.org/.* Accessed March 1, 2006.

10. Myers TW: Structural integration: developments in Ida Rolf's "recipe"—part 1, *J Bodywork Movementt Ther* 8(2):131-42, 2004.

11. Myers TW: Structural integration: developments in Ida Rolf's "recipe"—part 2, *J Bodywork Movement Ther* 8(3):189-98, 2004.

12. Myers TW: Structural integration: developments in Ida Rolf's "recipe"—part 3, an alternative form, *J Bodywork Movement Ther* 8(4):249-64, 2004.

13. Claire T: *Bodywork: what type of massage to get—and how to make the most of it,* 1995, William Morrow/HarperCollins.

14. Deutsch JE: The Ida Rolf method of structural integration. In Davis C, editor: *Complementary therapies in rehabilitation: evidence of efficacy in therapy, prevention and wellness,* 2004, SLACK, pp 99-105.

15. Deutsch JE: Structural integration (Rolfing). In Carlson J, editor: *Complementary therapies and wellness: practice essential for holistic care,* Upper Saddle River, NJ, 2004, Prentice-Hall, pp 256-67.

16. Urbanczik A: A tour of the first three sessions, *Guild News* 4:32-5, 1994.

17. Urbanczik A: A tour of the basic series—sessions 4, 5, and 6, *Guild News* 5:21-3, 1995.

18. Cottingham JT, Porges SW, Richmond K: Shifts in pelvic inclination angle and parasympathetic tone produced by Rolfing soft tissue manipulation, *Phys Ther* 68:1364-70, 1988.

19. Cottingham JT, Porges SW, Lyon T: Effects of soft tissue mobilization (Rolfing pelvic lift) on parasympathetic tone in two age groups, *Phys Ther* 68:352-6, 1988.

20. Structural Integration (Rolfing), osteopathic, chiropractic, Feldenkrais, Alexander, myofascial release and related methods. In Oschman JL, editor: *Energy medicine: the scientific basis,* Edinburgh, 2000, Churchill Livingstone, pp 165-74.

21. Kotzsch E: Restructure the body with Rolfing: deep massage that realigns the human form, *East West Natural Health* 35, 1999.

22. Silverman J, Rappaport M, Hopkins K et al: Stress intensity control and the structural integration technique, *Confinia Psychiatrica* 16:201-19, 1973.

23. Hunt VV, Massey WW: Electromyographic evaluation of structural integration techniques, *Psychoenergetic Systems* 2:199-210, 1977.

24. Cottingham JT, Maitland J: Integrating manual and movement therapy with philosophical counseling for treatment of a patient with amyotrophic lateral sclerosis: a case study that explores the principles of holistic intervention, *Altern Ther Health Medicine* 6(2):120-8, 2000.

25. Jones TA: Rolfing, *Phys Med Rehabil Clin North Am* 15(4):799-809, 2004.

26. Cottingham JT, Maitland J: A three-paradigm treatment model using soft tissue mobilization and guided movement-awareness techniques for a patient with chronic low back pain: a case study, *J Orthop Sports Phys Ther* 26(3):155-67, 1997.

27. Deutsch JE et al: Structural integration applied to patients with chronic pain, *Phys Ther Clin North Am* 9(3):411-27, 2000.

28. Osborn K: Lifespan. Rolfing children, *Massage & Bodywork* 19(6):138-41, 2004-2005.

29. Perry J, Jones M, Thomas L: Functional evaluation of Rolfing in cerebral palsy, *Develop Med Child Neurol* 23:717-29, 1981.

30. Talty C, DeMassi I, Deutsch JE: Structural Integration applied to patients with chronic fatigue syndrome: a retrospective chart review, *J Othop Sports Phys Ther* 27(1):83, 1998.

31. Deutsch JE, Judd P, DeMassi I: Structural integration applied to patients with a primary neurologic diagnosis: two case studies, *Neurol Report* 21(5):161-2, 1997.

32. Sackett D et al: *Evidence-based medicine: how to practice and teach EBM,* ed 2, Toronto, 2000, Churchill Livingstone.

33. Palisano R, Campbell S, Harris S: Evidence-based decision making in pediatric physical therapy. In Campbell S, Vander Linden D, Palisano R, editors: *Physical therapy for children,* ed 3, St. Louis, 2006, Elsevier, pp 3-32.

34. Guild for Structural Integration, Therapist Locator. Available at: *http://www.rolfguild.org/usa.html.* Accessed March 13, 2006.

35. Rolfing Institute, Therapist Locator. Available at: *http://www.rolf.org/find/locate.asp.* Accessed March 13, 2006.

# CHAPTER 20

## Feldenkrais

*James Stephens*

---

Jane Knowles is a 54-year-old woman who has been diagnosed with MS and has experienced a rapid progression of weakness in her legs in the last 2 years.

### Initial Examination

**Client Report:** Jane experienced weakness in her right leg as the first symptom of MS 15 years ago but did not receive a definitive diagnosis of MS until 4 years ago at the age of 50. In the last 2 years, she has experienced a rapid progression of weakness in her right leg and beginning weakness in her left leg. She is married and lives with her husband. She has been working with a physical therapist for 6 months for a basic stretching and strengthening program. She has heard of FM from a psychologist and was referred to the therapist by her neurologist for her rehabilitation evaluation and program.

**Client Goals:** To improve her walking distance and speed so that she could walk for exercise and with her husband; to improve her balance so that she can perform activities in the home and community without fear of falling; and to generally improve her strength, mobility, and quality of life

**Employment:** Before her diagnosis, Jane worked full time as an independent business consultant, which involved long hours and a lot of travel. She still does occasional consulting jobs, but she has reduced her work drastically.

**Recreational Activities:** Jane always has enjoyed a regular exercise program of stretching and aerobics that involved primarily walking with her husband. She and her husband have grown children, who live in another state.

**General Health:** Good

**Medications:** Avonex; Baclofen, 10 mg/day, under a nutritionists supervision B6 supplement

**Cardiopulmonary:** Resting blood pressure (BP) 120/76 and heart rate (HR) 80. After 3 minutes of walking terminated because of fatigue, BP 136/84 and HR 96

**Musculoskeletal:** Range of motion (ROM): within normal limits (WNL) throughout except dorsiflexion (df) −5 on the right (R). Posture: WNL except slight forward lean in standing

**Neuromuscular:** Strength: upper extremity (UE) grossly 5/5. Trunk flexion is 4−/5, extension 5/5. Left lower extremity (LLE) is grossly 4/5 except hip flexion 3/5, abduction and extension 3+/5. Right lower extremity (RLE): 3−/5 for hip flexion, extension, abduction, and rotation and knee flexion; 4−/5 for hip adduction, knee extension, and plantar flexion/df at the ankle. Motor control: modified Ashworth score was 0 for the UE, trunk, and LLE and 2 for the RLE. No clonus was noted. Fatigue was a problem affecting dorsiflexion after about 2 minutes of walking. Sensation: Intact to pin prick but slightly impaired to light touch both (LE), R>L.

## Function

Gait was deliberate and ataxic with foot drop B/L after 2 minutes, decreased trunk rotation, and increased hip flexion to initiate swing. Gait speed was approximately 1.0 mph (~1.5 ft/sec). Jane used a cane to help her balance but did not use an ankle foot orthosis (AFO). Balance was impaired, with single-leg stance 10 seconds on the L and 2 seconds on the R. She needed to hold a rail for balance and UE strength assist going up and down stairs. Getting up to standing from supine she rolled to prone, pushed up to her hands and knees, and pulled herself up on a chair. In a trial of half-kneel to standing she needed UE support for balance in half-kneel. Her score on the Berg Balance Scale (BBS) was 41/56. She is able to drive and is generally independent with mobility using assistive devices.

**Integumentary:** Unremarkable

**Cognitive and Communication:** Jane described cognition as a problem, and indicated that she needed to make lists and use other strategies to assist memory. She was able to follow directions to drive to the therapist's office 50 miles from her home without a problem and had no deficits in alertness.

## Evaluation

Jane appears to have a late-onset form of MS that has progressed slowly without exacerbations. The primary impact of the disease is at the level of strength and motor control, which manifests as weakness and poor differentiation and coordination of effort between the trunk and lower extremities. This causes significant impairments in balance and mobility. She has impaired endurance in functional activities. Her cognitive deficit impairs her ability to do the complex thinking required for her consulting job, but it does not appear to affect her balance and mobility significantly. Although the BBS has been used little with people with MS and they did not report a problem with falling, her low BBS score and her behavior of using a cane and holding onto walls and furniture suggest that she is at a high risk of falling.[1]

## Incorporating CAM into the Plan of Care

The therapist outlines a plan of care for Jane. First, the therapist refers her to an orthotist for measurement and construction of bilateral ankle foot orthosis, formal driving evaluation, and a full neuropsychological evaluation. The therapist then recommends small modifications of the daily stretching and strengthening exercise program Jane has been doing and develops an endurance component to her exercise program using walking as an activity. Last, the therapist develops a set of short Awareness Through Movement (ATM) lessons that are part of FM:

1. Movement of side-sit to kneeling to side-sit
2. Alternating movement of left and right half-kneeling
3. Movement side-lying leg-swing
4. Standing balance over one foot
5. Walking
6. Jumping on both feet

This chapter presents the case of a 54-year-old woman with multiple sclerosis (MS). The woman is being treated by a physical therapist, certified Feldenkrais practitioner (CFP), and researcher on outcomes of interventions using the Feldenkrais method (FM). The therapist determines upon meeting this client that she would be an excellent candidate for an intervention that integrates the use of FM and standard elements of physical therapy practice. His review of the evidence and clinical decision-making process are illustrated in this chapter.

## INVESTIGATING THE LITERATURE

The therapist uses two approaches to investigate the literature. The first is a detailed approach in which preliminary background reading is performed on the Feldenkrais (FM) method followed by a search of the databases and evaluation of the literature based on reviews and primary sources. The second is the use of the PICO format for a focused search to answer the clinical question generated by the case.

## Preliminary Reading

Many books provide introductory information about FM. They fall into three general categories: those dealing with the rationale and methodology behind the development of the method by Moshe Feldenkrais, the originator; those that are secondary interpretations and presentations of the method by Feldenkrais practitioners; and those that focus on specific applications to a variety of problems. The first group includes the classic *Body and Mature Behavior*,[2] which was Feldenkrais' first approximation of articulating his work, and the more recently published *The Potent Self*.[3] Each of these books details the anatomical, physiological, life-span developmental, and psychosocial thinking that informed the development of method. The underlying theme is that humans learn throughout their lifetime, that faulty learning can produce pathology of the mind and body, and that much of this pathology can be addressed by exploratory body movement lessons executed with careful attention to the details of the task-individual-environment constellation. Another book in this group is *The Elusive Obvious*,[4] which is the most accessible and conversational of Feldenkrais' writings. *Awareness Through Movement*[5] is the most practical; it details 12 movement lessons and the rationale behind their development and usefulness.

The second group contains books such as those by Rywerant[6] and Shafarman.[7] These books expand the rationale behind the method and include brief case examples and movement lessons. The case examples usually involve applications to the process of rehabilitation.

The third group of books deals with application to a specific problem, such as *Body Awareness as Healing Therapy: The Case of Nora*,[8] in which Feldenkrais talks about his work with a woman who had a stroke; Heggie's book on running[9]; Hutchinson's work on transforming body image for people with obesity[10]; and Jackson-Wyatt's[11] book on adapting to ergonomic problems in the workplace. This array of topics demonstrates that

FM has a wide application to issues of living in addition to specific applications to movement problems in rehabilitation.

Briefly, FM was created by Moshe Feldenkrais, who was trained as a mechanical and nuclear engineer and became a neurobehavioral scientist. He developed a method of attending to his own posture and movement to resolve the functional limitations associated with a medial meniscus tear he received while playing soccer as a young man in Paris in the 1920s. He later taught this method in two forms, ATM and functional integration (FI), to students who have carried it worldwide to be movement occurs that is absent in relation to normal movement organization expressing the intended movement used in many ways. One of these applications is in rehabilitation from injury and chronic disease.[12]

### *Assumptions Underlying the Feldenkrais Method*

In his book *Awareness Through Movement*[5] Feldenkrais stated, "Each of us acts according to the image of himself that he has built up over the years" (p. 10). This self-image has been constructed from movement, sensation, feeling, and thought. He continued, "In order to change our mode of action, we must change the image of ourselves we carry within us." The rest of the book presents, by example through 12 movement lessons, a method of changing self-image and subsequently the ability to act in the world.

Feldenkrais believed that an individual's self-image was a complex composite. For Massion,[13,14] self-image, which he calls *body schema*, is at the heart of the motor control process. Massion's body schema is a construct of the sensory/perceptual processes that represent the body's position and orientation in space, the organization of body segments, and the movement of those segments in terms of velocity, direction, and force. Feldenkrais believed that this self-image comprises sensation (and movement) and our emotional sense of ourselves, our thoughts about who we are and what we can do, and our sense of self-efficacy.

Little research has been done in this area to test the assumption that FM can change self-image. Using ATM as an intervention Dieg[15] reported increased accuracy of representation in blindfold-constructed clay models of self; Hutchinson[10] and Elgelid[16] reported improvements in description of body image using semantic differentiation scales;

Dunn and Rogers[17] reported changes in the sense of body size and weight; Ginsburg[18] argued for broad changes in self-image in his presentation of case studies; and Stephens et al[19] reported large, positive changes in self-efficacy in a group of people with MS. Feldenkrais created a method that uses movement to alter self-image with the understanding that the altered self-image allows generation of new movement. From a clinical perspective, this means that people gain a sense that they are able to do things that they were not able to do before.[20]

Writing in 1949, Feldenkrais[2] envisioned learning as a process by which the experience of life is recorded in the cortex by alteration of the connections between cells. This was accomplished by attending to the events in progress, discriminating among the actions and the resultant outcomes, and so producing new modes of action. Attending to the sensory, emotional, and thought processes and making real discriminations related to the actions in progress is therefore a method of modifying the self-image and laying the basis for generating new patterns of action. This process is closest to that described for motor skill acquisition by Newell.[21] It now appears that Feldenkrais' idea of learning is close to the process of active plasticity that goes on in the central nervous system as described by many current researchers using both animal and human models and in humans.[22-28] Currently preliminary evidence suggests changes occur in the brain activity associated with movement after work with FM that facilitated recovery of upper extremity functions after a stroke.[29]

Feldenkrais believed that in an ATM lesson, as people attended to and made discriminations among the effects of small movements, the central nervous system processes related to body schema or self-image would be refined and expanded. During this process of exploration using small movements, attention is paid to the organization, timing, and movement of body segments in relation to base of support and to the effort related to intention for the action and what Feldenkrais called "parasitic activity," which can be described as some aspect of the body organization that opposes the primary intention.[5,12] In an ATM lesson, a movement is repeated in many variations. One of the goals of the ATM lesson is to identify and integrate into function variations of movement that require the least amount of effort while still effectively achieving the intentions of the performer. This often may involve relearning strategies and patterns of use of the larger muscle groups, which provide more of the power of movement.[5]

### General Outline of a Session

The practitioner training process is informal and experientially based. No written, standard, accepted guidelines exist for how a lesson with an individual client should be conducted. As such, each practitioner's approach is somewhat different. For more insight into how approaches may differ, the reader is referred to Stephens and Miller,[12] who describe several client cases.

A session may begin with practitioners observing the postural configuration of the clients in one or more positions. When asked to stand, sit, or lie down, clients perform that activity according to the image and habit they have for doing it, incorporating any process of compensation that they may have developed. The practitioners then observe this habitual organization as it presents and further explore it by gently pushing or supporting through the skeleton of the clients to see how they respond to this perturbation. Practitioners approach this with an understanding of what a normal, unimpaired response to such a push or support may look and feel like. Practitioners look for postural alignment and a flow of mechanical energy through the skeleton that engages other segments of the body in a way appropriate in response to the direction and force of the push or support. Practitioners then use this process to identify some aspect of the postural or movement organization that appears unusual as a focus for work.

The practitioner's intent is to create an environment and an opportunity for learning related to the client's problem and attend to environmental factors such as lighting, temperature, and noise. Physical comfort is important. The client is asked to dress comfortably in clothes that do not restrict movement. Props are used to support clients in their preferred posture so that they may attend to the movements presented by the practitioner in addition to their responses to movements. Practitioners approach working with the client through FI, ATM, or some combination of the two.

In FI, practitioners work with clients first by continuing the ATM process or supporting the habitual postural configurations of the client to facilitate a good understanding of how this posture is achieved and controlled, allowing clients to relax and perform their spontaneous movement or posture. Then practitioners lead clients through small movements into patterns of organization slightly different from what is spontaneous and natural and help the client to realize that these patterns are different and are a choice for voluntary action.

In ATM the FI process is performed at the level of voluntary movement. Clients are asked initially to observe the feeling of their resting posture. Then they are asked to repeat a small movement (e.g., rolling the head to the side while in a supine position) and to begin observing how the rest of their body participates in this movement. Through this process the spatiotemporal pattern of control (coordination) can be observed. Attention is brought to areas of the body where unnecessary movement occurs or where movement is absent in relation to normal movement organization. Small exploratory movements are then done or artificial constraints applied (e.g., locking the head and shoulder together by placing the hand on the forehead) to give the client a clearer sense of how the body is or could be organized in movement. This small movement then is placed into other movement and postural configurations to see how other parts of the body can be integrated with this movement to make it smoother and easier. To illustrate using the example of the client rolling the head while in a supine position, the client would try turning the head while moving the arms or legs or while sitting or standing rather than supine. New options for movement are thus created from an exploratory process, and the client can begin to develop and expand the use of those new options in functional activities.

## Searching the Databases

Many approaches exist for a search on FM. For example, a search of the term *Feldenkrais* through the OVID Gateway, including the databases MEDLINE from 1966 to present, CINAHL, all evidence-based medicine (EBM) reviews, Health Star, Sport Discus, and PsychInfo, yields 148 hits. Removing duplicates reduces the number to 115. Selecting only those papers that have English abstracts and are either reviews of the use or process of the FM or experimental or case studies reduces the number to 39. These papers fall into three categories: (1) experimental or case studies involving patients with neurological diagnoses, five papers (four MS and one traumatic brain injury); (2)

experimental or case studies involving orthopedic or other diagnoses, 20 papers; and (3) review papers describing the process or general use of FM, 14 papers. This search turned up most of the relevant literature on FM. Because the author has been in contact with practitioners and researchers throughout the world for many years, he also refers to some papers that are not listed in any of the databases mentioned above.

### Critical and Primary Source Reviews

One Cochrane critical review of complementary therapies was found for people with MS.[30] This review included one paper that used FM. Although the sample size was small, the results suggested that FM was a promising treatment for people with MS in terms of psychological well-being. The study reviewed used 20 patients with MS in a crossover design, in which patients received eight weekly sessions of FI and eight weekly sessions of sham "non-therapeutic passive bodywork."[31] The results suggested improvements related to perceived stress and lowered anxiety related to the Feldenkrais intervention but no changes in measures of hand function or other measures of function. Another, more thorough review of FM in general was done by Ives and Shelley,[32] who concluded that despite serious methodological flaws in much of the research, a consistent direction of outcomes suggests that the work may be effective and that more research is needed.

### Evaluate the Literature

1. *What impairments that present in MS may cause postural control and balance problems?*

Postural control is understood to be a multifaceted, systemic process that involves the expression of the motor system, the functions of the sensory system, and their integrated action through the processes of intention, planning, anticipation, and adaptation within specific movements.[33] Rodgers et al[34] identified deficits in ROM, strength, spasticity, and sensory disturbances in people with MS who also had gait deficits. They followed up with a 6-month aerobic exercise program and failed to find any resulting changes in gait. Strength, spasticity, balance, and gait deficits in people with MS were addressed in studies by Lord, Wade, and Halligan[35] and Petajan and White[36] with use of broad intervention programs directed toward impairments. These programs were successful in improvement of balance and gait, but no specific parameters of impairment were identified as being of primary importance. Cattaneo et al[37] studied groups of people with MS who were either fallers or nonfallers based on their history. They were unable to develop a logistic regression model that effectively predicted who would be a faller based on measures of impairment such as strength or spasticity. In a similar effort, Kasser, McCubbin, and Hooker[38] studied the intrasubject variability in a range of physical measures, including strength and upright postural control; psychological measures including stress, mood, and self-efficacy; and functional assessment of performance of ADL. They observed covariation among physical measures (with high variability) and psychological measures (with lower variability) but no consistent correlations between these impairment measures and functional performance. They concluded that their findings suggested that the system places a high value on organization to preserve and optimize functional performance in the face of dynamically changing impairments. All these results suggest that an approach that addresses the integration and dynamics of many factors affecting performance is more likely to have an impact on function.

2. *Does evidence suggest that FM improves balance in any group of people?*

Seegert and Shapiro[39] investigated postural sway and alignment in a group of 25 healthy young adult women who performed three different ATM lessons and also served as their own supine resting controls. The ATM lessons also were done in the supine position and selected with the idea of changing the process of postural control and alignment of the neck, shoulders, and low back. Postural alignment and sway on a force platform were assessed in standing. Results indicated that although ATM and resting changed postural alignment of the neck, only ATM decreased the amount of postural sway. This suggests that a set of three supine ATM lessons carried out during 1 hour can improve standing stability. Bennett et al[40] used a set of ATM lessons done sitting with a group of 12 elderly women and found non-significant improvements in functional status and functional reach in addition to significant improvement in Timed Up and Go (TUG) compared with matched controls over a 6-week period of doing ATM three times per week. In a much larger study in Australia, 59 elderly women were assigned randomly to FM, tai chi, or control groups.[41] The ATM group participated in two classes per week over 16 weeks. Improved TUG and BBS scores and increased movement time to a limit of stability target were observed in the ATM group. These findings also suggest that ATM performed over a longer period of time can have a significant impact on measures of mobility and postural control.

3. *Does evidence suggest that FM is effective in improving function in people with MS, and more specifically, that FM improves balance in people with MS?*

In the first study using FM with people with MS, Bost et al[42] described increases in movement complexity (new movement strategies) and movement quality (smoothness of movement) over a period of 30 days. This study also described an improved general well-being, positive self-concept, and self-acceptance related to participation in ATM. These findings confirm the psychological effects noted earlier by Johnson et al.[31] In a small multiple-case study, Stephens et al[20] described large increases in sense of well-being and changes in speed and coordination of a supine-to-stand movement and gait, which may have contained explanations for participants' subjective reports of improved sense of balance and control in walking. In a follow-up RCT study with 12 people with MS, Stephens et al[19] found significant improvements in some measures of balance and large nonsignificant improvements in others. Performance on the Balance Master Modified Clinical Test of Sensory Integration and Balance (mCTSIB) and the Activities Balance Confidence scale improved significantly. Results included a prospective reduction in falls, an increase in self-efficacy, and balance performance using the Equiscale tests that were close to <0.05 but were nonsignificant.

In summary, some evidence suggests that FM may be used to address problems of postural control in people with MS. As with many other CAM therapies, only a few relevant studies exist, and the numbers of subjects in these studies are small. However, taken together, these studies give the therapist confidence to decide that ATM using functional movements that were initially difficult and poorly controlled could be used successfully as part of an intervention that would improve overall control of functional mobility and improve quality of life. The therapist may not always have time to do such an extensive search. Instead she may use a targeted PICO approach.

**Table 20-1** **Tests and Measures Outcomes**

| MEASURE | INITIAL VISIT | 3-MONTH FOLLOW-UP |
| --- | --- | --- |
| Posture | Forward lean in standing | Standing more erect |
| Strength: hip | L 3-3+/5; R 3–/5 | L 3+-4–/5; R 3+-·4–/5 |
| Fatigue | After 2 minutes of walking | After 15 minutes of walking |
| Gait speed | ~1.5 ft/sec | ~2.9 ft/sec |
| Gait | Decreased trunk rotation; foot drop; cane, no AFO | Increased trunk rotation, less and later foot drop; cane, no AFO |
| Balance: BBS score | 41/56 | 54/56 |
| Unilateral stand time | L 10 sec, R 2 sec | L 30 sec, R 10 sec |
| Transfer floor to stand | Climb furniture using hands | Transfer without using hands |
| Stairs | Up and down using rail for power assist | Up without rail; down rail only for safety |

## PICO BOX

For persons with MS does the use of FM improve balance, gait, and quality of life?

P: Persons with MS
I: Feldenkrais method
O: Balance
O: Gait
O: Quality of life

The search was performed in MEDLINE and CINAHL combining all of the search terms in the PICO and did not yield any articles. It was performed again using only one outcome term at a time. This process produced two articles, one each when using *gait* and *quality of life* as terms, in the CINAHL database. These articles are citations 19 and 20 in the reference list. This process is efficient but not as comprehensive as the one used by the author.

P = **Population** (patient/client, problem, person, condition, or group attribute)
I = **Intervention** (the CAM therapy or approach)
C = **Comparison** (standard care or comparison intervention)
O = **Outcome** (the measured variable of interest)

## CLINICAL DECISION MAKING

### Generate a Clinical Hypothesis

As a Feldenkrais practitioner and researcher, the therapist recognizes that a process of motor learning embodied in the FM may be used to help resolve some of the clients' functional problems. By her own report, Jane's strength and stretching program seem to be maintaining her level of strength and flexibility at a functional level. In some aspects of her clinical picture (e.g., balance, postural control, mobility, and even aspects of strength), as revealed by the initial examination, she demonstrated difficulties that could be addressed with use of ATM.

Clinical experience and the review of literature, including two RTCs that suggest improved balance performance that after ATM intervention (Hall et al,[41] elderly women; Stephens et al,[19] people with multiple sclerosis). Based on this, the therapist believes that ATM is appropriate as part of the intervention with the client, and therefore ATM is made part of Jane's intervention plan.

### Examine

The BBS and the timed unilateral stance test are selected as outcome measures for balance and postural control because they are widely used, easy to use, and highly correlated with function.[43] For Jane, it also is useful to have measures of endurance and mobility to compare pre-intervention and post-intervention performance. For this, gait speed and time/distance before fatigue are used (Table 20-1).

In retrospect, several other measures may have been useful to get some more general information about other dimensions of performance. One of the instruments now widely used and approved by the National MS Society is the Multiple Sclerosis Quality of Life Inventory (MSQLI).[44] This instrument is a compilation of 10 independently developed and validated measures, which assess fatigue, pain, cognition, and social support, among other areas. Some of these dimensions of life activity also have been suggested to improve as a result of ATM interventions.[45]

## Intervene

As noted earlier, the plan of care has four different elements. First, the client is referred to an orthotist for fabrication of bilateral molded AFOs. The initial test with generic AFOs during the evaluation suggests that she would benefit greatly from using MAFOs, especially for long-distance walking. She is evaluated and has a pair of MAFOs made, which she wears only for walking exercises, primarily for cosmetic reasons. They prove useful in this capacity because they allow her to build aerobic capacity and walk with her husband, which she enjoys. Second, the endurance component of her plan of care also includes Schwinn Airdyne bike and swimming as alternate activities.[46] Third, modifications in her stretching and strengthening program are addressed primarily through the ATM activities with which she is given to work. Fourth, the ATM activities are provided.

The initial session with the client lasted 2 hours. Because she has a long drive to the clinic, one long session is scheduled. Several shorter sessions would have been preferable. The first four of the following six lessons were developed in the initial session over the period of an hour. They are simultaneously audiotape recorded so that she can play the tapes at home as a guide through the exploratory process of the lessons. This particular set of lessons is developed individually for Jane. The first lesson is developed to address problems of hip weakness in a functional movement. The second lesson is a building block in development of the strength and postural control to stand from sitting on the floor without use of her hands to push off from anything. Lesson 3 addresses some of the issues of trunk stiffness and lack of control of the rotation needed for more efficient walking. Lesson 4 builds on lesson 3 in the upright position and develops control in the stance phase of gait. Lesson 5 combines what is learned in lessons 3 and 4 in actual walking. Lesson 5 is begun during the second session. Lesson 6, on jumping, is introduced in the second session. It was an attempt to further improve postural control in a dynamic upright activity while building the strength and endurance in the lower legs to support faster and more efficient gait.

These six lessons are described in more detail here. For a more detailed description of lesson 3 as a sample lesson, refer to Appendix 1. For information on how to find a practitioner, refer to Appendix 2.

### Lesson 1

Lesson 1 addresses movement of side-sit to kneeling to side-sit. This lesson begins with one leg crossed in front, and the other leg turned behind the body in a side-sitting position. Initially Jane did not have the strength or coordination to bring herself to kneeling from this position. The first approximation involves learning to slide the hands forward in front of the body on the floor to discover that bringing the center of mass forward far enough lifts the buttocks off the floor. This initially is done by bringing the hands forward on the floor almost to the point of being in a quadruped position. The next part of the lesson is to translate the forward movement into upward momentum. This is achieved by bringing the head upward during the forward movement and getting a sense for how the pressure on the hands could be transferred to the knees. As this is understood, the hands could move off the floor, still in front of the body but now moving upward to enhance the upward momentum. The legs are then slid along the floor to the other side, and the movement problem becomes one of controlling downward momentum back into a side-sitting position on the other side. At the impairment level, this lesson addresses strength deficits in hip extensors, abductors, rotators, and paraspinals in concentric and eccentric modes, along with coordination of this complex movement, including generation and control of momentum. At the functional level, this is the beginning of a way for the client to get up off the floor, which she had a great deal of trouble doing at the initial examination.

### Lesson 2

Lesson 2 addresses alternating movement from half-kneeling on the left to half-kneeling on the right. Half-kneel is part of the transition between kneeling and standing. Most people, when asked to come from kneeling to half-kneel, lift one foot off the floor and swing it forward to a standing position. This requires great stability and strength in both the standing and the swinging legs. The purpose of this lesson is to introduce the possibility of rotation of the body to accomplish this transition with almost no effort at all. This lesson begins in a kneeling position, where the first lesson ended.

The first movements involve exploration of shifting weight onto one knee while raising the other slightly and keeping that foot on the floor. Stability on one knee is explored. Then instead of lifting the moving leg to place it in standing position, the foot is treated like a hinge, and the moving leg is swung up to standing by rotating the body to face in the direction of the moving leg. Then again, stability on one knee is explored by slightly lifting the leg that has been moving.

This lesson works with strength and stability of the standing leg, coordination of doing multiple movements sequentially without losing balance, and introduces the idea of using a completely new strategy to perform a movement usually done in a different way.

### Lesson 3

Lesson 3 addresses the movement of side-lying leg swing. This series of movements begins simply lying on the side and sensing the stability of the body with the legs in different configurations: together straight, flexed slightly at the hip and knee, and to 90/90 degrees and separated. The point of this lesson is to play with the balance in a variety of ways as the movement becomes more difficult initially by raising and moving an arm, then a leg, then both the arm and leg from the side-lying position. The final phase of this movement lesson is performing a counterrotating movement through the trunk while swinging the arm and leg in opposite directions. This is the movement that the trunk and extremities do when walking fast and is a lead into doing this activity with walking in an upright position.

### Lesson 4

Lesson 4 addresses standing balance over one foot. This lesson starts out with use of a chair to assist balance. Attention is directed to the foot and the places where pressure is distributed on the foot as different parts of the body are moved in circles over the standing foot starting with the knee, then the hip, the chest, shoulder, and head. The idea is to bring a person's awareness to the many ways in which weight can be distributed on the foot and how this distribution can be controlled by organizing the posture of the body above the foot in different ways. These activities then are repeated on the other side. Then Jane was directed to explore weight shifting from side to side to see how patterns of weight bearing change with this activity. When the person is comfortable standing without the chair, it is moved out of the way so that more expansive movements can be done. Lateral weight shifting then is accompanied by a swing of the leg, which is the beginning of stepping in walking. This lesson begins to incorporate some of the trunk rotation from the previous lesson into the upright position. This lesson can be taken into stepping and turning-around activities in standing.

### Lesson 5

Lesson 5 addresses walking. This lesson incorporates an awareness of the movement of weight bearing across the stance foot during forward progression and integrates an awareness of the rotation of the trunk and movement of the shoulder and arm on one side then the other through a process of observation. The goal is to observe first what the body is doing and then feel the way into rotation through the trunk with rhythmic changes in weight bearing.

### Lesson 6

Lesson 6 addresses jumping on both feet. This activity is added as a higher-level, dynamic challenge to develop balance, strength, control, and a sense of quickness about movement, which did not exist before. At the beginning Jane could not do this at all. The lesson begins with Jane placing a hand on the wall for balance and going up on her toes. It progresses to an exploration of balancing on the toes with the hand only near the wall. This is followed by stepping and regaining balance while standing on the toes and then moving from a slight squat, knees-flexed position to knees extended on the toes, exploring the coordination of that movement, and then increasing its speed. Finally, jumping, while using the wall as needed, is added.

Janes is told to work with each of these lessons one at a time several times per day for 15 to 20 minutes or as her time and energy allowed until she had mastered the movement, then to move on to the next lesson in order. All movements are difficult and could be done only at a low level at the beginning. During the initial learning process, rests are naturally built in, and the client repeatedly is drawn back to development of the kinesthetic image of her body in the movement so that these elements of practice and discovery were built into the lessons as she worked with them on her own. Jane is given an audiotaped ATM walking lesson produced by Mark Reese to use at home.

## Evaluate

The client is followed by phone conversation 2 weeks after initial examination and seen for reevaluation and progression of her plan of care (check out of MAFOs and refinement of ATM lessons 1 through 4 and addition of lessons 5 and 6) after

1 month and again after 3 months for evaluation of her progress and refinement of her learning with all six lessons. Jane is seen for a total of three sessions (total of approximately 6 hours) over the course of 3 months. This schedule is decided upon in part because of the distance she had to travel, about 2 hours one way. She also needs time to have the MAFO fabricated and then checked for fit and effectiveness during the second session. Because she has audiotapes at home to guide her work, she could call if she needs further clarification and is conscientious with practice of her lessons. Therefore more frequent sessions are not necessary.

At her 3-month follow-up evaluation, Jane has made the following improvements (see also Table 20-1).

### Musculoskeletal Improvement

ROM: WNL throughout except dorsiflexion (+10 degrees) on the right. Posture: WNL now more erect in standing than previously. She is more erect and much more solid and relaxed by her own report, with this posture.

### Neuromuscular Improvement

Strength: LLE grossly 4/5 except hip flex 3+/5, abduction and extension 4–/5. RLE: 3+/5 for hip flex, 4–/5 for ext, ABD, rotation and knee flex; 4/5 for hip ADD, knee extension and pf/df at the ankle. Motor control: modified Ashworth score was 0 for the UE, trunk, and LLE and 2 for the RLE.

There is no clonus. Fatigue is a problem affecting df after about 10 minutes of walking. After 15 minutes walking was terminated because of fatigue. The Ashworth spasticity scores did not change, but Jane's strength levels in the lower extremities were increased greatly without doing any specifically focused PRE program. Therefore a logical conclusion is that the strength gains are a result of the particular activities designed into the ATM lessons, some process of neural adaptation enhancing coordination of movements and efficient timing of muscle contraction, and the increase in activity level facilitated by the whole process. Although fatigue is not addressed directly, her ability to perform at a higher level may be viewed as a reflection also of a reduced problem with fatigue.

### Functional Improvement

Gait is still slow and now only mildly ataxic but with improved speed (approximately 2 mph, or 2.9 ft/sec), and with increased rotation of her trunk. She continues to use a cane to help her balance but does not use MAFOs because of discomfort and cosmetic reasons. She is referred back to the orthotist for suggested cut-down modifications. Balance: single leg stance 30 seconds on the left and 10 seconds on the right. She continues to hold a rail for safety but is able to go up and down stairs without UE strength assist. She is able to come to half-kneel from sitting on the floor and from half-kneel to standing without UE assist for balance or push-off. Her score on the BBS is 54/56. Her postural control is enormously improved.

### Three Year Follow-Up

She recently has been seen for her third annual follow-up visit. Although some setbacks have occurred in the intervening years, she has returned to the 3-month post-initial exam functional level except that some stiffness has returned to her gait. This could be the focus of further training in this area. However, she has progressed to a level of endurance that she did not have before, now being able to walk for 30 minutes without significant fatigue, more than a mile. She continues to enjoy jumping, which she finds very exhilarating on a daily basis. At this time, the client has discontinued the use of MAFOs for cosmetic reasons. Interestingly, in her normal daily activities, Jane appears to get along fine now without the MAFOs and without any problems with foot drop. She does use the MAFOs for exercise.

## Report the Outcomes

The integration of ATM lessons into the plan of care for this client was used to address her motor control and functional problems. It also was used to provide her with a strategy for approaching daily difficulties and problem solving on her own. The fact that she required only once a year follow-up visits while maintaining and improving her level of function was an indication of positive results from the intervention.

This case was presented as a poster at the III STEP meeting in Salt Lake City in July 2005. This was a conference of physical therapists and movement scientists in which the management of clients with neurological conditions was discussed. It was attended by 650 participants from 25 countries.

## SUMMARY

In this chapter the case of a woman with MS who has difficulties with motor control and mobility was described. The evidence on ATM was evaluated by asking broad and specific questions about the case. Two articles found in the literature deal specifically with the case. These articles were identified through the author's search and the PICO approach. The author's broader search provided useful background information that could enrich this client's management but may not be readily available to all practitioners. Six ATM lessons were developed to assist the client, and the positive outcomes of the ATM management were presented.

Acknowledgments: I would like to acknowledge the invaluable assistance of Reena Gopinathan and Sandra Ustaris for their help in developing and writing rough draft materials for the literature review.

## REFERENCES

1. Teasell R et al: The incidence and consequences of falls in stroke patients during inpatient rehabilitation: factors associated with high risk, *Arch Phys Med Rehabil* 83(3):329-33, 2002.
2. Feldenkrais M: *Body and mature behavior: a study of anxiety, sex, gravitation and learning,* New York, 1949, International Universities Press, pp 31-40.
3. Feldenkrais M: *The potent self: dynamics of the body and the mind,* New York, 1985, Harper Collins.
4. Feldenkrais M: *The elusive obvious,* Cupertino, Calif, 1981, Meta Publications.
5. Feldenkrais M: *Awareness through movement,* New York, 1972, Harper Collins.
6. Rywerant J: *The Feldenkrais method: teaching by handling,* San Francisco, 1983, Harper & Row.
7. Shafarman S: *Awareness heals: the Feldenkrais method for dynamic health,* New York, 1997, Addison Wesley Publishing.
8. Feldenkrais M: *Body awareness as healing therapy: the case of Nora,* Berkeley, CA, 1994, North Atlantic Books.
9. Heggie J: *Running with the whole body,* Emmaus, Penn, 1986, Rodale Press.
10. Hutchinson MG: *Transforming body image: learning to love the body you have,* Freedom, Calif, 1985, The Crossing Press.
11. Jackson-Wyatt O: *Natural ease for work: can you move to get the job done?* New York, 1994, Viking Press.
12. Stephens J, Miller TH: Feldenkrais method: learning to move through your life with grace and ease (Or optimizing your potential for living). In Davis C, editor: *Complementary therapies in rehabilitation: evidence for efficacy, prevention and wellness,* Thorofare, NJ, 2004, Slack Publishers.
13. Massion J: Postural control system, *Curr Opin Neurobiol* 4(6):877-87, 1994.
14. Massion J, Alexandrov A, Frolov A: Why and how are posture and movement coordinated? *Prog Brain Res* 143:13-27, 2004.
15. Deig D: Self image in relationship to Feldenkrais awareness through movement classes, independent study project, Indianapolis, Ind, 1994, University of Indianapolis, Krannert Graduate School of Physical Therapy.
16. Elgelid HS: Feldenkrais and body image, unpublished master's thesis, Conway, Ark, 1999, University of Central Arkansas.
17. Dunn PA, Rogers DK: Feldenkrais sensory imagery and forward reach, *Percept Mot Skills* 91:755-7, 2000.
18. Ginsburg C: Body-image, movement and consciousness: examples from a somatic practice in the Feldenkrais method, *J Consciousness Studies* 6(2-3):79-91, 1999.
19. Stephens J et al: Use of awareness through movement improves balance and balance confidence in people with multiple sclerosis: a randomized controlled study, *Neurology Report* 25(2):39-49, 2001.
20. Stephens JL et al: Responses to ten Feldenkrais awareness through movement lessons by four women with multiple sclerosis: improved quality of life, *Phys Therapy Case Reports* 2(2):58-69, 1999.
21. Newell KM: Motor skill acquisition, *Ann Rev Psychol* 42:213-37, 1991.
22. Ioffe ME: Brain mechanisms for the formation of new movements during learning: the evolution of classical concepts, *Neurosci Behav Physiol* 34(1):5-18, 2004.
23. Butefisch CM: Plasticity in the human cerebral cortex: lessons from the normal brain and from stroke, *Neuroscientist* 10(2):163-73, 2004.
24. Wickens JR, Reynolds JN, Hyland BI: Neural mechanisms of reward-related motor learning, *Curr Opin Neurobiol* 13(6):685-90, 2003.
25. Daoudal G, Debanne D: Long-term plasticity of intrinsic excitability: learning rules and mechanisms, *Learn Mem* 10(6):456-65, 2003.
26. Nudo RJ: Adaptive plasticity in motor cortex: implications for rehabilitation after brain injury, *J Rehabil Med* (41 Suppl):7-10, 2003.
27. Schnupp JW, Kacelnik O: Cortical plasticity: learning from cortical reorganization, *Curr Biol* 12(4): R144-6, 2002.
28. Gilbert CD, Sigman M, Crist RE: The neural basis of perceptual learning, *Neuron* 31(5):681-97, 2001.
29. Nair DG et al: Assessing recovery in middle cerebral artery stroke using functional MRI, *Brain Inj* 19(13):1165-76, 2005.
30. Huntley A, Ernst E: Complementary and alternative therapies for treating multiple sclerosis symptoms: a

systematic review. [Review] [42 refs] *Complement Ther Med* 8(2):97-105, 2000.

31. Johnson SK et al: A controlled investigation of bodywork in multiple sclerosis, *J Altern Complement Med* 5(3):237-43, 1999.

32. Ives JC, Shelley GA: The Feldenkrais method in rehabilitation: a review, *WORK: A Journal of Prevention, Assessment and Rehabilitation* 11:75-90, 1998.

33. Shumway-Cook A, Woollocott M: *Motor control,* ed 2, Philadelphia, 2001, Lippincott, Williams and Wilkins.

34. Rodgers MM et al: Gait characteristics of individuals with multiple sclerosis before and after a 6-month aerobic training program, *J Rehabil Res Devel* 36(3):183-8, 1999.

35. Lord SE, Wade DT, Halligan PW: A comparison of two physiotherapy treatment approaches to improve walking in multiple sclerosis: a pilot randomized controlled study, *Clin Rehabil* 12(6):477-86, 1998.

36. Petajan JH, White AT: Recommendations for physical activity in patients with multiple sclerosis, *Sports Med* 27(3):179-91, 1999.

37. Cattaneo D et al: Risk of falls in subjects with multiple sclerosis, *Arch Phys Med Rehabil* 83(6):864-7, 2002.

38. Kasser SL, McCubbin JA, Hooker K: Variability in constraints and functional competence in adults with multiple sclerosis, *Am J Phys Med Rehabil* 82(7):517-25, 2003.

39. Seegert EM, Shapiro R: Effects of alternative exercise on posture, *Clin Kinesiol* 53(2):41-7, 1999.

40. Bennett JL et al: Effects of a Feldenkrais based mobility program on function of a healthy elderly sample, abstract in *Geriatrics,* publication of Geriatric section of APTA. Presented at CSM in Boston, February 1998.

41. Hall SE et al: Study of the effects of various forms of exercise on balance in older women, unpublished manuscript, Healthway Starter Grant, file 7672, Nedlands, Western Australia, 1999, Dept of Rehabilitation, Sir Charles Gardner Hospital.

42. Bost H et al: *Feldstudie zur wiiksamkeit der Feldenkrais-Methode bei MS—betroffenen,* Saarbrucken, Germany, 1994, Deutsche Multiple Sklerose Gesellschaft.

43. Smith PS, Hembree JA, Thompson ME: Berg Balance Scale and Functional Reach: determining the best clinical tool for individuals post stroke, *Clin Rehabil* 18(7):811-8, 2004.

44. Ritvo PG et al: *MSQLI: multiple sclerosis quality of life inventory: a users manual,* New York, 1997, The National Multiple Sclerosis Society.

45. Stephens JL et al: Psychosocial changes related to a series of ATM classes with people with multiple sclerosis. Presented at Feldenkrais Guild of North America, Annual Conference, Rhinebeck, NY, October, 2003.

46. Petajan JH et al: The impact of aerobic training on fitness and quality of life in multiple sclerosis, *Ann Neurol* 39(4):432-41, 1996.

47. Stephens J: *Feldenkrais method: background, research and orthopedic case studies,* Orthopedic Physical Therapy Clinics of North America: Complementary Medicine. 2000;9(3):375-394.

48. Batson G, Deutsch JE: Effects of Feldenkrais awareness through movement on balance in adults with chronic neurological deficits following stroke: a preliminary study, *Complement Health Pract Rev* 10(3):203-10, 2005.

49. Connors K, Grenough P: Redevelopment of the sense of self following stroke, using the Feldenkrais Method. Poster presented at the Feldenkrais Annual Research Forum, Seattle, Wash, August, 2004.

## ADDITIONAL RESOURCES

The Feldenkrais Guild of North America
*http://www.feldenkrais.com/profession/about the feldenkrais guild of north america/*

The International Feldenkrais Federation Academy Research Journal
*http://feldenkrais-method.org*

The International Feldenkrais Federation Academy Research Journal
*http://www.iffresearchjournal.org/*

The Feldenkrais Method of Somatic Education
*https://www.feldenkrais.com/*

The Intelligent Body-Improving with Age DVD
*http://www.feldenkraisinstitute.org/order/*

# APPENDIX 1

## Side-Lying Leg Swing (Lesson 3)

The focus of any activity of ATM is to create a process of sensory and perceptual experience of the body using movement as an experimental tool to manipulate the person's experience. The purpose is not to produce a particular movement outcome. By instead creating a process, clients can get a sense of what they are comfortable doing and discover ways of organizing movement to expand that range of activity but stay within the bounds of comfort and easy effort.

### LESSON

The following directions are given to the client: Begin lying on the side in a comfortable position, legs flexed at the hips and knees and resting one on the other, arm on the body, and head supported as needed. Scan the body to notice any excessive muscular effort and the ease of breathing. (This initial scan is used as a baseline to compare with changes that may occur with subsequent movement.) Raise the top leg and swing it a small distance forward, keeping the knee straight, and then swing back to the initial position in a smooth motion. Repeat this movement five to ten times, while noting each time the amount of effort used, the point at which balance may be lost, and any change in the breathing. Repeat these movements with the leg swinging backward from the initial position.

Many people tend to lock the trunk together with the swinging leg (especially with the backward movement) and roll forward or back as the leg moves. If this happens, the practitioner should note it, and an experiment is done to give the client an experience of moving the trunk and the leg separately. The arm elevated above the shoulder and the arm is swung slightly forward and behind the body, while any movement of the trunk or legs is noted. If this causes a balance problem also, the client is instructed to make smaller and simpler movements of the arm or leg until a sense of being able to move the limbs without the trunk following is developed.

These movements may cause fatigue either in the leg or through the body. Lessons are structured so that clients have frequent rests. This may be done by simply resting and scanning the body for any postural configuration changes noted in the side-lying position or the supine position. Or the client may roll to the other side and repeat the movements on that side. In any case, rest as needed is important.

When the client is able to separate limb from trunk movement, the complexity of the movement is increased by having the leg swing forward to back through the initial position in a continuous movement and repeating this multiple times, expanding the range over sets of repetitions as it becomes easier to do. Usually during this process the client begins to get a sense of how the upper trunk and shoulder may be moving in the opposite direction as the leg. As the client begins to expand this awareness, the arm may be added to the movement so that the arm is swinging forward as the leg swings back in a reciprocal movement. The client's attention should be brought back to effort, ease, and breathing as the movement becomes more complex. Situations in which control is produced by escalating the effort are avoided. The client's attention is directed to the pressure of the body against the floor as it changes with the movement. The client is asked to develop a sense of the floor supporting the movement. The client plays with these variables of support, effort, and speed of movement in the process of exploring the problem of balance that was noticed originally.

This process could take somewhere between 15 and 30 minutes (or longer as time permits). At the end of this time clients usually have a different sense of their body either lying in the initial side-lying position or in the supine position: much more relaxed, breathing easier, resting more heavily on the floor, movement, especially rotating much more fluid and easier. To apply this sense of the body to standing, it is useful to then bring the client to a standing position and begin with some simple trunk rotation standing and then move into walking. Often this is a difficult transition for the student. This is another problem and lesson and can be approached using the same process, although with different movements as described above.

# APPENDIX 2

## Selecting a Practitioner

1. *For whom is the method appropriate?*

   In a review of the use of FM with orthopedic patients in a physical therapy clinic, Stephens[47] described successful outcomes with 157 patients, age 12 to 83, representing 50 different IDC-9 diagnoses involving every area of the body. Reviews of the Feldenkrais literature by Ives[32] and the bibliography presented on the Feldenkrais website indicate that FM has been used with clients who have chronic pain, eating disorders, lengthening hamstrings, personality disorders, stuttering, rheumatoid arthritis, posture change, and neurological diagnoses including multiple sclerosis, traumatic brain injury, Parkinson's disease, and cerebral palsy. Recently, three pilot studies using ATM with people who are post-stroke have been presented.[29,48,49]

2. *How are practitioners trained?*

   Although many physical therapists have trained in FM, trainings are also open to people of other backgrounds. Dancers, actors, musicians, psychologists, physicians, physical educators, nurses, occupational therapists, organizational consultants, and systems engineers also have trained as Feldenkrais practitioners. Trainings take different formats but generally include the equivalent of 160 days (32 weeks) of experiential and didactic work organized in shorter periods over several years. A national (including Canada) organization, the Feldenkrais Guild of North America (FGNA), and an international organization, the International Feldenkrais Federation, have developed and maintain standards of practice and sanction official training programs according to established guidelines. These organizations also support research and provide services to members. The IFF recently has established an online journal for research on FM. For more information about training programs in North America, contact the FGNA (see additional resources).

3. *Where can certified practitioners be found?*

   To locate a practitioner for referral of a client or as a resource to learn more about FM, contact the FGNA. The FGNA maintains an online listing of practitioners along with schedules of their classes.

   As noted above, practitioners have widely different backgrounds and also widely different types of professional practice. Many practitioners are physical therapists and may specialize in work with a particular client population. Many practitioners have other kinds of backgrounds and work primarily with clients from that background, such as dance (dancers); theater (actors), education (people with learning disabilities), speech therapy (people with communication disorders), and music (musicians). It is a good idea to inquire about the practitioner's professional training, level of experience as a practitioner, most typical types of clients, and amount of experience with the client's specific functional issues.

# CHAPTER 21

## The Alexander Technique

*Glenna Batson*

---

Grace is a 53-year-old retired cell biologist diagnosed with OA of the left knee secondary to a traumatic injury sustained 4 years earlier. She reports mild functional restrictions in activities of daily living (ADL) because of pain, which results in movement compensation and limits on endurance. She has taken supplements and participated in physical therapy to reduce pain and increase participation in ADL. The client is interested in adding the Alexander Technique (AT) to her plan of care. The therapist who is treating Grace is trained as an AT practitioner and has an extensive library of resources on Alexander. She uses general references, her Alexander library, and further searches to evaluate the literature supporting the use of AT for this particular client.

### ■ Initial Examination

**Client Report:** Client reports a history of increasing pain and activity restriction over past 3 years. She has pursued no treatments to date and was referred by a colleague.

**Client Goals:** To garden 3 hours a day two times a week and increase walking distance to 1 mile without disabling pain

**Employment:** Retired cell biologist

**Recreational Activities:** Gardening, walking

**General Health:** Good: Chronic, activity-related pain from knee OA; episodic, recurrent respiratory infections

**Medications:** Self-directed supplements, e.g., glucosamine sulfate for OA and garlic oil to prevent her respiratory infections

**Cardiovascular:** Endurance in sit-to-stand and fast Timed Up and Go (TUG) limited by pain onset; paradoxical breathing

**Musculoskeletal:** PROM: left (L) hip flexion (120 degrees) and (L) knee flexion (110 degrees) restricted by pain, swelling, muscular tightness, and restricted patellar glide. Pain on terminal extension (L knee) with subpatellar crepitus in weight bearing (WB) and non-WB positions. Posture: symmetrical landmarks; greater WB on right; L knee in loose-packed position

**Neuromuscular:** Force generation: knee extension=3+/5 bilaterally, ankle df=4/5 bilaterally; sit to stand (5× average) at self-selected speed: 1.56 sec; as fast as possible 0.70 sec; TUG (3× average)=8.6 sec. Coordination: dyscoordinated sit-to-stand pattern. Sensory system intact.

**Function:** Pain: right (R) knee pain, at rest=1/10; standing=1/10; after walking 15 minutes=3/10; avoids running, kneeling, squatting, jumping, pivoting. Koos Knee Survey (KKS) (65% composite score of pain, activity restriction, quality of life) and West Haven-Yale Multidimensional Pain Inventory (WHYMPI) (2.94 out of 5 point scale).

**Integumentary:** Varicosity, L shin and dorsum of foot and R thigh, increasing with limb dependency, and fragile to bruising and abrasion. Thigh girth measures, R=16″, L=16.5″.

### ■ Plan of Care

The plan of care includes eight physical therapy sessions twice a week for patellar mobilization, vastus medialis oblique muscle strengthening, kinesthetic body scanning, breathing reeducation, and movement coaching in ADL using AT principles. A home program is instituted. The client refuses referral for further evaluation of reported respiratory infection. A follow-up is scheduled for 2 weeks post-intervention to reinforce efficient coordination patterns, reevaluate strength and joint mobility, and monitor pain.

***Reevaluation Post Two Weeks*** The client's pain profile continues to fluctuate daily depending on type and length of activity. Joint noise is subsiding with improved patellar mobility, body mechanics, and sit-to-stand coordination. The client expressed a sense of improved breathing and postural ease. Her average compliance with her home program is three times per week. Repetition and reinforcement of physical exercise and cognitive cues are needed to sustain improved movement coordination.

### Incorporating CAM into the Plan of Care

The client has been introduced to AT at a public workshop and is interested in pursuing a trial of AT for ongoing OA management. The therapist, a certified AT teacher, investigated the literature on AT as a possible adjunct to treatment.

## INVESTIGATING THE LITERATURE

The therapist uses two strategies to investigate the literature. The first is a detailed approach in which preliminary background reading is performed on AT and pain. This is followed by searching databases and evaluating the literature using reviews and primary sources on AT pain and arthritis. The second is the use of the PICO format for a focused search to answer the clinical questions generated by the case.

### Preliminary Reading

To determine the appropriateness of recommending AT for the client described in this case study, the therapist must evaluate the evidence supporting its use, particularly for clients whose diagnosis or impairments are similar to Grace's. More than 30 "trade" books exist about AT, geared to a general audience and prospective trainees. (See Additional Resources for references to books.) These are not evidence-based but rather give a broad overview of the technique and a guide to application. Several book chapters have been written for complementary medicine texts that reference case studies.[1-3] The most substantive of these chapters is by Stern, a physical therapist and an AT practitioner, with substantial experience in both fields, whose approach to the topic is evidence based and accessible to medical audiences.[1]

Of the many holistic approaches that proliferated in Western culture throughout the nineteenth century, AT is distinguished among body-based systems for promoting active self-care in everyday functioning.[4] For more than 100 years, AT has been used to help people promote personal well-being by altering stressful postures and movements that interfere with ease and efficiency.[1,5] An active process of neuromuscular reeducation, AT uses kinesthetic cues and cognitive guidance to decrease pain associated with stressful movement behaviors and to improve balance and coordination.[6]

Frederick Matthias Alexander (1869-1955) was the oldest of the generation of twentieth-century movement educators (along with Gerda Alexander, Charlotte Selver, Moshe Feldenkrais, and others),[7] who developed an approach to the study of human experience ("somatic learning")[8] by investigating his own physical problems. An actor by profession, Alexander suffered recurrent bouts of laryngitis early in his career, for which conventional medicine offered only temporary relief. A radical shift occurred in his thinking when he turned from a passive vantage point of self-inquiry ("What's wrong with my voice?") to a proactive one ("How am I using my voice?").[9] Alexander explains the 10-year evolution of his method in one of his five classic books, *The Use of the Self*, written in 1932.[10]

Through self-observation, he sensed that the source of his dysfunction was a small yet perceivable reaction to the stress of speaking, much like a startle reflex.[1,10] The startle reflex in humans is a stress response[11] associated with processing of novel or aversive stimuli and involves a wide range of responses in the autonomic and somatic nervous systems.[12] Alexander's reaction manifested as a global tightening of the spinal extensors, which caused increased postural fixation and associated chest wall depression, cranial extension, and exaggerated cervical lordosis (forward head posture). Increased effort of breathing and speech resulted. On closer reflection, Alexander noticed the startle reaction had habituated, namely that it was triggered by the intent to act, intensifying with performance anxiety. Alexander first tried to "correct" his problem using a co-contraction strategy of contracting the antagonists (the flexor muscles) to keep the extensor muscles from exerting the greater force. He did this by tucking the chin to alter forward head posture. This strategy resulted only in misdirected energy and greater movement fixation.[10] When he stopped trying to change his posture by sustained muscular force and instead responded to proprioceptive feedback from exploring head balance, he experienced a spontaneous redistribution of tension throughout his body that signaled an overall improvement in coordination and neuromuscular control. Alexander had discovered an inherent mechanism for dynamic self-organization and self-regulation. The crux of his discovery was that by "re-educating the kinesthetic systems associated with posture and respiration," Alexander could voluntarily alter this maladaptive response to stress and improve his coordination. Known initially as the "Founder of a Respiratory Method,"[5] Alexander first applied his work to reeducating dysfunctional patterns of breathing and speech. Among the doctors and scientists of Alexander's day who were intrigued by his discovery were Sir Charles Sherrington, George Coghill, Aldous Huxley, Raymond Dart, and John Dewey.[4,5] Alexander began training teachers in London in the 1930s, five of whom are still teaching today.

Two basic theoretical assumptions underlie AT: (1) use affects function and (2) noninterference with the natural, coordinated action of the head and back governs use.[10,13] Within the community of Alexander Technique teachers the term "good use" which refers to mental instructions for directing movement of different parts of the body is considered an expression of adaptive psychophysical behavior, not "posture."[5,9,10] "Good use" connotes balanced use of the tonic and phasic musculature of the spine as well as appropriate application of muscle force within the context of the environment and the task. Good use also is associated with freedom from conditioned reactions to life's stresses, of remaining openly adaptive to change, whatever the environmental demands.[1,4] Second,

good use is governed by natural postural responses that provide a state of renewable responsiveness of the neuromuscular system underlying dynamic postural control.[14] Alexander called this state of neuromuscular responsiveness the "primary control,"[10,13] or simply, "poise."[5,10] Good use implies efficient postural control and timely neuromuscular coordination for graded force output commensurate with the needs of the task: neither too floppy or unsupported nor too tense or restrictive.[15] Ongoing proprioceptive awareness (what Alexander called "the means whereby"[10]) is the key feature in engaging primary control. "Misuse" is associated with habituated, stressful reactions to environmental stimuli that result in inefficient neuromuscular patterns.[1,11,14] When stressful reactions become habituated, altered sensory perception and compensatory movement result, which can lead to movement dysfunction and injury.[1,5]

AT is an indirect method of motor learning. In AT people are not taught how to sit or stand. Rather, people learn to identify their own effortful patterns of use and avoid practicing them, which results in greater ease in activity. AT teachers help clients recognize, proprioceptively, the difference between good use and misuse by offering an experience of improved postural support and ways of avoiding stressful behaviors.[16] A hallmark of an AT lesson is the subjective experience of efficient movement: light, buoyant, and effortless movement of the body as a coordinated whole, in which extraneous or misdirected muscular effort has been eliminated.[16]

### Description of Alexander Technique

During a typical AT lesson clients come dressed in comfortable clothes to allow for full mobility. A lesson normally takes 45 minutes to 1 hour, in which ADL, such as sitting, standing, walking, and lying down, are practiced with the AT principles embedded. The goal is to enhance individuals' perceptual awareness of somatosensory feedback within the context of functional activities. Alexander was insistent that clients use his principles in everyday life so that persons would be able to direct their effort appropriately in activity, rather than simply learn to relax or release tension.[5]

AT teachers engage clients in an active verbal dialogue that addresses the degree of awareness of their body movement. Simultaneously, light touch focuses attention and trains kinesthetic perception, particularly around the head, neck, and back, which are key areas for activating primary control. Repetition of activities is gauged according to clients' levels of understanding of their movement and their ability to sustain attention to kinesthetic feedback. Teachers remain in a state of good use, avoiding forceful manual manipulation, so that their own good use can communicate kinesthetically about the nature and means of postural change.[17]

Alexander devised three major "steps" to the technique, which he called "the means-whereby," "inhibition," and "direction."[11] Although none of those steps truly can be isolated from the whole process of motor learning, Alexander teachers may follow a stepwise process to apply Alexander's principles and to assess and guide a client's patterns of use. First, teachers direct clients to form an image of how they move (the "means whereby"). This is referred to as a client's "body map,"[15] which represents a body image or schema. Second, the practitioner uses "inhibition" to redirect a client away from patterns of effort in simple, functional activities, such as sitting, standing, walking, talking, and reaching, to modify them. Inhibition is not the suppression of habits associated with misuse but rather the ability to reorganize the motor system.[5,13] The goal is not to correct the client or point out what is "wrong" but to promote curiosity and self-awareness in activity so that the client can begin to make more informed choices about movement. Misdirected efforts emerge in the conception and execution of the action. Enhanced sensory feedback is believed to help clients expand their sense of their "body map"[15] and to distinguish between misuse and an experience of greater support within task demands. Clients are taught to pause between intending to move and initiating the movement, to observe and reorganize a habitual response, and to choose a more optimal, coordinated course of action. Inhibition at once helps people learn to avoid excessive and superfluous effort, while making room for more adaptive movement options to be brought to conscious awareness.[1,4]

The third step, "direction," naturally evolves out of intentional, voluntary action. Alexander developed four "directives,"[10] thought patterns that through repetition serve as kinesthetic cues to maintain optimal joint movements in response to gravity and muscle forces shaping movement. These directives are to "let the neck be free," so that the head will "balance forward and up," so that the back will "lengthen and widen," and the "knees free out and away."[10]

AT teachers use light manual guidance to provide feedback about the status of neuromuscular tensions interfering with activation of the primary control. Energy medicine proponents[18,19] explain that light touch allegedly influences the energy field of the body through induction of fascial plasticity, energy flow, and expansion of previously fixed and contracted tissues. Further, touch activates spindles and Golgi tendon organs that influence neural feedback systems to regulate muscle tone throughout the body and increase the overall integration of neuromuscular balance.[18,19] Preliminary research from cognitive neuroscience has shown that light touch helps preserve postural support and balance in young and elderly persons,[20] those congenitally blind,[21] and persons with vestibular disorders.[22] The proposed mechanism is that light touch stimulates the "graviceptors" of the spinal muscles,[20] proprioceptors in the deep spinal muscles responsible for orienting the spine in gravity. This theory appears to support the type of manual guidance used in AT.

## Searching the Databases and Evaluating the Literature

After the preliminary reading is completed, a search of five databases is conducted (MEDLINE, CINAHL, PsycInfo, SportsDiscus, and CAM on PubMed), using the keyword *Alexander Technique*. A scan of the articles suggests that AT has been investigated for use in the areas of improving posture; relieving breathing dysfunctions; decreasing performance anxiety and stress; relieving back pain; improving performance in speech, singing, athletics, performing arts, riding, and swimming; ergonomics (sitting posture and repetitive strain injury); and managing Parkinson's disease (see Additional Resources at the end of the chapter). Additional terms searched were *complementary, alternative medicine, integrative medicine, body-based, osteoarthritis, osteoarthrosis,* and *pain,* because of their pertinence to the client. Key words were then combined to identify studies in which AT is applied in subjects with either pain or arthritis. Duplicate references were removed. Search results did include general articles mentioning AT among multiple body-based therapies or other complementary therapies (Table 21-1).

The therapist first reads a systematic review[23] in which the authors suggest that outcomes research in AT can be divided into three broad categories: self-efficacy in reduction of stress and anxiety,[24] reduction of pain,[25,26] and postural improvement in persons with[27] and without neurological impairments.[28-30] Although a dearth of clinical trials exists, other types of uncontrolled studies can

## Table 21-1 Literature Search Results

|  | MEDLINE (1966-JUNE 2004) | CINAHL (1982-JULY 2004) | EBM REVIEWS | PSYCHINFO (1872-JUNE 2004) | SPORTSDISCUS (1830-2004) | CAM ON PUB MED (2004) |
|---|---|---|---|---|---|---|
| Introductory articles | 4 | 8 | 1 | 10 | 16 | 15 |
| Reviews | 3 | 3 | 0 | 1 | 0 | 0 |
| RCTs | 2 | 1 | 0 | 0 | 0 | 0 |
| Clinical trials | 3 | 1 | 0 | 2 | 2 | 1 |
| Case studies | 3 | 2 | 0 | 1 | 0 | 0 |
| Dissertations | 0 | 0 | 0 | 0 | 1 | 1 |
| Arthritis, arthrosis | 0 | 0 | 0 | 0 | 0 | 1 |
| Pain, stress, relaxation | 1 | 0 | 0 | 0 | 0 | 1 |
| Low back pain | 2 | 0 | 0 | 0 | 0 | 0 |

provide limited, but useful, insight into the benefits of AT,[23] such as the EMG studies on neck muscle tension,[28] reduction in anxiety,[24,26] and improved coordination among performing artists.[31,32] Although no evidence exists to warrant any strict contraindications for use of AT,[23,33] further investigation and more rigorous controlled trials are needed to establish a solid body of evidence of its effectiveness.[23,27,31]

Applying the research findings of AT directly to this client's plan of care is somewhat limited because of the lack of research on the efficacy of AT for OA. Nevertheless, several controlled studies were found in which subjects experienced reduction in musculoskeletal pain after the application of AT.[25,34] OA of the knee is associated with significant losses in mobility in ADL,[35] although controversy exists as to whether pain is the major limiting factor,[36,37] even when the OA is severe.[36] Therefore applying the AT literature to functional improvement helps substantiate its efficacy for this client. The long-term effects of AT were examined in a case study on a client with mechanical low back pain,[36] in which therapeutic gains were maintained only when AT was added to the protocol of manual therapy and therapeutic exercise. AT trains proprioceptive awareness to promote appropriate postural responses to movement perturbations.[30] Altered proprioception is a factor associated with the etiology of knee osteoarthritis,[37-40] and proprioceptive training is useful to promote kinesthetic awareness and joint stability for timely neuromuscular control in joint loading.[38,40] Finally, the literature on AT can be applied to self-efficacy to promote self-care strategies.[24] Complementary approaches, such as AT, have effectively helped persons with rheumatic diseases be proactive in self-care.[41] In treating OA, active approaches to treatment and continued education and self-care

have been shown to be more effective than palliative approaches.[42,43]

An alternative searching strategy would be to use PICO approach. This approach is summarized below.

### PICO BOX

For persons with OA of the knee does the use of the Alexander Technique reduce pain and increase walking, participation in ADL, and coordination?

P: Persons with OA of the knee
I: Alexander Technique
O: Pain
O: Walking
O: ADL
O: Coordination

A MEDLINE search conducted in July 2006 using all of the search terms did not yield any citations. Combining Alexander Technique and pain (9) and coordination (2) did provide some references. Most of the references related to the use of AT for people with low back pain. One article, a case report, published after the therapist conducted her search[44] deals with both pain and coordination.

In this instance a targeted search using a PICO approach does not yield enough information because the literature on AT is small. Because the client has expressed an interest in AT the therapist's strategy of using preliminary reading and other resources is an approach to answering the client's questions. The therapist then combines her clinical experience and makes inferences about the theory of the approach to recommend AT to her client.

P = **Population** (patient/client, problem, person, condition, or group attribute)
I = **Intervention** (the CAM therapy or approach)
C = **Comparison** (standard care or comparison intervention)
O = **Outcome** (the measured variables of interest)

## CLINICAL DECISION MAKING

### Generate a Clinical Hypothesis

The therapist (a certified AT teacher) feels that her 22 years of clinical experience combined with information found in the literature suggest that AT may be helpful to decrease the client's arthritic knee pain, improve functional mobility, promote more comfortable breathing, and provide tools for sustained self-care. The decision to include AT in the plan of care was based on the client's history of trauma, the chronic nature of the primary problem (knee OA), the secondary expressed problem of breathing dysfunction, the client's lack of self-care strategies employed to date, and her willingness to try a holistic approach to preserving mobility in her chosen recreational activities of gardening and walking. The client had not been proactive in pursuing any physical intervention for maintaining joint health. She had admitted to limiting her activity, particularly movements involving rapid, repetitive, and/or impulsive loading,[39] and to self-medicating periodically for swelling. The therapist therefore feels that AT is a reasonable recommendation in that it may help in pain management and improvement of coordination in ADL (avoidance of maladaptive movement patterns) and foster more responsibility for self-care.

### Examine

Before the client begins training in AT, the therapist conducts an examination that includes standardized tools for assessing activity-related knee pain: the Knee Injury and Osteoarthritis Outcome Score (KOOS).[45] The KOOS assesses five domains: pain, other symptoms, ADL function, sport and recreation, and knee-related quality of life.[46] Using a Likert scale of 0 (no problems) to 4 (extreme problems), scores are summated for all domains using a 0 to 100 scale. It has been validated in several populations and has greater responsiveness compared with other generic instruments, such as the Western Ontario and McMaster Universities Osteoarthritis Index (WOMAC).[47] It is easier to administer (10 minutes) and easier to score than the Multidimensional Pain Inventory[48] and is available free of charge. Standardized timed tests (TUG and Five Times Sit-to-Stand tests)[49,50] also were employed in the neuromuscular exam to evaluate for balance,[51] pain onset[36,39] (effect on endurance), postural malalignment,[52] and observable limb kinematics at different velocities[53,54] (self-selected and fast).

### Intervene

Based on the evaluation, the therapist develops a plan of care that includes body "mapping,"[15] breathing education,[5,31] joint mobilization, functional strengthening,[55] and coaching of activities in ADL using AT principles.[1,34] The physical therapist encouraged the client to ask questions and participate in the decisions regarding adding AT to her plan of care. Verifying the AT practitioner's credentials was not necessary in this case. In general, however, therapists referring clients for AT should verify the credentials of the AT teacher and receive written permission to contact the teacher for updates on AT sessions. (See Box 21-1 for basic credentials and Figure 21-1 for a sample letter of referral.) Reevaluation and follow-up, with possible referral to community resources for further AT study, should be routine after the initial intervention phase is completed.

---

### Box 21-1   Identifying an AT Practitioner

Licensed health care providers and consumers should be aware of credentialing. To become an AT teacher, a minimum of 3 years of full-time attendance (1600 hours) at an approved teacher-training course is required. Training emphasis is on "observation and modification of human movement patterns to identify and eliminate sources of movement dysfunction" (National Center for Complementary and Alternative Medicine http://www.nccam.nih.gov). Credentialing bodies exist that maintain standards of certification and professional ethics. These governing organizations hold annual meetings, maintain standards of practice, and support continuing professional development. In the United States, the American Society for the Alexander Technique (AmSAT) is the largest professional association of certified teachers, followed by Alexander Technique International (ATI). Board-certified teachers must meet curriculum requirements to be certified by either AmSAT or ATI to practice. More than 2000 teachers currently teach worldwide, with more than 25% in the United States. Teachers are employed in a variety of settings, such as university music, dance, and drama departments; heath care clinics; fitness centers; and ergonomic settings. A select number of AT teachers are also physical or occupational therapists or hold another allied health degree. Teachers with medical licenses can bill as third-party providers in accordance with their state laws and receive reimbursement by select insurance plans.

Dear Dr. _____,

I would like to refer _____ to you for evaluation of the condition A.
Mr/Ms/Mrs. _____ is a 45-year-old secretary with a history of conditions B, C, and
D. He has been followed here for condition E for the past 6 months, and has responded well to Y
therapy.  Most of _____'s remaining symptoms appear to be aggravated by postural
stress.  At this stage, I believe _____would benefit from Alexander Technique to
promote postural support and ease of movement.

Thank you for seeing _____ at your earliest convenience. I've asked him/her to call your
office in a few days to set up an appointment.  Please do not hesitate to contact me should you
need additional information.  I would also appreciate a brief report within one month of your
seeing the client to ensure proper follow-up.  All reports will remain in a confidential file.

Sincerely,

Name, title,

office contacts

**Figure 21-1** Sample referral letter.

The following exercise program was followed:

1. Body mapping in the supine position: 15 minutes of verbally directed body scanning to establish awareness of body schema (relationships of the torso to legs and to facilitate improved breathing pattern)
2. Patellar mobilization and adductor and hamstring stretching are followed by quadriceps setting and bilateral vastus medialis (VMO) strengthening, with kinesthetic, visual, and verbal cueing to optimize muscle recruitment timing and sequencing; progressive resistance straight leg raises SLRs in all directions is initiated, with weights strapped onto foot to avoid bruising the client's skin and increasing leg varicosity
3. Sit-to-stand coaching on a bar stool to avoid excessive knee flexion, using AT principles of sensory awareness, inhibition, and direction to optimize motor control
4. A verbal and kinesthetic dialogue assessing Grace's strategies for managing pain and coaching her in avoiding stressful behaviors at home
5. Home program consisting of self-cueing in activity, balanced with constructive rest with attention to body mapping, kinesthetic imagery, and breathing

The 4-week intervention is tolerated well. The client reports a greater sense of lightness and ease in transitioning through various postural and level changes. She is able to distinguish between good and poor movement mechanics. Client needs encouragement to carry out home program and considerable kinesthetic feedback to understand how to move efficiently to gain benefits from the home exercises. She will be seen twice a month to continue with AT coaching in ADL along with mobilization and strengthening.

## Reevaluate

After eight sessions, Grace has a better understanding of how to care for a chronic problem. She is better able to contain knee swelling by using ice, muscle pump, and proper mechanics. She feels she has learned how to avoid injurious postures and movements. She reports that her experience with AT has resulted in improved breathing and consequently an improved sense of calm and well-being. She believes AT also has been helpful to assist her understanding of her limitations of comfort in prolonged or awkward postures and how sit-to-stand can be achieved without joint pain, joint noise, and maladaptive coordination. Although the intervention was too brief to result in a lasting change in her pain profile, Grace is optimistic in and more proactive with her self-care. She also is interested in pursuing AT lessons once a month to help maintain gains.

A follow-up evaluation is conducted 1 month after the termination of therapy. The client reports that the AT body mapping and breathing exercises are helpful. She experiences less pain in the left knee and is able to garden up to 6 hours on a good day. She still avoids long walks and continues to use compensatory postures to garden. She uses AT cueing in bending and squatting. She experiences sharp peripatellar pain with the quadriceps strengthening exercises and therefore has not been compliant.

Post-intervention KOOS score is essentially unchanged (65%), except in one domain, in which the client had reintroduced modified squatting into her gardening, reporting mild pain as a consequence. Timed score changes also are insignificant: TUG score (three trials) averaged 11 seconds (self-selected) and 8.5 seconds (fast as possible). Five Times Sit-to-Stand (two trials) average 1.7 seconds (self-selected), and 0.8 second (as fast as possible), with pain and joint noise increasing on the second trial. The client appeared to benefit most from the technique when activities are conducted slowly enough and with enough awareness to avoid stressful impact on the osteoarthritic knee.[56] Continued training in AT is recommended to continue to maintain the gains in altering injurious movement habits.

## Report the Outcomes

Dissemination of these findings can add to the AT literature and its potential use to reduce pain and to increase mobility in persons with arthritis. In addition, case reports in which a complementary therapy has been integrated into a plan of care can encourage a dialogue about the use of these therapies in the management of pain in a client population frequently encountered by rehabilitation professionals. Possible venues for papers of this type may be *The Journal of Alternative and Complementary Therapies, Journal of the American Geriatric Society, Arthritis Care and Research, Journal of Orthopedic and Sports Physical Therapy, Journal of Bodywork and Manual Therapy,* and the *Alternative and Complementary Medicine Journal.*

## SUMMARY

The case of a 53-year-old woman who had knee pain and limitation in function resulting from osteoarthritis is described. The therapist, who is a trained Alexander practitioner, assists the client in determining if AT should be added to her plan of care. After searching the literature, the therapist determines that some support exists for use of AT with this client because it has been shown to reduce musculoskeletal pain. The therapist also uses some of the literature on how the relationship among knee mechanics, aging, and proprioceptive deficits in the knee may produce knee pain. Because AT is a technique with a strong basis in proprioceptive

retraining, she uses indirect evidence from mechanistic studies in addition to direct evidence from outcome studies on musculoskeletal pain as the basis for including AT in her plan of care. Outcomes of the intervention, which for this client were successful in achieving her mobility goals, were tracked with standardized outcome measures. Dissemination of the findings to a variety of audiences is proposed.

## REFERENCES

1. Stern J: The Alexander technique. In Novey DW, editor: *Clinician's complete reference to complementary/alternative medicine,* St Louis, 2000, Mosby.
2. Zuck D: The Alexander technique. In David CM, editor: *Complementary therapies in rehabilitation: holistic approaches for prevention and wellness,* Thorofare, NJ, 1997, Slack.
3. Batson G: The Alexander technique. In Wainapel SF, Fast A, editors: *Alternative medicine and rehabilitation,* New York, 2003, Demos Medical Publishing.
4. Gelb M: *Body learning: an introduction to the Alexander technique,* New York, 1994, Henry Holt & Company.
5. Alexander FM: *Articles and letters,* London, 1995, Mouritz.
6. American Society for Alexander Technique: Discover the Technique. Available at: *http://www.alexandertech.org.* Accessed February 7, 2005.
7. Murphy M: *The future of the body: explorations into the further evolution of human nature,* Los Angeles, 1992, Jeremy P Tarcher.
8. Hanna T: Clinical somatic education: a new discipline in the field of health care, *SOMATICS, Magazine-Journal of the Bodily Arts and Sciences.* Available at: *http://www.somatics.com/hannart.htm.* Accessed February 7, 2005.
9. De Alcantara P: *Indirect procedures: a musician's guide to the Alexander technique,* Oxford, 1997, Clarendon Press.
10. Alexander FM: *The use of the self,* California, 1986, Centerline Press.
11. Selye H: *Stress without distress,* New York, 1994, Lippincott.
12. Bradley MM, Lang PJ, Cuthbert BN: Emotion, novelty, and the startle reflex: habituation in humans, *Behav Neurosci* 107:970-80, 1993.
13. Alexander FM: *Conscious constructive control of the individual,* Long Beach, California, 1985, Centerline Press.
14. Dennis R: Defining primary control, *AmSAT News* 64:14-5, 2004.
15. Conable B, Conable W: *The Alexander technique: a manual for students,* ed 3, Columbus, Ohio, 1998, Andover Press.

16. Brennan R: *The Alexander technique: natural poise for health,* Shaftesbury, Dorset, 1991, Element Books.

17. Zahn R: Francisco Varela's three gestures of becoming aware and its relevance to the Alexander Technique. Presented at the World Congress of the Alexander Technique. Oxford, UK, 2004.

18. Oschman JL: Structural integration (Rolfing), osteopathic, chiropractic, Feldenkrais, Alexander, myofascial release, and related methods. In *Energy medicine: the scientific basis,* New York, 1999, Churchill Livingstone.

19. Cottingham JT: *Healing through touch,* Boulder, Colo, 1985, Rolf Institute.

20. Jeka J: Light touch as a balance aid, *Phys Ther* 77:476-87, 1997.

21. Jeka JJ et al: Haptic cues for postural control in sighted and blind individuals, *Percept Psychophys* 58:409-23, 1996.

22. Lackner JR et al: Precision contact of the fingertip reduces postural sway in individuals with bilateral vestibular loss, *Exp Brain Research* 126:459-66, 1999.

23. Ernst E, Canter PH: The Alexander technique: a systematic review of controlled clinical trials, *Research in Complementary and Classical Medicine* 10:325-9, 2003.

24. Valentine ER et al: The effect of lesson in the Alexander technique on music performance in high and low stress situations, *Psychology of Music* 23:129-41, 1995.

25. Vickers AP, Ledwith F, Gibbens AO: The impact of the Alexander technique on chronic mechanical low back pain, unpublished report, 2000.

26. Elkayam O et al: Multidisciplinary approach to chronic back pain: prognostic elements of the outcome, *Clin Experimental Rheumatol* 14:281-8, 1996.

27. Stallibrass C, Chalmers C: Randomized controlled trial of the Alexander technique for idiopathic Parkinson's disease, *Clin Rehabil* 16:705-18, 2002.

28. Pierce Jones F: Method for changing stereotyped response patterns by the inhibition of certain postural sets, *Psychol Rev* 72:196-214, 1956.

29. Abehaim L et al: The role of activity in the therapeutic management of back pain. Report on the International Paris Task Force on Back Pain, *Spine* 25(Suppl 4):S1-S33, 2000.

30. Dennis RJ: Functional reach improvement in normal older women after Alexander technique instruction, *J Gerontol* 54(a):M8-11, 1999.

31. Dennis J: Alexander technique for chronic asthma, *Cochrane Database Syst Rev* CD000995:2, 2002.

32. Batson G: Traditional and nontraditional approaches to performing arts physical therapy: the dance medicine perspective, *Orthop Phys Ther Clin North Am* 6:207-30, 1997.

33. Jain S, Janssen K, DeCelle S: Alexander technique and Feldenkrais method: a critical overview, *Phys Med Rehabil Clin North Am* 15:811-25, 2004.

34. Cottingham JT, Maitland J: Three-paradigm treatment model using soft tissue mobilization and guided movement-awareness techniques for a client with chronic low back pain: a case study, *J Othop Sports Phys Ther* 26:155-67, 1997.

35. Messinger-Rapport BJ, Thacker HL: Prevention for the older woman. Mobility: a practical guide to managing osteoarthritis and falls. Part 6, *Geriatrics* 58:22-9, 2003.

36. Thomas SG, Pagura SM, Kennedy D: Physical activity and its relationship to physical performance in patients with end stage knee osteoarthritis, *J Orthop Sports Phys Ther* 33:745-54, 2003.

37. Rollin M, Gallagher MD: Biopyschosocial pain medicine and mind-brain-body science, *Phys Med Rehabil Clin North Am* 15:854-71, 2004.

38. Radin EL et al: Relationship between lower limb dynamics and knee joint pain, *J Orthop Res* 9(3):398-405, 1991.

39. Skinner HB, Barrack RL, Cook SD: Age-related decline in proprioception, *Clin Orthop Relat Res* 184:208-11, 1986.

40. Solomonow M, Krosgaard M: Sensorimotor control of knee stability: a review, *Scand J Med Sci Sports* 11:64-80, 2001.

41. Neims AH: Complementary and alternative therapies for rheumatic diseases. Part I. Issues, *Rheum Dis Clin North Am* 25:401-12, 1999.

42. Harrison AL: The influence of pathology, pain, balance, and self-efficacy on function in women with osteoarthritis of the knee, *Phys Ther* 84:822-31, 2004.

43. Loring K, Laurin J, Holman HR: Arthritis self-management: a study of the effectiveness of patient education for the elderly, *Gerontologist* 24:455-7, 1984.

44. Cacciatore TW, Horak FB, Henry SM: Improvement in automatic postural coordination following Alexander Technique lessons in a person with low back pain, *Phys Ther* 85(6):565-78, 2005.

45. Roos EM et al: Knee injury and osteoarthritis outcome score (KOOS): development of a self-administered outcome measure, *J Orthop Sports Phys Ther* 28:88-96, 1988.

46. Roos EM, Lohmander LS: The Knee Injury and Osteoarthritis Outcome Score (KOOS): from joint injury to osteoarthritis, *Health Qual Life Outcomes.* 1:64, 2003. Available at: *http://www.hqlo.com/content/1/1/64.*

47. Roos EM, Roos HP, Lohmander LS: WOMAC Osteoarthritis Index: additional dimensions for use in subjects with post-traumatic osteoarthritis of the knee, *Osteoarthr Cartil* 7:216-21, 1999.

48. Bernstein IH, Jaremko ME, Hinkley BS: On the utility of the West Haven-Yale Multidimensional Pain Inventory, *Spine* 20(8):956-63, 1995.

49. Howe T, Oldham J: Functional tests in elderly osteo-arthritic subjects: variability of performance, *Nurs Stand* 9:35-8, 1995.

50. Stratford PW et al: The relationship between self-report and performance-related measures: questioning the content validity of timed tests, *Arthritis Rheum* 49:535-40, 2003.

51. Noren AM et al: Balance assessment in patients with peripheral arthritis: allocation and reliability of some clinical assessments, *Physiother Res Int* 6:193-204, 2001.

52. Hirose D et al: Posture of the trunk in the sagittal plane is associated with gait in community-dwelling elderly population, *Clin Biomech* 19:57-63, 2004.

53. Childs JD et al: Alterations in lower extremity movement and muscle activation patterns in individuals with osteoarthritis, *Clin Biomech* 19:44-9, 2004.

54. Pai YC et al: Alteration in multijoint dynamics in patients with bilateral knee osteoarthritis, *Arthritis Rheum* 37:1297-304, 1994.

55. McCool JF, Schneider JK: Home-based leg strengthening for older adults initiated through private practice, *Prev Med* 28:105-10, 1999.

56. Pereira MI, Gomes PS: Movement velocity in resistance training, *Sports Med* 33:427-38, 2003.

## ADDITIONAL RESOURCES

### Alexander Technique Books

Alexander FM: *The universal constant in living*, Long Beach, California, 1986, Centerline Press.

Maisel E, editor: *The resurrection of the body: the writing of F. Matthias Alexander*. Shaftesbury, UK, 1997, Shambhala Publications.

Brennan R: *The Alexander Technique manual: a step-by-step guide to improve breathing, posture and well-being*. Boston, 1996, Charles Tuttle.

Brown R: *Authorised summaries of FM Alexander's four books*, London, 1992, STAT Books.

Caplan D: *Back trouble: a new approach to prevention and recovery*, Gainesville, Fla, 1987, Triad Publishing Company.

Conable B: *What every musician needs to know about the body: the practical application of body mapping and the Alexander Technique to making music*, Columbus, Ohio, 1998, Andover Press.

Cranz GJ: The *chair: rethinking culture, body, and design*, New York, 1999, WW Norton.

Drake J: Body know-how: a practical guide to the use of the Alexander Technique in everyday life, London, 1991, Thorsons.

Jones FP: *Freedom to change*, London, 1996, Mouritz.

Kodish BI: *Back pain solutions: how to help yourself with posture-movement therapy and education*, Pasadena, Calif, 2001, Extensional Publishing.

Maisel E: *The Alexander Technique: the essential writings of F Matthias Alexander*, London, 1990, Thames and Hudson.

Nielsen M: A study of stress amongst professional musicians. In Stevens C, editor: *The Alexander Technique: medical and physiological aspects*, London, 1994, STAT Books.

Rickover RM: *Fitness without stress: a guide to the Alexander technique*, Portland, Ore, 1988, Metamorphous Press.

### Research Studies and Reviews

Austin JHM: Enhanced respiratory muscular function in normal adults after lessons in proprioceptive musculoskeletal education without exercises, *Chest* 102:486-90, 1992.

Batson G: Conscious use of the human body in movement: the peripheral neuroanatomic basis of the Alexander Technique, *Med Probl Performing Artists* 11:3-11, 1996.

Cranz GJ: The Alexander Technique in the world of design: posture and the common chair: part II: body-conscious design for chairs, interiors and beyond, *Body Movement Ther* 4:155-65, 2000.

Deane KHO et al: Physiotherapy versus placebo or no intervention in Parkinson's disease, *Cochrane Database Syst Rev* 00075320, 2, 2000.

Emerich KA: Nontraditional tools helpful in the treatment of certain types of voice disturbances, *Curr Opin Otolaryngol Head Neck Surg* 11:149-53, 2003.

Fisher K: Early experiences of a multidisciplinary pain management programme, *Holistic Med* 3:47-56, 1988.

Gilman MJ: Stuttering and relaxation: applications for somatic education in stuttering treatment, *Fluency Disord* 25:59-76, 2000.

Hertzberg E: Using the Alexander technique to combat osteoarthritis, *J Altern Complement Med* 8:27-9, 1990.

Hudson B: The effects of the Alexander Technique on the respiratory system of the singer/actor: part 1: F.M. Alexander and concepts of his technique that affect respiration in singer/actors, *J Sing* 59:9-17, 2002.

Krim D: Multiple perspectives on the experience and effectiveness of the Alexander Technique in relation to athletic performance enhancement: a qualitative study, dissertation, Ann Arbor, Mich, 1993, University Microfilms International.

Kristl MJ: The Alexander technique as a management tool of a connective tissue disorder, *Bodywork Movement Ther* 5:181-90, 2001.

Machonochie KJ: Changing the pattern of behavior: outline of a therapy for criminal reform, *J Criminal Law Criminol* 47:162-73, 1956.

Maitland S: An exploration of the application of the Alexander technique for people with learning disabilities, *Br J Learn Disabil* 24:70-6, 1996.

Oliver SK: Case study: The Alexander Technique as an intervention in lower back dysfunction in dancers, *Kines Med Danc* 15:80-7, 1993.

Oschman JL: Structural integration (Rolfing), osteopathic, chiropractic, Feldenkrais, Alexander, myofascial release and related methods: an energy review part 5B, *J Bodywork Manual Ther* 1:305-9, 1997.

Reiser S: Stress reduction and optimal psychological functioning, Alexander Technique Sixth International Montreux Congress on Stress, 1994.

Stallibrass C, Hampson M: The Alexander technique: its application in midwifery and the results of preliminary research into Parkinson's, *Complement Ther Nurs Midwifery* 7(1):13-8, 2001.

Stallibrass C, Sissons P, Chalmers C: Randomized controlled trial of the Alexander Technique for idiopathic Parkinson's disease, *Clin Rehabil* 16:695-708, 2002.

Stevens C: The development of the Alexander technique and evidence for its effects, *Br J Ther* 2:621-6, 1995.

Tinbergen N: Ethology of stress diseases, Nobel Laureate Lecture. *England Science* 185:20-7, 1974.

Wasley D, Taylor A: Changes in psycho-physiological response to a musical performance after 16 weeks of aerobic exercise and Alexander technique training, *J Sports Sci* 21:292-3, 2003.

# CHAPTER 22

## Craniosacral Therapy

*Ellen Zambo Anderson, Perry Wolk-Weiss*

---

### CASE

Karen is a 48-year-old woman with a history of insulin-dependent diabetes mellitus (IDDM) and a new onset of upper thoracic pain. She sees her physician on a regular basis for management of her health status and IDDM. Having had prior success with chiropractic care for low back pain, she seeks chiropractic treatment for discomfort and thoracic pain between her scapulae.

### ■ Initial Examination

**Client Goals:** Decrease her thoracic pain and discomfort
**Employment:** Assists at daughter's school
**Recreational Activities:** Walking
**General Health:** Generally good with the exception of diabetes
**Medications:** Insulin
**Neuromusculoskeletal:** Standing posture (anteroposterior): balanced shoulders and hips. Standing posture (lateral): balanced. Cervical spine ROM: pain-free and WNLs. Strength: WNLs. Thoracic pain: 3/10 at rest, 7/10 with movement, 8/10 with sneezing. Palpation: moderate suboccipital tenderness; cervical paraspinals, scalenes, and upper trapezius did not show marked signs of trigger points or hypertonicity. Palpation for vertebral subluxation revealed aberrant motion at C1-C3 and T4-T7.

### ■ Evaluation

The chiropractor determined that the client's examination findings reflected a chiropractic diagnosis of cervical and thoracic vertebral subluxation with aberrant motion at C1-C3 and T4-T7.

### ■ Plan of Care

Karen's plan of care included spinal manipulation to the cervical and thoracic spine to reduce the presence of vertebral subluxations and restore normal spinal alignment and stability of the thoracic spine.

### ■ Reevaluation

After several sessions the client's pain, ROM, posture, and spine were reexamined. The client reported that her thoracic pain was reduced to 0/10 at rest, 4/10 with movement, 6/10 with sneezing. Palpation revealed less suboccipital tenderness and improved alignment and movement at C1-C3 and T4-T7.

During the reevaluation the client revealed that she had a history of Ménière's disease and frequently suffered from nausea, vertigo, and tinnitus. She asked if spinal manipulations ever helped Ménière's disease or if the chiropractor knew of any techniques that may help reduce her symptoms. Given this new information and request, the chiropractor reexamined the client.

### ■ Reexamination

Symptoms experienced by Karen during exacerbation of Ménière's disease are vertigo, nausea, and tinnitus. These exacerbations occur about once a week. For the first 5 to 6 hours during an exacerbation, Karen's symptoms are severe, and she is unable to perform activities such as walking, working, reading, and driving. After 6 hours, she can perform sedentary activities with moderate dizziness and minimal tinnitus. After 12 hours, Karen reports that her symptoms of vertigo are minimal and that she can resume

driving. The chiropractor examines Karen's cranium and documents a left sphenobasilar cranial fault.

### Incorporating CAM into the Plan of Care

The chiropractor, who is trained in CST, believes that CST may change the relationship of the cranium with the structures of the inner ears and positively affect some of the symptoms the client experiences from Ménière's disease. He decides to investigate the scientific literature to determine if CST may be helpful in Ménière's disease and asks the client to consider adding CST to the standard chiropractic plan of care. The client agrees to continue with spinal manipulation to further decrease her thoracic pain. CST will be added if the literature supports it use.

The scenario presented in this chapter includes a client with thoracic pain and Ménière's disease whose care is managed by a chiropractor. Although chiropractics is considered by the National Center for Complementary and Alternative Medicine (NCCAM) to be a complementary practice (see Chapter 18) the same clinical decision-making process described in Chapter 2 can be used by any licensed health care provider who considers providing an intervention not traditionally taught in their professional curriculum. Regardless of the discipline, all heath care providers are encouraged to be knowledgeable about one's own professional scope of practice before the integration of a complementary therapy. This knowledge, along with information about other legal, ethical, and cultural issues (see Chapter 3), will be helpful for managing patients and professional liability.

The client in this chapter did not initially report a history of Ménière's disease. After she informed the chiropractor of this condition and inquired about spinal manipulation for Ménière's disease, the chiropractor considered inclusion of craniosacral therapy (CST) into her plan of care.

## INVESTIGATING THE LITERATURE

The chiropractor uses two strategies to investigate the literature. The first is a detailed approach in

which preliminary background reading is performed on Ménière's disease and CST. This is followed by a search of the databases and evaluation of the literature using reviews and primary sources for Ménière's disease and CST. The second is the use of the PICO format for a focused search to answer the clinical question generated by the case.

### Preliminary Reading

In this case, the client presents with Ménière's disease, a condition that may be unfamiliar to health care providers who do not specialize in vestibular rehabilitation. An overview of the symptoms and impairments associated with Ménière's disease can be found in resources listed in the references at the end of this chapter. They include books[1-4] and reputable medical websites.[5-7]

### *Ménière's Disease*

Ménière's disease is an idiopathic inner ear disorder. Also known as *endolymphatic hydrops,* this condition is characterized by episodic attacks of fluctuating hearing loss, a sensation of "fullness" in the ear, tinnitus, rotatory vertigo, postural imbalance, nystagmus, nausea, and vomiting. Although severe vertigo can persist from 30 minutes to 24 hours, less severe symptoms can last 72 hours. Residual instability and hearing loss may continue for several more days or weeks and then return to their pre-attack status. As the disease progresses, hearing may fail to return, whereas the symptoms of vertigo may diminish in severity and frequency.[2]

Several factors have been attributed to Ménière's disease, but a clear etiology of the condition remains elusive. The presence of endolymphatic hydrops in persons with Ménière's disease is considered to be a function of malabsorption of endolymph in the endolymphatic duct and sac. This condition can create obstructions and increased hydraulic pressure within the inner ear's endolymphatic system, which potentially affects the anatomical relationships between the temporal bone, the organ of Corti, the utricle, and the saccule.[6] Of note are observations that lesions of the temporal bone associated with hydrops include temporal bone fractures, atrophy of the sac, and narrowing of the lumen in the endolymphatic duct, which prompts some health professionals to "postulate a cause-and-effect relationship between constricted anatomy in the temporal bone and malabsorption of the endolymph."[2]

### Diagnosis

No specific, definitive test for Ménière's disease exists. The diagnosis of Ménière's disease is by differential diagnosis and is based on the clinical findings and longitudinal course of the disease rather than on a single attack. Because many of the symptoms of Ménière's disease mimic symptoms of other conditions and diseases, these conditions must be ruled out before a diagnosis can be made.

A panel of blood tests, for example, may be helpful to rule out infection and metabolic and hormonal imbalances, which can present symptoms similar to those of Ménière's disease. Imaging studies, including magnetic resonance imaging (MRI) and computed tomography (CT) scans, can be used to identify the presence of anatomical abnormalities and lesions that may cause Ménière's disease–like symptoms. Other tests, such as audiometry, can be helpful for documenting fluctuations in hearing acuity, a common finding in Ménière's disease, whereas transtympanic electrocochleography (ECoG) can be used to detect distortion of the inner ear and the likely presence of hydrops, an observation consistent with Ménière's disease.[5,6]

In keeping with the recommendation to follow the longitudinal course of the disease and exclude

conditions that may mimic the symptoms of Ménière's disease, the American Academy of Otolaryngology–Head and Neck Surgery's Committee on Hearing and Equilibrium developed a diagnostic guideline for Ménière's disease that can be found in Box 22-1.[7]

### Treatment

Because the etiology of Ménière's disease is unclear, medical treatment for it is focused primarily on relief of the client's symptoms. Vertigo sometimes can be managed with medications considered to be vestibulosuppressants, such as meclizine (Antivert), diazepam (Valium), lorazepam (Ativan), and alprazolam (Xanax), whereas prochlorperazine (Compazine) or dimenhydrinate (Dramamine) may be prescribed for nausea. A short course of steroids appears to be helpful to treat acute attacks of Ménière's disease, whereas diuretics have been

---

**Box 22-1  Guidelines for the Diagnosis of Ménière's Disease**

**CERTAIN MÉNIÈRE'S DISEASE**
Definite Ménière's disease, plus histopathological confirmation

**DEFINITE MÉNIÈRE'S DISEASE**
Two or more definitive spontaneous episodes of vertigo (20 minutes or longer)
Audiometrically documented hearing loss on at least one occasion
Tinnitus or aural fullness
Other causes excluded

**PROBABLE/DEFINITE MÉNIÈRE'S DISEASE**
One definitive episode of vertigo
Audiometrically documented hearing loss on at least one occasion
Tinnitus or aural fullness
Other causes excluded

**POSSIBLE MÉNIÈRE'S DISEASE**
Episodic vertigo without documented hearing loss
Sensorineural hearing loss (fluctuating or fixed) with disequilibrium, but without definitive episodes
Other causes excluded

From Committee on Hearing and Equilibrium, American Academy of Otolaryngology-Head and Neck Surgery Committee on Hearing and Equilibrium guidelines for the diagnosis and evaluation of therapy in Meniere's disease.

used prophylactically to reduce endolymphatic pressure. Clients also are advised to make dietary changes that may help manage their condition. Avoidance of salt is one of the primary recommendations because sodium appears to play a role in increased fluid retention of the inner ear. In addition, clients often are asked to limit food and substances that appear to be "triggers" for acute attacks. These trigger substances include caffeine, nicotine, alcohol, and foods with high cholesterol and carbohydrate content.[5,6]

Surgical treatment for Ménière's disease is reserved for clients for whom conservative medical treatment has failed and attacks are frequent and severe. Even with these conditions, surgical intervention is controversial. During one procedure, the petrous bone is removed so that the endolymphatic reservoir sac can expand and dissipate pressure. A shunt also can be provided so that fluid can drain from the endolymphatic space to the mastoid or subarachnoid space. Success rates are reported to be 60% to 80%, although critics argue that this surgery is no more effective than sham surgery, which suggests that the benefits are due to the placebo effect. A vestibular nerve section is the most common surgery for persons with unilateral Ménière's disease and severe vertigo. Vertigo control with hearing preservation occurs in 95% of the surgeries. Postoperative vestibular rehabilitation frequently is required to ensure accommodation to unilateral vestibular functioning. A labyrinthectomy, which is less invasive than a vestibular section, is indicated only for clients whose hearing has been destroyed by the disease. The success rate for labyrinthectomy is better than 95%, with recovery enhanced by postsurgical vestibular rehabilitation. The newest treatment approach for severe Ménière's disease is transtympanic perfusion of gentamicin, in which the medication is applied through a myringotomy into the middle ear cavity, where it is then absorbed through the membrane of the inner ear. Early success rates appear to be favorable, although long-term studies have yet to be completed.[8]

In the case described at the beginning of this chapter, Karen does not initially seek treatment from her chiropractor for Ménière's disease. Rather, she is receiving chiropractic treatments to manage her upper thoracic pain. When the chiropractor becomes aware of Karen's history of Ménière's disease, he considers the possibility, based on his knowledge and training in CST, that she may benefit from this approach to health and healing. A brief history and description of CST is followed by a review of the scientific literature available on CST and its application in Ménière's disease.

### Cranial Osteopathy

Dr. Andrew Taylor Still (1828-1917), considered to be the founder of osteopathy (refer to Chapter 18) believed that the body is a self-regulating, self-healing, integrated unit. He theorized that most diseases and pathological conditions were either directly or indirectly caused by vertebral misalignment. Therefore manipulation of the spine, with the intent to correct vertebral displacement, would help to ameliorate abnormal conditions elsewhere in the body.[9] This theory and Still's approach to medicine were controversial during the late nineteenth century. Nevertheless, Still's successes in treatment of clients using manual therapy or what was then being called "osteopathy" brought him notoriety, and in 1892 he established the American School of Osteopathy in Kirksville, Missouri.

A student of Still's, William G. Sutherland, DO, was fascinated with the design of the human skull and believed that the cranial sutures were actually joints that did not calcify or fuse completely during maturation. Sutherland proposed that interosseous cranial motion was rhythmic and constant throughout life and, in fact, was crucial to maintaining health. When the interosseous cranial motion was abnormal or restricted, then abnormal symptoms or conditions would emerge.[10] Sutherland experimented with his own head by palpating and restricting cranial movement. He then began gently palpating the heads of others and claimed that he could sense subtle rhythmic movement of the cranium. Sutherland also proposed, based on his palpations and observations, that the sacrum had palpable movement that was in synchrony with cranial motion.[10] Sutherland argued that these structures were linked by the spinal dura mater, which allowed the motion at the occiput to influence the motion at the sacrum, and vice versa. Disruption of the synchronicity could be represented by physiological or anatomical abnormalities.

### Craniosacral Therapy

Sutherland's concepts and theories were known in the osteopathic community of health care providers but were not even considered in the practice of traditional medicine. In the 1970s, osteopathic physician John E. Upledger worked with a team of physicians and scientists at Michigan State University to investigate Sutherland's concepts of cranial bone movement and a craniosacral system. From their work, Upledger developed CST, a manual method to evaluate and treat the craniosacral system consisting of the cranium, brain, dura mater, arachnoid membrane, pia mater, spinal cord, cerebrospinal fluid (CSF), and sacrum.[10]

Two key assumptions or beliefs underpin CST. The first belief is that the cranium is not fixed. Rather, subtle movements can and do occur at the articulations between the cranial bones. The second assumption is that the dural membranes move rhythmically in response to the absorption and production of the CSF and that this movement influences the movement of the cranial bones, the vertebral column, and the sacrum.

Upledger and Vredevoogd[10] have suggested that, based on its anatomical structure, the craniosacral system is a distinct physiological system and is intimately associated with the central and autonomic nervous systems and the neuromuscular and endocrine systems. They describe the craniosacral system as a semi-closed hydraulic system formed by the dura mater, in which the choroid system within the brain ventricles acts as the CSF intake component and the arachnoid system serves as the outflow component (Figure 22-1). This continuous, rhythmic flow of fluid creates subtle movement of the dura mater membranes, which, because they are attached to the skull, vertebral column, and sacrum, can affect the functioning of multiple systems.[11] Restrictions in normal physiological motion of the craniosacral system have been associated with a wide range of conditions including, but not limited to, neck and back pain, headache, autism, scoliosis, fibromyalgia, posttraumatic stress disorder, and temporomandibular joint syndrome.[11]

CST includes examination of the craniosacral system through gentle palpation at multiple sites, including the cranium, the thoracic and lumbar spine, the sacrum, and the feet. Through this palpation, practitioners assess the craniosacral rhythm in terms of flow or restriction of flow, speed, and amplitude (Figures 22-2 to 22-4). Treatment based on this assessment includes gentle mobilization of the cranium, spine, and sacrum to release restrictions in the craniosacral system to restore and improve functioning of the nervous system. Through this subtle mobilization, CST practitioners believe they are able to enhance the body's natural healing processes by improving the craniosacral rhythm or flow. Although this intervention is considered gentle, contraindications include conditions in which an increase in intracranial

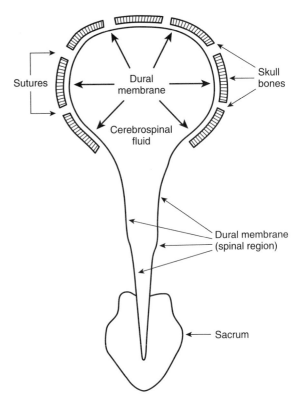

**Figure 22-1** The craniosacral system as a semi-closed hydraulic system of the cerebrospinal fluid and the dura mater.

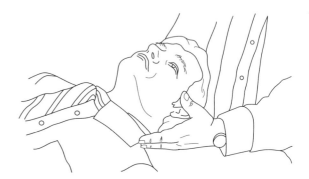

**Figure 22-2** Palpation of the cranium to assess craniosacral rhythm.

pressure should be avoided. Examples of such conditions include cerebral hemorrhage, intracranial aneurysm, subdural or subarachnoid bleeding, and brain stem herniation.

Most practitioners of CST have a medical or health care background, but not all schools or training programs require licensure or registration as a health care provider to become a craniosacral therapist. The Upledger Institute, Inc., the most well-known American training institute in CST,

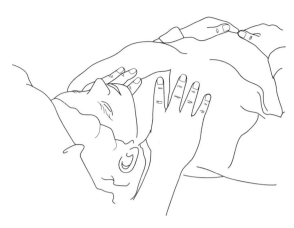

**Figure 22-3** Palpation of the thorax to assess craniosacral rhythm.

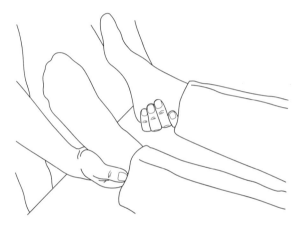

**Figure 22-4** Palpation of the feet to assess craniosacral rhythm.

does, however, require licensure or registration as a health care practitioner as a prerequisite for the required course CranioSacral I. Coursework in craniosacral therapy includes lecture and laboratory experiences, during which students learn to examine and treat clients using craniosacral techniques developed by John Upledger. The Upledger Institute, Inc., offers two levels of certification. Level One—Techniques requires successful completion of CranioSacral Therapy I and II and three exams, including a practical/oral examination. CranioSacral Therapy I and II typically are taught over 4 consecutive days, which include lectures and opportunities to practice examination and treatment techniques. Level Two—Diplomat requires completion of Level One plus successful completion of Advanced I Upledger CranioSacral Therapy, three different examinations, a 20-hour preceptor-

ship, five written case histories, and either a publication or 6 hours of presentation on CST.

## Searching the Databases
### Critical Reviews

The chiropractor considers the possibility that Ménière's disease can affect the anatomy of the temporal bone and the endolymph[2] and that CST may be a helpful intervention for improvement of the alignment of the cranium, including the temporal bone. He therefore hypothesizes that CST may be beneficial in addressing some of the symptoms associated with Ménière's disease. The medical and health-related databases were searched using the key words *Ménière's disease, craniosacral, craniosacral therapy,* and *cranial osteopathy* as seen in Table 22-1. When Ménière's disease was searched in the Cochrane Collection of Evidence-Based Medicine (EBM) databases, nine systematic reviews and four reviews of effects were obtained. However, none of the reviews included CST or cranial osteopathy as an intervention for Ménière's disease. Most of the reviews focused on pharmacological or surgical treatment for Ménière's disease or tinnitus.

Continuing to search for review articles, the key words *craniosacral* and *craniosacral therapy* and *cranial osteopathy* were searched in the EBM, MEDLINE, CINAHL, and CAM on PubMed databases. One potentially helpful systematic review by Green et al[12] was obtained and read. For this review the authors conducted a systematic search and critical appraisal of research on craniosacral therapy. Although the search was not limited to specific study designs, client population, or measured outcomes, the quality of the studies and the reported outcomes were assessed using standard tools and accepted methods. The review included 34 studies that were divided into one of three categories: craniosacral interventions and health outcomes; the pathophysiological mechanisms of craniosacral dysfunction; and the validity of craniosacral assessment.

Studies within the intervention and health outcomes category included two case reports,[13,14] considered by Green et al[12] to be the lowest grade of evidence, one retrospective study of persons with temporomandibular joint dysfunction,[15] and a prospective study of children with neurological impairments.[16] Concerns also were raised by a study[17] in which subjects with traumatic brain injury incurred adverse events from CST. Green's[12] category of

**Table 22-1   Literature Search Results**

| TERMS ENTERED | ALL EBM REVIEWS (MAY 2006) | MEDLINE (1966-MAY 2006) | CINAHL (1982-MAY 2006) | CAM ON PUBMED (MAY 2006) |
|---|---|---|---|---|
| Ménière's disease (MD) | 145* | 4955 | 277 | 204 |
| and craniosacral | 0 | 0 | 0 | 0 |
| and craniosacral therapy | 0 | 0 | 0 | 0 |
| and cranial osteopathy | 0 | 0 | 0 | 0 |
| Craniosacral | 9 | 35 | 127 | 28 |
| and nausea | 1 | 0 | 1 | 0 |
| and vertigo | 0 | 0 | 1 | 0 |
| and tinnitus | 0 | 0 | 0 | 0 |
| Craniosacral therapy | 4 | 16 | 118 | 25 |
| and nausea | 0 | 0 | 0 | 0 |
| and vertigo | 0 | 0 | 0 | 0 |
| and tinnitus | 0 | 0 | 0 | 0 |
| Cranial osteopathy | 1 | 7 | 11 | 176 |
| and nausea | 0 | 0 | 0 | 1 |
| and vertigo | 0 | 0 | 0 | 3 |
| and tinnitus | 0 | 0 | 0 | 1 |

*Cochrane Database of Systematic Reviews=9; Database of Abstracts of Reviews of Effects=4; Cochrane Central Register of Controlled Trials=132.

pathophysiological mechanisms of craniosacral dysfunction[12] included a few studies in which the researchers directly investigated the relationship between craniosacral mobility restrictions and health.[18-20] Rather than measure health outcomes after CST, the researchers sought to determine the association between health and the state of functioning of the craniosacral system. According to Green's critical review,[12] these studies were conducted using weak research designs and had severely limited content and face validity because of a lack of classification criteria for health status and subject characteristics. Other researchers who addressed pathophysiology and craniosacral dysfunction investigated the fusion or potentially available movement between the cranial bones.[21-23] Although the outcomes of these studies support the theory that the adult cranium is not always rigid and fused, limited support exists for the assumption that manual manipulation can induce motion at the cranial sutures. Green[11] also found that the validity of craniosacral assessment had been investigated by several researchers, and except for Upledger's study,[24] which has a number of limitations, all determined that assessment of craniosacral rhythm is unreliable.[25-27]

Hartman and Norton's review[28] of interexaminer and cranial osteopathy included many of the same studies reviewed by Green[12] and drew similar conclusions. They further suggested that based on

poor diagnostic reliability and scant evidence of treatment efficacy, the teaching and practice of cranial osteopathy should be severely limited.

### Primary Sources

A scarcity of systematic review articles typically reflects a limited number of case studies, quasi-experimental studies, and experimental studies. This is true for CST. Despite the search results (see Table 22-1), which identify many citations about CST avail-able through the CINAHL and CAM on PubMed databases, many of these citations are descriptive articles written by Upledger and published in non–peer-reviewed periodicals.[29-31] The other articles, many of which were included in the Green[11] review, are case reports and quasi-experimental studies.

The chiropractor obtains and reads these primary sources to determine their potential relevancy to Karen's case and to perhaps verify the observations and conclusions offered by Green.[12] Arguably, the most relevant question is one of treatment outcomes. Does any evidence support CST as an efficacious intervention or modality, and, more specifically, has CST been investigated as a treatment for Karen's complaints of upper thoracic spine pain or symptoms associated with Ménière's disease? Equally important is whether any reports of harm or risk exist with CST for persons with Ménière's disease. A more targeted

Derby Hospitals NHS Foundation
Trust
Library and Knowledge Service

search of the literature is conducted by combining terms related to CST with Ménière's disease and the symptoms experienced by Karen, but only one article is revealed.[32] The article, written by McPartland,[32] reviewed nine cases in which clients who received CST experienced adverse events that included but were not limited to confusion, headaches, vertigo, nausea, and vomiting. The author also reported that the majority of the adverse events were experienced when nonlicensed practitioners performed the CST and were resolved after CST treatment with trained licensed clinicians.

Because the targeted search revealed no other outcome studies, the articles retrieved with the search terms *craniosacral, craniosacral therapy,* and *cranial osteopathy* were scanned by title and abstract to identify studies that may be relevant for Karen's case. CST or cranial osteopathy has been investigated as treatment for gastroesophageal reflux in an infant,[14] auditory/vestibular (A/V) symptoms and facial/cervical pain and paresthesias after a closed head injury,[33] enhancement of neurological performance in children with developmental delay,[16] and as a component of prenatal care.[34] Researchers also have investigated the effect CST may have on sleep latency and muscle sympathetic nerve activity[35] in healthy subjects.

The only article relevant to Karen's concern of tinnitus is the case report[33] of a 52-year-old woman who suffered a blunt head trauma to her right parietooccipital area during a motor vehicle accident. Her symptoms included A/V symptoms including hearing loss, aural fullness, and tinnitus. Her dizziness was described as disequilibrium rather than vertigo, and she complained of visual disturbances consistent with vestibular ocular reflex (VOR) abnormality. In addition to the A/V symptoms, the client had cranial nerve (CN) VII palsy, hypoesthesia throughout the right-sided distribution of CN V, cervical spine tenderness and pain, decreased cervical range of motion, and a right "mouth droop." After 10 physical therapy sessions, which included heat, gentle soft tissue mobilization, and attempts at cervical spine mobilizations, the client's condition and complaints were unchanged. At that point, the client reported that she felt her "skull needed to move" and so a cranial examination was conducted and CST was initiated. After four sessions of CST, the client was found to have improvement in the hypoesthetic sensation of CN V. After eight visits, the facial symptoms were remarkably improved according to the client's subjective reports and she has been asymptomatic for right-sided

hemi-facial paresis for at least 8 months. A blink-reflex nerve conduction study was conducted to obtain additional objective data regarding the client's improvements, but the test results were used to suggest an etiology for the client's symptoms rather than measure her clinical improvement with CST. In addition, the amelioration of the client's other symptoms such as dizziness, tinnitus, and pain was not well described.

A targeted search of the literature using the PICO method is not helpful in this case. The combination of key words yields zero citations.

---

### PICO BOX

For clients with Ménière's disease does craniosacral therapy (CST) decrease nausea, vertigo, and tinnitus?

P: People with Ménière's disease
I: CST
C: No comparison
O: Nausea
O: Vertigo
O: Tinnitus

A search performed in MEDLINE on September 12, 2007, combining all of the terms yielded zero references. Searches performed with each of the outcome measures separately also yielded zero references. In this case, it is necessary to scan all the references found with the search term *craniosacral therapy* for articles relevant to the client's status and goals.

P = **Population** (patient/client problem, patient, condition, or group attribute)
I = **Intervention** (the CAM therapy or approach)
C = **Comparison** (standard care or comparison intervention)
O = **Outcome** (the measured variables of interest)

---

### Evaluating the Literature

Most of the research reports on CST have addressed concerns and questions about craniosacral assessment[25-27] and the pathophysiology of craniosacral dysfunction,[18-20] including whether movement between the cranial bones is possible.[21-23] Research investigating the effectiveness or outcomes of CST is limited to a handful of published reports. All the studies, except for the case study by Elliot,[33] included subjects that were very dissimilar to Karen. In one case report, the researchers described how an infant with gastroesophageal reflux benefited from CST.[14] In a prospective study,[16] health care providers rendered six to 12 individual osteopathic treatments, including cranial manipulation, to children who were diagnosed with either neurological problems or medical conditions. The investigators reported significant improvement of sensory and motor performance in the children with neurological problems. Although performance was assessed using Houle's Profile of Development (POD), a standardized assessment tool, the authors did not clearly specify the criterion by which the determination and classification of "neurological problems" and "medical diagnosis" were made. Other research design concerns include a poor explanation of the independent variable, which was described as osteopathic manipulation that may be administered to any part of the body and limited controls for confounding variables such as nutrition and environmental exposure.

In a block design with repeated measures experiment, healthy subjects were exposed to cranial manipulation, specifically compression of the fourth ventricle (CV4)—a common intervention in CST, simple touch (sham CV4), and no treatment (control).[35] Significant reduction ($p < 0.05$) in sleep latency was found in subjects after CV4 treatment as compared with post-sham and post-control conditions. Muscle sympathetic nerve activity (MSNA), measured using standard microneurographic technique, also was found to be significantly decreased after CV4 treatment ($p < 0.01$). The researchers were explicit about their assumptions regarding the existence of primary respiratory movement (PRM) and a CST practitioner's ability to detect a cranial rhythmic impulse (CRI) and addressed possible confounding effects of circadian cycles. Although the subject size was small, the study provides some preliminary information about the possible physiological effects of CST.

Unfortunately, all of the studies that have been described include subjects who are dissimilar to Karen and do not include outcome measures for pain or common complaints of Ménière's disease, such as vertigo, tinnitus, or nausea. The best available evidence appears to be the case report of the woman who experienced a closed head injury and experienced symptoms that included aural fullness, dizziness, tinnitus, paresthesias, and cervical pain and tenderness. Only after CST was included in her physical therapy plan of care did her A/V symptoms and paresthesias begin to dissipate and resolve. The subject's reports of improvement were not, however, documented using standardized outcome measures, and so it is difficult to quantify the changes she experienced.

In Karen's case, the health care provider was a chiropractor who, in addition to regularly attending advanced continuing education seminars, received training through the Upledger Institute and is experienced in cranial osteopathy and CST. His knowledge of cranial and cervical anatomy and alignment in combination with his clinical experience of treating clients with Ménière's disease leads him to suggest CST as an intervention for treatment of Karen's symptoms associated with Ménière's disease. Although no clear evidence exists that an examination of craniosacral rhythm or impulse is reliable or that CST is efficacious in the treatment of Ménière's disease, it seems plausible that abnormalities in cranial and spinal alignment could be palpated and that misalignment may contribute to Karen's condition. Given the fact that few pharmacological or other noninvasive interventions effectively treat or cure Ménière's disease, it is not surprising that complementary or alternative approaches would be considered. The case report by Elliot et al[33] offers some suggestion that CST may help in decreasing paresthesias and A/V symptoms, but this isolated case should not be interpreted as providing adequate evidence to support the use of CST as an intervention for Ménière's disease. Rather, the practitioner would need to inform the client that, although no documented cases exist in the scientific literature regarding the application of CST in persons with Ménière's disease, his advanced knowledge, training, and clinical experience lead him to believe that CST may be helpful for relief of her vertigo and other symptoms. Although Karen does not have the same medical history as the clients who experienced adverse events from CST in the published studies by Greenman and McPartland,[17,32] the practitioner should raise the issue of risk versus benefits when discussing complementary therapies with his client. Like many persons with chronic conditions, Karen is interested in trying an alternative or complementary approach to manage her symptoms because standard care has not been helpful.

## CLINICAL DECISION MAKING

### Generate a Clinical Hypothesis and Relevant Outcome Measures

The chiropractor hypothesizes that the addition of CST into Karen's plan of care would decrease the frequency and intensity of her symptoms from Ménière's disease.

To test the hypothesis, the chiropractor would need to identify and use appropriate tools that could be used to measure the frequency and intensity of Karen's symptoms. He consults with a physical therapist colleague who specializes in vestibular rehabilitation and learns that the Rhodes Index of Nausea, Vomiting and Retching (INVR),[36] is an eight-item self-report that uses a five-point Likert scale to measure frequency and degree of nausea, vomiting, and retching over a 12-hour period. The Dizziness Handicap Inventory (DHI)[36] has been used widely to quantify the symptoms of clients who experience dizziness and has been used by Cunha, Settanni, and Gananca[38] to examine the effect of dizziness in clients with Ménière's disease. To quantifiably assess the impact of tinnitus on daily living, a self-report tool called the Tinnitus Handicap Inventory (THI)[39] can be administered. An instrument that measures symptom occurrence and symptom distress across a wide range of symptoms including but not limited to pain, nausea, fatigue, breathing, fear, and appearance is the Adapted Symptom Distress Scale-2 (SDS-2).[40] This 31-item, five-point self-report may be helpful in quantifying symptoms not typically associated with Ménière's disease, but its usefulness in Karen's case is probably limited.

### Intervene and Evaluate

The chiropractor can integrate CST into the plan of care by explaining the state of the CST literature to Karen so that she is made aware of the limited investigations regarding the outcomes and possible risks and benefits of this approach. In this case, the client signed an informed consent before CST was added to her treatment sessions. After 22 sessions over 3.5 months, which included CST and spinal manipulation, the client reports complete relief of her thoracic pain and improvement in her symptoms from Ménière's disease as follows: She experiences symptoms once every 7 weeks instead of weekly. The duration of intense symptoms has decreased from 4-6 hours to 2-3 hours. After 3 hours, she is able to perform sedentary activities with only minimal dizziness and tinnitus and is able to drive within 8 hours, as opposed to 12 hours before therapy. The chiropractor notes that the two exacerbations of Ménière's disease symptoms the client experienced in 14 weeks of treatment were associated with cranial distortion.

Unfortunately, the chiropractor was unable to administer INVR, DHI, or THI before integrating CST into the client's plan of care. Although the chiropractor is able to document the client's subjective reports that her symptoms have improved with the addition of CST, not having data from these standardized measurements tools limits support of his hypothesis.

### Report the Outcomes

Even though the chiropractor did not use standardized measurement tools to measure the client's outcomes, he believes the addition of CST into her plan of care has positively affected the frequency and severity of her symptoms from Ménière's disease. Using this clinical observation to document or advance the practice of CST will be difficult, however, because the pretreatment status and meaningful posttreatment outcomes were not identified quantitatively. A detailed description of the CST intervention also would need to be documented so that clinicians could have a clear understanding of the actual treatment that was provided so that comparisons to other CST outcome studies could be initiated. With some modification and inclusion of measurable outcomes, a case report of this type may be of interest to the readers of the *Journal of Bodywork and Movement Therapies;* the *Journal of Manipulative and Physiological Therapeutics* the *Journal of the American Osteopathic Association; Otology & Neurotology; Ear, Nose and Throat Journal;* and *Alternative Therapies in Health and Medicine.*

### SUMMARY

In this chapter, the client seeks chiropractic services for thoracic pain and discomfort. After a few sessions of standard chiropractic care, the client demonstrates improvement in her cervical and thoracic alignment and mobility. She mentions to her chiropractor that she has Ménière's disease and often experiences exacerbation of her symptoms, which include vertigo, nausea, and tinnitus. Based on his clinical experience working with clients who have Ménière's disease and his training in CST, the chiropractor considers the possibility that CST may be helpful in addressing Karen's symptoms. The chiropractor determines that although CST has not been investigated in clients with Ménière's disease, a published case report exists of a subject's A/V symptoms that appeared to improve with CST. The chiropractor discusses the limited scientific literature and reports of adverse events with the client, who agrees to the addition of CST into her plan of care and reports a reduction in the frequency and intensity of the symptoms associated with Ménière's disease after treatment. Given the scarcity of outcome studies of CST, clear documentation in the client record of the intervention and quantifiable outcome measures can add substantially to the usefulness of this clinical experience for future clinical decision making.

## REFERENCES

1. Haybach PJ, Underwood J: *Ménière's disease: what you need to know,* Portland, Ore, 1998, Vestibular Disorders Association.
2. Herdman SJ: *Vestibular rehabilitation,* Philadelphia, 1994, FA Davis, p 84.
3. Beers MH, Berkow R, editors: *The Merck manual of diagnosis and therapy,* ed 18, Hoboken, NJ, 2006, John Wiley & Sons.
4. Johnson J, Lalwani AK: Vestibular disorders. In Lalwani AK, editor: *Current diagnosis & treatment in otolaryngology—head & neck surgery,* Columbus, Ohio, 2004, McGraw-Hill, p 766.
5. Li J: E-medicine. *Inner Ear, Ménière Disease, Medical Treatment.* Available at: *http://www.imedicine.com/DisplayTopic.asp?bookid=4&topic=232.* Accessed May 1, 2006.
6. Li J: E-medicine. *Endolymphatic Hydrops.* Available at: *http://www.imedicine.com/DisplayTopic.asp?bookid=7&topic=412.* Accessed May 1, 2006.
7. Committee on Hearing and Equilibrium, American Academy of Otolaryngology-Head and Neck Surgery. Committee on hearing and equilibrium guidelines for the diagnosis and evaluation of therapy in Ménière's disease, *Otolaryngol Head Neck Surg* 113:181-5, 1995.
8. Li J: E-medicine. Inner Ear, Ménière Disease, Surgical Treatment. Available at: *http://www.imedicine.com/DisplayTopic.asp?bookid=4&topic=233.* Accessed May 1, 2006.
9. Getitz N: *The DOs: osteopathic medicine in America,* ed 2, Baltimore, 2004, The Johns Hopkins University Press.
10. Upledger, JE, Vredevoogd JD: *Craniosacral therapy,* Seattle, 1983, Eastland Press.
11. Upledger JE: *Your inner physician and you,* Berkeley, Calif, 1991, North Atlantic Books.
12. Green C et al: A systematic review of craniosacral therapy: biological plausibility, assessment reliability and clinical effectiveness, *Complement Ther Med* 7:201-7, 1999.
13. Baker EG: Alteration in width of maxillary arch and its relation to sutural movement of cranial bones, *J Am Osteopath Assoc* 70:559-64, 1971.
14. Joyce P, Clark C: The use of craniosacral therapy to treat gastoesophageal reflux in infants, *Inf Young Children* 9:51-8, 1996.
15. Blood SD: The craniosacral mechanism and the temporomandibular joint, *J Am Osteopath Assoc* 86:512-9, 1986.
16. Frynmann VM, Carney RE, Springall P: Effect of osteopathic medical management on neurologic development in children, *J Am Osteopath Assoc* 92:729-44, 1992.
17. Greenman PE, McPartland JM: Cranial findings and iatrogenesis from craniosacral manipulation in patients with traumatic brain syndrome, *J Am Osteopath Assoc* 95:182-8, 1995.
18. Upledger JE: The relationship of craniosacral examination findings in grade school children with developmental problems, *J Am Osteopath Assoc* 77:760-76, 1978.
19. Frymann VM: Relation of disturbances of craniosacral mechanisms to synptomatology of the newborn: study of 1,250 infants, *J Am Osteopath Assoc* 65:1059-75, 1966.
20. White WK, White JE, Baldt G: The relation of the craniofacial bones to specific somatic dysfunctions: a clinical study of the effects of manipulation, *J Am Osteopath Assoc* 85:603-4, 1985.
21. Kokich VG: Age changes in the human frontozygomatic suture from 20-95 years, *Am J Orthod* 69:411-30, 1976.
22. Frymann VM: A study of the rhythmic motions of the living cranium, *J Am Osteopath Assoc* 70:928-45, 1971.
23. Hubbard R, Melvin JW, Baradawala IT: Flexure of cranial sutures, *J Biomech* 4:491-6, 1971.
24. Upledger JE: The reproducibility of craniosacral examination findings: a statistical analysis, *J Am Osteopath Assoc* 76:890-9, 1977.
25. Wirth-Pattullo VM, Hayes KW: Interrater reliability of craniosacral rate measurements and their relationship with subjects' and examiners' heart and respiratory rate measurements, *Phys Ther* 74:908-20, 1994.
26. Hanten WP et al: Craniosacral rhythm: reliability and relationships with cardiac and respiratory rates, *J Orthop Sports Phys Ther* 27:213-8, 1998.
27. Rogers JS et al: Simultaneous palpation of the craniosacral rate at the head and feet: intrarater and interrater reliability and rate comparisons, *Phys Ther* 78:1175-85, 1998.
28. Hartman SE, Norton JM: Interexaminer reliability and cranial osteopathy, *Sci Rev Altern Med* 6:23-34, 2002.
29. Upledger JE: CranioSacrally speaking. The potential impact of orthodontia on whole-body health, *Massage Today* 6:161-7, 2006.
30. Upledger JE: CranioSacrally speaking: no more earaches, *Massage Today* 5:21, 2005.

31. Upledger JE: CranioSacrally speaking: taming osteoporosis, *Massage Today* 5:8, 2005.

32. McPartland JM: Craniosacral iatrogenesis: side-effects from cranial-sacral treatment, *J Bodywork Movement Ther* 1(1):2-8, 1996.

33. Elliott JM et al: Cranial manipulation with possible neurovascular contact injury at the cerebello-pontine angle: a case report, *Altern Ther Health Med* 9:108-12, 2003.

34. Phillips CJ, Meyer JJ: Chiropractic care, including craniosacral therapy, during pregnancy: a static-group comparison of obstetric interventions during labor and delivery, *J Manipulative Physiol Ther* 18:525-9, 1995.

35. Cutler MJ et al: Cranial manipulation can alter sleep latency and sympathetic nerve activity in humans: a pilot study, *J Altern Compl Med* 11:103-8, 2005.

36. Rhodes VA, McDaniel RW: The index of nausea, vomiting, and retching: a new format of the index of nausea and vomiting, *Oncol Nurs Forum* 26:889-94, 1999.

37. Jacobson GP, Newman CW: The development of the dizziness handicap inventory, *Arch Otolaryngol Head Neck Surg* 116:424-7, 1990.

38. Cunha F, Settanni FA, Gananca FF: What is the effect of dizziness on the quality of life for patients with Ménière's disease? *Rev Laryngol Otol Rhinol* 126:155-8, 2005.

39. Newman CW, Jacobson GP, Spitzer JB: Development of the Tinnitus Handicap Inventory. *Arch Otolaryngol Head Neck Surg.* 122:143-8, 1996.

40. Rhodes VA et al: An instrument to measure symptom experience: symptom occurrence and symptom distress, *Cancer Nurs* 23:49-54, 2000.

# CHAPTER 23

## Pilates

*Ellen Zambo Anderson, Chantel Dickinson*

Elizabeth is a 40-year-old attorney who was involved in a motor vehicle accident (MVA) 5 years ago. She sustained a lumbar disc herniation at L5-S1. Nonoperative management was unsuccessful and an anterior/posterior interbody lumbar fusion was performed 2 years after the MVA. A second procedure to remove hardware from the right lumbar spine was performed 2 months after the fusion secondary to the onset of radicular signs. After her surgery, she was instructed by her physician to exercise by "walking as much as possible." She was referred to physical therapy 1 month after her second surgery (3 months after the first surgery) for general range of motion (ROM) and strengthening.

### ■ Initial Examination

*Client Report:* The client described a constant "ache" in her low back of 5-6/10 with intermittent tingling down her entire right leg. She stated that she did not have the right lower extremity symptoms before the surgery. She continued to wear the lumbar brace as directed by her physician. She reported that sitting and standing tolerance is limited to less than 10 minutes.

*Client Goals:* To return to full-time work and a regular exercise program and to be able to travel in a car for 2 to 3 hours so that she can get to her vacation home in the mountains on the weekends

*Employment:* Personal injury attorney

*Recreational Activities:* Walking, hiking

*General Health:* Good

*Medications:* Percocet, Neurontin

*Musculoskeletal:* ROM: Trunk not tested because of surgical precautions. Bilateral upper extremities, left lower extremity (LLE)=WNLs throughout. Posture: standing: decreased cervical lordosis and thoracic kyphosis, increased lumbar lordosis, pelvic obliquity with right posterior superior iliac spine (PSIS) lower and anterior superior iliac spine (ASIS) higher, right hip in extreme external rotation as compared with the left; supine: right lower extremity $1/2$ inch shorter than left. Palpation: tenderness at right quadratus lumborum, piriformis belly, sciatic notch; left PSIS, posterior iliac crest border, paraspinals.

*Neuromuscular:* Force generation: Trunk not tested because of surgical precautions. Transversus abdominis activation in supine=poor. LLE=4/5 throughout; right hip flexors, abductors, extensors, adductors=3/5; right hip internal and external rotators=4/5; right knee extensors=4/5 within available range; right knee flexors=4/5; right ankle=3/5 throughout; great toe extensors=3/5. Neurodynamic tests: right straight-leg raise test was positive at 40 degrees; left was negative to 85 degrees. LLE nonsignificant. Deep tendon reflexes: decreased right Achilles; bilateral knee and left Achilles normal

**Function:** Pain: low back pain, at rest=4/10; sitting and standing 10 minutes=7/10; walking 10 minutes=7/10

**Integumentary:** Surgical scars healed well. Palpation to anterior and right posterior scar revealed limited soft tissue mobility.

### Evaluation

The therapist determined that the client's examination findings were consistent with her medical diagnosis of lumbar radiculopathy. The therapist believed the client's symptoms could be managed with specific exercises to address impairments in posture, strength, and movement/mobility, plus soft tissue mobilization and ice to decrease pain and improve mobility.

### Plan of Care

Elizabeth's plan of care included progressive lumbopelvic stabilization exercises, gentle range of motion and stretching, soft tissue mobilization, and ice. Elizabeth walked daily as directed by her physician and was instructed in a home lumbar stabilization exercise program to be done on the days she did not attend therapy.

### Reevaluation

After 18 sessions over 6 weeks a reexamination demonstrates an improvement in the client's lower extremity strength and reduction of pain at rest (3/10), sitting and standing (5/10), and walking after 10 minutes (5/10). Her right straight-leg raise remains positive but improved to 54 degrees; however, she states that the "buzzing" and "tingling" in the right leg persists throughout the day. The client also reports that she "can't feel" her lower abdominals working during the exercises and that she's frustrated with "gaining weight and getting flabby."

## Incorporating CAM into the Plan of Care

A 6-week course of physical therapy that included a variety of exercises, soft tissue mobilization, and ice has been helpful in reducing the client's pain and increasing lower extremity strength, but her radicular symptoms have persisted, and her lumbopelvic region continues to be weak. The therapist, who has been practicing Pilates, knows that Pilates focuses on improving trunk and lumbopelvic strength, correcting faulty movement patterns, and realigning posture. She believes it might be a reasonable adjunctive therapy activity to hasten the client's recovery. Based on her readings and knowledge about Pilates, the therapist refers the client to a certified Pilates instructor for a one-to-one supervised Pilates program that will be integrated into the client's current therapy program.

## INVESTIGATING THE LITERATURE

The therapist is familiar with the Pilates method of exercise through her own personal exercise program and has begun to hear that physical therapists are starting to incorporate principles of Pilates into rehabilitation programs. Her personal experiences of practicing Pilates do support the claims that Pilates can increase core strength and improve awareness of postural alignment and so she is considering becoming a certified instructor. Before making this commitment, however, the therapist decided to investigate the scientific literature about Pilates to better understand its assumptions and principles and to identify any research studies that may have been conducted to measure or test Pilates' outcomes in rehabilitation. Knowledge the therapist gained from reading the literature informs her decision to pursue certification as a Pilates instructor and the recommendation that Elizabeth add Pilates to her current therapy program. The process of investigating the literature, which included preliminary background reading, searching databases, and evaluating the literature, is described.

### Preliminary Reading

#### Joseph H. Pilates (1880-1967)

Many books have been written about Pilates and are useful resources for learning about its history as an approach to fitness and health.[1-10] Joseph Hubertus Pilates was born in Germany in 1880. As a child, he suffered from asthma and many other illnesses, which resulted in fragility and weakness.[1,2] Determined to overcome his ailments, Pilates became passionate about physical exercise and fitness. He studied many forms of exercise including yoga and martial arts during his young adulthood and began to develop his own philosophy and method of training and fitness. While interned in a prison camp for German nationals during World War I, Pilates taught his exercises to inmates and began developing equipment that could be used to rehabilitate clients who were restricted to their hospital beds.[1,2,4,8] In 1923 Pilates left Germany and emigrated to the United States. On the crossing, he fell in love with a woman named Clara, who became his wife. Together, they opened an exercise studio in New York City. Within a few years, Pilates' unique method of physical and mental conditioning caught the attention of professional dancers and choreographers who sought to maintain or regain strength and flexibility as they recovered from a variety of performance-related injuries. Dance artists such as ballet master George Balanchine and modern dance notable Martha Graham supported Pilates' method of body conditioning and exercise and studied with him for many years.[1,4,9]

Pilates' original program consisted of a series of mat exercises designed to build abdominal strength and develop control of the body. Then he designed and built several pieces of equipment to enhance the exercises and substitute for the manual assistance he was providing for his clients. Pilates also trained the first generation of teachers in his New York studio, including Romana Kryzanowska, Kathy Grant, Ron Fletcher, and several others. Although many of the original teachers have branched out to different areas of the country and have incorporated their own experiences and style into the Pilates method of exercise, the original principles of Pilates have been maintained and continue to be passed down through several generations of Pilates instructors.[1]

### Contrology

Perhaps the best way to learn about Pilates' philosophy of fitness and approach to exercise is to read a book written by Pilates entitled *Return to Life Through Contrology*, which originally was published in 1945. In this text, Pilates explains that, "Physical fitness is the first requisite of happiness . . . (and that) physical fitness is the attainment

and maintenance of a uniformly developed body with a sound mind fully capable of naturally, easily, and satisfactorily performing our many and varied daily tasks with spontaneous zest and pleasure" (p. 6).[10] *Contrology*, the term Pilates used to describe his method of exercise, was designed to develop coordination of the mind, body, and spirit through purposeful and repetitive exercises. These exercises, according to Pilates,[10] would strengthen muscles and correct abnormal postures while encouraging flexibility and graceful movement. By mindfully attending to the breath and the body's posture and movement of each repetition of every exercise, the exercises of Contrology were proposed to "correct wrong postures, restore physical vitality, invigorate the mind and elevate the spirit" (p. 9).[10] Central to the Pilates method of body conditioning and exercise is the "powerhouse," located between the bottom of the rib cage and the hips. Here muscles, including the rectus abdominis, transversus abdominis (TA), obliques, multifidus, erector spinae, gluteals, and quadratus lumborum, support the spine and trunk. When strong, the powerhouse improves alignment and posture and provides a base from which all movements can be generated.[1] Most of the more than 500 exercises described by Pilates focus on strengthening the powerhouse or what some exercise and rehabilitation professionals now call the *core*, while training the mind and the body to work together. Proponents of Pilates suggest that the Pilates method of body conditioning and exercise can improve strength, endurance, balance, and coordination[3] and address respiratory problems and chronic pain.[2] Other claims include improved sexual enjoyment, better sleep, and the elimination of "love handles."[1,9]

### Principles

Most contemporary teachers of the Pilates method of exercise and conditioning ascribe to the principles or concepts outlined by Pilates in his writings. Although the terminology used to name these principles may vary from instructor to instructor (Table 23-1), their explanations of the underlying concepts as originally described by Pilates are consistent. The terms most commonly used to identify Pilates' principles and concepts are provided below.

### Control

Pilates' method of exercise requires control of every movement. Strength is developed by moving slowing against and with gravity, avoiding momentum as a means to complete a movement. Each exercise is executed with breath, concentration, and control.

### Breath

Every exercise described in Pilates' text[10] includes instructions for a specific breathing pattern of when to inhale and when to exhale. According to Pilates, correct breathing requires a full inhalation and complete exhalation so that the blood can receive "vitally necessary life-giving oxygen" and the muscles can be stimulated into greater activity (p. 13).[10]

### Flow

Pilates' method of exercise encourages flowing movements rather than static postures. Emphasis is placed on graceful performance of each exercise with flowing transitions so that elongation, flexibility, and strength are promoted and achieved.

### Precision

Precision goes beyond simple control of a movement to include temporal and spatial awareness. Pilates detailed expectations of how each exercise is initiated, the degree and speed of movement through space that should be achieved, and how the movement should reach completion before the next movement is initiated.

### Centering

Proper execution of the exercises recommended by Pilates requires participants to intend for their bodies to be centered in space. Participants must be able to strongly contract their deep abdominal muscles to be able to maintain a center of control. A strong center of control is considered necessary for precise and flowing movements.

### Concentration

The Pilates method of exercise requires mental focus and attention to each component of every exercise. All movement is associated with a thought process so that the individual experiences kinesthetic and mental awareness of the body's alignment and movement at any given moment during exercise.

Some Pilates instructors and authors have identified coordination, opposition, isolation, stabilization, visualization, and relaxation as additional principles of the Pilates method of exercise. Explanations of these principles seem to overlap with the principles of control, breath, flow, precision, centering, and concentration. The concepts of precision and control, for example, include the expectation that the exercises are performed in a coordinated manner, in which some muscles are active in performing a movement, while other muscles, such as the abdominals, contract to main-

| Table 23-1 | Principles of the Pilates Method of Body Conditioning and Exercise | | | | | | | |
|---|---|---|---|---|---|---|---|---|
| PRINCIPLE | HERMAN (1) | WINSOR (2) | ALPERS (3) | SILER (4) | UNGARO (5) | ACKLAND (6) | BRIGNELL (7) | GALLAGHER (9) |
| Control | ✓ | ✓ | | ✓ | ✓ | ✓ | ✓ | ✓ |
| Breath | ✓ | ✓ | ✓ | ✓ | ✓ | ✓ | ✓ | ✓ |
| Flow | ✓ | ✓ | ✓ | ✓ | ✓ | | ✓ | ✓ |
| Precision | ✓ | | ✓ | ✓ | ✓ | | ✓ | ✓ |
| Centering | ✓ | | | ✓ | ✓ | ✓ | ✓ | ✓ |
| Concentration | | ✓ | ✓ | ✓ | ✓ | | ✓ | ✓ |
| Opposition | ✓ | | ✓ | | | | | |
| Relaxation | | ✓ | | | | | | |
| Coordination | | | | | | ✓ | | |
| Realignment | | | | | | ✓ | | |
| Visualization | | ✓ | | | | ✓ | | |
| Routine | | | | | ✓ | ✓ | | |
| Isolation | | | | | | ✓ | | |
| Imagination | | | | ✓ | | | | |
| Intuition | | | | ✓ | | | | |
| Integration | | | | ✓ | | | | |
| Stability | ✓ | | | | | | | |
| Range of motion | ✓ | | | | | | | |

tain stability of the torso. The exercises also require the ability to isolate certain muscles to contract and shorten, while opposing muscles are relaxed and lengthened so that movement can flow with ease and precision.

Probably the most accessible form of Pilates is a group of floor exercises often referred to as the *mat program*. This collection of exercises is the focus of most books written about Pilates[1-10] and for which clear descriptions and illustrations or photographs are available. Exercisers are encouraged to perform an abdominal scoop and achieve and maintain a neutral spine while performing the exercises. Adherence to these positions helps ensure the building of strength and length of the powerhouse musculature and helps guard against injury.[10] A sample of three mat exercises can be seen in Figures 23-1 to 23-3.

Many mat exercises recommended by Pilates also can be performed using a variety of exercise apparatus first designed by Pilates himself. Pilates realized from his experience working with hospitalized clients and injured dancers that many people required physical assistance to either initiate or complete some of the exercises he thought were imperative for health and physical fitness. In an effort to help people who were weak, deconditioned, or injured and replace himself as their spotter and physical assistant, Pilates developed exercise equipment such as the roll-back bar, which consisted of a dowel and two fairly strong springs. The roll-back bar could assist clients in performing a roll-up (or sit-up) in a controlled and fluid manner.[1] Eventually, as abdominal strength developed, need for the roll-back bar would be eliminated. Today, the roll-back bar has been incorporated into a piece of equipment designed by Ellie Herman, called the *Pilates Spring Board*.[1] Pilates designed other pieces of exercise equipment using springs so that muscles could be worked against variable amounts of resistance and through shortened and elongated positions. The recoiling nature of a spring also requires control of a movement in both directions if the exercise or movement is to be balanced and precise, yet flowing and rhythmic. Popular Pilates-designed exercise equipment that can assist with achieving proper alignment and control while providing appropriate resistance for strengthening and muscular endurance includes the Reformer, the Cadillac, the Wunda Chair, and the Barrel. Based on clients' needs, Pilates instructors can use these pieces of

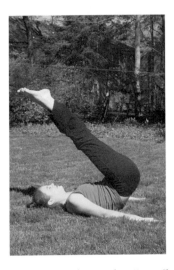

**Figure 23-2** Hip-up. Photographer: Karen Clarkson.

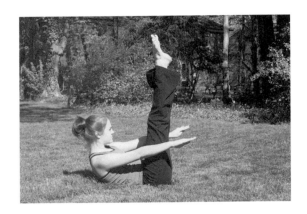

**Figure 23-1** The hundred. Photographer: Karen Clarkson.

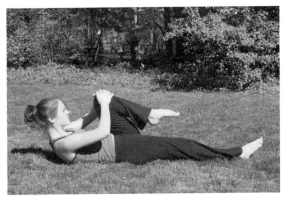

**Figure 23-3** Single leg stretch. Photographer: Karen Clarkson.

equipment to assist the performance or completion of an exercise for persons who have pain or are recovering from an injury. Conversely, the instructor also can use the features of the equipment to place the client in different positions, reduce the amount and type of support, and increase resistance to movements in an effort to make the exercises more challenging.

## Searching the Databases

### Critical Reviews and Primary Sources

After reading about the assumptions and principles of Pilates and taking a look at the range of exercises included in the Pilates mat program, the therapist searches the Cochrane Collection of Evidence-Based Medicine Databases for critical reviews of Pilates. No reviews are identified, and so the MEDLINE, CINAHL, and CAM on PubMed databases are searched to determine if any research has been done on the application of Pilates in a client population (Table 23-2). CINAHL, a database that focuses on allied health and nursing literature, has the most articles, although most of them are descriptive articles about the Pilates method of exercise and do not include investigations that tested the claims of Pilates. When the key word *Pilates* is limited to research articles, five articles remained, including studies that compared Pilates with other forms of exercise[11,12] and assessed the effects of Pilates on flexibility, body composition, posture, and leaping.[13-15]

The key word *Pilates* identified 13 articles in the MEDLINE database and 16 articles in the CAM on PubMed database that can be accessed online without a subscription. Of these citations, five were identified previously in CINAHL and the rest, with the one exception,[16] were descriptive. Because the results of the literature search were so limited, the key word *Pilates* also was searched using Google Scholar, a free search engine. According to Google, Google Scholar provides access to scholarly literature, including peer-reviewed journals and papers, abstracts, and books found across many disciplines and sources, some of which may not be indexed in medical and health-related databases. Search results are ordered by relevance as determined by Google's ranking system. Using Google Scholar, a scientific study of Pilates was found. The full text article was available online in English, although the original publication was in a Brazilian sports medicine journal.[17]

## Evaluating the Literature

Herrington and Davies[11] have suggested that abdominal muscle strengthening exercises have been used widely for enhancing spinal stability and managing low back pain. In their study they evaluated the effect of abdominal curls, Pilates, and no exercise on subjects' ability to contract the transversus abdominus muscle, a muscle regarded as critical for spinal stability. After 6 months of training, the healthy female subjects (mean age=34.6 years; SD=8.2 years) were tested for the ability to isolate and contract the TA and their ability to maintain lumbopelvic stability. No subjects in the abdominal curl group (n=12) or the control group (no exercise) (n=12) passed the lumbopelvic stability test after 6 months of training. Five or 42% of the subjects in the Pilates group (n=12) passed the test. TA isolation was achieved by four subjects (33%) in the abdominal curls group and the three subjects (25%) in the control group, whereas 85% or 10 subjects in the Pilates group were able to isolate and contract the TA. The authors concluded the subjects who trained using Pilates were better able to contract the TA and maintain lumbopelvic control than subjects who performed standard abdominal curl exercises or no exercise.

Petrofsky et al[12] measured electromyographic (EMG) activity of several lower extremity and back muscles in six healthy subjects as they exercised in

| Table 23-2 | Literature Search Results | | | |
|---|---|---|---|---|
| | COCHRANE COLLECTION OF EBM DATABASES (CDSR, ACP JOURNAL CLUB, DARE, CTTR) FEB. 2006 | CINAHL 1982-FEB. 2006 | MEDLINE 1966-FEB. 2006 | CAM ON PUBMED |
| Pilates | 0 | 109 | 13 | 16 |
| Limit to research | Not valid | 5 | Not valid | Not valid |

three different conditions: (1) using resistive exercise machines; (2) performing Pilates exercises; and (3) performing Pilates exercises with a resistive elastic band. The authors reported that muscle activity of the abdominals and paraspinal muscles was greater with exercise performed on exercise machines as compared with Pilates. However, when performed with a resistive elastic band, Pilates exercises were equal to a medium intensity workout on the resistive exercise machines.

Kolyniak, Cavalcanti, and Aoki[17] investigated the effect of Pilates exercises on trunk flexor and extensor strength. Twenty healthy subjects (ages 27 to 41 years of age) were measured for peak torque (PT), total work (TT), and power and set total work performed (QTT) of their trunk extensors and flexors at baseline and after 3 months of intermediate-advanced level Pilates training. Significant increases in all parameters were observed for the trunk extensors. Significant increases also were noted for trunk flexion in QTT and TT, although the percentage of increase was less for the flexors (10%) than for the extensors (21%, 29%, respectively). Analysis of the ratios of trunk flexors to extensors revealed significant reductions in all parameters. The authors concluded that Pilates may be an effective strategy for strengthening trunk flexors and extensors and may be helpful in attenuating muscle imbalances, which may contribute to spinal instability and back pain.

Segal, Hein, and Basford,[13] McMillian, Proteau, and Lebe,[14] and Jago et al[16] also conducted studies of the effects of Pilates exercises. The researchers assessed claims that Pilates training can improve flexibility,[13] posture,[13,14] and body composition.[13,16] Segal, Hein, and Basford[13] found that persons (n=47) who enrolled in a weekly Pilates program had significantly improved flexibility as measured by the fingertip-to-floor distance at 2, 4, and 6 months. Despite the subjects' reports that they felt their posture had improved, Segal, Hein, and Basford[13] found no significant difference in standing posture. In trained dancers, however, McMillan, Proteau, and Lebe[14] found that dancers who participated in Pilates training twice a week for 3 months had improved upper trunk posture during pliés when compared with dancers who did not receive Pilates instruction.

Segal, Hein, and Basford[13] also assessed claims that Pilates training can have positive effects on body composition. No significant changes in truncal lean body mass or weight were observed

after healthy adults trained weekly for 6 months. Jago et al[16] found, however, that young girls (n=16; mean age=11.2 years +/−0.6 years) who participated in Pilates training 5 days per week for 4 weeks had significantly lowered BMI (body mass index) percentiles as compared with girls (n=14) who performed traditional after-school activities.

Although some research has been conducted to measure potential benefits of Pilates, the research designs and subject selection and assignment of many studies limit their application to a client population. A few investigators have conducted research[12,13,17] in which proposed outcomes of Pilates training such as flexibility, body composition, and core stability and strength were tested. These were observational studies, however, and did not include a control or comparison group. Sampling bias also may be an issue: one investigation did not include a description of subject recruitment,[12] one included subjects who were already performing Pilates exercises before the study began, and one included subjects who had already signed up for Pilates classes before they were recruited for the study.

McMillan, Proteau, and Lebe[14] and Jago et al[16] conducted clinical trials in which they included a comparison group, although neither researcher satisfied the requirements for random assignment, and selection bias is noted as a limitation for both studies. McMillan measured dancers' dynamic upper spine posture before and after Pilates training and found improvement when compared with a group who continued to dance but did not perform Pilates. Jago et al compared 11-year-old girls from one YMCA after-school program with 11-year-old girls from another YMCA in the same city. Pilates was offered at one YMCA, five times per week as part of an after-school program. Traditional, non-Pilates activities were offered at the other facility. No significant differences existed between the two groups at baseline, nor did differences exist in attendance rate. Measures of BMI percentiles suggested that Pilates may be helpful for lowering BMI percentiles in girls who participate in Pilates training as compared with those who do not. The authors did note, however, that the sample size was small (n=14, n=16) and that they did not monitor dietary or metabolic variables. In addition, the researchers reported that the results should be interpreted cautiously because the results may have been influenced by a small number of subjects whose BMI fell considerably and that greater changes occurred in participants with low initial values, which resulted in a larger drop in BMI percentile.

The only clinical trial to include control and comparison groups found in the Pilates literature was conducted by Herrington and Davies.[11] The researchers reported that subjects who were in the Pilates group were better able to isolate the TA and maintain lumbopelvic control than the other two groups and suggested that further investigation is warranted to determine why so many Pilates-trained subjects (42%) and all the other subjects (100%) failed the lumbopelvic stability test yet remained pain-free for the 6-month study.

Scientific investigations of the Pilates method have included subjects that are similar to Elizabeth for gender and age,[11,13,17] but none have included subjects with neuromuscular conditions and pain. In addition, two of the studies have included subjects whose status was very different than Elizabeth. In one, the subjects were dancers,[14] presumed to be strong and flexible. In the other, the subjects were capable of performing intermediate-advanced level Pilates training.[17] The limited rigor of the studies also must be considered when attempting to apply findings to particular clients and their impairments.

After reviewing the literature, the therapist believes that the Pilates method of body conditioning and exercise may be a valuable intervention for some patients who require physical rehabilitation, but she is not encouraged that Pilates will positively affect Elizabeth's posture or her complaints of "feeling flabby." The therapist does acknowledge, however, that some evidence suggests that Pilates can be beneficial for increasing core strength and lumbopelvic stability, two impairments that may be contributing to Elizabeth's pain and paresthesias. Not being able to feel the abdominals work was a complaint of Elizabeth's even after 6 weeks of standard therapy that included stabilization exercises, so the therapist also is encouraged that at least in one study with healthy subjects, practicing Pilates appeared to help subjects isolate the TA, a deep abdominal muscle.

What concerns the therapist most about the literature is that Pilates has not been investigated in persons with back pain, radicular symptoms, or postsurgery. Based on the background readings and the therapist's own personal experience with Pilates, the therapist believes the Pilates mat program will promote positions and movements that will benefit Elizabeth. The therapist decides that Elizabeth should take a few private sessions with the Pilates instructor before she enrolls in a class. In addition, the therapist asks Elizabeth and the Pilates instructor if she could attend a session or two with Elizabeth so that she can observe Elizabeth perform the movements and make periodic inquiries about her pain and radicular symptoms. Knowing the exercises Elizabeth is performing with the Pilates instructor also would help the therapist develop a therapy plan of care that would complement the Pilates practice and address Elizabeth's goal of reducing her pain.

The therapist realizes that given her client population, which includes many persons with back pain, and her inclination to become a certified Pilates instructor, she should remain knowledgeable about the most current information on this topic. She decides to periodically search the literature using the PICO method by combining the key words *Pilates* and *back pain*.

---

### PICO BOX

For a person with back pain does Pilates reduce back pain?

P: Persons with low back pain
I: Pilates
C: No comparison
O: Back pain

On October 23, 2006, a CINAHL search combining *Pilates* and *back pain* rendered two additional citations, which were not available at the time of the original search in February 2006. Both references are clinical trials that investigated the efficacy of Pilates in persons with low back pain. One citation is a published report in a peer-reviewed journal,[18] in which the researchers report a significant reduction of functional disability and pain in the Pilates exercise group compared with the control group. The other citation is a doctoral dissertation,[19] in which subjects who performed Pilates did as well in pain reduction, function, and core stability as subjects who performed traditional lumbar stabilization exercise.

P = **Population** (patient/client, problem, person, condition, or group attribute)
I = **Intervention** (the CAM therapy or approach)
C = **Comparison** (standard care or comparison intervention)
O = **Outcome** (the measured variables of interest)

## CLINICAL DECISION MAKING

### Generate a Clinical Hypothesis

The therapist hypothesized that Pilates training will address Elizabeth's concern of not being able to feel her abdominal muscles working when she performs lumbopelvic stabilization exercises. The therapist also hypothesized that the addition of Pilates to the therapy plan of care will help Elizabeth increase her core strength and lumbopelvic stability, which the therapist believes is necessary if Elizabeth is to have less pain and radicular symptoms.

### Relevant Outcome Measures

On initial evaluation, the therapist found that Elizabeth had pain and paresthesias, which interfered with her functioning, and weakness of the right lower extremity and transversus abdominus. After 18 sessions of therapy, Elizabeth's strength and pain had improved, but she still had complaints of paresthesias and she continued to rate her pain as 5/10 after 10 minutes of standing and walking. Taking objective and reliable measures of isolated muscle contraction and strength and lumbopelvic stability can be challenging yet important, particularly in this case, because the therapist wants to determine if Pilates training could help to augment the effects of Elizabeth's current therapy program.

To address this issue, the therapist conducts a reexamination of Elizabeth that includes measurement of TA contraction and isolation and lumbopelvic stability using the stabilizer pressure biofeedback unit (Chattanooga Group, Inc.) as used and described by Herrington and Davies.[11]

### Intervene and Evaluate

The physical therapist summarizes and explains the state of the Pilates literature to Elizabeth so that she is able to participate in the decision about whether to exercise using the Pilates method. The physical therapist is specific when she describes the outcomes of the research and informs Elizabeth that none of the research included subjects who had complaints similar to hers and that none of the subjects had a history of back surgery.

From her preliminary reading the therapist has learned that although the authors of books about Pilates suggest that the mat exercises can be done safely at home using a book or video as a guide, they strongly recommend that persons who want to experience the full benefits of Pilates should take a class or obtain individual instruction with a qualified Pilates instructor.[1-9] Two international organizations dedicated to the teaching of Joseph Pilates are the Pilates Method Alliance (PMA) and the Pilates Guild. The PMA maintains an international registry of Pilates teachers and training organizations. Although the PMA does not offer training programs, they do offer recommendations for evaluating teacher training programs. For example, the PMA suggests that Pilates program directors have at least 10 years of experience teaching Pilates and that facilitators have a minimum of 5 years of teaching experience. In addition, Pilates training programs should require that participants have a personal Pilates practice and receive at least 400 hours of training including lectures, observations, and supervised teaching. Written and practical final examinations also are highly recommended.

The Pilates Guild provides referral services for certified instructors and studios and seeks to promote consistent and high-quality Pilates instruction through education and certification. The Pilates Guild requires that participants in a Pilates certification program complete two phases of training. The first phase comprises a series of academic seminars that may be completed in 12-day intensives. The second phase is focused on experiential training and is done through a 600-hour apprenticeship, during which a candidate observes and practices Pilates, assists a certified instructor, and then teaches solo with direct supervision. Satisfactory completion of a final examination also is required to become a certified Pilates instructor through the Pilates Guild.

The PMA offers the following questions to help identify a qualified Pilates instructor:

1. Are the instructors trained through a comprehensive training program?
2. Did that training program require a written and practical test, lecture, observation, practice, and apprentice hours?
3. How many total hours were spent in the training program?
4. Does the instructor have any other movement-related teaching experience?
5. How long have the instructors been teaching Pilates?

6. What are the instructor's/studio's philosophy and specialty? Are they able to handle special needs, injuries, and rehabilitation?

7. Does the instructor or studio teach the full repertoire of Pilates on all pieces of apparatus?

Because Elizabeth was agreeable to trying Pilates, the therapist verified the credentials of the Pilates instructor and received written permission from the client to contact the instructor. Elizabeth and the instructor agreed to allow the therapist to attend Elizabeth's first session so that she could consult with both during the session. The therapist also received permission from the client and the instructor that would allow her to publish a case report that would describe the client's status, the rehabilitation program including the Pilates method of exercise, and the client's outcomes.

## Report the Outcomes

The therapist is aware that many physical therapy practices are beginning to use the Pilates method of exercise with clients who require physical rehabilitation for a variety of conditions, yet few peer-reviewed articles have been published on this topic. The therapist can potentially add to the Pilates and rehabilitation literature by writing a case report that describes (1) why and how the Pilates method of body conditioning and exercises was considered as an adjunct to a client's rehabilitation program and (2) whether the client's outcomes supported the therapist's clinical hypothesis. A case report of this nature may encourage further research into specific exercise programs that may be helpful in addressing core strength and stability in clients with histories of back surgery, pain, and paresthesias. A possible venue for this type of paper may be *The Journal of Orthopedic and Sports Physical Therapy* and the *Journal of Bodywork and Movement Therapies.*

## SUMMARY

In this chapter, Elizabeth, a client with a history of L5-S1 disc herniation, spinal surgery, weakness, pain, and radicular symptoms, improves with 6 weeks of physical therapy, but the pain and radicular symptoms persist. In addition, the client complains of feeling flabby and not knowing when her abdominal muscles are working during her exercises. Given the proposed claims of the Pilates

method of body conditioning and exercise, the therapist considers Pilates as an approach to exercise that may be beneficial for Elizabeth. The therapist investigates and evaluates the available literature on the Pilates method and determines that Pilates may be worth trying, although the method has not been investigated with persons who have had back surgery or who complain of neuromuscular symptoms. The therapist recommends a trial of Pilates with a qualified instructor and receives permission to attend the Pilates session with her client.

## REFERENCES

1. Herman E: *Pilates for dummies,* Hoboken, NJ, 2002, Wiley Publishing.
2. Winsor M, Laska M: *The Pilates powerhouse,* Cambridge, Mass, 1999, DeCapo Books.
3. Alpers AT, Segel RT, Gentry L: *The everything Pilates book,* Avon, Mass, 2002, Adams Media.
4. Siler B: *The Pilates book,* New York, 2000, Broadway Books.
5. Ungaro A: *The Pilates promise,* New York, 2004, DK Publishing.
6. Ackland L, Paton T, Halas M: *10-Step Pilates,* London, 1999, Thorsons.
7. Brignell R: *Pilates: a beginner's guide,* New York, 2000, Sterling Publishing.
8. Karter K: *The complete idiot's guide to the Pilates method,* Indianapolis, Ind, 2001, Alpha Books.
9. Gallagher SP, Kryzanowska R: *The Pilates method of body conditioning,* Philadelphia, 1999, BainBridge Books.
10. Pilates JH, Miller WJ: *Return to life through contrology,* Nevada, 1998 Presentation Dynamics Inc.
11. Herrington L, Davies R: The influence of Pilates training on the ability to contract the transversus abdominis muscle in asymptomatic individuals, *J Bodywork Movement Ther* 9:52-7, 2005.
12. Petrofsky JS et al: Muscle use during exercise: a comparison of conventional weight equipment to Pilates with and without a resistive exercise device, *J Appl Res* 5:160-73, 2005.
13. Segal NA, Hein J, Basford JR: The effects of Pilates training on flexibility and body composition: an observational study, *Arch Phys Med Rehabil* 85:1977-81, 2004.
14. McMillan A, Proteau L, Lebe R: The effect of Pilates-based training on dancers' dynamic posture, *J Dance Med Sci* 2:101-7, 1998.
15. Hutchinson MR et al: Improving leaping ability in elite rhythmic gymnasts, *Med Sci Sports Exer* 30:1543-7, 1998.
16. Jago R et al: Effect of 4 weeks of Pilates on the body composition of young girls, *Prev Med* 42:177-80, 2006.

17. Kolyniak IEGG, Cavalcanti SMB, Aoki MS: Isokinetic evaluation of the musculature involved in trunk flexion and extension: Pilates method effect, *Rev Bras Med Esporte* 10(6):491-3, 2004.

18. Rydeard R, Leger A, Smith D: Pilates-based therapeutic exercise: effect on subjects with nonspecific chronic low back pain and functional disability: a randomized controlled trial, *J Ortho Sports Phys Ther* 36:472-84, 2006.

19. Gagnon LH: Efficacy of Pilates exercises as therapeutic intervention in treating patients with low back pain, (The University of Tennessee) 2005; PhD dissertation.

# Index

WITHDRAWN

Derby Hospitals NHS Foundation
Trust
Library and Knowledge Service